New Frontiers in Gastroenterology and Hepatology

New Frontiers in Gastroenterology and Hepatology

Edited by Jonas Dexter

hayle medical

New York

Hayle Medical,
750 Third Avenue, 9th Floor,
New York, NY 10017, USA

Visit us on the World Wide Web at:
www.haylemedical.com

ISBN: 978-1-63241-608-7

The publisher's policy is to use permanent paper from mills that operate a sustainable forestry policy. Furthermore, the publisher ensures that the text paper and cover boards used have met acceptable environmental accreditation standards.

Printed in China.

Cataloging-in-Publication Data

New frontiers in gastroenterology and hepatology / edited by Jonas Dexter.
p. cm.
Includes bibliographical references and index.
ISBN 978-1-63241-608-7
1. Gastroenterology. 2. Hepatology. 3. Digestive organs--Diseases. I. Dexter, Jonas.
RC801 .N49 2019
616.33--dc23

Table of Contents

Preface

The world is advancing at a fast pace like never before. Therefore, the need is to keep up with the latest developments. This book was an idea that came to fruition when the specialists in the area realized the need to coordinate together and document essential themes in the subject. That's when I was requested to be the editor. Editing this book has been an honour as it brings together diverse authors researching on different streams of the field. The book collates essential materials contributed by veterans in the area which can be utilized by students and researchers alike.

The branch of medicine concerned with the functioning of the digestive system along with the disorders affecting it is known as gastroenterology. Hepatology is concerned with the functioning of the liver, pancreas, gallbladder and biliary tree. It studies the diseases and disorders related to them. Hepatology and gastroenterology are closely related fields of medicine. Colonoscopy, endoscopy, endoscopic ultrasound, liver biopsy are some of the common diagnostic and therapeutic procedures performed by gastroenterologists. This book unfolds the innovative aspects of gastroenterology, which will be crucial for the progress of this field in the future. It also unravels the recent studies in the field of hepatology. This book is a vital tool for all researching or studying gastroenterology and hepatology as it gives incredible insights into emerging trends.

Each chapter is a sole-standing publication that reflects each author´s interpretation. Thus, the book displays a multi-facetted picture of our current understanding of application, resources and aspects of the field. I would like to thank the contributors of this book and my family for their endless support.

Editor

1

A Comparison of Endoscopic Ultrasound-Guided Fine-Needle Aspiration and Fine-Needle Biopsy in the Diagnosis of Solid Pancreatic Lesions

Lachlan R. Ayres,[1] Elizabeth K. Kmiotek,[2] Eric Lam,[3] and Jennifer J. Telford[3]

[1] *Poole Hospital NHS Foundation Trust, Poole, UK*
[2] *Jagiellonian University Medical College, Krakow, Poland*
[3] *Division of Gastroenterology, St. Paul's Hospital, University of British Columbia, Vancouver, BC, Canada*

Correspondence should be addressed to Lachlan R. Ayres; lachlanayres@hotmail.com

Academic Editor: Qi Chen

Background and Aims. Endoscopic ultrasound (EUS) guided fine-needle aspiration (FNA) is the method of choice for sampling pancreatic lesions. This study compares the diagnostic accuracy and safety of FNB using a novel core needle to FNA in solid pancreatic lesions. *Methods.* A retrospective review of patients in whom EUS FNA or FNB was performed for solid pancreatic lesions was conducted. Diagnostic performance was calculated based upon a dual classification system: classification 1, only malignant pathology considered a true positive, versus classification 2, atypical, suspicious, and malignant pathology considered a true positive. *Results.* 43 patients underwent FNB compared with 51 FNA. Using classification 1, sensitivity was 74.0% versus 80.0%, specificity 100% versus 100%, and diagnostic accuracy 77.0% versus 80.0% for FNB versus FNA, respectively (all $p > 0.05$). Using classification 2, sensitivity was 97% versus 94.0%, specificity 100% versus 100%, and diagnostic accuracy 98.0% versus 94.0% for FNB versus FNA, respectively (all $p > 0.05$). FNB required significantly fewer needle passes (median = 2) compared to FNA (median = 3; $p < 0.001$). Adverse events occurred in two (4.5%) FNB patients compared with none in the FNA group ($p > 0.05$). *Conclusion.* FNA and FNB have comparable sensitivity and diagnostic accuracy. FNB required fewer passes.

1. Introduction

Endoscopic ultrasound (EUS) guided fine-needle aspiration (FNA) is the method of choice for evaluating and sampling solid pancreatic lesions [1–3]. EUS can detect cancers less than 10 mm in size and is more sensitive than computed tomography (CT) [4]. It has a safe, cost-effective, and highly accurate method to diagnose solid pancreatic mass lesions [2, 4–7].

There is uncertainty relating to the optimal needle gauge, number of needle passes, presence of an on-site pathologist, and more recently whether the ability to procure core samples using fine-needle biopsy (FNB) is advantageous [3, 8–11]. Several core biopsy needles are available which have the potential to preserve tissue architecture and morphology which is helpful for the characterization of some lesions such as stromal tumors and lymphomas [12–14]. Generally, FNB is comparable to FNA in terms of diagnostic accuracy for solid pancreatic lesions [13–17].

The recently developed SharkCore™ FNB needle is designed with six cutting edge surfaces and an opposing bevel to trap core tissue which preserves architecture and limits tissue fracturing in addition to including a passively activated safety sheath to prevent needle stick injuries. A recently published pilot study demonstrated comparable diagnostic performance compared to FNA [18].

The aim of this study was to compare the sensitivity, specificity, and safety of SharkCore FNB to conventional FNA in evaluating solid pancreatic masses.

2. Methods

A retrospective review was performed on consecutive patients who underwent index EUS guided FNB of solid

Table 1: Patient demographics.

	FNA (n = 51)	FNB (n = 43)	p
Sex n (%)			0.147
Female	29 (56.9)	18 (41.9)	
Male	22 (43.1)	25 (58.1)	
Age			0.756
Median (IQR)	66.0 (55.0–75.0)	66.0 (56.0–75.0)	
Mean (SD)	64.8 (12.2)	65.9 (12.7)	
Range	33.0–83.0	36.0–88.0	

FNA = fine needle aspiration; FNB = fine needle biopsy; IQR = interquartile range; SD = standard deviation.

pancreatic lesions by two experienced endosonographers at St. Paul's Hospital, Vancouver, BC, using the Covidien Shark-Core platform (Shark Core®, Covidien, Dublin, Leinster, Ireland) using 19 G, 22 G, or 25 G needles. When the study was conceived 50 FNB had been performed on solid pancreatic lesions (November 2014 to July 2015). Thus a similar number of consecutive patients undergoing FNA using a 22 G or 25 G needle (Expect, Boston Scientific, Natick, MA, USA) of solid pancreatic lesions were taken for comparison (from October 2013 to October 2014). There was no on-site pathologist present for either cohort. The number of needle passes and needle throws was not standardized and was at the discretion of the endosonographer. Assessment of an adequate specimen was also at the discretion of the endosonographer generally using a crude visual assessment of the material expressed from the needle.

Patients were excluded when there was a predominantly cystic component to the mass or if adequate follow-up was not available: either surgical pathology or six months' clinical follow-up. The study was approved by the University of British Columbia Ethics Board.

Electronic medical records were interrogated and demographic data recorded. The size of the lesion was documented based on the largest dimension reported in millimeters. The location of the lesion was categorized as falling within the head, uncinate, genu, body, or tail of pancreas. Technical failures, number of needle passes, and needle gauge were recorded.

The pathological diagnosis by EUS was categorized as nondiagnostic, benign, atypical, suspicious, or malignant (i.e., classes 1–5, resp.). Diagnostic accuracy, positive predictive value, negative predictive value, sensitivity, and specificity were calculated using a dual classification system employed in a meta-analysis of EUS FNA by Hewitt et al. 2012 [2]. Under this approach malignancy status was established as follows:

(i) Classification 1: nondiagnostic, benign, atypical, and suspicious are considered negative for malignancy. Only the designation "malignant," that is, class 5, is considered a true positive.

(ii) Classification 2: nondiagnostic and benign are negative for malignancy. Atypical and suspicious are also considered positive for malignancy.

Diagnostic accuracy was compared to gold standard surgical pathology, subsequent EUS FNA/FNB, or six-month clinico-radiological follow-up. It was computed as the ratio between the sum of true positive and true negative values divided by the total number of lesions. Neuroendocrine tumors which have a range of malignant potential were all regarded as a "positive" diagnosis and grouped with adenocarcinoma and lymphoma for the purposes of the analysis. Adverse events, as determined by interrogating electronic medical records, were also recorded and compared.

2.1. Statistical Analysis. Statistical analysis was performed using the chi-square test, Fisher's exact test, or Wilcoxon rank sum test as appropriate using SAS 9.4 and R 3.2.0. A p value of ≤ 0.05 was considered statistically significant.

3. Results

3.1. Patient Demographics. Patients ranged from 33 to 88 years of age (median = 66 years of age for both groups). There were 22 (43.1%) versus 25 (58.1%) males in the FNA and FNB groups, respectively. Demographic data of the study population is reported in Table 1.

3.2. Lesion Characteristics. There was no difference in location, size, or pathological class (all $p > 0.05$) between the two groups. Lesion characteristics are shown in Table 2. Most lesions were located in the head of pancreas (61.7%) followed by the body (13.8%), tail (10.6%), uncinate (7.4%), and genu (6.4%). The mean lesion size was 27 mm (± 12.2 (SD)), 72.3% were malignant, 10.6% suspicious, 6.4% atypical, 8.5% benign, and 2.1% nondiagnostic. The majority of lesions (68%) were pancreatic ductal adenocarcinoma with neuroendocrine lesions the second most common. The two groups differed significantly in terms of the final diagnosis (p = 0.018) in that there were more neuroendocrine tumors (NET) in the FNA group and more inflammatory lesions and lymphomas in the FNB group.

3.3. Diagnostic Accuracy: Classification 1. The diagnostic performance of FNA and FNB is presented in Table 3. In the FNA group 39/51 (77%) specimens were positive for malignancy compared to 29/43 (67%) in the FNB group. Of 12 samples negative for malignancy in the FNA group, ten were false negatives (14 and ten for FNB). This translates to a

Table 2: Lesion characteristics.

	FNA ($n = 51$)	FNB ($n = 43$)	p
Location of lesion in pancreas, n (%)			0.275
Head	27 (52.9)	31 (72.1)	
Uncinate	5 (9.8)	2 (4.7)	
Genu	3 (5.9)	3 (7.0)	
Body	8 (15.7)	5 (11.6)	
Tail	8 (15.7)	2 (4.7)	
Lesion size (largest dimension, mm)			0.787
Missing, n (%)	1 (2.0)	5 (11.6)	
Median (IQR)	26.0 (18.0, 34.0)	26.0 (18.0, 36.0)	
Mean (SD)	26.8 (12.8)	27.4 (11.5)	
Range	(5.0, 70.0)	(9.0, 55.0)	
Cytologic/histologic diagnosis			0.468
Nondiagnostic	2 (3.9)	0 (0.0)	
Benign	3 (5.9)	5 (11.6)	
Atypical	2 (3.9)	4 (9.3)	
Suspicious	5 (9.8)	5 (11.6)	
Malignant	39 (76.5)	29 (67.4)	
Final diagnosis			0.018
Pancreatic adenocarcinoma	37 (72.5)	31 (72.1)	
Neuroendocrine tumour	12 (23.5)	4 (9.3)	
Inflammatory	0 (0.0)	4 (9.3)	
Lymphoma	0 (0.0)	1 (2.3)	
Benign/normal	2 (3.9)	1 (2.3)	
Other	0 (0.0)	2 (4.7)	

FNA = fine needle aspiration; FNB = fine needle biopsy; IQR = interquartile range; SD = standard deviation.

Table 3: Diagnostic performance: classification 1.

	FNA	FNB	p
Sensitivity	0.80 (0.66, 0.90)	0.74 (0.58, 0.87)	0.615
Specificity	1.00 (0.09, 1.00)	1.00 (0.28, 1.00)	1.000
PPV	1.00 (0.87, 1.00)	1.00 (0.83, 1.00)	1.000
NPV	0.17 (0.02, 0.48)	0.29 (0.08, 0.58)	0.652
Accuracy	0.80 (0.67, 0.90)	0.77 (0.61, 0.88)	0.801

Values in brackets are 95% confidence interval. p value is based on Fisher's exact test; FNA = fine needle aspiration; FNB = fine needle biopsy.

sensitivity of 80% versus 74%, specificity of 100% versus 100%, positive predictive value (PPV) of 100% versus 100%, negative predictive value (NPV) of 17% versus 29%, and an accuracy of 80% versus 77% for FNA and FNB, respectively (all $p > 0.05$).

3.4. Diagnostic Accuracy: Classification 2. Using the less stringent classification 2 (see Table 4), the sensitivity, NPV, and accuracy all increased as compared to classification 1, but there was still no statistically significant difference between FNA and FNB in any of these measures. In the FNA group 46/51 (90%) were malignant versus 38/43 (88%) in the FNB group. Of five samples negative for malignancy three were false negatives for FNA (compared to five and one for FNB). Thus sensitivity was 94% versus 97%, specificity 100% versus 100%, PPV 100% versus 100%, NPV 40% versus 80%, and accuracy 94% versus 98% for FNA and FNB, respectively.

3.5. Technical Outcomes. In the FNB group, 35 (81%) lesions were sampled using a 25 G needle, six (14%) lesions were sampled using 22 G, and one (2%) lesion was sampled using 19 G (needle gauge not reported in one case). Technical outcomes are reported in Table 5. Fewer needle passes were performed in the FNB group: median two (mean 2.1) compared to a median of three (mean 3.2) in the FNA group ($p < 0.001$). In the FNA group five (9.8%) patients required a repeat EUS compared to eight (18.6%) in the FNB group ($p = 0.218$). Two adverse events were reported (one gastrointestinal bleed, no blood transfusion or endoscopic therapy required, and one self-limiting episode of mild acute pancreatitis) in the FNB group compared to none in the FNA group $p > 0.05$. No technical failures were reported in either group.

In the FNA group four (7.8%) specimens were paucicellular/inadequate, three of which required repeat EUS versus

TABLE 4: Diagnostic performance: classification 2.

	FNA	FNB	p
Sensitivity	0.94 (0.83, 0.99)	0.97 (0.87, 1.00)	0.626
Specificity	1.00 (0.09, 1.00)	1.00 (0.28, 1.00)	1.000
PPV	1.00 (0.89, 1.00)	1.00 (0.87, 1.00)	1.000
NPV	0.40 (0.05, 0.85)	0.80 (0.28, 0.99)	0.524
Accuracy	0.94 (0.84, 0.99)	0.98 (0.88, 1.00)	0.623

Values in brackets are 95% confidence interval. p value is based on Fisher's exact test; FNA = fine needle aspiration; FNB = fine needle biopsy

TABLE 5: Technical outcomes.

	FNA (n = 51)	FNB (n = 43)	p
Passes			<0.001
Unknown	1	0	
1	1 (2.0)	0 (0.0)	
2	5 (10.0)	36 (83.7)	
3	27 (54.0)	6 (14.0)	
4	16 (32.0)	1 (2.3)	
5	1 (2.0)	0 (0.0)	
Required a repeat EUS/FNA, n (%)			0.218
No	46 (90.2)	35 (81.4)	
Yes	5 (9.8)	8 (18.6)	
Adverse events, n (%)	0 (0)	2 (4.65)	0.207

FNA = fine needle aspiration; FNB = fine needle biopsy; EUS = endoscopic ultrasound.

three (7.0%) specimens in the FNB group of which two required repeat EUS (p = 1.00).

4. Discussion

In this study comparing FNA to FNB, both needles demonstrate similar diagnostic performance, with FNB requiring significantly fewer needle passes to obtain sufficient diagnostic material regardless of the classification system used. To our knowledge this is the largest study comparing SharkCore FNB to conventional FNA in the diagnosis of solid pancreatic masses.

The dual classification system used in this investigation was adapted from Hewitt et al. 2012 who conducted a meta-analysis of EUS FNA in the diagnosis of pancreatic masses. Their pooled findings for sensitivity, specificity, PPV, and NPV were 85%, 98%, 99%, and 64% under classification I and 91%, 94%, 98%, and 72% under classification 2 [2]. These data are comparable to the findings presented here.

Our experience with SharkCore is similar to the findings described in a North American multicenter study using SharkCore for the diagnosis of various solid lesions. Of 250 lesions sampled, 88% were diagnostic with a median of two passes. Subgroup analysis showed that for pancreatic masses 86% were diagnostic [19]. They found a trend towards superior pathologic yield when compared to cytologic yield (87% versus 68%) but this was not statistically significant. Similarly, the Newcastle group (UK) found that SharkCore had a 90.1% sensitivity compared to ProCore™ 71.1% in a cohort of 201 patients with solid pancreatic lesions [20].

Various studies demonstrate that ProCore FNB requires fewer passes to obtain a pathologic diagnosis [13, 15–17, 19, 21]. Similarly, a recent pilot study by Adler et al. found that the SharkCore FNB required fewer passes compared to standard FNA (1.5 passes versus three passes, resp.) in a 30-patient cohort [18]. This finding supports the results of this study where a median number of two passes was needed for FNB versus three for FNA.

Of the studies investigating ProCore FNB, most did not identify a significant difference in diagnostic sensitivity between FNA and FNB for solid pancreatic masses [13–16, 19, 22]. Furthermore, when other lesions were analyzed in conjunction with pancreatic masses such as lymph nodes and gastrointestinal mass lesions, both needles still exhibited comparable levels of accuracy [17, 21, 23]. FNA sensitivity ranged within 72–92% versus 90–97.8% for FNB, and specificity ranged within 80%–100% versus 100%, respectively [13, 16, 17, 21]. This is similar to our own findings where FNA sensitivity was 80%–94% compared to 74%–97% for FNB in classification systems 1 and 2, respectively. Two studies found FNB (ProCore) to be inferior to FNA in the diagnosis of pancreatic masses [24, 25]. However both studies were small and one used a different number of passes for FNA and FNB.

Accuracy ranged within 90–94.8% for FNA and 84.6–98.3% for FNB in previously published comparative studies [15–17, 21, 24]. Not all investigations examined in this paper specified the criteria establishing malignancy; thus stringent comparisons using the two classification systems are not possible. As with most studies of EUS FNA/FNB false positives are rare and none occurred in either cohort in our study yielding specificities of 100% for both FNA and FNB under both classification systems.

Despite reports of FNB providing improved tumor type discrimination, histopathological quality, and preservation of architecture [13, 14], other studies, including our own, have not demonstrated that it increases sensitivity, although we speculate that this could be borne out if the number of needle passes was increased for FNB.

Interestingly we found that with FNA five of ten false negatives (using classification I) were neuroendocrine tumors. For FNB, seven of ten false negatives (using classification I) were pancreatic adenocarcinoma and none were eventually proven to be neuroendocrine tumors. The number of cases is too small to draw strong conclusions but this may indicate that FNB is advantageous in neuroendocrine tumors which have a spectrum of malignant potential and where a core specimen may be more important.

Although we retrospectively applied two classifications to the data, it is interesting to observe how cases were managed in reality. In the FNB group, eight patients (18.2%) required a second EUS (six pancreatic adenocarcinomas, one hemangioendothelioma, and one benign). This compares to five (9%) in the FNA group (three pancreatic adenocarcinomas and two neuroendocrine tumors). This trend is not statistically significant.

It is perhaps intuitive that, for a needle designed to obtain a core, the trade-off for obtaining more tissue comes at the expense of more adverse events. The only adverse events that occurred in the study population (a gastrointestinal bleed and an episode of pancreatitis) were in the FNB group although this was not statistically significant. To date, studies using other FNB needles have reported a similar safety profile to FNA [22] and many reported no adverse events at all [13, 14, 19, 25]. Studies with larger sample sizes are required to assess the safety profile of the SharkCore FNB.

This study was retrospective and so has inherent limitations. Other limitations are that tissue sampling was not standardized in terms of number of passes, number of needle throws, and use of suction or "slow-pull" technique. Secondly the FNA group differs significantly from the FNB group in terms of the final diagnosis; however the majority of lesions were pancreatic adenocarcinoma and neuroendocrine tumors for both groups and this is unlikely to have had a material effect on diagnostic performance. Thirdly pathological specimens were not always reported in a strict categorical format. Finally, the FNB cohort dates from when the SharkCore needle was introduced, whereas the FNA cohort represents data taken at a time when both endosonographers were very familiar with that needle. There is inevitably a learning curve with new equipment and it is possible that, with more experience and familiarity, performance could improve slightly for FNB. Lastly, the sample size reported here is relatively small.

5. Conclusions

In summary, the study found FNA and FNB to have comparable diagnostic accuracy and safety, with FNB requiring fewer passes. A prospective, randomized trial is warranted to establish whether FNB has an advantage over FNA.

Disclosure

This data was presented in abstract format at DDW 2016 (http://www.giejournal.org/article/S0016-5107(16)01175-5/fulltext).

References

[1] H. Uehara, K. Ikezawa, N. Kawada et al., "Diagnostic accuracy of endoscopic ultrasound-guided fine needle aspiration for suspected pancreatic malignancy in relation to the size of lesions," *Journal of Gastroenterology and Hepatology*, vol. 26, no. 8, pp. 1256–1261, 2011.

[2] M. J. Hewitt, M. J. W. McPhail, L. Possamai, A. Dhar, P. Vlavianos, and K. J. Monahan, "EUS-guided FNA for diagnosis of solid pancreatic neoplasms: a meta-analysis," *Gastrointestinal Endoscopy*, vol. 75, no. 2, pp. 319–331, 2012.

[3] B. R. Weston and M. S. Bhutani, "Optimizing diagnostic yield for EUS-guided sampling of solid pancreatic lesions: A technical review," *Journal of Gastroenterology and Hepatology*, vol. 9, no. 6, pp. 352–363, 2013.

[4] K. Hanada, A. Okazaki, N. Hirano et al., "Diagnostic strategies for early pancreatic cancer," *Journal of Gastroenterology*, vol. 50, no. 2, pp. 147–154, 2014.

[5] M. A. Eloubeidi, D. Jhala, D. C. Chhieng et al., "Yield of endoscopic ultrasound-guided fine-needle aspiration biopsy in patients with suspected pancreatic carcinoma: emphasis on atypical, suspicious, and false-negative aspirates," *Cancer*, vol. 99, no. 5, pp. 285–292, 2003.

[6] S. Yoshinaga, H. Suzuki, I. Oda, and Y. Saito, "Role of endoscopic ultrasound-guided fine needle aspiration (EUS-FNA) for diagnosis of solid pancreatic masses," *Digestive Endoscopy*, vol. 23, no. 1, pp. 29–33, 2011.

[7] M. S. Bhutani, P. Koduru, V. Joshi et al., "The role of endoscopic ultrasound in pancreatic cancer screening," *Endoscopic Ultrasound*, vol. 5, no. 1, pp. 8–16, 2016.

[8] P. Thomas Cherian, P. Mohan, A. Douiri, P. Taniere, R. K. Hejmadi, and B. S. Mahon, "Role of endoscopic ultrasound-guided fine-needle aspiration in the diagnosis of solid pancreatic and peripancreatic lesions: Is onsite cytopathology necessary?" *HPB*, vol. 12, no. 6, pp. 389–395, 2010.

[9] A. R. Schneider, A. Nerlich, T. Topalidis, and W. Schepp, "Specialized clinical cytology may improve the results of EUS (endoscopic ultrasound)-guided fine-needle aspiration (FNA) from pancreatic tumors," *Endoscopy International Open*, vol. 03, no. 02, pp. E134–E137, 2015.

[10] C. Fabbri, A. M. Polifemo, C. Luigiano et al., "Endoscopic ultrasound-guided fine needle aspiration with 22- and 25-gauge needles in solid pancreatic masses: A prospective comparative study with randomisation of needle sequence," *Digestive and Liver Disease*, vol. 43, no. 8, pp. 647–652, 2011.

[11] M. F. Madhoun, S. B. Wani, A. Rastogi et al., "The diagnostic accuracy of 22-gauge and 25-gauge needles in endoscopic ultrasound-guided fine needle aspiration of solid pancreatic lesions: A meta-analysis," *Endoscopy*, vol. 45, no. 2, pp. 86–92, 2013.

[12] M. J. Levy, "Endoscopic ultrasound-guided trucut biopsy of the pancreas: Prospects and problems," *Pancreatology*, vol. 7, no. 2-3, pp. 163–166, 2007.

[13] A. Alatawi, F. Beuvon, S. Grabar et al., "Comparison of 22G reverse-beveled versus standard needle for endoscopic ultrasound-guided sampling of solid pancreatic lesions," *United European Gastroenterology Journal*, vol. 3, no. 4, pp. 343–352, 2015.

[14] M. J. Yang, H. Yim, J. C. Hwang et al., "Endoscopic ultrasound-guided sampling of solid pancreatic masses: 22-gauge aspiration versus 25-gauge biopsy needles," *BMC Gastroenterology*, vol. 15, pp. 1–8, 2015.

[15] Y. N. Lee, J. H. Moon, H. K. Kim et al., "Core biopsy needle versus standard aspiration needle for endoscopic ultrasound-guided sampling of solid pancreatic masses: A randomized parallel-group study," *Endoscopy*, vol. 46, no. 12, pp. 1056–1062, 2014.

[16] R. L. Ganc, A. P. Carbonari, R. Colaiacovo et al., "Mo1414 EUS-FNA of Solid Pancreatic Lesions: a Prospective, Randomized, Single Blinded, Comparative Study Using the 22-Gauge EchoTip®Procoretm HD and the 22-Gauge EchoTip® Ultra HD Endoscopic Ultrasound Needles," *Gastrointestinal Endoscopy*, vol. 79, no. 5, pp. AB427–AB428, 2014.

[17] T. Hucl, E. Wee, S. Anuradha et al., "Feasibility and efficiency of a new 22G core needle: A prospective comparison study," *Endoscopy*, vol. 45, no. 10, pp. 792–798, 2013.

[18] D. G. Adler, B. Witt, B. Chadwick et al., "Pathologic evaluation of a new endoscopic ultrasound needle designed to obtain core tissue samples: A pilot study," *Endoscopic Ultrasound*, vol. 5, no. 3, pp. 178–183, 2016.

[19] B. L. Witt, D. G. Adler, K. Hilden, and L. J. Layfield, "A comparative needle study: EUS-FNA procedures using the HD ProCore™ and EchoTip® 22-gauge needle types," *Diagnostic Cytopathology*, vol. 41, no. 12, pp. 1069–1074, 2013.

[20] M. K. Nayar, B. Paranandi, M. F. Dawwas et al., "Comparison of the diagnostic performance of 2 core biopsy needles for EUS-guided tissue acquisition from solid pancreatic lesions," *Gastrointestinal Endoscopy*, vol. 85, no. 5, pp. 1017–1024, 2017.

[21] M. Lin, C. D. Hair, L. K. Green et al., "Endoscopic ultrasound-guided fine-needle aspiration with on-site cytopathology versus core biopsy: a comparison of both techniques performed at the same endoscopic session," *Endoscopy International Open*, vol. 02, no. 04, pp. E220–E223, 2014.

[22] J. Y. Bang, S. Hebert-Magee, J. Trevino, J. Ramesh, and S. Varadarajulu, "Randomized trial comparing the 22-gauge aspiration and 22-gauge biopsy needles for EUS-guided sampling of solid pancreatic mass lesions," *Gastrointestinal Endoscopy*, vol. 76, no. 2, pp. 321–327, 2012.

[23] G. Mavrogenis, B. Weynand, A. Sibille et al., "25-gauge histology needle versus 22-gauge cytology needle in endoscopic ultrasonography-guided sampling of pancreatic lesions and lymphadenopathy," *Endoscopy International Open*, vol. 03, no. 01, pp. E63–E68, 2015.

[24] G. Vanbiervliet, B. Napoléon, M. C. Saint Paul et al., "Core needle versus standard needle for endoscopic ultrasound-guided biopsy of solid pancreatic masses: A randomized crossover study," *Endoscopy*, vol. 46, no. 12, pp. 1063–1070, 2014.

[25] D. S. Strand, S. K. Jeffus, B. G. Sauer, A. Y. Wang, E. B. Stelow, and V. M. Shami, "EUS-guided 22-gauge fine-needle aspiration versus core biopsy needle in the evaluation of solid pancreatic neoplasms," *Diagnostic Cytopathology*, vol. 42, no. 9, pp. 751–758, 2014.

2

The Effectiveness of Antiviral Treatments for Patients with HBeAg-Positive Chronic Hepatitis B: A Bayesian Network Analysis

Zhang Hao,[1] Zhu Biqing,[2] Yang Ling,[1] and Zeng Wenting[1]

[1]*Department of Infectious Diseases, The First Affiliated Hospital of Guangzhou Medical University, Guangzhou Medical University, Yanjiang Road 151, Guangzhou 510120, China*
[2]*Guangzhou Kingmed Center for Clinical Laboratory Co., Ltd., Guangzhou International Biological Island, Spiral Three Road 10, Guangzhou 510330, China*

Correspondence should be addressed to Zeng Wenting; 13609645855@163.com

Academic Editor: Kevork M. Peltekian

This network analysis is to determine the most effective treatment in HBeAg-positive patients. PubMed databases were searched for randomized controlled trials. Bayesian network meta-analysis was used to calculate the pairwise hazard ratios, 95% credible intervals, and ranking of surrogate outcomes. 9 studies were identified. The results show that NA add-on PEG IFN might be a better antiviral approach for HBeAg-positive patients in end point of treatment, with a comparable results of nucleoside/nucleotide analogs (NA), PEG IFN, PEG IFN add-on NA, PEG IFN combined NA, and PEG IFN combined placebo in alanine aminotransferase (ALT) normalization and HBV DNA undetectable. Cumulative probabilities of being the most efficacious treatment were NA add-on PEG IFN (30%) for HBeAg loss. The second efficacious (23%) is HBeAg seroconversion. This network analysis shows that NA add-on PEG IFN might be a better antiviral approach for HBeAg-positive patients in end point of treatment. But the long-term efficiency should be further determined.

1. Introduction

Hepatitis B virus (HBV) infection is one of the most common persistent viral infections in human beings. Over 240 million people worldwide are estimated to currently be chronically infected with HBV [1]. Chronic infection of HBV leads to serious medical complications, such as cirrhosis, hepatocellular carcinoma, and liver failure. The number of deaths from liver cirrhosis, liver cancer, and acute hepatitis due to HBV infection has greatly increased [2]. This highlights the need for effective treatments for chronic hepatitis B (CHB).

Currently, two sets of treatments are available for the treatment of HBV infection, which are the nucleoside/nucleotide analogs (NA) or PEGylated interferon (PEG IFN)[3]. With currently available treatment, HBsAg loss is uncommon; approximately 3–5% of the patients treated with PEG IFN, and 0 to 3% of patients treated with NA, lose HBsAg [4]. In order to improve response to antiviral treatment, different studies have used add-on therapy in various combinations. These include the simultaneous administration of the two drugs in naïve patients, "add-on" or "switch to" strategies in patients already on therapy [5–7]. However, the results are inconsistent. Therefore, we are performed the evidence base by conducting a network analyses of all published trials of different antiviral treatments (monotherapy, combination, adding on, or switching). Our aim is to determine which treatment is the most effective in treating CHB patients by analyzing surrogate outcomes in CHB.

2. Methods

2.1. Eligibility Criteria. The eligibility criteria for inclusion into this network analyses are studies involving adults with HBeAg-positive CHB in randomized, controlled trials (RCTs) that investigated a combination of the following therapies (such as monotherapy, combination, add-on, or switching): placebo (PLA), lamivudine (LAM), adefovir (ADV), entecavir (ETV), lamivudine (LdT), tenofovir (TDF), and PEG IFN. The following exclusion criteria were excluded in this study: (1) non-RCTs; (2) coinfection with hepatitis A, C, D, or E, cytomegalovirus, or HIV; (3) patients who were children; (4) patients who were not with HBeAg-positive; (5) patients who had liver failure, HCC, or other liver related complications caused by autoimmune diseases, drugs, or alcoholism.

2.2. Literature Search. PubMed were searched for potential references along with citation searching of relevant articles. The search was limited to English language publications. The original review conducted up to 15th January 2018. The search was conducted using the key words 'HBV or hepatitis B or CHB' and 'IFN or interferon' and 'random*'. Potentially relevant papers were reviewed by two authors (Zhang H and Zhu BQ) and a third author (Yang L) addressed disagreements. Papers from the original review were also retrieved and reviewed. Meeting abstracts and unpublished data were not included.

2.3. Efficacy Measures. Efficacy was evaluated based on the following criteria: alanine aminotransferase (ALT) normalization: ALT levels < 40 IU/ml; undetectable HBV DNA: HBV DNA levels < 1,000 copies/ml or less; HBeAg loss; HBeAg seroconversion: HBeAg loss and occurrence of HBeAb at the end of treatment (EOT).

2.4. Data Extraction. Data extraction was carried out by two independent reviewers (Zhang H and Zhu BQ). We recorded the following for each study: (1) trial characteristics (the first author's name, published year, country of study, sum of each group, and quality of RCT); (2) patient characteristics (mean age, ethnicity of patients); (3) the details of each regimen (i.e., the antiviral drug used and treatment duration); and (4) observation time and outcomes. We contacted the authors of the eligible publications that had inadequate information; if effective data were still not obtained, those papers were excluded. All the data were reviewed to eliminate duplicate reports of the same trial.

2.5. Assessment for Risk of Bias. We used the Jadad scale to evaluate the quality of the RCTs [15]. The quality of each trial was assessed independently by two study investigators (Zhang H and Zhu BQ). Discrepancies were resolved by discussion with a third person (Zeng WT).The Jadad scale was used to score the methodological quality of RCTs based on the following items: randomization (0–1 points), blinding (0–1 points), and dropouts and withdrawals (0–1 point).

2.6. Statistical Analysis. First, we conducted pairwise meta-analyses to synthesize studies comparing the same pair of treatments with STATA 11.0 software. The results were reported as pooled hazard ratios (HRs) with the corresponding 95% confidence interval (CI). Regression analyses were performed to estimate funnel plot asymmetry. Heterogeneity was explored by the chi-squared test and I^2 test with significance limit set at a P value of 0.10.

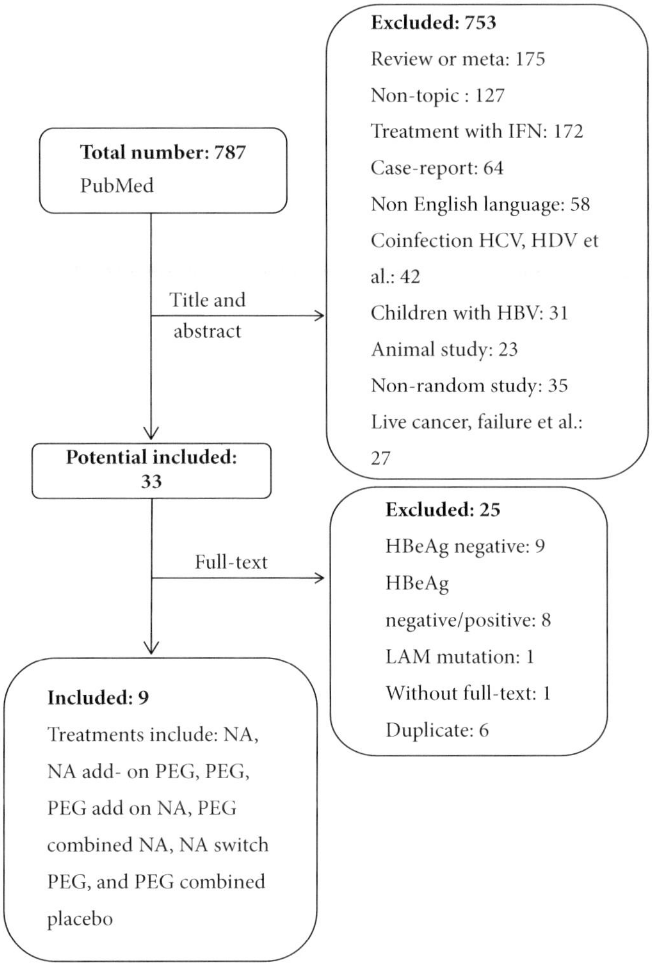

Figure 1: Flow chart of study selection and exclusion.

Second, we built a fixed-effects network within a Bayesian framework, which were burned-in for 5000 Markov Chain Monte Carlo iterations and convergence was based on the Gelman-Rubin-Brooke statistic. A further 25 000 iterations were run and the sampled values were used to estimate response probabilities and HRs. The analysis was performed using in Gemtc software. We networked the translated binary outcomes within studies and specified the relations among the HRs across studies making different comparisons. This method combined direct and indirect evidence for any given pair of treatments. We used P < 0.05 and 95% CIs to assess significance.

3. Results

3.1. Study Characteristics. Figure 1 describes the literature search and exclusion of studies. In total, 9 studies were identified (2 023 patients). We identified 7 trials were designed as two-arm trials analyzing [6–9, 11, 13, 14], whereas the other 2 were three-arm trials [10, 12] (Table 1). Of these, 590 received NA (29.2%), 129 received NA add-on PEG IFN (6.4%), 237 received PEG IFN (11.7%), 137 received PEG IFN add-on NA (6.8%), 431 received PEG IFN combined NA (21.3%), 92

Table 1: Main characteristics of studies included.

Study	Country	Year	Project	Initial Treatment	Include patients	End point	Randomized Treatment	Jada Scores
Chi H et al. [8]	Netherlands, China	2017	NCT01532843	≥12wk ETV or TDF	HBV DNA <2 000 IU/mL, ALT<5 times the upper limit of normal	ALT normalization, HBV DNA undectable, HBeAg loss and HBeAg seroconversion	NA, NA add-on PEG IFN	2
Sun J et al. [9]	China	2016	NCT01086085	24wk PEG IFN	Non early responders	ALT normalization, HBV DNA undectable, HBeAg loss and HBeAg seroconversion	PEG IFN, PEG IFN add- on NA	2
Brouwer WP et al. [6]	Europe, Asia	2015	NCT00877760	24wk ETV	ALT >1.3 times the upper limit of normal	ALT normalization, HBV DNA undectable, HBeAg loss and HBeAg seroconversion	NA, NA add-on PEG IFN	2
Xie Q et al. [10]	China	2014	NCT00614471	NA	HBV DNA ≥100 000 copies/mL, ALT >2 but ≤10 times the upper limit of normal	ALT normalization, HBV DNA undectable, HBeAg loss and HBeAg seroconversion	PEG IFN, NA and PEG IFN add-on NA	2
Liu YH et al. [11]	China	2014	-	NA	HBV DNA ≥100 000 copies/mL, ALT >2 but ≤10 times the upper limit of normal	ALT normalization, HBV DNA undectable, HBeAg loss and HBeAg seroconversion	PEG IFN, PEG IFN combined NA	1
Ning Q et al. [7]	China	2014	OSST	9-36 months ETV	HBV DNA <1000copies/mL, HBeAg<100PEIU/L	ALT normalization, HBV DNA undectable, HBeAg loss and HBeAg seroconversion	NA, NA switch PEG IFN	2
Lau GK et al. [12]	16 countries	2005	-	NA	HBsAg negative, HBV DNA ≥500 000 copies/mL, ALT >1 but ≤10 times the upper limit of normal	ALT normalization, HBV DNA undectable, HBeAg loss and HBeAg seroconversion	NA, PEG IFN combined PLA, and PEG IFN combined NA	3
Chan HL et al. [13]	Hong Kong	2005	-	-	HBV DNA ≥500 000 copies/mL, ALT >1.3 but ≤5 times the upper limit of normal	ALT normalization, HBV DNA undectable, and HBeAg seroconversion	PEG IFN add-on NA, NA	2
Janssen HL et al. [14]	15 countries	2005	-	-	ALT >2 times the upper limit of normal	ALT normalization, HBV DNA undectable, HBeAg loss and HBeAg seroconversion	PEG IFN combined NA, PEG IFN combined PLA	3

Note: NA, nucleoside/nucleotide analogs; PEG IFN, PEG IFNylated interferon; PLA, placebo; ETV, entecavir; TDF, tenofovir; wk, week

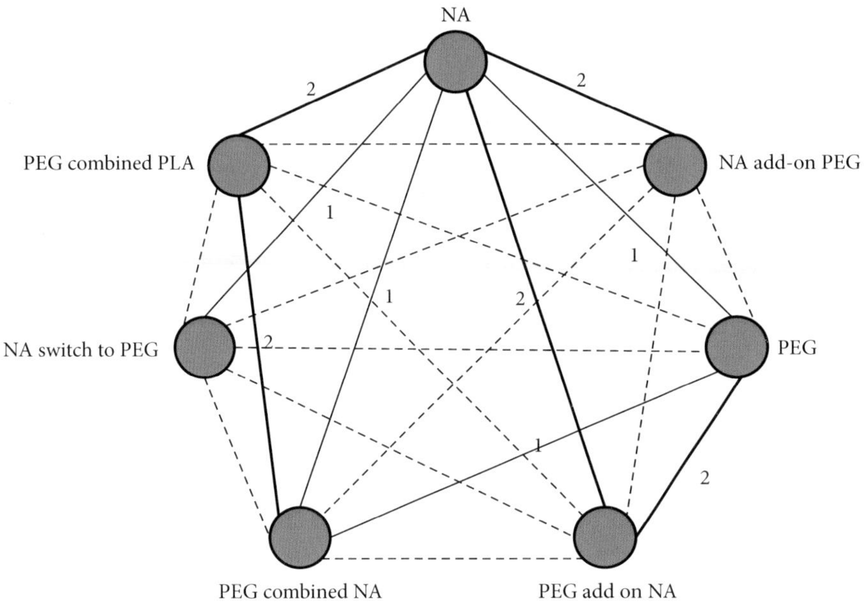

Figure 2: Network of trial comparisons for NA, NA add-on PEG IFN, PEG IFN, PEG IFN add-on NA, PEG IFN combined NA, NA switch to PEG IFN, PEG IFN combined PLA. NA, nucleoside/nucleotide analogs; PEG IFN, pegylated interferon; PLA, placebo. Numbers represent that number of direct comparisons available. Dashed lines indicate indirect treatment comparisons.

received NA switch PEG IFN (4.5%), and 407 received PEG IFN combined Placebo (20.1%).

3.2. Direct Meta-Analyses

ALT Normalization. All the included trials reported the rate of ALT normalization. The significant difference was found in the treatment of NA versus NA switch PEG IFN (Pooled HR 1.392, p=0.019) and NA versus PEG IFN combined PLA (Pooled HR 1.367, p=0.002). That means patients with NA treatment could achieve high rate of ALT normalization compared with the above two treatments. However, no significant differences were found among the treatments: NA versus NA add-on PEG IFN, PEG IFN versus PEG IFN add-on NA, PEG IFN versus NA, PEG IFN add-on NA versus NA, PEG IFN versus PEG IFN combined NA, NA vs. PEG IFN combined NA, and PEG IFN combined versus PEG IFN combined PLA (Table 2). As the combined analyses were no more than three studies, the heterogeneity cannot be performed.

HBV Undetectable. All the included trials also reported the rate of HBV undetectable. The significant difference was found in the treatment of PEG IFN versus PEG IFN combined NA (Pooled HR 0.518, p=0.048), NA versus PEG IFN combined NA (Pooled HR 0.698, p<0.001), NA versus PEG IFN combined PLA (Pooled HR 1.417, p=0.01), and PEG IFN combined NA versus PEG IFN combined PLA (Pooled HR 2.153, p<0.001). No significant differences were found among the treatments: NA versus NA add-on PEG IFN, PEG IFN versus PEG IFN add-on NA, PEG IFN versus NA, PEG IFN add-on NA versus NA, and NA versus NA switch PEG IFN (Table 2). As the combined analyses were no more than three studies, the heterogeneity cannot be performed.

HBeAg Loss and Seroconversion. All the included trials also reported the rate of HBeAg seroconversion. Seven of them reported the rate of HBeAg loss. No significant differences were in all the treatments under the direct analyses (Table 2).

3.3. Network Meta-Analyses. The structure of the network analysis is reported in Figure 2. Table 3 summarizes the results of the network meta-analysis for ALT normalization, HBV undetectable, HBeAg loss, and seroconversion. The significant differences of ALT normalization were found in the treatment of NA (HR 9.68, 95% CI 2.59-41.22), PEG IFN (HR 9.00, 95% CI 1.83-51.79), PEG IFN add-on NA (HR 18.05, 95% CI 3.64-109.82), and PEG IFN combined NA (HR 6.76, 95% CI 1.49-43.48) versus NA switch PEG IFN, respectively. As expected, a significant low rate of HBV undetectable was found in the treatment of NA (HR 21.11, 95% CI 2.90-262.11), NA add-on PEG IFN (HR 36.56, 95% CI 3.27-567.15), PEG IFN (HR 17.12, 95% CI 1.47-248.25), PEG IFN add-on NA (HR 28.39, 95% CI 2.31-404.85), PEG IFN combined NA (HR 82.47, 95% CI 8.49-1406.85), and PEG IFN combined PLA (HR 13.49, 95% CI 1.21-236.27) versus NA switch PEG IFN, respectively.

As no significant differences of HBeAg loss and seroconversion existed in the treatments (Table 3), the rank probability to be the best treatment should be showed in Figure 3. Cumulative probabilities of being the most efficacious treatment were as follows: NA add-on PEG IFN (30%) for HBeAg loss and NA switch PEG IFN (37%) for HBeAg seroconversion. The followed approach is NA

Table 2: The results of direct analysis estimates of efficacy (hazard ratio).

Treatment	Study	ALT normalization			HBV DNA undetectable			HBeAg loss			HBeAg seroconversion		
		HR	95% CI	p	HR	95% CI	p	HR	95% CI	p	HR	95% CI	p
NA vs. NA add-on PEG IFN	Chi H et al. [8] Brouwer WP et al. [6]	0.89	0.71-1.12	0.31	0.94	0.76-1.15	0.53	0.62	0.35-1.10	0.10	0.52	0.25-1.06	0.07
PEG IFN vs. PEG IFN add-on NA	Sun J et al. [9] Xie Q et al. [10]	0.83	0.64-1.07	0.16	0.82	0.61-1.11	0.21	0.76	0.54-1.09	0.13	0.83	0.55-1.25	0.37
PEG IFN vs. NA	Xie Q et al. [10]	1.03	0.67-1.59	0.88	1.07	0.73-1.55	0.74	0.78	0.48-1.29	0.34	0.96	0.49-1.86	0.89
PEG IFN add-on NA vs. NA	Xie Q et al. [10] Chan HL et al. [13]	1.14	0.89-1.47	0.30	0.74	0.53-1.03	0.08	1.21	0.85-1.73	0.29	1.31	0.86-1.99	0.21
PEG IFN vs. PEG IFN combined NA	Liu YH et al. [11]	0.89	0.48-1.64	0.70	**0.52**	**0.27-1.00**	**0.04**	NA	NA	NA	0.77	0.34-1.70	0.51
NA vs. NA switch PEG IFN	Ning Q et al. [7]	**1.39**	**106-1.84**	**0.02**	1.18	0.93-1.51	0.18	0.91	0.50-1.64	0.75	0.46	0.19-1.16	0.10
NA vs. PEG IFN combined NA	Lau GK et al. [12]	1.20	1.00-1.45	0.05	**0.70**	**0.58-0.85**	**<0.01**	0.84	0.62-1.14	0.27	0.88	0.64-1.22	0.45
NA vs. PEG IFN combined PLA	Lau GK et al. [12]	**1.37**	**1.12-1.67**	**<0.01**	**1.42**	**1.09-1.85**	**0.01**	1.34	0.95-1.90	0.09	0.80	0.58-1.10	0.17
PEG IFN combined NA vs. PEG IFN combined PLA	Lau GK et al. [12] Janssen H et al. [14]	1.20	1.00-1.43	0.05	**2.15**	**1.73-2.69**	**<0.01**	NA	NA	NA	1.12	0.72-1.75	0.82

Note: NA, nucleoside/nucleotide analogs; PEG IFN, PEG IFNylated interferon; PLA, placebo; HR, hazard ratio.

Table 3: League table presenting network meta-analysis estimates of efficacy (hazard ratio).

ALT normalization						
NA						
2.59 (0.70, 6.09)	*NA add-on PEG IFN*					
1.07 (0.41, 2.82)	0.42 (0.11, 2.32)	*PEG IFN*				
0.55 (0.22, 1.32)	0.21 (0.06, 1.07)	0.51 (0.21, 1.14)	*PEG IFN add-on NA*			
1.47 (0.46, 3.22)	0.56 (0.14, 2.52)	1.34 (0.39, 3.54)	2.64 (0.72, 7.73)	*PEG IFN combined NA*		
9.68 (2.59, 41.22)	3.80 (0.84, 27.37)	**9.00 (1.83, 51.79)**	**18.05 (3.64, 109.82)**	**6.76 (1.49, 43.48)**	*NA switch PEG IFN*	
2.49 (0.80, 6.49)	0.95 (0.26, 4.86)	2.32 (0.65, 7.42)	4.59 (1.26, 15.25)	1.71 (0.80, 4.32)	0.26 (0.04, 1.26)	*PEG IFN combined PLA*
HBV DNA undetectable						
NA						
0.59 (0.17, 2.27)	*NA add-on PEG IFN*					
1.25 (0.40, 5.05)	2.09 (0.38, 13.95)	*PEG IFN*				
0.74 (0.26, 3.21)	1.24 (0.25, 8.88)	0.59 (0.20, 2.04)	*PEG IFN add-on NA*			
0.26 (0.07, 0.91)	0.44 (0.07, 2.52)	0.21 (0.04, 0.74)	0.35 (0.06, 1.38)	*PEG IFN combined NA*		
21.11 (2.90, 262.11)	**36.56 (3.27, 567.15)**	**17.12 (1.47, 248.25)**	**28.69 (2.31, 404.85)**	**82.47 (8.49, 1406.85)**	*NA switch PEG IFN*	**13.49 (1.21, 236.27)**
1.64 (0.37, 6.51)	2.71 (0.36, 17.18)	1.30 (0.20, 5.62)	2.16 (0.29, 9.75)	6.23 (1.91, 19.45)		*PEG IFN + Placebo*
HBeAg loss						
NA						
0.52 (0.10, 2.73)	*NA add-on PEG IFN*					
0.63 (0.11, 3.29)	1.21 (0.11, 11.91)	*PEG IFN*				
0.68 (0.15, 2.75)	1.31 (0.14, 11.60)	1.09 (0.25, 4.64)	*PEG IFN add-on NA*			
0.75 (0.10, 5.48)	1.46 (0.11, 19.44)	1.19 (0.09, 17.27)	1.11 (0.10, 13.48)	*PEG IFN combined NA*		
0.81 (0.10, 6.95)	1.57 (0.11, 22.91)	1.31 (0.09, 21.36)	1.19 (0.10, 16.22)	1.08 (0.06, 21.17)	*NA switch PEG IFN*	
1.47 (0.08, 25.96)	2.83 (0.11, 76.01)	2.37 (0.08, 64.49)	2.15 (0.08, 52.38)	1.93 (0.26, 15.12)	1.80 (0.05, 62.85)	*PEG IFN combined PLA*
HBeAg seroconversion						
NA						
0.39 (0.08, 1.86)	*NA add-on PEG IFN*					
0.53 (0.13, 2.25)	1.34 (0.16, 12.44)	*PEG IFN*				
0.81 (0.21, 3.14)	2.09 (0.27, 16.73)	1.52 (0.39, 5.86)	*PEG IFN add-on NA*			
0.55 (0.12, 2.26)	1.40 (0.15, 12.65)	1.04 (0.20, 4.88)	0.69 (0.11, 3.79)	*PEG IFN combined NA*		
0.37 (0.04, 2.91)	0.94 (0.07, 13.35)	0.69 (0.05, 8.63)	0.45 (0.04, 5.23)	0.67 (0.05, 9.14)	*NA switch PEG IFN*	
0.62 (0.11, 3.00)	1.55 (0.16, 15.37)	1.17 (0.17, 7.39)	0.76 (0.10, 5.06)	1.12 (0.30, 4.32)	1.68 (0.10, 24.88)	*PEG IFN combined PLA*

Note: NA, nucleoside/nucleotide analogs; PEG IFN, PEG IFNylated interferon; PLA, placebo

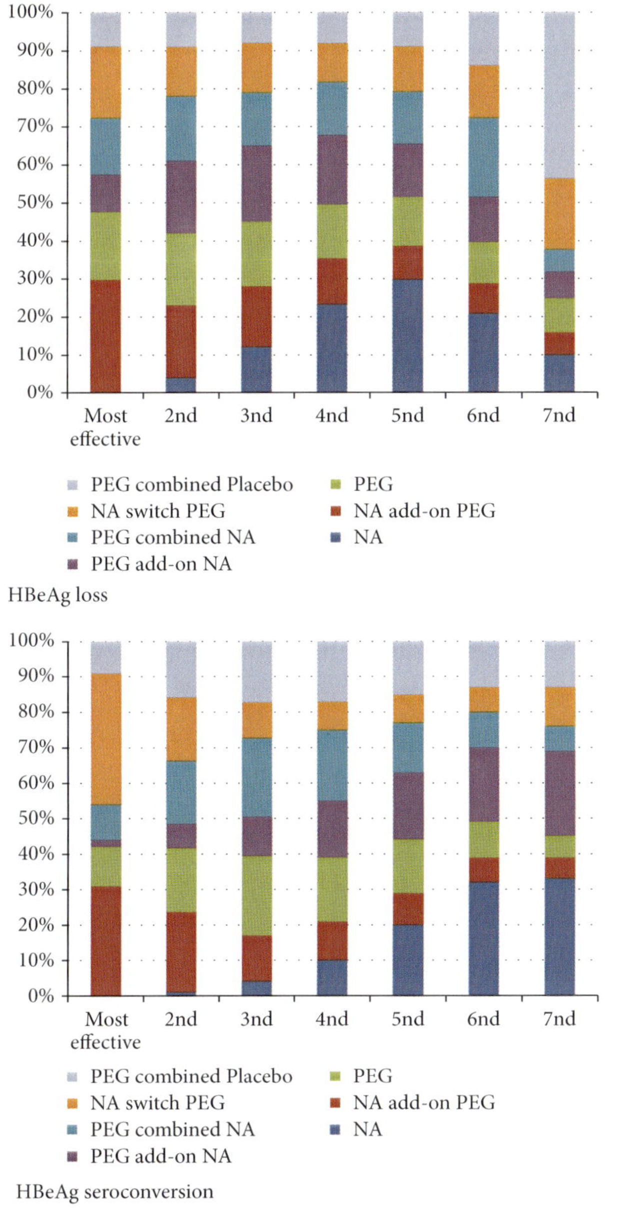

FIGURE 3: Rankogram reporting the probabilities of being the best treatment (reflective of the length in stacked bar for each drug in given column) in terms of HBeAg loss and HBeAg seroconversion.

add-on PEG IFN for HBeAg seroconversion (23%). There was no significant inconsistency within the network meta-analysis.

4. Discussion

Conventional meta-analysis cannot compare the relative effect of one drug to another unless they were compared to each other in the same study. In network meta-analysis, multiple treatment comparisons for a specific disease, which were not compared to each other, can be made simultaneously through a common comparator treatment [16–19]. This network analysis of 9 clinical trials shows that NA add-on PEG IFN is more effective in HBeAg-positive patients based on the goal of loss of HBV DNA, loss of HBeAg, and development of anti-HBeAg antibodies. Also, to the best of our knowledge, this is the first study that provides both direct and indirect evidence in terms of comparative effectiveness of antiviral treatments (monotherapy, combination, adding on, or switching) by included RCTs studies.

Theoretically, a combined NA and PEG IFN approach may provide advantages by combining the potent antiviral effect of NA plus the immune modulation of IFN [5, 20]. However, the evidence of such a combined approach is lacking. In our network analysis, this combined approach was not better than other antiviral approaches in the ALT normalization, HBV undetectable, HBeAg loss, and HBeAg seroconversion, except in the treatment of NA switch PEG IFN. Also, this combined antiviral treatment costs more than other approaches.

Our network analysis showed that NA add-on PEG IFN might be a better antiviral approach for HBeAg-positive patients based on the HBV DNA undetectable, HBeAg loss, and HBeAg seroconversion. As we all know, All NAs are competitive inhibitors of the natural endogenous intracellular nucleotide, which means NAs are effective in suppressing HBV replication [21]. However, the challenge of antiviral therapy is to clear the HBV covalently closed circular DNA (cccDNA) pool. NA has been reported to reduce intrahepatic as well as serum cccDNA [22]. But it is unknown whether long-term NAs have a greater effect on HBV intrahepatic cccDNA decline. As reported, low quantitative hepatitis B surface antigen (qHBsAg) and HBV DNA were strong predictive stopping rule in HBV patients treated with PEG IFN [23]. Serum qHBsAg appears to be more strongly correlated with cccDNA levels in HBeAg-positive patients [24]. Thus, patients first with NA treatment achieved undetectable HBV DNA, followed by adding on PEG IFN which might get a better efficiency.

Our analyses have some strengths, including the use of an exhaustive search strategy, use of RCTs studies, and treatment comparisons by Bayesian networks. However, the results need to be interpreted with caution for the following reasons.

First, the initial treatment for patients with HBeAg-positive was different among the included studies. Table 1 has shown the results. Second, the criteria of included patients were different, and the heterogeneity cannot performed because no more studies were included. Third, most of the studies were performed in China. Forth, HBsAg loss and/or seroconversion which are the major end points of successful HBV therapy were not analyzed, because the data of HBsAg loss and/or seroconversion is limited in the included studies. Therefore, more clinical studies performed in different populations are necessary to access the generalizability of the results. Finally, the efficiency of the network study was based on the end point of treatments. The long-term efficiency should be further determined.

5. Conclusion

This network analysis shows that NA add-on PEG IFN might be a better antiviral approach for HBeAg-positive patients in end point of treatment. Studies of combination therapy with

PEG IFN and NA are still ongoing in a large cohort of patients with a long-term follow-up, and it is possible that this add-on approach may be a future option that may be considered in individual patients, when more robust data will provide definitive evidence of efficacy and clinical benefits.

Authors' Contributions

Zhang Hao and Zhu Biqing collected the data and the statistical analysis. Zhang Hao wrote the article. Yang Ling retrieved the data and disposed of the disagreements. Zeng Wenting is guarantor of the article. All authors approved the final version of the manuscript.

Acknowledgments

This study was supported by Science and Technology Planning Project of Guangdong Province to Wenting Zeng (2013B022000101)

References

[1] J. J. Ott, G. A. Stevens, J. Groeger, and S. T. Wiersma, "Global epidemiology of hepatitis B virus infection: new estimates of age-specific HBsAg seroprevalence and endemicity," *Vaccine*, vol. 30, no. 12, pp. 2212–2219, 2012.

[2] R. Lozano, M. Naghavi, and K. Foreman, "Global and regional mortality from 235 causes of death for 20 age groups in 1990 and 2010: a systematic analysis for the Global Burden of Disease Study 2010," *The Lancet*, vol. 380, no. 9859, pp. 2095–2128, 2012.

[3] N. A. Terrault, N. H. Bzowej, K.-M. Chang, J. P. Hwang, M. M. Jonas, and M. H. Murad, "AASLD guidelines for treatment of chronic hepatitis B," *Hepatology*, vol. 63, no. 1, pp. 261–283, 2016.

[4] Liver EAFT, "EASL clinical practice guidelines: Management of chronic hepatitis B virus infection," *Journal of Hepatology*, vol. 57, no. 1, pp. 167–185, 2012.

[5] P. Marcellin, S. H. Ahn, X. Ma et al., "Combination of tenofovir disoproxil fumarate and peginterferon α-2a increases loss of hepatitis B surface antigen in patients with chronic hepatitis B," *Gastroenterology*, vol. 150, no. 1, pp. 134–144, 2016.

[6] W. P. Brouwer, Q. Xie, M. J. Sonneveld et al., "Adding pegylated interferon to entecavir for hepatitis B e antigen-positive chronic hepatitis B: a multicenter randomized trial (ARES study)," *Hepatology*, vol. 61, no. 5, pp. 1512–1522, 2015.

[7] Q. Ning, M. Han, Y. Sun et al., "Switching from entecavir to PegIFN alfa-2a in patients with HBeAg-positive chronic hepatitis B: a randomised open-label trial (OSST trial)," *Journal of Hepatology*, vol. 61, no. 4, pp. 777–784, 2014.

[8] H. Chi, B. E. Hansen, S. Guo et al., "Pegylated interferon Alfa-2b add-on treatment in hepatitis b virus envelope antigen-positive chronic hepatitis B patients treated with nucleos(t)ide analogue: A randomized, controlled trial (PEGON)," *The Journal of Infectious Diseases*, vol. 215, no. 7, pp. 1085–1093, 2017.

[9] J. Sun, H. Ma, Q. Xie et al., "Response-guided peginterferon therapy in patients with HBeAg-positive chronic hepatitis B: A randomized controlled study," *Journal of Hepatology*, vol. 65, no. 4, pp. 674–682, 2016.

[10] Q. Xie, H. Zhou, X. Bai et al., "A randomized, open-label clinical study of combined pegylated interferon alfa-2a (40KD) and entecavir treatment for hepatitis B 'e' antigen-positive chronic hepatitis B," *Clinical Infectious Diseases*, vol. 59, no. 12, pp. 1714–1723, 2014.

[11] Y.-H. Liu, T. Wu, N. Sun et al., "Combination therapy with pegylated interferon alpha-2b and adefovir dipivoxil in HBeAg-positive chronic hepatitis B versus interferon alone: A prospective, randomized study," *Journal of Huazhong University of Science and Technology (Medical Sciences)*, vol. 34, no. 4, pp. 542–547, 2014.

[12] G. K. K. Lau, T. Piratvisuth, X. L. Kang et al., "Peginterferon Alfa-2a, lamivudine, and the combination for HBeAg-positive chronic hepatitis B," *The New England Journal of Medicine*, vol. 352, no. 26, pp. 2682–2695, 2005.

[13] H. L. Chan, N. W. Leung, A. Y. Hui et al., "A Randomized, Controlled Trial of Combination Therapy for Chronic Hepatitis B: Comparing Pegylated Interferon-α2b and Lamivudine with Lamivudine Alone," *Annals of Internal Medicine*, vol. 142, no. 4, p. 240, 2005.

[14] H. L. A. Janssen, M. Van Zonneveld, H. Senturk et al., "Pegylated interferon alfa-2b alone or in combination with lamivudine for HBeAg-positive chronic hepatitis B: a randomised trial," *The Lancet*, vol. 365, no. 9454, pp. 123–129, 2005.

[15] A. R. Jadad, R. A. Moore, D. Carroll et al., "Assessing the quality of reports of randomized clinical trials: Is blinding necessary?" *Controlled Clinical Trials*, vol. 17, no. 1, pp. 1–12, 1996.

[16] M. J. Sweeting, A. J. Sutton, and P. C. Lambert, "What to add to nothing? Use and avoidance of continuity corrections in meta-analysis of sparse data," *Statistics in Medicine*, vol. 23, no. 9, pp. 1351–1375, 2004.

[17] J. Wetterslev, K. Thorlund, J. Brok, and C. Gluud, "Estimating required information size by quantifying diversity in random-effects model meta-analyses," *BMC Medical Research Methodology*, vol. 9, article no 86, 2009.

[18] L. Govan, O. Wu, Y. Xin, S. J. Hutchinson, and N. Hawkins, "Comparative effectiveness of antiviral treatment for hepatitis B: a systematic review and Bayesian network meta-analysis," *European Journal of Gastroenterology & Hepatology*, vol. 27, no. 8, pp. 882–894, 2015.

[19] B. Njei, N. Gupta, O. Ewelukwa, I. Ditah, M. Foma, and J. K. Lim, "Comparative efficacy of antiviral therapy in preventing vertical transmission of hepatitis B: A network meta-analysis," *Liver International*, vol. 36, no. 5, pp. 634–641, 2016.

[20] P. Marcellin, S. H. Ahn, W.-L. Chuang et al., "Predictors of response to tenofovir disoproxil fumarate plus peginterferon alfa-2a combination therapy for chronic hepatitis B," *Alimentary Pharmacology & Therapeutics*, vol. 44, no. 9, pp. 957–966, 2016.

[21] C. S. Coffin and S. S. Lee, "New paradigms in hepatitis B management: Only diamonds are forever," *British Medical Bulletin*, vol. 116, no. 1, pp. 79–91, 2015.

[22] M.-F. Yuen, D. K.-H. Wong, S. S.-M. Sum et al., "Effect of lamivudine therapy on the serum covalently closed-circular (ccc) DNA of chronic hepatitis B infection," *American Journal of Gastroenterology*, vol. 100, no. 5, pp. 1099–1103, 2005.

[23] M. J. Sonneveld, V. Rijckborst, C. A. B. Boucher, B. E. Hansen, and H. L. A. Janssen, "Prediction of sustained response to peginterferon alfa-2b for hepatitis B e antigen-positive chronic hepatitis B using on-treatment hepatitis B surface antigen decline," *Hepatology*, vol. 52, no. 4, pp. 1251–1257, 2010.

3

Primary Prophylaxis to Prevent the Development of Hepatic Encephalopathy in Cirrhotic Patients with Acute Variceal Bleeding

Fátima Higuera-de-la-Tijera,[1] Alfredo I. Servín-Caamaño,[2] Francisco Salas-Gordillo,[1] José L. Pérez-Hernández,[1] Juan M. Abdo-Francis,[1] Jaime Camacho-Aguilera,[2] Sai N. Alla,[3,4] and Fiacro Jiménez-Ponce[3,4]

[1] *Gastroenterology and Hepatology Department, Mexico's General Hospital, Mexico City 06726, Mexico*
[2] *Internal Medicine Department, Mexico's General Hospital, Mexico City 06726, Mexico*
[3] *Research Department, Chief of the Medical Direction of "Instituto de Seguridad y Servicios Sociales de los Trabajadores del Estado" (ISSSTE), Mexico City 14050, Mexico*
[4] *Cognitive Science A.C., Mexico City 10700, Mexico*

Correspondence should be addressed to Fátima Higuera-de-la-Tijera; fatimahiguera@yahoo.com.mx

Academic Editor: Olivier Barbier

Background and Aim. Variceal bleeding is the second most important precipitating factor related to the development of episodic hepatic encephalopathy; but to date there are no recommendations to prevent this complication. The aim of this study was to compare if primary prophylaxis with lactulose or L-ornithine L-aspartate or rifaximin, in cirrhotic patients with variceal bleeding, is better than placebo for avoiding the development of hepatic encephalopathy. *Methods.* A randomized, double-blind, placebo-controlled clinical trial (ClinicalTrials.gov identifier: NCT02158182) which included cirrhotic patients with variceal bleeding, without minimal or clinical hepatic encephalopathy at admission. *Findings.* 87 patients were randomized to one of four groups. The basal characteristics were similar between groups. Comparatively with placebo, the frequency with regard to the development of hepatic encephalopathy was as follows: lactulose (54.5% versus 27.3%; OR = 0.3, 95% CI 0.09-1.0; $P = 0.06$); L-ornithine L-aspartate (54.5% versus 22.7%, OR = 0.2, 95% CI 0.06-0.88; $P = 0.03$); rifaximin (54.5% versus 23.8%; OR = 0.3, 95% CI 0.07-0.9; $P = 0.04$). There was no significant difference between the three groups receiving any antiammonium drug ($P = 0.94$). In the group receiving lactulose, 59.1% had diarrhea, and 45.5% had abdominal discomfort, bloating, and flatulence. Two patients (10%) treated with lactulose and a patient (4.5%) in the placebo group developed spontaneous bacterial peritonitis due to *E. coli*; one of them died due to recurrent variceal bleeding. There were no other adverse effects. *Conclusions.* Antiammonium drugs, particularly L-ornithine L-aspartate and rifaximin, proved to be effective in preventing the development of hepatic encephalopathy in those cirrhotic patients with variceal bleeding.

1. Introduction

Hepatic encephalopathy (HE) is a neurological disorder caused by the accumulation of toxic substances in the blood due to the inability of liver to perform its detoxification functions [1]. Ammonium plays an important role in the pathophysiology of this disorder, and even the currently available treatments for HE are designed to reduce the production and intestinal absorption of ammonium or to promote the metabolism thereof in extrahepatic tissues. Treatments that have proven to be effective in both minimal HE (MHE), detected through changes in neuropsychometric tests, and in overt HE (OHE) include nonabsorbable disaccharides such as lactulose, antibiotic that acts in intestinal lumen such as rifaximin, and drugs favoring extrahepatic metabolism of ammonium such as L-ornithine L-aspartate (LOLA) [2–5].

It is well known that the development of HE deteriorates the cognitive function in cirrhotic patients and also predisposes to risks such as increased frequency of falls. This cognitive impairment has a significant negative impact on the quality of life of these patients [6, 7].

Severe cases of HE can lead to coma and death [7]. In patients with acute on chronic liver failure it has been shown that the development of HE independently predicts higher mortality [8, 9]. In this clinical context, studies show extremely high mortality in patients who develop HE with cerebral edema [10]. In 2009, in a period of one year, Fichet reported a 54% mortality-rate in patients with severe HE admitted in intensive care units [11].

Acute variceal bleeding (AVB) occurs in 25 to 30% of patients with cirrhosis [12]. The development of HE in patients with AVB is a well-known complication and the incidence of this complication ranges from 16.9 to 40% [13, 14]. The absorption of toxic products such as ammonium is the main mechanism involved in the development of HE after an episode of AVB. In order to favor the elimination of blood from the gastrointestinal tract various treatment strategies had been used such as bulking enemas and intestinal irrigation with mannitol [15–19]. However, currently these therapies are not recommended and therefore not used routinely.

To date, only two nonblinded studies have evaluated oral administration of lactulose versus placebo, demonstrating that lactulose is an effective therapy to prevent the development of HE after an AVB [13, 14].

The aim of this study was to compare whether the clinical effect of primary prophylaxis with lactulose or LOLA or rifaximin in cirrhotic patients with AVB is better than placebo for preventing the development of HE.

2. Methods

A randomized, double-blinded, controlled clinical trial (ClinicalTrials.gov number NCT02158182) was performed at "*Hospital General de México*". The selection criteria included cirrhotic patients, both genders, admitted to hospital for AVB, without MHE assessed by the Psychometric Hepatic Encephalopathy Score (PHES) and critical flicker frequency (CFF) or OHE according to West-Haven criteria [20]. Exclusion criteria were patients under 18 years and over 65 years; patients with any type of dementia or any manifestation of neurological disease; patients with any type of bacterial infection at admission; patients who were receiving secondary prophylaxis for spontaneous bacterial peritonitis (SBP) with norfloxacin or another antibiotic because we thought it could be a bias for our investigation since infections are the main precipitating factor of episodic HE; patients with a previous diagnosis of MHE or OHE and who were receiving treatment with specific therapies for HE; patients whose aetiology of AVB and portal hypertension were distinct from cirrhosis; patients with serum creatinine $\geq$ 2.0 mg/dL or previously diagnosed with chronic renal failure; patients treated in the previous 6 months with any of the drugs used in this clinical trial. Patients with severe AVB who were hemodynamically unstable or who required orotracheal intubation at admission were not eligible for this trial. Patients who withdrawn their informed consent to participate in the study and who have not completed at least one evaluation after treatment were eliminated.

2.1. Sample Size. We used the formula for contrasting hypotheses of two proportions. We considered a one-sided level of significance of 5% ($\alpha = 0.05$) hypothesizing that any of the prophylactic manoeuvres employed would be superior to placebo and also considering noninferiority between the antiammonium therapies. We considered a statistical power of 80% ($1\text{-}\beta = 0.80$) acceptable. As at the time of design this study there were no previous clinical trials about preventing the development of HE in cirrhotic patients with AVB treated with rifaximin or with LOLA, we based our sample size calculation on the assumption that an acceptable difference would be to find 40% less development of HE in those treated with lactulose or with rifaximin or with LOLA, each group by itself compared to the placebo group. With these data the sample size was 18 patients per group but we considered an additional 20%, because of possible losses (4 patients per group). Hence the sample size of 22 patients per group was assigned.

2.2. Definition of Terms

Primary Prophylaxis. It is also called "primary prevention" which is defined as those measures directed to prevent a condition or disease [21]. For this study, primary prophylaxis strategies were the administration of lactulose or rifaximin or LOLA, aimed at preventing the development of OHE in cirrhotic patients admitted for AVB.

Overt Hepatic Encephalopathy (OHE). It was defined according to the American Association for the Study of Liver Diseases (AASLD) and European Association for the Study of the Liver (EASL) guideline as "brain dysfunction caused by liver insufficiency and/or portosystemic shunting, and manifests as a wide spectrum of neurological/psychiatric abnormalities ranging from mild clinical alterations to coma". OHE can encompass a wide spectrum of mental and motor disorders and may arise episodically over a period of hours of days in a previously stable patient [22]. Clinically we assessed patients daily through the West-Haven criteria [20]. Clinical diagnosis was performed by carrying out a systemic neurological exploration by a blinded expert neurologist.

Minimal Hepatic Encephalopathy (MHE). It means absence of evident clinical manifestations, but with alterations in neuropsychometric tests, such as PHES and/or CFF [20, 22].

Acute Variceal Bleeding (AVB). Cirrhotic patients were admitted to hospital for hematemesis and/or melena and demonstrated endoscopically the presence of esophageal or esophagogastric varices with active bleeding or red signs suggesting inactive, but recent bleeding. The AVB was handled specifically according to the recommendations of practice guidelines of the AASLD [19].

Spontaneous Bacterial Peritonitis (SBP). This diagnosis was clinically suspected in those who developed symptoms and/or signs of peritoneal irritation, but also in those who developed HE, since several cases of SBP are oligosymptomatic. In all these cases, we performed a diagnostic paracentesis to obtain a polymorphonuclear count (PMN) and ascites culture. The diagnosis was confirmed by a PMN ≥ 250 cells/mm3 in ascites and a positive ascites culture. It was first empirically treated according to the recommendations of the AASLD practical guidelines [23], and then the antibiotic treatment was adjusted according to the report of ascites culture.

2.3. Study Endpoints. The primary endpoint was the development of OHE in the first week (7 days) after an AVB. Secondary endpoints were as follows: The time in days for the development of OHE after an AVB; also the late occurrence of OHE on the first 28 days after an AVB; finally, the development of adverse effects during therapy. Specifically, for the group receiving rifaximin, a secondary endpoint was to verify the frequency of development of SBP in comparison with the other groups.

2.4. Procedure and Randomization

Preinclusion Phase. Informed consent was obtained for all participants in this study; medical history along with neurological examination of every patient was performed, to rule out OHE; the West-Haven criteria were applied [20]. Likewise, the mini-mental test was performed; if the result was normal, then the PHES was applied and finally the CFF was performed in order to detect those patients with MHE. Patients with OHE or MHE at admission were excluded from this study.

At admission laboratory studies were taken: urea, creatinine, sodium, chlorine, potassium, total bilirubin, albumin, hemoglobin levels, leukocytes count, platelets count, prothrombin time, and international normalized ratio (INR).

In case of ascites diagnostic paracentesis was performed for PMN count and culture; moreover urinalysis, blood and urine cultures, and chest X-ray were performed to exclude infections at admission. Endoscopy was performed within the first 12 hours after admission to determine the source of bleeding. Number of red cells units transfused, hemodynamic parameters such as cardiac frequency and mean arterial pressure at admission, and recurrence of AVB were recorded.

Randomization. A person was the monitor who made the black bags for containing the medications and the corresponding placebos, for all different groups, and this person did not participate in allocation or clinical evaluation of patients.

After the initial assessment by a blinded investigator, patients who met selection criteria and signed the informed consent were allocated to one of four possible groups by another investigator; also he was blinded to the drugs administered in each group; he only knew the name of the group by the letter (A, B, C, or D) but he did not know which medication corresponded to the letter of the group. Randomization was carried out using a table of random numbers considering four groups of equal size, constructed with the Epidat 3.1 statistic program (Galicia, Spain 2006), to evenly distribute patients to each treatment groups. The investigator, who allocated patients to the treatment groups, never had contact with them.

Group A was treated with lactulose (Lactulax®) orally, 30 mL every 8 hours, while patients had residual melena; then it was adjusted by increasing or reducing the dose to 10 ml every day according to the dose response to achieve two to three daily soft stools. Group B was treated with LOLA (Hepa-Merz®) intravenous infusion (500 ml of saline solution containing 10 grams of LOLA for 24 hours). Group C was treated with rifaximin (Flonorm®) administered at a standard dose of 400 mg orally every 8 hours. Group D was the control group that received all the corresponding placebos to achieve blinding of the study; patients in this group received an intravenous glucose solution of 5% for 24 hours, dextrose solution of 30 ml orally every 8 hours, adjusted equally as mentioned for lactulose dose, and 2 dextrose tablets orally every 8 hours in similar size, color, and shape to the rifaximin tablets. Groups A, B, and C also received treatment corresponding to the complementary placebos to ensure that both the investigator and the patient were blind towards the prophylaxis maneuver they were receiving. In all groups treatment duration was 7 days.

2.5. AVB Treatment. Hemodynamic stabilization, as well as vasopressors (octreotide or terlipressin), was administered following the recommendations of the AASLD practical guidelines [19]. Endoscopic study was conducted in the first 12 hours after admission. In case of AVB by esophageal varices band ligation was performed, and in case of AVB by gastric varices sclerotherapy was used.

2.6. Primary Prophylaxis of Infections. Quinolones or cephalosporins were administered during a period of 7 days according to the recommendations of practice guidelines from the AASLD [19, 23]. In group C patients, rifaximin was the only antibiotic administered, because a specific secondary endpoint in this group was to verify the frequency of development of SBP in comparison with the other groups. This group received saline solution intravenously instead of the systemic antibiotics to try blinding the study correctly.

2.7. Follow-Up. Patients were reassessed daily through West-Haven scale and systematic neurological exploration searching for OHE [20]. Laboratory controls were taken on day 3 and on day 7; these included urea, creatinine, sodium, chlorine, potassium, bilirubin, albumin, also hemoglobin, leukocytes count, platelets count, prothrombin time, and INR.

In case of clinical suspicion of infection development, a control diagnostic paracentesis for PMN count and ascites culture and urine and blood cultures and chest X-ray were taken.

After 7 complete days of therapy and follow-up, stable patients without additional complications were discharged for outpatient follow-up. Only those patients who required treatment due to development of OHE or any other complications stayed in hospital for management. Thereafter, all patients were reassessed every week until 28-day follow-up searching for late complications.

2.8. Statistical Analysis. Quantitative variables were expressed as mean and standard deviation or median and range according to their parametric or nonparametric distribution. The qualitative variables were expressed as a ratio and percentage. To compare among groups, Student's t-test or Mann–Whitney U test and one-way ANOVA with post hoc contrasts were applied using LSD test or T2 Tamhane according to the homogeneity of variances; Kruskal-Wallis, Chi-square, and Fisher's exact tests were applied as appropriate. To estimate the risk, odds ratios and their respective 95% confidence interval were calculated. For the multivariate analysis, binary logistic regression was performed. Additionally we constructed Cox regression models. Epidat 3.1 statistical package (Galicia, Spain 2006) and SPSS version 19.0 (Chicago, IL 2010) were used.

2.9. Ethical and Biosafety Aspects. All patients signed the written informed consent to participate in the study. This study was approved by Institutional Ethics and Investigation Committees.

3. Results

103 cirrhotic patients were evaluated and admitted for AVB; of them 15 met some exclusion criteria (4 were older than 65 years, 3 were receiving secondary prophylaxis with norfloxacin for SBP, 3 had recent intake of alcohol, and 5 did not agree to participate). 88 patients were randomized to one of four possible groups, but one in group C finally withdrew his consent to participate in the study. See Figure 1. The baseline characteristics of patients included in the study are summarized in Table 1.

3.1. Development of Overt Hepatic Encephalopathy (OHE). In the placebo group 12/22 patients (54.5%) developed OHE after the AVB episode; in the lactulose group this occurred in 6/22 patients (27.3%); in the group receiving LOLA this occurred in 5/22 patients (22.7%); and in the group receiving rifaximin this occurred in 5/21 patients (23.8%). Comparatively with placebo, the frequency regarding the development of OHE was as follows: lactulose (54.5% versus 27.3%, OR 0.3, 95% CI 0.09 to 1.1; $P = 0.06$); LOLA (54.5% versus 22.7%, OR 0.2, 95% CI 0.06 to 0.88; $P = 0.03$); rifaximin (54.5% versus 23.8%, OR 0.3, 95% CI 0.07 to 0.9; $P = 0.04$). When we compared the three groups that received antiammonium therapies, we found no significant differences between the three groups ($P = 0.94$).

The time in days from admission to the development of OHE among those who developed it was as follows: lactulose, median 2.5 (range: 2-4); LOLA, median 3 (range: 1-3); rifaximin, median 3 (range: 1-4); placebo, median 2 (range 1-4); $P = 0.88$. Nobody developed OHE beyond day 4 on 28-day follow-up.

Regarding the degree of OHE according to the West-Haven criteria, the degree of OHE was more severe in those who received placebo (median 3, range 2-4) compared to those who received any antiammonium prophylactic measure: LOLA (median 1, range 1-2) ($P = 0.04$); rifaximin (median 2, range 1 to 3) ($P = 0.05$); and lactulose (median 2, range: 1 to 3) ($P = 0.02$).

3.2. Adverse Effects. In the group receiving lactulose 12/22 patients (54.5%) had diarrhea and required a dose reduction to 50% (15 ml orally every 8 hours); also 2/22 patients (9.1%) required reducing the dose to 10 ml every 12 hours to achieve the goal of two to three soft stools a day but without diarrhea. Moreover 10/22 (45.5%) reported bloating, abdominal discomfort, and flatulence.

Two patients (9.1%) in the lactulose group developed SBP secondary to *E. coli*; one died on day 10 of follow-up as a consequence of the recurrence of AVB. One patient (4.5%) in the placebo group also developed SBP (*E. coli*); this person improved with adjusted antibiotic treatment according to the results of bacteriological culture.

One patient (4.8%) in rifaximin group had nausea and dyspepsia, no other adverse events were recorded in this group, and no patient in this group developed SBP at 1-month follow-up. One patient in this group died at day 15 of follow-up due to recurrence of the AVB. In the group of LOLA no adverse events or deaths were registered.

3.3. Comparison between Characteristics of Patients Who Developed OHE versus Those Who Did Not Develop OHE. Patients who developed OHE subsequent to the AVB episode recorded a lower mean arterial pressure on admission compared to patients who did not develop encephalopathy (64.1 ± 10.8 versus 69.6 ± 10.2; $P = 0.02$). The serum albumin was lower among patients who developed OHE versus those who did not develop OHE (2.7 ± 0.7 versus 3.2 ± 0.5; $P < 0.0001$). Prothrombin time (19.3 ± 9.3 versus 15.4 ± 3.6; $P = 0.03$) and INR (1.6 ± 0.8 versus 1.3 ± 0.3; $P = 0.03$) were longer among those who developed OHE versus those who did not develop OHE. See Table 2.

In the univariate analysis the recurrence of AVB and decompensated (Child B or C) cirrhosis were identified as predisposing factors associated with the development of OHE. On the other hand, receiving prophylaxis with some antiammonium therapy was a protective factor that prevented the development of OHE following an AVB episode. Neither the development of SBP nor the origin (esophageal or gastric) of variceal bleeding influenced the development of OHE. See Table 3. The multivariate analysis confirmed that the recurrence of AVB is the main risk factor for the development of OHE (OR = 12.1; 95% CI 3.5-42.5; $P < 0.0001$). The multivariate analysis also confirmed that receiving prophylaxis with any antiammonium therapy was a protective factor to avoid the development of OHE in cirrhotic patients following an episode of AVB (OR = 0.2; 95% CI 0.05 to 0.6; $P = 0.006$). See Table 4.

Additionally, with the variables that showed statistical significance in the univariate analysis, we constructed two distinct Cox regression models, the dependent variable was the

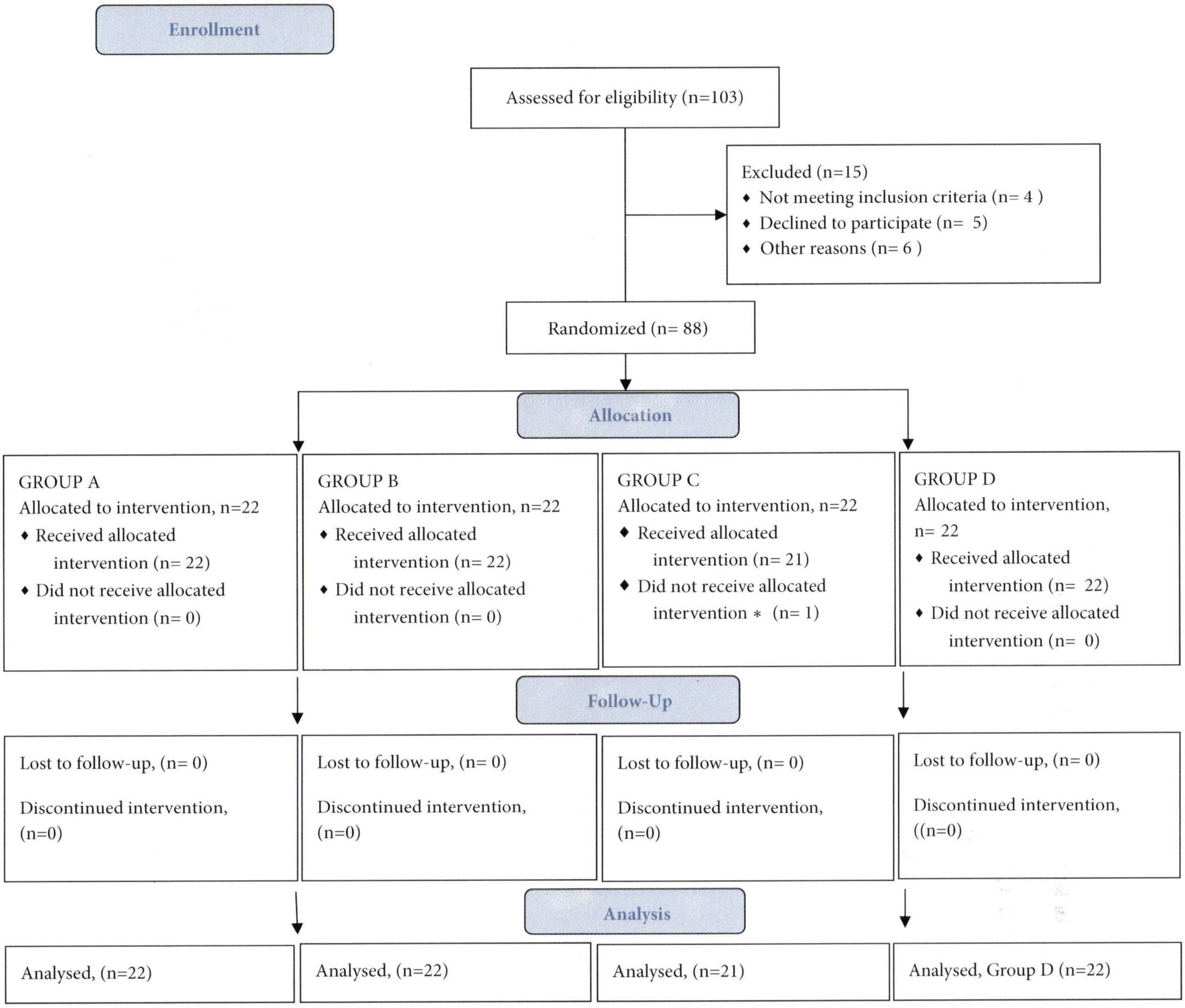

FIGURE 1: Group A was treated with lactulose orally, 30 mL every 8 hours; meanwhile it was adjusted according to the dose response to achieve two to three daily soft stools. Group B was treated with LOLA administered at a standard dose of 10 grams intravenously diluted with saline solution of 500 ml with a continuous infusion for 24 hours. Group C was treated with rifaximin administered at a standard dose of 400 mg orally every 8 hours. Group D was the control group that received all the corresponding placebos to achieve blinding of the study; patients in this group received an intravenous glucose solution of 5% for 24 hours, dextrose solution of 30 ml orally every 8 hours, and 2 dextrose tablets orally every 8 hours in similar size, color, and shape to the tablets of rifaximin. Groups A, B, and C received also the other corresponding placebos in other double-blind study. The duration of therapy was 7 days in all groups. *Withdrawn his informed consent.

development of OHE, and the time for occurrence of OHE was determined in days. In the first model we introduced dichotomous variables: recurrence of bleed, decompensated cirrhosis, and receiving or not an antiammonium therapy. In the second model we introduced categorical variables: recurrence of bleed, cirrhosis stratified according to Child (A, B, or C), and group of treatment (A, B, C, or D). None of the two models demonstrated statistical significance for any variable. See Table 5.

4. Discussion

The AVB is recognized as the second most important factor triggering episodic HE [24, 25], but to date, there are no recommendations or sufficient evidence regarding which strategies could prevent this complication.

Our study shows that primary prophylaxis with anti-ammonium drugs, started early in cirrhotic patients admitted due to AVB, is a strategy which is effective in avoiding the

TABLE 1: Basal characteristics of patients.

Characteristic	Lactulose n = 22	LOLA n = 22	Rifaximin n = 21	Placebo n = 22	*P*
Age (years)	50.1 ± 11.3	54.3 + 7.7	53.0 + 10.9	49.3 ± 9.5	0.31
Male gender, n (%)	14 (63.6)	14 (63.6)	10 (47.6)	17 (77.3)	0.25
CHILD A/B/C	7/10/5	7/13/2	9/10/2	5/15/2	0.54
Units of red cells concentrates	1.1 ± 1.4	1.4 + 1.2	1.0 + 1.1	1.4 ± 1.1	0.51
Cause of cirrhosis (n)					
Alcohol	8	11	9	11	0.65
Hepatitis C	6	4	3	4	
NASH	4	7	5	4	
Other	4	0	4	3	
MAP (mmHg)	70.4 ± 10.3	68.4 ± 11.6	67.8 ± 10.3	65.7 ± 10.5	0.50
Cardiac frequency (beats/min)	90.9 ± 15.6	95.4 ± 12.3	88.8 ± 7.8	94.9 ± 10.4	0.47
Time before endoscopy (hours)	8.0 ± 1.9	7.0 ± 1.0	7.6 ± 1.6	7.0 ± 1.0	0.07
Urea (mg/dl)	41.4 ± 20.6	39.5 ± 18.6	41.9 ± 22.2	44.8 ± 22.2	0.86
Creatinine (mg/dl)	0.92 ± 0.26	0.81 ± 0.18	0.83 ± 0.21	0.93 ± 0.22	0.20
Sodium (mEq/L)	137.6 ± 3.7	138.2 ± 4.6	138.5 ± 3.1	136.6 ± 3.7	0.39
Potassium (mEq/L)	4.0 ± 0.5	3.9 ± 0.5	4.0 ± 0.5	3.9 ± 0.4	0.62
Chlorine (mEq/L)	104.9 ± 4.0	101.9 ± 4.2	103.2 ± 5.6	104.3 ± 6.2	0.24
Albumin (mg/dl)	3.0 ± 0.7	3.2 ± 0.5	3.0 ± 0.6	2.9 ± 0.7	0.47
Bilirubin (mg/dl)	1.7 ± 1.4	1.7 ± 1.2	1.7 ± 1.3	2.1 ± 1.8	0.69
Hemoglobin (g/dl)	9.9 ± 4.7	8.6 ± 2.9	8.8 ± 2.7	8.3 ± 2.7	0.46
Hematocrit (%)	30.1 ± 14.6	26.3 ± 8.3	26.7 ± 7.9	25.7 ± 7.9	0.50
Platelets (10^9cells/mcl)	130.6 ± 95.3	107.3 ± 34.4	131.1 ± 69.7	127.5 ± 71.9	0.65
Leucocytes (10^3cells/mcl)	8.1 ± 5.4	7.6 ± 2.8	6.8 ± 2.6	9.0 ± 5.1	0.39
Neutrophils (10^3cells/mcl)	6.0 ± 4.0	5.7 ± 2.3	5.2 ± 2.3	7.0 ± 4.6	0.41
Prothrombin time (sec)	17.3 ± 5.9	15.6 ± 3.9	17.8 ± 10.7	16.7 ± 4.0	0.73
INR	1.5 ± 0.5	1.3 ± 0.4	1.5 ± 0.9	1.4 ± 0.3	0.64
Variceal bleeding source Esophageal/Gastric (n)	19/3	20/2	16/5	20/2	0.46
Rebleeding, n (%)	3 (13.6)	7 (31.8)	7 (33.3)	5 (22.7)	0.39

INR: international normalized ratio; LOLA: L-ornithine L-aspartate; MAP: mean arterial pressure; NASH: nonalcoholic steatohepatitis.
Statistical significance: $P \leq 0.05$.

development of OHE, globally decreasing the incidence of OHE in 25.9% when compared with the placebo group; this is consistent with what other authors have previously reported, such as P. Sharma et al. [14], who in an open clinical trial compared the prophylactic effect of lactulose with placebo in preventing the development of OHE in cirrhotic patients with AVB and found a difference, between groups, of 26% in favor of the group treated with lactulose.

Our study highlights that lactulose was the antiammonium drug that did not strictly reach statistical significance to prevent the development of OHE in cirrhotic patients with AVB compared with placebo ($P = 0.06$). However, when its effectiveness was compared with LOLA and rifaximin, there was no significant difference between the three antiammonium measures ($P = 0.08$). In comparison to LOLA and rifaximin, lactulose recorded multiple gastrointestinal adverse effects that were not severe; this is similar to a previous report by Als-Nielsen B, in a systematic review [26]. It is important to note that our results can be unpowered because this was a pilot study with a hypothetical sample size calculation based on a formula for contrasting hypothesis of two proportions. We recognize that we could make a mistake because we finally include four different treatment groups. With this in mind, we calculate again the sample size, this time using the statistical program G Power 3.1.9.2 to compare proportions between four groups, using as main

TABLE 2: Comparison between the characteristics of patients who develop and those who did not develop encephalopathy after acute variceal bleeding.

Characteristic	With HE (n = 59)	Without HE (n = 28)	*P*
Age (years)	50.8 ± 10.4	53.4 ± 8.9	0.25
Male gender, n (%)	35 (59.3)	20 (71.4)	0.27
CHILD A/B/C	24/29/6	4/19/5	0.03
Units of red cells concentrates	1.1 ± 1.1	1.5 ± 1.3	0.15
Cause of cirrhosis (n)			
Alcohol	24	15	0.48
Hepatitis C	14	3	
NASH	14	6	
Other	7	4	
MAP (mmHg)	69.6 ± 10.2	64.1 ± 10.8	0.02
Cardiac frequency (beats/min)	91.2 ± 12.6	95.3 ± 10.5	0.12
Time before endoscopy (hours)	7.6 ± 1.6	6.9 ± 1.1	0.02
Urea (mg/dl)	39.3 ± 19.4	47.4 ± 22.5	0.09
Creatinine (mg/dl)	0.87 ± 0.21	0.88 ± 0.22	0.75
Sodium (mEq/L)	137.9 ± 3.3	136.8 ± 4.7	0.22
Potassium (mEq/L)	4.0 ± 0.4	3.9 ± 0.6	0.75
Chlorine (mEq/L)	103.3 ± 4.5	103.3 ± 6.1	0.99
Albumin (mg/dl)	3.2 ± 0.5	2.7 ± 0.7	<0.0001
Bilirubin (mg/dl)	1.6 ± 1.3	2.1 ± 1.5	0.09
Hemoglobin (g/dl)	8.7 ± 3.1	9.0 ± 3.7	0.74
Hematocrit (%)	26.5 ± 9.1	27.8 ± 11.3	0.59
Platelets (10^9cel/mcl)	120.1 ± 69.7	128.4 ± 65.9	0.60
Leucocytes (10^3cel/mcl)	7.3 ± 3.7	8.7 ± 4.8	0.14
Neutrophils (10^3cells/mcl)	5.4 ± 2.8	6.7 ± 4.4	0.16
Prothrombin time (sec)	15.4 ± 3.6	19.3 ± 9.3	0.03
INR	1.3 ± 0.3	1.6 ± 0.8	0.03
Variceal bleeding source Esophageal/Gastric (n)	50/9	25/3	0.74

HE: hepatic encephalopathy; INR: international normalized ratio; MAP: mean arterial pressure; NASH: nonalcoholic steatohepatitis.
Statistical significance: $P \leq 0.05$.

TABLE 3: Factors related to the development of hepatic encephalopathy in patients with cirrhosis after an acute episode of variceal bleeding. Univariate analysis.

Characteristic	Without HE (n = 59)	With HE (n = 28)	OR (95% CI)	*P*
Rebleeding, n (%)	7 (11.9)	15 (53.6)	8.6 (2.9 - 25.3)*	<0.0001
Decompensated cirrhosis CHILD B/C, n (%)	35 (59.3)	24 (85.7)	4.1 (1.3 - 13.4)*	0.01
SBP development, n (%)	2 (3.4)	1 (3.6)	1.1 (0.09 - 12.2)	1.00
Primary prophylaxis with any anti-ammonium drug, n (%)	49 (83%)	16 (57.1%)	0.2 (0.09 - 0.7)**	0.009
Gastric variceal bleeding source, n (%)	9 (15.3%)	3 (10.7%)	0.7 (0.2 - 2.7)	0.74

CI: confidence interval; HE: hepatic encephalopathy; OR: odds ratio; SBP: spontaneous bacterial peritonitis.
Statistical significance: $P \leq 0.05$. * Risk factor. ** Protective factor.

TABLE 4: Factors related to the development of hepatic encephalopathy in patients with cirrhosis after an acute episode of variceal bleeding. Multivariate analysis by binary logistic regression.

Characteristic	OR (95% CI)	*P*
Recurrence of bleeding (yes)	12.1 (3.5 - 42.5)*	<0.0001
Decompensated cirrhosis (CHILD B ó C)	3.0 (1.0 - 15.1)*	0.05
Primary prophylaxis with any anti-ammonium drug	0.2 (0.05 - 0.6)**	0.006

CI: confidence interval; OR: odds ratio.
Statistical significance: $P \leq 0.05$. *Risk factor. **Protective factor.

TABLE 5: Factors related to the development of hepatic encephalopathy in patients with cirrhosis after an acute episode of variceal bleeding. Multivariate analysis by Cox regression models.

MODEL 1		
Characteristic	**OR (95% CI)**	***P***
Recurrence of bleeding (yes)	1.9 (0.8 – 4.5)	0.17
Decompensated cirrhosis (Child-Pugh B or C)	1.0 (0.4 – 3.0)	0.96
Primary prophylaxis with any anti-ammonium drug	0.6 (0.2 – 1.5)	0.28
MODEL 2		
Characteristic	**OR (95% CI)**	***P***
Recurrence of bleeding (yes)	1.6 (0.6 – 4.4)	0.39
Cirrhosis (Child-Pugh A)	-	0.50
(i) Child-Pugh B	0.8 (0.2 – 2.8)	0.76
(ii) Child-Pugh C	1.7 (0.4 – 7.3)	0.46
Group of Treatment (Placebo)	-	0.69
(i) LOLA	0.6 (0.2 – 2.3)	0.47
(ii) Lactulose	0.5 (0.2 – 1.7)	0.26
(iii) Rifaximin	0.6 (0.2 – 2.0)	0.41

CI: confidence interval; LOLA: L-ornithine L-aspartate; OR: odds ratio.
Statistical significance: $P \leq 0.05$.

statistical test X2 considering the command "goodness of fit tests: contingency tables" with a priori effect size of 0.40, alpha error of 0.05, statistical power of 80% ($1-\beta = 0.80$), and 4 degrees of freedom, obtaining a total sample size of 75 patients. However, if we increase the statistical power to 95% ($1-\beta = 0.95$), the total sample size increases to 117 patients. We consider that future clinical studies must be conducted to validate our findings.

In addition to a lower incidence in patients who received primary prophylaxis with some antiammonium therapy, it is noteworthy that in patients who did develop OHE the severity of the clinical HE determined by West-Haven scale was significantly lower in those who received some anti-ammonium drug, in comparison with the placebo group.

Bacterial infections, such as SBP, are recognized as a factor with a dominant role as a risk factor associated with the development of episodic HE [24]. However, in our study, very few patients (only 3) developed SBP, which explains the fact that, in the univariate analysis, this variable did not behave as a risk factor associated with development of HE. Interestingly, none of them were in the rifaximin group; therefore, this suggests the importance of designing specific clinical trials to validate if rifaximin can be an effective prophylactic therapy not only in avoiding the development of HE, but also in preventing the development of SBP in cirrhotic patients with AVB; if this finding is confirmed by future studies, it could be the most cost-effective strategy in this specific clinical scenario. Some previous studies suggest that rifaximin has an important role in regulating the intestinal microbiota [2, 27–29]. A recent meta-analysis, which included five studies with 555 patients, comparing rifaximin (295 patients) with systemic antibiotics (260 patients), found a potential protective effect of rifaximin (OR for SBP was 0.34; 95% CI 0.11-0.99; $P < 0.05$), with the advantage that rifaximin is a nonabsorbable drug compared to systemic antibiotics [30].

In our study, the recurrence of the AVB was the most important factor associated with the risk of developing OHE. Patients presenting with an episode of AVB have a risk higher than 60% of recurrence within the next year [25]. After the recurrence of the AVB, decompensated cirrhosis (Child B or C) was in our study the second most important factor which contributed to development of OHE. Similarly, Rattanasupar A et al. found that main risk factors for developing HE after an AVB were as follows: being Child C class, serum potassium < 3.5 mmole/L, leucocytes count > 10,000 cells/mm3, and hemoglobin level < 8 g/dL. Also, they found that cirrhotic patients with AVB who developed HE had high morbidity and mortality rates [31]. Based on the logistic regression model, our study suggests the introduction of any antiammonium drug could be a protective factor to prevent the development of OHE. However, this fact was not confirmed by the Cox regression models, maybe because of a small sample size in our study.

A limitation of our clinical trial is that we did not include patients with severe AVB who were hemodynamically unstable or who required orotracheal intubation at admission; it can compromise the external validity of our findings, which would be recommendable to perform new clinical trials to address the impact of primary prophylaxis with antiammonium drugs in this specific clinical context. Other interesting studies in hemodynamically unstable patients would be those conducted in "real life cohorts".

Another important limitation of our study is that although it was a double-blind clinical trial, the blinding was imperfect because lactulose exerts a cathartic effect difficult to go unnoticed. In fact, the main adverse effects registered in our patients were gastrointestinal and were present in the group receiving lactulose.

5. Conclusions

In conclusion, our study shows that early primary prophylaxis with antiammonium drugs, particularly LOLA and rifaximin, seems to be a promising clinical strategy, effective and safe to avoid the development of OHE in cirrhotic patients with AVB. The most important risk factor associated with the development of OHE was the recurrence of the AVB.

Abbreviations

AASLD: **American Association for Study of Liver Disease**
AVB: **Acute variceal bleeding**
CCF: Critical flicker frequency
EASL: European Association for the Study of the Liver
HE: Hepatic encephalopathy
INR: International normalized ratio
LOLA: L-Ornithine L-aspartate
MHE: Minimal hepatic encephalopathy
NASH: Nonalcoholic steatohepatitis
OHE: Overt hepatic encephalopathy
PHES: Psychometric Hepatic Encephalopathy Score
PMN: Polymorphonuclear cells
SBP: Spontaneous bacterial peritonitis.

Disclosure

The results of this study were presented orally at the Parallel Session of Portal Hypertension and Hepatic Encephalopathy, at the International Liver Congress 2017, held in Amsterdam, The Netherlands. An abstract was published in the Congress Supplement of Journal of Hepatology (DOI: https://doi.org/10.1016/S0168-8278(17)30362-8).

Acknowledgments

This research received grant and funding from "Estímulo Ángeles Espinosa Yglesias 2014" provided to **Fátima Higuera-de la Tijera** for support of her Ph.D. by "*Fundación Mexicana para la Salud Hepática A.C.*" (FUNDHEPA). Alfasigma Inc. supported the authors with the pay of publication fee.

References

[1] P. Ferenci, A. Lockwood, K. Mullen, R. Tarter, K. Weissenborn, and A. T. Blei, "Hepatic encephalopathy—definition, nomenclature, diagnosis, and quantification: final report of the Working Party at the 11th World Congresses of Gastroenterology, Vienna, 1998," *Hepatology*, vol. 35, no. 3, pp. 716–721, 2002.

[2] V. Khungar and F. Poordad, "Hepatic Encephalopathy," *Clinics in Liver Disease*, vol. 16, no. 2, pp. 301–320, 2012.

[3] M. Luo, L. Li, C.-Z. Lu, and W.-K. Cao, "Clinical efficacy and safety of lactulose for minimal hepatic encephalopathy: A meta-analysis," *European Journal of Gastroenterology & Hepatology*, vol. 23, no. 12, pp. 1250–1257, 2011.

[4] J. P. Ong, G. Oehler, C. Krüger-Jansen, J. Lambert-Baumann, and Z. M. Younossi, "Oral L-ornithine-L-aspartate improves health-related quality of life in cirrhotic patients with hepatic encephalopathy: An open-label, prospective, multicentre observational study," *Clinical Drug Investigation*, vol. 31, no. 4, pp. 213–220, 2011.

[5] N. M. Bass, K. D. Mullen, A. Sanyal et al., "Rifaximin treatment in hepatic encephalopathy," *The New England Journal of Medicine*, vol. 362, no. 12, pp. 1071–1081, 2010.

[6] E. Román, J. Córdoba, M. Torrens, C. Guarner, and G. Soriano, "Falls and cognitive dysfunction impair health-related quality of life in patients with cirrhosis," *European Journal of Gastroenterology & Hepatology*, vol. 25, no. 1, pp. 77–84, 2013.

[7] J. Bustamante, A. Rimola, P.-J. Ventura et al., "Prognostic significance of hepatic encephalopathy in patients with cirrhosis," *Journal of Hepatology*, vol. 30, no. 5, pp. 890–895, 1999.

[8] C. A. Stewart, M. Malinchoc, W. R. Kim, and P. S. Kamath, "Hepatic encephalopathy as a predictor of survival in patients with end-stage liver disease," *Liver Transplantation*, vol. 13, no. 10, pp. 1366–1371, 2007.

[9] H. Garg, A. Kumar, V. Garg, P. Sharma, B. C. Sharma, and S. K. Sarin, "Clinical profile and predictors of mortality in patients of acute-on-chronic liver failure," *Digestive and Liver Disease*, vol. 44, no. 2, pp. 166–171, 2012.

[10] O. Detry, A. De Roover, P. Honoré, and M. Meurisse, "Brain edema and intracranial hypertension in fulminant hepatic failure: Pathophysiology and management," *World Journal of Gastroenterology*, vol. 12, no. 46, pp. 7405–7412, 2006.

[11] J. Fichet, E. Mercier, O. Genée et al., "Prognosis and 1-year mortality of intensive care unit patients with severe hepatic encephalopathy," *Journal of Critical Care*, vol. 24, no. 3, pp. 364–370, 2009.

[12] G. Garcia-Tsao, A. J. Sanyal, N. D. Grace et al., "Prevention and management of gastroesophageal varices and variceal hemorrhage in cirrhosis," *Hepatology*, vol. 46, no. 3, pp. 922–938, 2007.

[13] J. Wen, Q. Liu, J. Song, M. Tong, L. Peng, and H. Liang, "Lactulose is highly potential in prophylaxis of hepatic encephalopathy

in patients with cirrhosis and upper gastrointestinal bleeding: Results of a controlled randomized trial," *Digestion*, vol. 87, no. 2, pp. 132–138, 2013.

[14] P. Sharma, A. Agrawal, B. C. Sharma, and S. K. Sarin, "Prophylaxis of hepatic encephalopathy in acute variceal bleed: A randomized controlled trial of lactulose versus no lactulose," *Journal of Gastroenterology and Hepatology*, vol. 26, no. 6, pp. 996–1003, 2011.

[15] A. Rolachon, J. P. Zarski, J. M. Lutz, J. Fournet, and J. Hostein, "Is the intestinal lavage with a solution of mannitol effective in the prevention of post-hemorrhagic hepatic encephalopathy in patients with liver cirrhosis? Results of a randomized prospective study," *Gastroentérologie Clinique et Biologique*, vol. 18, pp. 1057–1062, 1994.

[16] R. Bockel and M. Doffoel, "Whole-gut irrigation with mannitol in cirrhotic patients with gastro-intestinal bleeding. Changes in blood ammonia and amino acids levels," *La Nouvelle presse médicale*, vol. 10, pp. 33–36, 1981.

[17] G. Champault, F. Psalmon, and J. C. Patel, "Post-haemorrhagic encephalopathy in cirrhosis. Prevention by digestive irrigation with 100 mg/L mannitol," *La Nouvelle presse médicale*, vol. 7, pp. 2455–2458, 1978.

[18] G. H. Micklefield, U. Schwegler, D. Hüppe, H. D. Kuntz, and B. May, "Orthograde intestinal irrigation with a mannitol solution in reducing hepatic encephalopathy in patients with liver cirrhosis and gastrointestinal haemorrhage," *Z Gastroenterol*, vol. 27, pp. 374–377, 1989.

[19] G. Garcia-Tsao and J. Bosch, "Management of varices and variceal hemorrhage in cirrhosis," *The New England Journal of Medicine*, vol. 362, no. 9, pp. 778–832, 2010.

[20] A. Torre-Delgadillo, F. J. Bosques-Padilla, C. A. Cortez-Hernßndez, J. F. Rivera-Ramos, M. Uribe-Esquivel, and C. A. Cortez-Hernández, "Gastroenterology diagnosis and treatment guidelines of hepatic encephalopathy. Physiopathology and diagnosis," *Revista de Gastroenterología de México*, vol. 74, pp. 164–169, 2009.

[21] B. Starfield, J. Hyde, J. Gérvas, and I. Heath, "The concept of prevention: A good idea gone astray?" *Journal of Epidemiology and Community Health*, vol. 62, no. 7, pp. 580–583, 2008.

[22] N. Dharel and J. S. Bajaj, "Definition and Nomenclature of Hepatic Encephalopathy," *Journal of Clinical and Experimental Hepatology*, vol. 5, no. 1, pp. S37–S41, 2015.

[23] B. A. Runyon, "Management of adult patients with ascites due to cirrhosis: an update," *Hepatology*, vol. 49, no. 6, pp. 2087–2107, 2009.

[24] H. Vilstrup, P. Amodio, J. Bajaj et al., "Hepatic encephalopathy in chronic liver disease: 2014 Practice Guideline by the American Association for the Study Of Liver Diseases and the European Association for the Study of the Liver," *Hepatology*, vol. 60, no. 2, pp. 715–735, 2014.

[25] A. Berzigotti and J. C. García-Pagán, "Prevention of recurrent variceal bleeding," *Digestive and Liver Disease*, vol. 40, no. 5, pp. 337–342, 2008.

[26] B. Als-Nielsen, L. L. Gluud, and C. Gluud, "Nonabsorbable disaccharides for hepatic encephalopathy," *Cochrane Database of Systematic Reviews*, no. 2, Article ID CD003044, 2004.

[27] L. Gerard, K. W. Garey, and H. L. DuPont, "Rifaximin: a nonabsorbable rifamycin antibiotic for use in nonsystemic gastrointestinal infections," *Expert Review of Anti-infective Therapy*, vol. 3, no. 2, pp. 201–211, 2005.

[28] Z. D. Jiang and H. L. Dupont, "Rifaximin: In vitro and in vivo antibacterial activity - A review," *Chemotherapy*, vol. 51, no. 1, pp. 67–72, 2005.

[29] E. A. Debbia, E. Maioli, S. Roveta, and A. Marchese, "Effects of rifaximin on bacterial virulence mechanisms at supra- and sub-inhibitory concentrations," *Journal of Chemotherapy*, vol. 20, no. 2, pp. 186–194, 2008.

[30] A. Goel, U. Rahim, L. H. Nguyen, C. Stave, and M. H. Nguyen, "Systematic review with meta-analysis: rifaximin for the prophylaxis of spontaneous bacterial peritonitis," *Alimentary Pharmacology & Therapeutics*, vol. 46, no. 11-12, pp. 1029–1036, 2017.

[31] A. Rattanasupar, N. Tiawijit, and B. Rachatapantanakorn, "Predictive factor for hepatic encephalopathy in cirrhotic patients who presented with acute variceal bleeding," *Journal of the Medical Association of Thailand*, vol. 97, no. 6, pp. 567–573, 2014.

4

The Continental Divide: Anti-TNF use in Pediatric IBD Is Different in North America Compared to Other Parts of the World

Peter C. Church,[1] **Jeffrey Hyams**,[2,3] **Frank Ruemmele**,[4] **Lissy de Ridder**,[5] **Dan Turner**,[6] **and Anne M. Griffiths**[1,7]

[1] *Division of Gastroenterology, Hepatology & Nutrition, The Hospital for Sick Children, Department of Paediatrics, University of Toronto, Toronto, Canada*
[2] *Division of Digestive Diseases, Hepatology, and Nutrition, Connecticut Children's Medical Center, Hartford, CT, USA*
[3] *University of Connecticut School of Medicine, Farmington, CT, USA*
[4] *Université Sorbonne Paris Cité, Université Paris Descartes, and Assistance Publique-Hôpitaux de Paris, Hôpital Necker-Enfants malades, Service de Gastroentérologie Pédiatrique, Paris, France*
[5] *Department of Pediatric Gastroenterology, The Erasmus MC Sophia Children's Hospital, Rotterdam, Netherlands*
[6] *The Juliet Keidan Institute of Pediatric Gastroenterology and Nutrition, Shaare Zedek Medical Center, The Hebrew University of Jerusalem, Jerusalem, Israel*
[7] *Sick Kids Inflammatory Bowel Disease Centre, The Hospital for Sick Children, Toronto, Canada*

Correspondence should be addressed to Peter C. Church; peter.church@sickkids.ca

Academic Editor: Salvatore Oliva

Background and Aims. Use of anti-TNF therapies varies internationally. As an initiative of the international Pediatric IBD Network (PIBDNet), we compared global pediatric IBD anti-TNF practice patterns. *Methods.* Physicians were surveyed about anti-TNF use in Crohn's disease (CD) and ulcerative colitis (UC). Chi-squared, independent samples Mann–Whitney *U*, or related samples Wilcoxon signed rank tests were used to compare groups. *Results.* 344 physicians treating pediatric IBD responded from 43 countries (54% North America, 29% Europe, 6% Oceania, 6% Asia, 3% Africa, and 2% South America). Respondents treated a median 40 IBD patients. CD was more commonly treated with anti-TNF than UC (40% vs. 10%, p<0.001). North Americans more often used anti-TNF (median 50% vs. 30%, p<0.001) and before immunomodulator (80% vs. 35% CD, p<0.001; 76% vs. 43% steroid-dependent UC, p<0.001). Anti-TNF monotherapy was more common in North America. Anti-TNF in combination with methotrexate, instead of thiopurine, characterized North American practices. North Americans more often continued immunomodulator indefinitely and less often adhered to standard infliximab induction dosing. Access limitations were more common outside North America and Europe for both CD (67% vs. 31%, p<0.001) and UC (62% vs. 33%, p<0.001). *Conclusions.* Anti-TNF use in North America varies significantly from elsewhere.

1. Introduction

Anti-TNF antibodies are highly effective therapies for treating pediatric inflammatory bowel disease (IBD). Industry-initiated multicentre clinical trials involving open-label induction followed by randomized dose-ranging maintenance therapy support the efficacy of infliximab and adalimumab in luminal inflammatory pediatric Crohn's disease (CD) and of infliximab in pediatric ulcerative colitis (UC) [1–3]. The ability of anti-TNF therapy to heal the intestine, thereby improving long-term outcomes, makes these biologics particularly important for children [4, 5], among whom IBD is occurring increasingly frequently globally [6]. As an initiative of the international Pediatric IBD Network (PIBDNet), we aimed to explore regional differences in anti-TNF therapy practice patterns in pediatric IBD. Examining the variation in anti-TNF use among children internationally is important for understanding the timing, dosing, and attention to maintaining durability of response. Understanding regional differences in practice could aid in interpretation of studies reporting outcomes and safety data which sometimes vary by country. Also, allocated resources depend on local needs and existing routine practices. Identifying differences in practice is the first step to studying the effect these differences have on outcomes of interest, with the goal of optimizing care among children with long lives ahead during which effective IBD therapy is required.

2. Materials and Methods

PIBDNet was established in 2015 as a worldwide network of pediatric IBD specialists with the overall aim of improving outcomes in children with IBD globally, as new therapies emerge, through facilitation of investigator-initiated and industry-sponsored pediatric clinical trials, monitoring of drug safety, and advocacy with regulatory bodies. Membership is open to all physicians, who treat children and adolescents with IBD.

An electronic survey (Supplemental Digital Content) was developed by the PIBDNet executive through an iterative, consensus process and sent to all PIBDNet members. Other potential respondents were ascertained using national membership lists provided by PIBDNet members (from Belgium, Brazil, Canada, the Czech Republic, Finland, France, Italy, Malaysia, Portugal, and Singapore). In addition, subscribers to the Pediatric GI Bulletin Board hosted at the University of Vermont were included. Participants were asked to complete the survey if they currently treated any number of children with IBD.

There were 8 questions related to demographics. Respondents identified their country and type of practice (university-based vs. community-based) and number of years in practice. We used the "composition of macro geographical (continental) regions" database maintained by the United Nations Statistics Division to associate each chosen country with its corresponding continent [7]. We characterized the respondents' patient population by number and percentage of current patients actively being followed with IBD, the proportion of CD to UC, and the age of the oldest IBD patient ever treated.

There were 23 questions which explored practice patterns in CD including percentage of patients treated with anti-TNF therapy (separating infliximab (IFX) and adalimumab (ADA) for both luminal and perianal fistulizing CD) and percentage of time anti-TNF therapy is used first line without a trial of immunomodulator (IM). With respect to luminal inflammatory CD, respondents were asked how often an IM is started with IFX or ADA in different scenarios, choice of IM (methotrexate (MTX) vs. thiopurines), and for how long they continue concomitant IM. Next, we asked how often standard induction dosing regimens were followed for IFX (5mg/kg/dose at weeks 0, 2, and 6) and ADA (160mg/80mg followed by 40mg every other week, if >40kg; 80mg/40mg followed by 20mg every other week, if <40kg) and we explored how the dosing regimens are modified. Respondents were asked how often anti-TNF therapy was discontinued for patients with luminal inflammatory CD in continuous remission and how often anti-TNF therapy was started after surgical resection as postoperative preventive therapy.

There were 14 questions which explored ulcerative colitis (UC). We examined the percentage of patients with UC treated with anti-TNF therapy (IFX vs. other) and how often it was used without a trial of IM in steroid-dependent patients. As with CD, we explored deviation from the standard IFX induction regimen for patients with both steroid-refractory and steroid-dependent UC. Respondents reported their use of combination IM (MTX vs. thiopurine) in IM-naïve patients and after IM failure and the usual duration of combination therapy. Finally, we asked about stopping anti-TNF therapy for patients with UC in continuous remission.

We included 5 questions about routine safety testing before and during anti-TNF therapy. Finally, we explored access limitations (3 questions).

The survey was open to responses between September and November 2015. Potential respondents were invited by email to complete an electronic survey hosted on the REDCap platform [8]. After the initial invitation, 4 further email reminders were sent.

2.1. Analysis. Results are presented as N (%), or median and interquartile range (IQR) as appropriate. To facilitate analyses, we planned to categorize respondents into 6 regions: North America, Europe, Asia, Oceania, Africa, and South America. However, there were relatively few respondents from the last 4 continents, and so they were combined. Our main analysis thus compared respondents from North America, Europe, and elsewhere. Additional subanalyses included comparisons of respondents from Canada compared to the USA, those in university-based practice vs. community-based practice, and those early in practice (<10 years) vs. later in practice (≥10 years).

Differences between groups were assessed by Chi-square or Fisher's exact test (depending on cell sizes) for categorical variables and Mann–Whitney U test (independent samples) or related samples Wilcoxon signed rank test (paired samples) for continuous variables.

Statistical analyses were performed using SPSS Statistics for Windows, Version 23.0 (Armonk, NY: IBM Corp). In all analyses, p values <0.05 were considered significant.

3. Results

PIBDNet members contributed 404 names. Another 1396 potential respondents, representing at least 52 countries, came from the pediatric gastroenterology bulletin board, after eliminating gastroenterology fellows/trainees, surgeons, pathologists, nurses, nurse practitioners, or dietitians. This left a maximum of 1800 potential respondents. However, several of these would be practicing primarily hepatology, pancreatology, and/or nutrition, making the true denominator much lower.

There were 344 complete responses (estimated response rate 19%), and 115 (33%) were from PIBDNet. A total of 182 (53%) were from North America, most of whom (72%) were from a university-based practice, with 53% (182 of all

TABLE 1: Demographics for the 344 respondents who completed the survey. Results are presented as N (%) or median (interquartile range) as appropriate.

Characteristic	N=344
Continent	
North America	183 (53%)
Europe	103 (30%)
Asia	20 (6%)
Oceania	21 (6%)
Africa	10 (3%)
South America	7 (2%)
Primary practice type	
University-based	248 (72%)
Community-based	96 (28%)
Years in practice following fellowship	
<10	184 (53%)
10-20	92 (27%)
20-40	68 (20%)
Percentage of practice devoted to IBD	20 (10-40)
Number of IBD patients in practice	40 (20-90)
Percentage of patients with CD	60 (50-70)
Oldest IBD patient ever treated (years)	
≤18	147 (43%)
18-21	93 (27%)
21-25	82 (24%)
25-75	21 (6%)

IBD: inflammatory bowel disease; CD: Crohn's disease.

344 respondents) relatively new to practice (Table 1). Respondents had a median of 40 IBD patients in their practice, representing a median of 20% of their total number of patients seen. However, there were 84/344 (24%) for whom IBD patients made up the majority (>50%) of their practice. There was a predominance (median 60%) of patients with CD.

3.1. Crohn's Disease. Respondents reported a median of 40% (IQR 25-60%) of their CD patients to be treated with anti-TNF therapy. This was higher in North America (median 50% vs. 30% Europe vs. 30% elsewhere, p<0.001) (Table 2). IFX was most frequently the initial anti-TNF drug used for both luminal (median 90% (IQR 50-100%)) and perianal fistulizing CD (median 100% (IQR 90-100%)).

North Americans more often (80% vs. 38% Europe vs. 30% elsewhere, p<0.001) used anti-TNF therapy without a trial of IM (Table 2). However, they used IFX (but not ADA) in combination with concomitant IM less often in both IM-naïve patients (median 50% of time vs. 90% Europe vs. 100% elsewhere, p<0.001) and after IM failure (median 80% of time vs. 98% Europe vs. 90% elsewhere, p<0.001). For both IFX and ADA, North Americans were less likely to choose thiopurines as their combination IM (24% vs. 94% Europe vs. 79% elsewhere for IFX, p<0.001; 20% North America vs. 93% Europe vs. 69% elsewhere for IM-naïve on ADA, p<0.001; and 25% North America vs. 76% Europe vs. 68% elsewhere for ADA used after IFX secondary loss of response, p<0.001) but were likely to continue combination therapy for a longer period of time.

North Americans were less likely than physicians elsewhere in the world to strictly adhere to standard IFX induction protocols (42% vs. 66% Europe vs. 84% elsewhere, p<0.001), although similar ADA induction protocols were followed (Table 2). Respondents from all regions had similar approaches to regimen intensification, with most preferring to increase the dose of IFX and/or shorten the dosing interval depending on the individual patient (64%), rather than uniformly increasing the dose (27%) or shortening the interval (9%).

Almost half of respondents (45%) had ever stopped anti-TNF therapy for a patient with luminal CD in continuous remission, and this was more common in Europe (59% vs. 38% North America vs. 42% elsewhere, p=0.003). North Americans were also more likely to initiate anti-TNF therapy as early preventive therapy after an ileal resection for internal penetrating disease (median 80% (IQR 40-100%) vs. 50% (IQR 0-100%) in both Europe and elsewhere, p=0.011).

We also compared the practice of respondents from Canada and the USA (Supplemental Table 1). Canadians treated a smaller percentage of patients with CD with anti-TNF therapy (median 36% vs. 50%, p=0.004) and used more combination IM therapy with IFX (median 85% vs. 30%, p=0.001 for IM-naïve, median 98% vs. 75%, and p= 0.027 after IM failure) and ADA (median 50% vs. 20%; p=0.043 for IM- and IFX-naïve and median 100% vs. 70%; p=0.046 after IFX loss of response).

Comparing those in university-based practice to those in community-practice (Supplemental Table 2), there were few significant differences. Those in university-based practice more often used combination IM for IFX (median 80% vs. 25%, p=0.003 for IM-naïve patients, median 90% vs. 75%, and p=0.027 after IM failure). They also used combination IM more frequently with ADA, but only after loss of response to IFX (median 90% vs. 50%, p=0.009).

Finally, there were no significant differences between those new to practice (<10 years after fellowship training) compared to others (≥10 years after training) (Supplemental Table 3).

3.2. Ulcerative Colitis. UC patients were less often treated with anti-TNF therapy compared to patients with CD (median 10% (IQR 5-25%) vs. median 40% (IQR 25-60%), p<0.001). As with CD, anti-TNF use was higher in North America (median 20% of UC treated with anti-TNF therapy vs. 10% Europe vs. 5% elsewhere, p<0.001) (Table 3). Some respondents (15% overall) restricted their use of anti-TNF therapy to hospitalized, steroid-refractory UC patients. This was more frequent outside of North America (10% vs. 18% Europe vs. 28% elsewhere, p=0.021). Infliximab was most often used as the first anti-TNF agent (median 100% (IQR 80-100%)), and this did not vary by geography (p=0.735).

North Americans sometimes used anti-TNF therapy for patients with UC more frequently without a preceding trial of IM (76% vs. 47% Europe vs. 36% elsewhere, p<0.001) and more frequently as monotherapy (Table 3). However, similar to practice patterns with CD, North Americans less often

TABLE 2: Practice patterns in luminal Crohn's disease with infliximab (IFX) and adalimumab (ADA). Results are presented as percentages or median (interquartile range) as appropriate.

		North America N=183	Europe N=103	Elsewhere N=58	p-value
Percentage of patients treated with anti-TNF therapy		50 (30-65)	30 (20-50)	30 (20-50)	<0.001
Anti-TNF sometimes used without IM trial		80%	38%	30%	<0.001
Percentage of time combination IM used with anti-TNF					
IFX	IM-naïve	50 (10-90)	90 (20-100)	100 (60-100)	<0.001
	After IM failure	80 (40-100)	98 (68-100)	90 (50-100)	0.003
ADA	IM- and IFX-naïve	25 (0-90)	80 (10-100)	20 (0-90)	0.056
	after IFX LoR	75 (10-100)	90 (20-100)	55 (0-100)	0.510
Thiopurine always or usually chosen as combination IM					
IFX		24%	94%	79%	<0.001
ADA	IM-naïve	20%	93%	69%	<0.001
	after IFX LoR	25%	76%	68%	<0.001
Combination IM continued indefinitely					
IFX		48%	16%	32%	<0.001
ADA	IM-naïve	49%	14%	11%	<0.001
	after IFX LoR	54%	14%	27%	<0.001
Always adhere to standard induction					
IFX		42%	66%	84%	<0.001
ADA		66%	64%	70%	0.932

anti-TNF: anti-tumour necrosis factor; IM: immunomodulator; LoR: loss of response.

TABLE 3: Practice patterns in ulcerative colitis with infliximab. Results are presented as percentages or median (interquartile range) as appropriate.

	North America N=183	Europe N=103	Elsewhere N=58	p-value
Percentage of the time Anti-TNF used	20 (5-30)	10 (5-23)	5 (2-10)	<0.001
Anti-TNF sometimes used without IM trial				
Steroid-dependent	76%	47%	36%	<0.001
Percentage of time combination IM used with anti-TNF				
IM-naïve	50 (0-90)	85 (15-100)	90 (25-100)	0.002
After IM-failure	80 (20-100)	95 (50-100)	100 (50-100)	0.003
Thiopurine always or usually chosen as combination IM	35%	100%	86%	<0.001
Combination IM continued indefinitely	44%	15%	29%	0.004
Always adhere to standard induction				
Steroid-refractory	46%	73%	61%	0.002
Steroid-dependent	70%	90%	78%	0.002

used thiopurines (35% vs. 100% Europe vs. 86% elsewhere, p<0.001) and more often continued combination IM indefinitely (44% vs. 15% Europe vs. 29% elsewhere, p=0.004).

Standard IFX induction protocols were strictly followed less often by North Americans than colleagues elsewhere for both steroid-refractory (46% vs. 73% Europe vs. 61% elsewhere, p=0.002) and steroid-dependent patients (70% vs. 90% Europe vs. 78% elsewhere, p=0.002) (Table 3). North Americans were more likely to increase induction doses to 10 mg/kg for steroid-refractory disease (40% vs. 18% Europe vs. 17% elsewhere, p<0.001). Europeans were less likely to increase to 10 mg/kg for steroid-dependent patients (8% vs. 25% North America vs. 22% elsewhere, p=0.046).

One-third of respondents (33%) had stopped anti-TNF therapy for a UC patient in continuous remission, and this was more common in Europe (51% vs. 26% North America vs. 22% elsewhere, p<0.001). For UC patients with secondary loss of response to IFX due to antibody formation, respondents have gone on to use alternative anti-TNF therapies a median of 20% (IQR 0-91%) of the time. This was significantly more common in Europe (50% (IQR 0-100%) vs. 20 % (IQR 0-93%) North America vs. 0% (IQR 0-10%) elsewhere, p=0.001).

In comparing respondents from Canada to those in the USA (Supplemental Table 4), Canadians treated a larger percentage of patients with UC with combination therapy in both the IM-naïve (median 90% vs. 45%, p=0.004) and IM

TABLE 4: Access limitations identified by respondents. Results are presented as N (%).

	North America N=183	Europe N=103	Elsewhere N=58	p-value
Access never limited for CD	103 (56%)	79 (77%)	16 (28%)	<0.001
Access never limited for UC	99 (54%)	76 (74%)	18 (31%)	<0.001
Access is sometimes limited in newly diagnosed CD	35 (19%)	12 (12%)	19 (33%)	0.005
Access is sometimes limited before failure of steroids or EEN followed by IM in CD	42 (23%)	13 (13%)	29 (50%)	<0.001
Access is sometimes limited except in hospitalized, steroid-refractory UC	20 (11%)	9 (9%)	12 (21%)	0.067
Access is sometimes limited in steroid-dependent UC before failure of steroids followed by an immunomodulator	41 (22%)	12 (12%)	23 (40%)	<0.001
Dosing regimen is sometimes limited	32 (17%)	9 (9%)	20 (34%)	<0.001
Duration of anti-TNF therapy is sometimes limited	5 (3%)	8 (8%)	5 (9%)	0.083
Access to day clinics for infusion is sometimes limited	14 (8%)	5 (5%)	6 (10%)	0.418

failure settings (median 100% vs. 70%, p=0.006). Canadians also less often adhered to standard IFX induction regimens (13% vs. 45%, p=0.001 for steroid-refractory disease, 31% vs. 55%, p=0.016 for steroid-dependent disease).

Similar to CD, the only difference between those in university-based practice compared to those in community-based practice was the frequency of combination IM use (Supplemental Table 5). Those in university-based practice used IM more frequently for IM-naïve patients (median 75% vs. 40%, p=0.027) but the difference for patients after IM failure did not reach statistical significance (median 90% vs. 75%, p=0.070).

Those with ≥10 years of experience after fellowship had more patients on anti-TNF therapy (median 15% (IQR 5–30) vs. 10 % (IQR 3–20), p = 0.010). (Supplemental Table 6).

3.3. Routine Testing. The vast majority of respondents (90%) performed some kind of routine testing before starting anti-TNF therapy. More testing was done in Europe (95%) compared to North America (90%) and elsewhere (83%) (p=0.039). Some type of testing for tuberculosis was performed by 90% overall (90% in North America vs. 95% Europe vs. 83% elsewhere, p=0.039. Chest X-ray was done relatively infrequently in North America (38% vs. 81% Europe vs. 76% elsewhere, p<0.001). QuantiFERON gold testing was more common in Europe (75% vs. 53% North America vs. 38% elsewhere, p<0.001). Rates of tuberculin skin testing were similar in all areas (68% North America vs. 57% Europe vs. 57% elsewhere, p=0.101). Once patients started on anti-TNF therapy, annual TB screening was more often done by North Americans (39% vs. 14 % Europe vs. 16% elsewhere, p<0.001). A majority of respondents in all locations routinely check varicella (54% North America vs. 59% Europe vs. 50% elsewhere, p=0.500) and Hepatitis B serology (72% North America vs. 70% Europe vs. 64% elsewhere, p=0.482). Epstein-Barr virus titres were checked less often in North America (25% vs. 61% Europe vs. 38% elsewhere, p<0.001).

Performance of some type of tuberculosis screening was similar across North America (94% Canada vs. 90% USA, p=0.447). However, compared to respondents from the USA, Canadians were more likely to perform TB skin testing (91% vs. 64%, p=0.003) and chest X-ray (84% vs. 29%, p<0.001). However, Canadians less often performed QuantiFERON gold testing (9% vs. 63%, p<0.001). Canadians more often checked varicella serology (78% vs. 49%, p=0.003) and EBV titres (50% vs. 19%, p<0.001). Respondents from the USA performed routine TB testing in follow-up frequently compared to Canadians (47% vs. 6%, p<0.001).

University-based respondents generally performed screening tests more frequently. TB screening was requested routinely by 93% of university-based respondents, compared to 83% of their community counterparts (p=0.009). Tuberculin skin testing and QuantiFERON gold testing rates were similar between groups, but chest X-rays were more common in the university setting (63% vs. 42%, p<0.001). Varicella screening and EBV screening were both more common in the university-based practices (59% vs. 46%, p=0.035; 42% vs. 26%, p=0.005, respectively).

Those newer to practice (<10 years after fellowship) were more likely to perform QuantiFERON gold testing (63% vs. 52%, p=0.040). All other preinduction testing and ongoing monitoring were similar between groups.

3.4. Access Limitations. The percentages of respondents reporting being limited in their use of anti-TNF therapy were 36% for CD and 37% for UC. However, perceived restriction of use was much more common in areas outside of North America or Europe. This was true for almost all scenarios for patients with CD and UC presented to respondents (Table 4).

When examining those within North America, Canadians generally identified more access restrictions (Supplemental Table 7). Canadians reported more often being limited in their use of anti-TNF therapy in newly diagnosed patients with CD (41% vs. 19% USA, p=0.009). They also reported more difficulty initiating anti-TNF therapy in patients with steroid-dependent UC without first trying an immunomodulator (41% vs. 29%, p=0.007). Lastly, Canadians more often reported not being able to use their desired dosage (31% vs. 15%, p=0.025).

The only difference between those in university-based vs. community-based practices (Supplemental Table 8) was decreased limitation for UC in university-based practices (59% vs. 73% never limited, p=0.029).

Those new to practice (<10 years following fellowship) reported more frequently being limited in their access to anti-TNF therapy for newly diagnosed CD patients (24% vs. 15%, p=0.026).

4. Discussion

Pediatric IBD specialists worldwide are attempting within PIBDNet to facilitate collaborative studies which will guide optimal pediatric care of children with CD and UC. Our PIBDNet survey of practice patterns with respect to anti-TNF use identifies significant differences between pediatric gastroenterologists in North America, Europe, and elsewhere. Identifying and characterizing these differences is the first step in studying their effect on outcomes of interest.

Compared to colleagues elsewhere, North American pediatric gastroenterologists treat a higher percentage of pediatric CD and UC with anti-TNF antibodies and more often prescribe anti-TNF agents without a prior trial of IM. The optimal positioning of anti-TNF therapy relative to other therapies in both CD and UC is still debated. Our North American pediatric data are very different from adult surveys of the American Gastroenterological Association in 2009 and of gastroenterologists in Maryland and Washington, DC in 2007, where 70% and 48% of respondents, respectively, said they would use IM prior to prescribing IFX. [9, 10]. Similarly, 90% of Swiss adult gastroenterologists reported that they use a conventional step-up strategy, first prescribing thiopurines before using anti-TNF therapy [11].

In all parts of the world pediatric CD was reported to be more often treated with anti-TNF therapy compared to UC. Similarly, the Canadian Child Inflammatory Bowel Disease Network has reported that 61% of patients with CD are maintained on an anti-TNF therapy, compared with 31% of UC patients [12].

In this survey we found IFX to be the overwhelming first choice anti-TNF drug for both CD and UC, which is consistent with previous adult reports and our clinical experience [11, 13]. What drives this choice is unclear. Others have cited the ability to monitor patients regularly and increased familiarity with IFX given that it has been available for IBD treatment for longer [13].

North American respondents (especially in the USA) reported using anti-TNF antibodies as monotherapy more often than their global counterparts, perhaps in part because of the dominant practice elsewhere of adding anti-TNF in patients already receiving but responding unsatisfactorily to IM. The common initiation in North America of infliximab as monotherapy is concerning, given the now substantial body of evidence, including adult randomized controlled trial and pediatric observational data, documenting the importance of concomitant IM in reducing the likelihood of secondary loss of responsiveness related to anti-infliximab antibodies [5, 14, 15].

Choice of combination IM was also different between North America and elsewhere, for both CD and UC. There is no prospective study directly comparing thiopurine to methotrexate combination therapy for any anti-TNF drug for either CD or UC. The SONIC study demonstrated improvement in multiple outcomes comparing adults treated with IFX and azathioprine combination therapy to those treated with either therapy alone [14]. The adult COMMIT study, whilst not demonstrating a treatment benefit to combination therapy with methotrexate, did demonstrate less immunogenicity and higher drug levels at trough [16]. In our sample, North Americans preferred methotrexate, whereas practitioners elsewhere more often chose thiopurines. The reasons underlying this difference are unknown. Certainly, the risk of hepatocellular T-cell lymphoma associated with use of thiopurines is well known. The same risk has not been associated with methotrexate in patients with IBD [17]. As recently reported, data from the prospective DEVELOP safety registry of pediatric IBD demonstrated an increased incidence of malignancy compared to age- and gender-matched healthy controls in the SEER database in children with IBD treated with thiopurines with or without biologics [18]. However, the use of methotrexate is presently not evidence-based and thus carries a slightly lower recommendation than thiopurines by the European Society for Pediatric Gastroenterology, Hepatology and Nutrition (ESPGHAN) [19].

Our respondents, especially from North America, preferred to continue combination IM for longer when used with IFX, for both CD and UC patients. Although there are adult data to support significant benefit of combination azathioprine with IFX for CD up to 12 months [14], no such prospective evidence exists to specifically guide pediatric practice. ESPGHAN and European Crohn's and Colitis Organization (ECCO) joint guidelines suggest discontinuing combination IM therapy after 6 months for CD and 4-8 months for UC, especially in males and those who are not at high risk for a severe disease course [19, 20].

Standard induction therapy with IFX was less often adhered to by North Americans. This difference was largest in CD but was also observed in steroid-refractory and steroid-dependent UC. Recognition of the need for customized dosing of IFX and ADA is not new. Escalating IFX doses beyond 5 mg/kg every 8 weeks in the setting of unsatisfactory response has been practised for years, especially in the adult population [21] and has also been reported in pediatric practice [5]. Similar practice with ADA (prescribing more than 40 mg every 2 weeks) has also been described in both adult and pediatric IBD populations [22, 23]. Current guidelines for management of children with IBD also endorse this practice [19, 20].

More recently, an intensified IFX induction regimen, with 3 doses given over a median of 24 days (instead of the usual 6 weeks), was studied for adult patients with acute severe UC [24]. These investigators found significantly decreased risk of colectomy during induction therapy. Many adult gastroenterologists are already practicing this way. A survey of 123 members from Crohn's and Colitis Foundation of America Clinical Research Alliance and the International Organization for Inflammatory Bowel Disease demonstrated that only 24% of respondents used standard IFX induction dosing for severe UC [25]. Individualized dosing based on therapeutic drug monitoring (TDM) seems logical, but prospective controlled trials confirming efficacy of TDM are hitherto lacking and access to TDM remains inconsistent in clinical practice [10].

Most respondents reported performing some screening investigations prior to starting anti-TNF therapy. However, considering the well-known risk of tuberculosis with anti-TNF therapy [26], it is surprising that only 90% screened for tuberculosis. This rate was lower in North America compared with Europe. The reasons for this are unclear, although it may be related to the very low prevalence of tuberculosis infection in this part of the world [27]. Pediatric guidelines for Crohn's disease from ECCO and ESPGHAN are clear that testing for tuberculosis prior to starting an anti-TNF agent should by mandatory [19]. They also suggest screening for hepatitis B virus and varicella zoster virus immunity, with consideration of immunization in those at risk of infection prior to starting anti-TNF therapy. The high rate of yearly TB testing during follow-up was surprising, since this does not appear to be based on guideline recommendations.

Our study's results should be interpreted with some limitations in mind. Respondents most likely answered our questions based on recall, rather than a detailed audit of their actual practice. We had 344 respondents who completed the entire survey, for a conservative estimated response rate of 19%. However, many of the 1800 potential respondents from the Pediatric GI Bulletin Board likely do not treat pediatric IBD (they may be hepatologists, nutritionists, surgeons, nurses, dieticians, etc.), making a realistic response rate much higher. A systematic review and meta-analysis of general practitioner response rates to postal surveys estimated an average response rate of 61% (95% CI 59%-63%) [28]. Email surveys have been shown to be less effective than postal surveys, with 1.82 times lower odds of response [29]. Taken together, these data suggest that our response rate of 19% is acceptable. Another limitation is the low response rate from Asia, Oceania, Africa, and South America, limiting our study's generalizability. This is particularly important when interpreting access limitations, as these parts of the world likely have the most inadequate access to anti-TNF therapy. Also, our investigation of the reasons behind the reported differences in practice, including access limitations, was brief in order to keep the survey length manageable for respondents. Elucidating the reasons behind the differences reported here is an important area for future study.

The use of anti-TNF therapies is significantly different in North America compared to Europe and other parts of the world. In North America, anti-TNF therapy is used earlier and more aggressively. Combination therapy with an IM is less common, and when it is used, thiopurines are avoided.

Disclosure

This work was presented as poster presentation at the 11th Congress of ECCO, Amsterdam, March 16-19, 2016, and Digestive Diseases Week, San Diego, May 21-24, 2016.

Authors' Contributions

All authors approved the final version of the manuscript. Peter C. Church developed the study concept and protocol, collected data, performed statistical analysis, and wrote the manuscript. Jeffrey Hyams, Frank Ruemmele, Lissy de Ridder, Dan Turner, and Anne M. Griffiths developed the study concept and protocol and assisted in writing the manuscript.

Acknowledgments

This research is presented on behalf of the International Pediatric IBD Network (PIBDNet).

References

[1] J. Hyams, L. Damaraju, M. Blank et al., "Induction and Maintenance Therapy With Infliximab for Children With Moderate to Severe Ulcerative Colitis," *Clinical Gastroenterology and Hepatology*, vol. 10, no. 4, pp. 391–399, 2012.

[2] J. Hyams, W. Crandall, S. Kugathasan et al., "Induction and maintenance infliximab therapy for the treatment of moderate-to-severe Crohn's disease in children," *Gastroenterology*, vol. 132, no. 3, pp. 863–873, 1165–1166, 2007.

[3] J. S. Hyams, A. Griffiths, J. Markowitz et al., "Safety and efficacy of adalimumab for moderate to severe Crohn's disease in children," *Gastroenterology*, vol. 143, no. 2, pp. 365–374, 2012.

[4] C. Topf-Olivestone and D. Turner, "How effective is the use of long-term anti-TNF for paediatric IBD? Clues from real-life surveillance cohorts," *Archives of Disease in Childhood*, vol. 100, no. 4, pp. 391-392, 2015.

[5] P. C. Church, J. Guan, T. D. Walters et al., "Infliximab maintains durable response and facilitates catch-up growth In luminal pediatric Crohn's disease," *Inflammatory Bowel Diseases*, vol. 20, no. 7, pp. 1177–1186, 2014.

[6] E. I. Benchimol, K. J. Fortinsky, P. Gozdyra, M. Van Den Heuvel, J. Van Limbergen, and A. M. Griffiths, "Epidemiology of pediatric inflammatory bowel disease: a systematic review of international trends," *Inflammatory Bowel Diseases*, vol. 17, no. 1, pp. 423–439, 2011.

[7] Division UNS, Composition of macro geographical (continental) regions, geographical sub-regions, and selected economic and other groupings, 2016.

[8] P. A. Harris, R. Taylor, R. Thielke, J. Payne, N. Gonzalez, and J. G. Conde, "Research electronic data capture (REDCap): a metadata-driven methodology and workflow process for providing translational research informatics support," *Journal of Biomedical Informatics*, vol. 42, no. 2, pp. 377–381, 2009.

[9] M. St. Charles, S. R. Weiss Smith, R. Beardsley, D. O. Fedder, O. Carter-Pokras, and R. K. Cross, "Gastroenterologists' prescribing of infliximab for Crohn's disease: A national survey," *Inflammatory Bowel Diseases*, vol. 15, no. 10, pp. 1467–1475, 2009.

[10] M. Donovan, K. Lunney, O. Carter-Pokras, and R. K. Cross, "Prescribing patterns and awareness of adverse effects of infliximab: A health survey of gastroenterologists," *Digestive Diseases and Sciences*, vol. 52, no. 8, pp. 1798–1805, 2007.

[11] S. R. Vavricka, S. Radivojevic, C. N. Manser et al., "Addressing current treatment challenges in Crohn's disease in real life: A physician's survey," *Digestive and Liver Disease*, vol. 46, no. 12, pp. 1066–1071, 2014.

[12] P. Church, T. Walters, E. Benchimol et al., "Steroid-free remission among Canadian pediatric inflammatory bowel disease patients," *Canadian Journal of Gastroenterology and Hepatology*, 2016.

[13] A. Oussalah, X. Roblin, D. Laharie et al., "Tumour necrosis factor antagonists and inflammatory bowel diseases: A national practice survey," *Alimentary Pharmacology & Therapeutics*, vol. 30, no. 8, pp. 854–863, 2009.

[14] J. F. Colombel, W. J. Sandborn, and W. Reinisch, "Infliximab, azathioprine, or combination therapy for Crohn's disease," *The New England Journal of Medicine*, vol. 362, no. 15, pp. 1383–1395, 2010.

[15] V. Grossi, T. Lerer, A. Griffiths et al., "Concomitant Use of Immunomodulators Affects the Durability of Infliximab Therapy in Children With Crohn's Disease," *Clinical Gastroenterology and Hepatology*, vol. 13, no. 10, Article ID 54359, pp. 1748–1756, 2015.

[16] B. G. Feagan, J. W. D. McDonald, R. Panaccione et al., "Methotrexate in combination with infliximab is no more effective than infliximab alone in patients with Crohn's disease," *Gastroenterology*, vol. 146, no. 3, pp. 681.el–688.el, 2014.

[17] T. Gabbani, S. Deiana, S. Lunardi, N. Manetti, and V. Annese, "Safety profile of methotrexate in inflammatory bowel disease," *Expert Opinion on Drug Safety*, vol. 15, no. 10, pp. 1427–1437, 2016.

[18] J. S. Hyams, M. C. Dubinsky, R. N. Baldassano et al., "Infliximab Is Not Associated With Increased Risk of Malignancy or Hemophagocytic Lymphohistiocytosis in Pediatric Patients With Inflammatory Bowel Disease," *Gastroenterology*, vol. 152, no. 8, pp. 1901–1914.e3, 2017.

[19] F. M. Ruemmele, G. Veres, K. L. Kolho et al., "Consensus guidelines of ECCO/ESPGHAN on the medical management of pediatric Crohn's disease," *Journal of Crohn's and Colitis*, vol. 8, no. 10, pp. 1179–1207, 2014.

[20] D. Turner, A. Levine, J. C. Escher et al., "Management of pediatric ulcerative colitis: joint ECCO and ESPGHAN evidence-based consensus guidelines," *Journal of Pediatric Gastroenterology and Nutrition*, vol. 55, no. 3, pp. 340–361, 2012.

[21] G. G. Kaplan, C. Hur, J. Korzenik, and B. E. Sands, "Infliximab dose escalation vs. initiation of adalimumab for loss of response in Crohn's disease: A cost-effectiveness analysis," *Alimentary Pharmacology & Therapeutics*, vol. 26, no. 11-12, pp. 1509–1520, 2007.

[22] M. C. Dubinsky, J. Rosh, W. A. Faubion et al., "Efficacy and safety of escalation of adalimumab therapy to weekly dosing in pediatric patients with Crohn's disease," *Inflammatory Bowel Diseases*, vol. 22, no. 4, pp. 886–893, 2016.

[23] V. Billioud, W. J. Sandborn, and L. Peyrin-Biroulet, "Loss of response and need for adalimumab dose intensification in Crohn's disease: A systematic review," *American Journal of Gastroenterology*, vol. 106, no. 4, pp. 674–684, 2011.

[24] D. J. Gibson, Z. S. Heetun, C. E. Redmond et al., "An accelerated infliximab induction regimen reduces the need for early colectomy in patients with acute severe ulcerative colitis," *Clinical Gastroenterology and Hepatology*, vol. 13, no. 2, pp. 330–335.el, 2016.

[25] H. H. Herfarth, G. Rogler, and P. D. R. Higgins, "Pushing the pedal to the metal: Should we accelerate infliximab therapy for patients with severe ulcerative colitis?" *Clinical Gastroenterology and Hepatology*, vol. 13, no. 2, pp. 336–338, 2015.

[26] J. Keane, S. Gershon, R. P. Wise et al., "Tuberculosis associated with infliximab, a tumor necrosis factor alpha-neutralizing agent," *The New England Journal of Medicine*, vol. 345, no. 15, pp. 1098–1104, 2001.

[27] WHO, *Global Tuberculosis Report*, World Health Organization, Geneva, Switzerland, 2016.

[28] S. T. Creavin, A. L. Creavin, and C. D. Mallen, "Do GPs respond to postal questionnaire surveys? A comprehensive review of primary care literature," *Journal of Family Practice*, vol. 28, no. 4, pp. 461–467, 2011.

[29] S. W. Pit, T. Vo, and S. Pyakurel, "The effectiveness of recruitment strategies on general practitioner's survey response rates—a systematic review," *BMC Medical Research Methodology*, vol. 14, article 76, 2014.

5

Transient Elastography for Significant Liver Fibrosis and Cirrhosis in Chronic Hepatitis B

Xiaolong Qi,[1,2] Min An,[3] Tongwei Wu,[2] Deke Jiang,[2] Mengyun Peng,[4] Weidong Wang,[5] Jing Wang,[4] Chunqing Zhang,[1] and on behalf of the CHESS Study Group[2]

[1] *Department of Gastroenterology, Shandong Provincial Hospital Affiliated to Shandong University, Jinan, China*
[2] *CHESS, Hepatic Hemodynamic Lab, Institute of Hepatology, Nanfang Hospital, Southern Medical University, Guangdong Provincial Research Center for Liver Fibrosis, Guangzhou, China*
[3] *The Second School of Clinical Medicine, Southern Medical University, Guangzhou, China*
[4] *Department of Hepatobiliary Disease, The Affiliated (T.C.M) Hospital of Southwest Medical University, Luzhou, China*
[5] *Department of Hepatobiliary Surgery, Shunde Hospital, Southern Medical University, Foshan, China*

Correspondence should be addressed to Weidong Wang; wangweidong1968@126.com and Jing Wang; lywj68@126.com

Academic Editor: Mingyu Sun

Background. The hepatitis B virus infection is a global health issue and the stage of liver fibrosis affects the prognosis in patients with chronic hepatitis B (CHB). We performed the meta-analysis describing diagnostic accuracy of transient elastography (TE) for predicting CHB-related fibrosis. *Methods.* We performed an adequate literature search to identify studies that assessed the diagnostic accuracy of TE in CHB patients using biopsy as reference standard. Hierarchical summary receiver-operating curves model and the bivariate mixed-effects binary regression model were applied to generate summary receiver-operating characteristic curves and pooled estimates of sensitivity and specificity. *Results.* The area under the summary receiver-operating curve for significant fibrosis and cirrhosis was 0.86 (95% confidence interval (CI): 0.83–0.89) and 0.92 (95% CI: 0.90–0.94), respectively. The sensitivity, specificity, and diagnostic odds ratio of TE for significant fibrosis were 0.78 (95% CI: 0.73–0.81, $p < 0.01$; $I^2 = 85.59\%$), 0.81 (95% CI: 0.77–0.84, $p < 0.01$; $I^2 = 88.20\%$), and 14.44 (95% CI: 10.80–19.31, $p < 0.01$; $I^2 = 100\%$) and for cirrhosis were 0.84 (95% CI: 0.80–0.88, $p < 0.01$; $I^2 = 76.67\%$), 0.87 (95% CI: 0.84–0.90, $p < 0.01$; $I^2 = 90.89\%$), and 36.63 (95% CI: 25.38–52.87, $p < 0.01$; $I^2 = 100\%$), respectively. The optimal cut-off values of TE were 7.25 kPa for diagnosing significant fibrosis and 12.4 kPa for diagnosing cirrhosis, respectively. *Conclusion.* TE is of great value in the detection of patients with CHB-related cirrhosis but has a suboptimal accuracy in the detection of significant fibrosis.

1. Introduction

Chronic hepatitis B virus infection continues to be a major public health issue worldwide with the prevalence of 3.61% [1]. As well known, liver fibrosis, one of the main prognostic factors in chronic hepatitis B (CHB), was associated with the risk of developing cirrhosis and cirrhosis-related complications [2, 3]. Therefore, liver fibrosis stage plays one of the most important roles in diagnostic and prognostic assessments in patients with CHB.

Liver biopsy (LB), as invasive in nature with related risks, is the gold standard for fibrosis assessment. However, LB is associated with obvious patient discomfort and risk of complications ranging from pain to more serious events with hospitalization rate of 1.4–3.2% [4] and mortality varying from 0.0088 to 0.3% [5]. Besides, LB provides only a quite small part of the organ, and thus there is a risk that the small part might not be representative for the live fibrosis in the whole liver [6].

Noninvasive methods of assessing fibrosis and cirrhosis were urgently needed, and serologic tests and novel imaging techniques were recently developed [7, 8]. Most of these studied focused on whether noninvasive methods can accurately detect minimal (F0-1), significant (≥F2), or advanced (≥F3-4) fibrosis based on the METAVIR score [9]. Transient elastography (TE), also known as FibroScan, was a device and a well-validated method with advantages of a short procedure time (<5 min), immediate results, and the ability to perform the test at the bedside or in an outpatient clinic [10]. Compared with blood tests, TE has a similar performance to predict significant fibrosis (SF) and higher accuracy to identify cirrhosis [11]. Measurement of liver fibrosis without biopsy is very tempting. In spite of the fact that recommendations suggested that noninvasive tests were still not ready to replace LB [12, 13], TE has become widely present in clinical practice. The accuracy of TE for detection of fibrosis has been assessed extensively in a variety of liver diseases [14–17]. However, it was reported that the presence of an IQR/M > 30% and liver stiffness median ≥7.1 kPa lead to a lower accuracy determined by the area under receiver-operating curve (AUROC) and these cases were considered "poorly reliable" [18]. Another study also indicated that there was a significant discrepancy in up to 20% of cases cirrhosis between different TE devices [19].

In the study, we performed an independent meta-analysis of the diagnostic accuracy of TE for predicting significant liver fibrosis (F2–4 versus F0-1) and cirrhosis (F4 versus F0–3) in CHB patients.

2. Methods

2.1. Literature Search Strategy. PubMed, Web of Science, and EMBASE database were searched to October 10, 2016, as well as Wanfang database and China National Knowledge Infrastructure. The search strategy was "FibroScan or transient elastography" in combination with "liver fibrosis assessment," "significant fibrosis or cirrhosis or advanced liver fibrosis," and "liver stiffness measurement." All eligible studies were retrieved and their reference lists were checked for additional relevant publications.

2.2. Inclusion Criteria. All diagnostic cross-sectional studies, cohort studies, and randomized studies that compared TE accuracy with biopsy in diagnosis fibrosis grade were eligible for inclusion. Studies that met all the following criteria were included: (i) studies which reported that all patients had undergone biopsy and TE; (ii) having enough data to create 2 × 2 table of test performance (with numbers of true and false positives and negatives); and (iii) studies which reported the method of definition of the fibrosis grade.

2.3. Exclusion Criteria. The exclusion criteria were as follows: (i) the patients belonging to the pediatric population, hepatitis C/hepatitis B virus coinfected patients, mixed chronic liver disease patients (but not CHB and nonalcoholic fatty liver disease), and liver/kidney transplant patients; (ii) studies that were clearly extensions of previously published cohorts; and (iii) studies unable to obtain sufficient data for statistical analysis.

2.4. Methodological Assessment. Methodological quality was assessed by the Quality Assessment of Diagnostic Accuracy Studies-2 (QUADAS-2) tool. QUADAS-2 was designed to assess the internal and external validity. Any differences between two authors were resolved with discussion between the two review authors and the third author was final arbiter.

2.5. Data Extraction and Management. As for each study, the following information was extracted: year of publication, study design, sample size, presence of HIV coinfection, the QUADAS-2 methodological items, prevalence of each fibrosis stage on biopsy, along with total prevalence of SF and cirrhosis, interval between biopsy and TE, size of biopsy sample, type of scoring system used for histology (METAVIR versus other), and AUROC. Two authors performed the data extraction independently. Disagreement was resolved with discussion between the two review authors, with a third author as final arbiter.

2.6. Statistical Analysis and Data Synthesis. Initial analysis was performed with the Review Manager (RevMan) 5.0. Stata 12.0 was used for meta-analysis of diagnostic accuracy studies, to compute the pooled sensitivity and specificity and to plot the summary receiver-operating characteristics curve (SROC) with summary point and corresponding 95% confidence interval (CI). Regression analysis was performed by Stata 12.0, with each time point providing another covariate to verify the influence of the chosen covariate on the accuracy estimates. We used hierarchical SROC model and the bivariate random efforts model to produce SROC and pooled estimates of sensitivity and specificity. We performed Fagan test to detect clinical significant by Stata 12.0. Heterogeneity was assessed with the inconsistency index (I^2) and I^2 values over 50% indicated substantial heterogeneity. Heterogeneity from threshold effect was explored by meta-disc 1.4.

3. Results

3.1. Search Results. 1238 articles were obtained and 188 were excluded for duplicates. 882 were excluded based on title and abstracts, and full-text copies of 106 studies were obtained and assessed for eligibility. Furthermore, 62 were excluded for inappropriate methodology, duplicate sample, pediatric population, or inability to obtain data for at least 2 × 2 table. Finally, a total of 44 articles comprising 45 studies were enrolled in the meta-analysis (Figure 1).

3.2. Characteristics of Included Studies. The overall prevalence of SF (F2–4) and cirrhosis (F4) ranged from 14.8% to 92.3% and from 1.1% to 69.2%, respectively. Reported AUROCs for SF diagnosis ranged from 0.614 to 0.98 (Table 1).

As shown in Table 1, only Miailhes et al. ($N = 59$) reported HIV coinfected patients [20]. In sixteen studies ($N = 2664$), LB was assessed with a histological score other than METAVIR [21–36]. In eight studies ($N = 1109$), mean length of biopsy sample was ≥20 mm [22, 34, 37–42]. Besides, in nineteen studies ($N = 1358$), data on time interval between biopsy and TE were not obtained [11, 21, 23, 25, 27, 28, 32–34, 39, 40, 42–47]. Three studies did not report cirrhosis (F4) [24, 35, 48]. Only four studies were retrospective [31, 48–50].

As presented in Figure 2, the results of methodological quality assessment based on the QUADAS-2 scale were depicted for all of the 44 eligible studies. The majority of the methodological concern lies within the index test, because TE in ten studies interpreted with knowledge of the results of the biopsy [24, 29, 33, 39, 46, 48, 51–54] and TE in one study

Table 1: Characteristics of the included studies.

Author	Study type	Year	HIV/HBV	METAVIR	Biopsy size	Biopsy to TE time (days)	Sample	Prevalence F2–F4	Prevalence F4	TE cut-off	AUROC
Cao et al.	Prospective	2014	NO	YES	>=15 mm and >=6 portal tracts	NA	162	0.61	0.12	7.3/17.5	NA/NA
Cardoso et al.	Retrospective	2011	NO	YES	>=15 mm and/or >=6 portal tracts	1	202	0.421	0.079	7.2/11	0.867/0.935
Castéra et al.	Prospective	2010	NO	YES	>=16 mm	NA	60	0.73	0.25	7.1/9.6	0.76/0.89
Chan et al.	Prospective	2009	NO	YES	>=15 mm and >=6 portal tracts	28	136	NA	0.25	NA/9	NA/0.93
Chen et al.	Retrospective	2011	NO	YES	>=15 mm	7	213	0.479	0.15	7.0/13.0	0.916/0.971
Chen et al.	Prospective	2012	NO	YES	>=15 mm and >=10 portal tracts	7	315	0.771	0.235	NA/10.4	NA/0.88
Cheng et al.	Prospective	2015	NO	YES	>=10 mm and >=8 portal tracts	1	459	0.61	0.152	7.2/18.2	0.82/0.87
Cheng et al.	Prospective	2014	NO	NO	>=15 mm and >=6 portal tracts	1	99	0.54	NA	8.15/NA	0.896/NA
Cho et al.	Prospective	2011	NO	YES	>=15 mm	1	121	0.727	0.074	7.8/14.0	0.849/0.867
Degos et al.	Prospective	2010	NO	YES	>=18 mm	1	284	0.415	0.102	5.2/12.9	0.78/0.90
Dong et al.	Prospective	2015	NO	NO	>=15 mm and >=6 portal tracts	NA	81	0.604	0.098	10.3/9.4	0.753/0.873

TABLE 1: Continued.

Author	Study type	Year	HIV/HBV	METAVIR	Biopsy size	Biopsy to TE time (days)	Sample	Prevalence F2–F4	Prevalence F4	TE cut-off	AUROC
Gaia et al.	Prospective	2011	NO	YES	>=20 mm	120	70	0.53	0.31	7.2/10.6	0.674/0.763
Goyal et al.	Prospective	2013	NO	YES	>=15 mm and >=6 portal tracts	38	357	0.792	0.059	6.0/11.0	0.84/0.93
Huang et al.	Prospective	2016	NO	NO	>=15 mm	NA	263	0.148	0.011	8/NA	0.911/NA
Jia et al.	Prospective	2015	NO	YES	>=10 mm and >=8 portal tracts	NA	469	0.612	0.122	7.3/10.7	0.82/0.90
Kim et al. 1	Prospective	2012	NO	NO	>=20 mm	1	194	0.845	0.387	8.8/14.1	0.873/0.910
Kim et al. 2	Prospective	2012	NO	YES	>=20 mm	1	170	0.712	0.276	8.0/14.0	0.937/0.963
Kim et al.	Prospective	2009	NO	YES	>=10 mm and >=10 portal tracts	1	91	NA	0.692	NA/10.3	NA/0.803
Kim et al. 1	Prospective	2009	NO	YES	>=6 portal tracts	1	130	0.923	0.515	NA/10.1	NA/0.840
Kim et al. 2	Prospective	2009	NO	YES	>=15 mm	NA	91	0.868	0.396	NA/NA	0.837/0.913
Kim et al. 3	Prospective	2012	NO	NO	>=15 mm	1	150	0.847	0.453	6.0/9.4	NA/NA
Lesmana et al.	Retrospective	2011	NO	YES	>=15 mm and >=5 portal tracts	1	117	0.624	NA	5.85/NA	0.614/NA
liu et al.	Prospective	2015	NO	NO	>=8 portal tracts	NA	115	0.53	0.15	8.50/11.75	0.838/0.914
Liu et al.	Prospective	2012	NO	NO	>=10 mm	NA	134	0.43	0.11	7.60/13.20	0.93/0.96
Marcellin et al.	Prospective	2009	NO	YES	>=6 portal tracts	1	173	0.503	0.081	7.2/11.0	0.81/0.93

Table 1: Continued.

Author	Study type	Year	HIV/HBV	METAVIR	Biopsy size	Biopsy to TE time (days)	Sample	Prevalence F2–F4	Prevalence F4	TE cut-off	AUROC
Meng et al.	Prospective	2015	NO	YES	>=12 mm and >=6 portal tracts	2	287	0.488	0.157	8.85/17.05	0.909/0.815
Meng et al.	Prospective	2016	NO	NO	>=15 mm	7	168	NA	0.15	15.1	0.927
Miailhes et al.	Prospective	2011	YES	YES	>=10 mm	3	59	0.61	0.203	5.9/9.4	0.85/0.96
Osakabe et al.	Prospective	2011	NO	YES	>=15 mm and >=8 portal tracts	30	51	0.882	0.275	7.1/16.0	0.844/0.93
Qin et al.	Prospective	2015	NO	NO	NA	1	152	0.68	0.07	8.2/13.1	0.752/0.973
Seo et al.	Retrospective	2015	NO	NO	>=15 mm	90	567	0.72	0.2	7.8/11.6	0.774/0.902
Sporea et al.	Prospective	2010	NO	YES	>=20 mm and >=8 portal tracts	NA	140	0.764	0.05	7/13.6	0.658/0.974
Stibbe et al.	Prospective	2011	NO	YES	>=20 mm	NA	48	0.458	0.104	7.0/14.0	NA/0.89
Trembling et al.	Prospective	2013	NO	YES	>=20 mm	1	182	0.626	0.198	NA/11.85	NA/O.95
Vigano et al.	Prospective	2011	NO	YES	>=20 mm	NA	125	0.53	0.16	6.2/13.1	NA/NA
Wang et al.	Prospective	2015	NO	NO	>=15 mm and >=6 portal tracts	NA	142	0.585	0.092	8.15/13.95	0.897/0.968
Wang et al.	Prospective	2014	NO	NO	>=15 mm	NA	80	0.7	0.1125	7.3/12.4	0.865/0.944
Wang et al.	Prospective	2016	NO	NO	NA	NA	127	0.76	0.24	NA/15.2	NA/0.805
Wong et al.	Prospective	2009	NO	YES	>=15 mm and >=6 portal tracts	NA	134	0.78	0.24	NA/13.4	NA/0.89
Wong et al. Tr-c	Prospective	2014	NO	YES	>=15 mm and >=6 portal tracts	NA	238	0.693	0.235	NA/10	NA/0.9

Table 1: Continued.

Author	Study type	Year	HIV/HBV	METAVIR	Biopsy size	Biopsy to TE time (days)	Sample	Prevalence F2–F4	Prevalence F4	TE cut-off	AUROC
Wong et al. Va-c	Prospective	2014	NO	YES	>=15 mm and >=6 portal tracts	NA	85	0.565	0.259	NA/10	NA/0.87
Zhang et al.	Prospective	2016	NO	NO	>=22 mm	7	180	0.72	0.18	7.5/10.6	0.813/0.799
Zhang et al.	Prospective	2016	NO	NO	>=15 mm	NA	124	0.54	NA	6.95	0.732
Zhang et al.	Prospective	2011	NO	NO	>=15 mm and >=6 portal tracts	NA	88	0.671	0.159	7.25/12.40	0.857/0/948
Zhu et al.	Prospective	2011	NO	YES	>=15 mm and >=6 portal tracts	1	175	NA	0.166	7.9/13.8	NA/0.98

AUROC, area under the receiver-operating curve; TE, transient elastography; HIV/HBV, hepatitis B and HIV-coinfected patients; METAVIR, liver biopsy assessed according to METAVIR or not; TE cut-off, TE cut-off used to predict; NA, data not available.

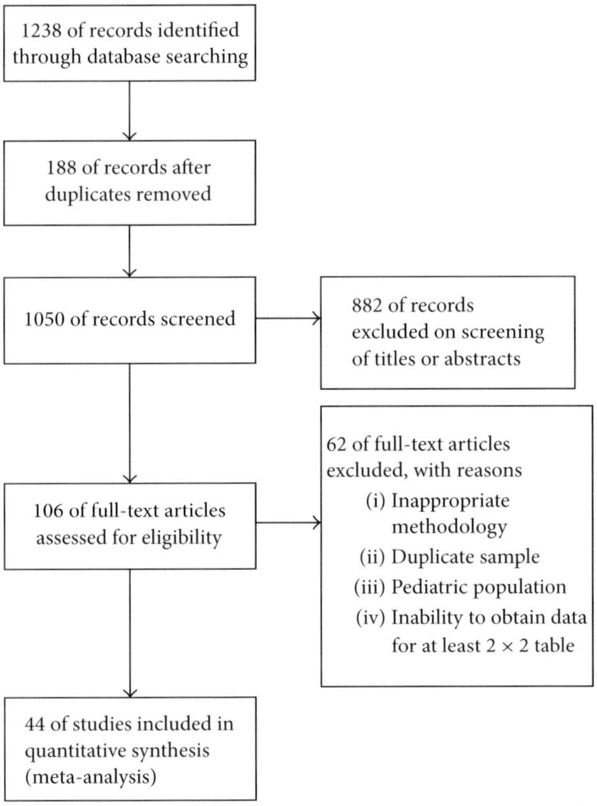

Figure 1: Flow diagram of study selection process.

was conducted with assistance by a time-motion ultrasound image [40]. Another possible issue was addressed in patient selection that participants might be enrolled consecutively with confirmed diagnosis in three studies [31, 50, 55]. Both of these concerns might be located in heterogeneity and sensitivity analyses.

3.3. Diagnosis of SF. We included 35 studies (N = 6,202) in the analysis for SF (F2–F4) [15–23, 25–27, 29–35, 37–40, 43, 56–59]. Summary representation of the overall analysis was presented in Figure 3(a) and Supplementary Figure 1. Sensitivity and specificity ranged from 51 to 97% and 38 to 100%, respectively (Supplementary Figure 1).

The area under SROC for SF was 0.86 (95% CI: 0.83–0.89) (Figure 3(a)). The meta-analysis summary estimate indicated pooled sensitivity of 0.78 (95% CI: 0.73–0.81, $p < 0.01$; $I^2 = 85.59\%$), specificity of 0.81 (95% CI: 0.77–0.84, $p < 0.01$; $I^2 = 88.20\%$) (Supplementary Figure 1(A)), positive likelihood ratio (LR+) of 4.01 (95% CI: 3.31–4.84, $p < 0.01$; $I^2 = 86.27\%$), negative likelihood ratio (LR−) of 0.28 (95% CI: 0.23–0.33, $p < 0.01$; $I^2 = 81.95\%$) (Supplementary Figure 1(B)), diagnostic score (DS) of 2.67 (95% CI: 2.38–2.96, $p < 0.01$; $I^2 = 71.57\%$), and diagnostic odds ratio (DOR) of 14.44 (95% CI: 10.80–19.30, $p < 0.01$; $I^2 = 100\%$) (Supplementary Figure 1(C)). However, it must be carefully considered as they were not pooled from studies with identical TE threshold. Overall, there was heterogeneity as graphically illustrated on the forest plot in Supplementary Figure 1. The cut-off value for SF (F2–4) ranged from 5.2 to 10.3 kPa with a mean value of 8.6 kPa and a median of 7.25 kPa.

As shown in Figure 3(b) and Table 2, in the analysis of LB-related factors with an impact on accuracy, there was no significant difference (joint p = 0.47 for classification criteria; joint p = 0.29 for interval time; joint p = 0.77 for average sample size). 26 studies conducted in Asian presented a better both pooled sensitivity (0.78, 95% CI: 0.73–0.82) and specificity (0.83, 95% CI: 0.79–0.87) than in Caucasian (joint $p = 0.03$).

As presented in Figure 3(c), it was indicated that posttest probability of LR+ increased to 86% and LR− decreased to 29% after TE was performed based on Fagan test.

3.4. Diagnosis of Cirrhosis. 41 studies were included in the cirrhotic analysis with a total of 7,205 patients, as four studies did not have any cases of liver cirrhosis (METAVIR F4) [21, 24, 35, 48]. The overall prevalence of METAVIR F4 and the AUROCs in the included studies ranged from 5% to 69.2% and from 0.80 to 0.98 (Table 1), respectively.

Summary representation of the overall analysis was shown in Figure 4(a). The area under the SROC for liver cirrhosis was 0.92 (95% CI: 0.90–0.94). Sensitivity ranged from 49% to 100%, much more widely than specificity which ranged from 62% to 99% (Supplementary Figure 2). The meta-analysis summary estimate covered the pooled sensitivity of 0.84 (95% CI: 0.80–0.88, $p < 0.01$; $I^2 = 76.67\%$), specificity of 0.87 (95% CI: 0.84–0.90, $p < 0.01$; $I^2 = 90.89\%$) (Supplementary Figure 2(A)), LR+ of 6.66 (95% CI: 5.34–8.31, $p < 0.01$; $I^2 = 84.77\%$), LR− of 0.18 (95% CI: 0.14–0.23, $p < 0.01$; $I^2 = 80.80\%$) (Supplementary Figure 2(B)), DS of 3.60 (95% CI: 3.23–3.97, $p < 0.01$; $I^2 = 66.54\%$), and DOR of 36.63 (95% CI: 25.38–52.87, $p < 0.01$; $I^2 = 100\%$), respectively (Supplementary Figure 2(C)). Again, these measures must be carefully considered without identical TE thresholds. The cut-off value for cirrhosis ranged from 9 kPa to 18.2 kPa with both a mean value and a median of 12.4 kPa.

As shown in Figure 4(b) and Table 3, although summary sensitivity was lower and summary specificity was higher in studies with METAVIR score (sensitivity: 0.82, 95% CI: 0.77–0.87; specificity: 0.88, 95% CI: 0.85–0.91), TE performed on the next day of LB (sensitivity: 0.79, 95% CI: 0.71–0.86; specificity: 0.88, 95% CI: 0.84–0.93), and average sample length $\geqslant 20$ mm (sensitivity: 0.79, 95% CI: 0.69–0.89; specificity: 0.88, 95% CI: 0.83–0.94), respectively, no statistical significance was detected (joint p = 0.17 for classification criteria; joint p = 0.21 for interval time; joint p = 0.47 for average sample size). Besides, pooled sensitivity and specificity were without significant difference (joint p = 0.12) between Caucasian (sensitivity: 0.78, 95% CI: 0.67–0.88; specificity: 0.91, 95% CI: 0.86–0.95) and Asian (sensitivity: 0.86, 95% CI: 0.81–0.90; specificity: 0.86, 95% CI: 0.83–0.89).

In addition, based on Fagan test, it was illustrated that posttest probability of LR+ and LR− rose and declined to 59% and 4%, respectively (Figure 4(c)).

3.5. Publication Bias. The results of publication bias analysis were performed with Stata in Supplementary Figure 3. No

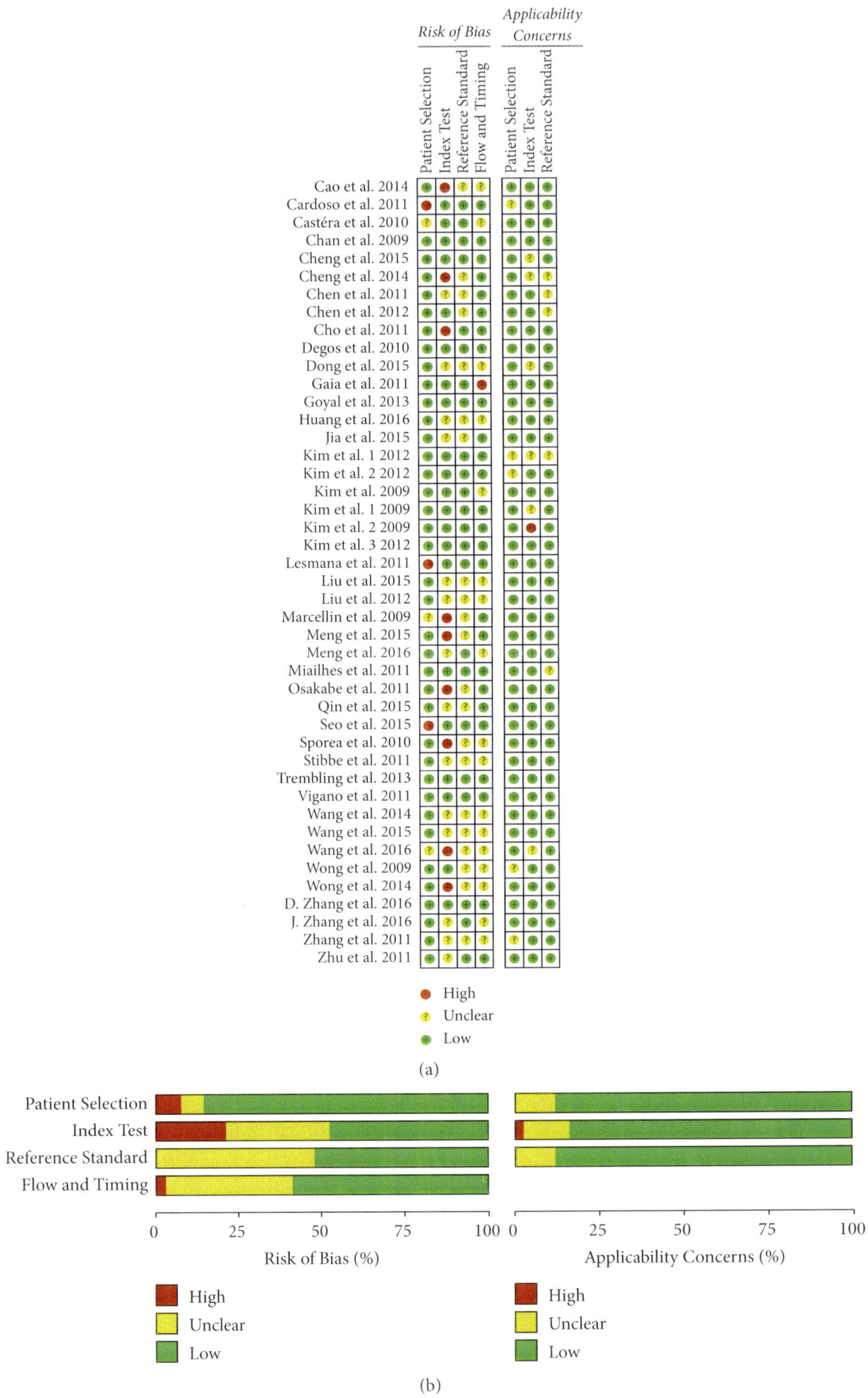

FIGURE 2: Summary of methodological quality of 44 studies according to Quality Assessment of Diagnostic Studies-2 (QUDAS-2) tool. (a) Overall and (b) study-level of bias.

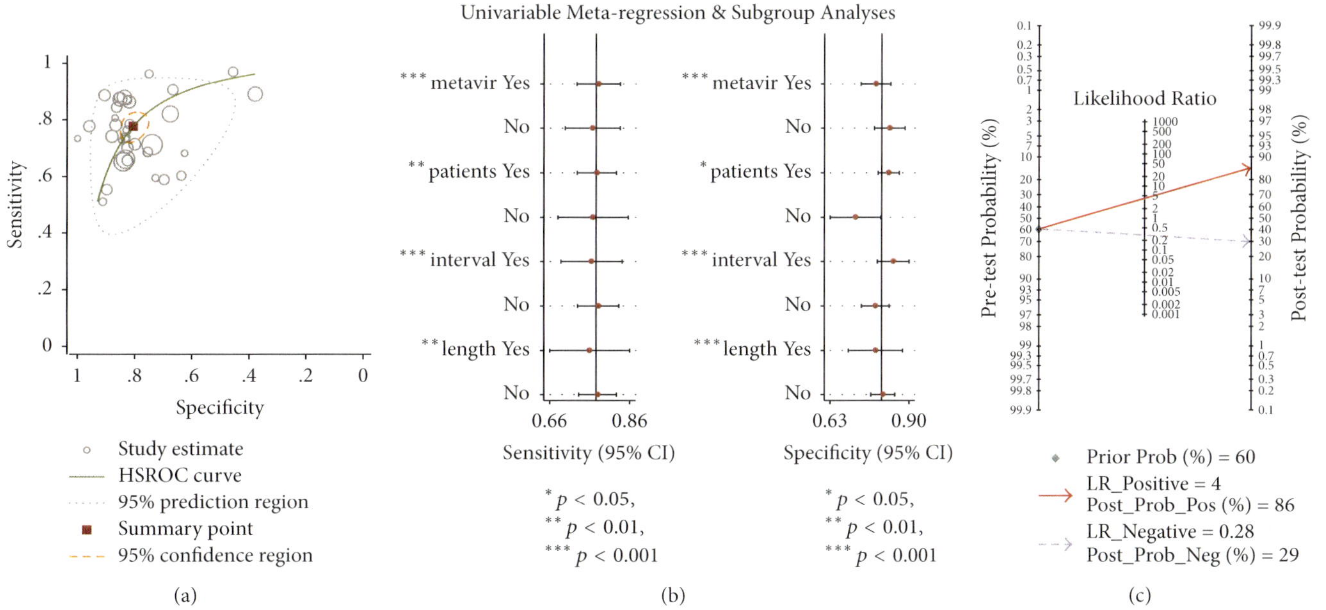

FIGURE 3: Meta-analysis of 32 studies that assessed the diagnosis accuracy of significant fibrosis based on transient elastography. (a) A summary receiver-operating characteristic (SROC) plot of transient elastography for detection of significant liver fibrosis (METAVIR F2–F4). (b) Regression analysis of studies whether reported with METAVIR score on the next day of biopsy or with sample size ≥ 20 cm for significant liver fibrosis. (c) Detection of clinical significance for significant liver fibrosis (METAVIR F2–F4) based on Fagan test. Heterogeneity was generated if $p < 0.01$ in sensitivity or specificity separately. However, joint p value was generated synthesisly for analysis of both sensitivity and specificity.

TABLE 2: Results of meta-regression for significant fibrosis.

Covariate	Number	Pooled sensitivity	p value	Pooled specificity	p value	Joint p value
Classification criteria						
METAVIR score	21	0.78 (0.75–0.83)	<0.01	0.79 (0.73–0.84)	<0.01	0.47
Non-METAVIR score	14	0.77 (0.70–0.83)		0.83 (0.78–0.89)		
Interval time						
On the next day of liver biopsy	11	0.76 (0.69–0.84)	<0.01	0.85 (0.79–0.90)	<0.01	0.29
More than one day after liver biopsy	24	0.78 (0.73–0.83)		0.78 (0.74–0.83)		
Average sample size						
⩾20 mm	7	0.76 (0.66–0.86)	<0.01	0.79 (0.69–0.88)	<0.01	0.77
Not ⩾ 20 mm	28	0.78 (0.74–0.82)		0.81 (0.77–0.85)		
Region						
Asian	26	0.78 (0.73–0.82)	<0.01	0.83 (0.79–0.87)	0.04	0.03
Caucasian	9	0.77 (0.68–0.85)		0.72 (0.63–0.80)		

significant publication bias was detected according to Deeks figures for SF ($p = 0.26$). However, there was bias among 41 studies enrolled in analysis of TE for cirrhosis ($p = 0.02$), which might result from the positive results of all 41 studies.

4. Discussion

TE can provide a reliable detection of liver fibrosis in patients with CHB and thus has been recommended by the American Association for the Study of Liver Diseases (AASLD) and European Association for the Study of the Liver (EASL) [60, 61]. This meta-analysis was conducted in a total of 7,808 CHB patients to summarize the diagnostic accuracy of TE for CHB-related SF, with optimal statistical method SROC. In addition, regression analysis was carried out to further explore sources of heterogeneity.

In our study, TE performed well in both SF (F2–4) and cirrhosis (F4) with pooled sensitivity of 78% and 84%, summary specificity of 81% and 87%, DOR of 14.44 and 36.63, LR+ of 4.01 and 6.66, LR− of 0.28 and 0.18, respectively. Study by Li et al. [62] with hierarchical SROC model was also performed in CHB patients, with summary sensitivity and specificity for SF (F2–4) and cirrhosis (F4) of 80% and 86%, 82%, and 88%, however, without DOR, LR+ and LR−. Interestingly, the pooled specificity for diagnosis SF (F2–4) and cirrhosis (F4) in both studies were higher than

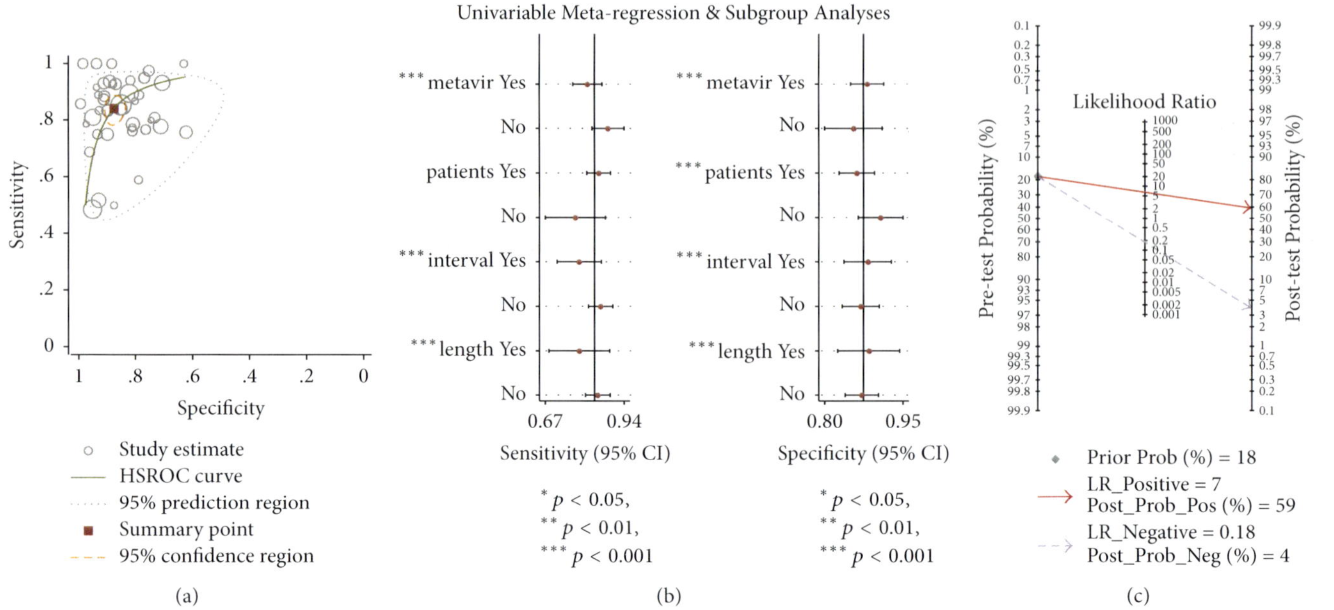

FIGURE 4: Meta-analysis of 37 studies that assessed the diagnosis accuracy of cirrhosis based on transient elastography. (a) A summary receiver-operating characteristic (SROC) plot of transient elastography for detection of cirrhosis (METAVIR F4). (b) Regression analysis of studies whether reported with METAVIR score on the next day of biopsy or with sample size ≥ 20 cm for cirrhosis. (c) Detection of clinical significance for cirrhosis (METAVIR F4) based on Fagan test.

TABLE 3: Results of meta-regression for cirrhosis.

Covariate	Number	Pooled sensitivity	p value	Pooled specificity	p value	Joint p value
Classification criteria						
METAVIR score	28	0.82 (0.77–0.87)	<0.01	0.88 (0.85–0.91)	<0.01	0.17
Non-METAVIR score	13	0.89 (0.83–0.94)		0.86 (0.80–0.91)		
Interval time						
On the next day of liver biopsy	13	0.79 (0.71–0.86)	<0.01	0.88 (0.84–0.93)	<0.01	0.21
More than one day after liver biopsy	28	0.86 (0.82–0.90)		0.87 (0.83–0.90)		
Average sample size						
⩾20 mm	8	0.79 (0.69–0.89)	<0.01	0.88 (0.83–0.94)	<0.01	0.47
Not ⩾ 20 mm	33	0.85 (0.81–0.89)		0.87 (0.84–0.90)		
Region						
Asian	31	0.86 (0.81–0.90)	<0.01	0.86 (0.83–0.89)	<0.01	0.12
Caucasian	10	0.78 (0.67–0.88)		0.91 (0.86–0.95)		

summary sensitivity, which suggested that the currently cut-off values of TE performed better in excluding diseases rather than confirming diseases. Furthermore, the areas under the SROC were 0.86 for SF (F2–4) and 0.92 for cirrhosis (F4), respectively, which indicated that TE was performed well in staging fibrosis in CHB patients. In addition, TE performed better for cirrhosis than SF with a higher value of AUC, sensitivity, specificity, DOR, LR+, and a lower value of LR−. Although the diagnostic accuracy was higher for cirrhosis, TE could also increase the diagnostic accuracy for SF based on Fagan test with increased LR+ and decreased LR−.

The higher TE values were used to confirm diagnosis, while the lower one was used to exclude the false positive diagnosis. However, if the TE value located between the values for rule in and rule out, biopsy was then recommended. Based on the descriptive statistics of enrolled studies, the cut-off values for diagnosing SF (F2–4) and cirrhosis (F4) ranged from 5.2 to 10.3 kPa and 9 to 18.2 kPa, respectively. The optimal cut-off values of TE in CHB patients in our study were 7.25 kPa for SF (F2–4) and 12.4 kPa for cirrhosis (F4). In the previous meta-analysis by Li et al., the weighted mean cut-off values of TE were comparable with 7.2 kPa for SF (F2-4) and 12.2 kPa for cirrhosis (F4) [62]. However, since there was no optimal statistical method to pool different cut-off values in individual studies, the optimal cut-off values in our meta-analysis were simply summarized as median, which could eliminate the impact resulting from the maximum and minimum values that was better than the mean value in previous study [62].

Elevated ALT levels might affect the predictive accuracy of TE [16, 24, 45, 50, 55, 56]; however, the study by Cardoso et al. reported that the use of TE cut-off values adjusted to ALT level did not improve the performance of liver stiffness in CHB patients [49]. Although elevated ALT might be the most important confounder on liver stiffness measurement, the synthesis analysis of ALT elevation could not be conducted due to insufficient data. Therefore, it would be beneficial if more clinical studies focused on the correlation between ALT elevation and TE in CHB patients.

One of the main limitations in this meta-analysis was the significant heterogeneity of the included studies. Spearman correlation coefficient for SF and cirrhosis were 0.055 (p = 0.755) and 0.057 (p = 0.723), and no threshold effect was presented. Therefore, regression analysis was carried out. Besides, TE value could be applied as diagnosis criteria for both SF and cirrhosis in Asian. However, for Caucasian, it was noted that TE was valid to diagnosis of cirrhosis, while it was less precise for SF. Unfortunately, the regression analysis was not conducted owing to the small size of HIV- and non-HIV-coinfected patients. It should be noted that the overlapped cut-off values from included studies might also result in the heterogeneity.

In conclusion, TE is of great value for detection CHB-related cirrhosis, however, with a suboptimal performance in detection of SF. Further studies should focus on the TE cut-off value and the effect of ALT elevation in patients with CHB.

Abbreviations

CHB:	Chronic hepatitis B
CI:	Confidence interval
DOR:	Diagnostic odds ratio
LB:	Liver biopsy
LR:	Likelihood ratio
QUADAS-2:	Quality Assessment of Diagnostic Accuracy Studies-2
SF:	Significant fibrosis
SROC:	Summary receiver-operating curves
TE:	Transient elastography
AUROC:	Area under receiver-operating curve.

Authors' Contributions

Xiaolong Qi, Weidong Wang, Jing Wang, and CHESS Study Group contributed to study concepts and design; Min An and Tongwei Wu performed literature search; Min An and Jing Wang conducted data extraction; Min An, Tongwei Wu, Deke Jiang, Mengyun Peng, and Chunqing Zhang performed data analysis: Tongwei Wu, Weidong Wang, Chunqing Zhang, and CHESS Study Group were responsible for manuscript preparation and revision. All authors and CHESS Study Group have participated sufficiently in the study and approved the final version. Xiaolong Qi, Min An, and Tongwei Wu contributed equally to this work.

Acknowledgments

Collaborators of CHESS Study Group are as follows: Zhiwei Li, Department of General Surgery, 302 Hospital of PLA, Beijing, China; Fuquan Liu, Department of Interventional Therapy, Beijing Shijitan Hospital, Capital Medical University, Beijing, China; Guofeng Chen, Liver Cirrhosis Diagnosis and Treatment Center, 302 Hospital of PLA, Beijing, China; and Qingge Zhang, Department of Hepatology, Xingtai People's Hospital, Xingtai, China. This work was supported by the grants from the National Natural Science Foundation of China (81600510), Guangzhou Industry-Academia-Research Collaborative Innovation Major Project (201704020015), and President Foundation of Nanfang Hospital, Southern Medical University (2017Z012).

References

[1] A. Schweitzer, J. Horn, R. T. Mikolajczyk, G. Krause, and J. J. Ott, "Estimations of worldwide prevalence of chronic hepatitis B virus infection: a systematic review of data published between 1965 and 2013," *The Lancet*, vol. 386, no. 10003, pp. 1546–1555, 2015.

[2] X. Lu, X. Li, Z. Yuan et al., "Assessment of liver fibrosis with the gamma-glutamyl transpeptidase to platelet ratio: a multicentre validation in patients with HBV infection," *Gut*, 2017.

[3] X. Qi, X. Zhang, Z. Li et al., "HVPG signature: A prognostic and predictive tool in hepatocellular carcinoma," *Oncotarget* , vol. 7, no. 38, pp. 62789–62796, 2016.

[4] C. H. Janes and K. D. Lindor, "Outcome of patients hospitalized for complications after outpatient liver biopsy," *Annals of Internal Medicine*, vol. 118, no. 2, pp. 96–98, 1993.

[5] D. H. Van Thiel, J. S. Gavaler, H. Wright, and A. Tzakis, "Liver biopsy: Its safety and complications as seen at a liver transplant center," *Transplantation*, vol. 55, no. 5, pp. 1087–1090, 1993.

[6] A. Regev, M. Berho, L. J. Jeffers et al., "Sampling error and intraobserver variation in liver biopsy in patients with chronic HCV infection," *American Journal of Gastroenterology*, vol. 97, no. 10, pp. 2614–2618, 2002.

[7] G. Shiha, A. Ibrahim, A. Helmy et al., "Asian-Pacific Association for the Study of the Liver (APASL) consensus guidelines on invasive and non-invasive assessment of hepatic fibrosis: a 2016 update," *Hepatology International*, vol. 11, no. 1, 2017.

[8] X. Qi, Z. Li, J. Huang et al., "Virtual portal pressure gradient from anatomic CT angiography," *Gut*, vol. 64, no. 6, pp. 1004-1005, 2015.

[9] M. Pinzani, F. Vizzutti, U. Arena, and F. Marra, "Technology Insight: noninvasive assessment of liver fibrosis by biochemical scores and elastography," *Nature Clinical Practice Gastroenterology & Hepatology*, vol. 5, no. 2, pp. 95–106, 2008.

[10] European Association for Study of Liver and Asociacion Latinoamericana para el Estudio del Higado, "EASL-ALEH Clinical Practice Guidelines: non-invasive tests for evaluation of liver disease severity and prognosis," *Journal of Hepatology*, vol. 63, no. 1, pp. 237–264, 2015.

[11] L. Castéra, J. Vergniol, J. Foucher et al., "Prospective comparison of transient elastography, fibrotest, APRI, and liver biopsy for the assessment of fibrosis in chronic hepatitis C," *Gastroenterology*, vol. 128, no. 2, pp. 343–350, 2005.

[12] G. Sebastiani and A. Alberti, "Non invasive fibrosis biomarkers reduce but not substitute the need for liver biopsy," *World Journal of Gastroenterology*, vol. 12, no. 23, pp. 3682–3694, 2006.

[13] D. C. Rockey and D. M. Bissell, "Noninvasive measures of liver fibrosis," *Hepatology*, vol. 43, no. 2, pp. S113–S120, 2006.

[14] S. Singh, L. L. Fujii, M. H. Murad et al., "Liver stiffness is associated with risk of decompensation, liver cancer, and death in patients with chronic liver diseases: a systematic review and meta-analysis," *Clinical Gastroenterology and Hepatology*, vol. 11, no. 12, pp. 1573–1584, 2013.

[15] A. Berzigotti, M. Reig, J. G. Abraldes, J. Bruix, J. Bosch, and J.-C. García-Pagán, "Value of transient elastography measured with fibroscan in predicting the outcome of hepatic resection for hepatocellular carcinoma," *Annals of Surgery*, vol. 261, no. 4, p. e105, 2015.

[16] C. Corpechot, A. El Naggar, A. Poujol-Robert et al., "Assessment of biliary fibrosis by transient elastography in patients with PBC and PSC," *Hepatology*, vol. 43, no. 5, pp. 1118–1124, 2006.

[17] C. S. Pavlov, G. Casazza, D. Nikolova, E. Tsochatzis, and C. Gluud, "Systematic review with meta-analysis: Diagnostic accuracy of transient elastography for staging of fibrosis in people with alcoholic liver disease," *Alimentary Pharmacology & Therapeutics*, vol. 43, no. 5, pp. 575–585, 2016.

[18] J. Boursier, J.-P. Zarski, V. de Ledinghen et al., "Determination of reliability criteria for liver stiffness evaluation by transient elastography," *Hepatology*, vol. 57, no. 3, pp. 1182–1191, 2013.

[19] J. Parra-Ruiz, C. Sanjuán, L. Muñoz-Medina, D. Vinuesa, M. A. Martínez-Pérez, and J. Hernández-Quero, "Letter: Accuracy of liver stiffness measurement - A comparison of two different FibroScan devices," *Alimentary Pharmacology & Therapeutics*, vol. 39, no. 12, pp. 1434-1435, 2014.

[20] P. Miailhes, P. Pradat, M. Chevallier et al., "Proficiency of transient elastography compared to liver biopsy for the assessment of fibrosis in HIV/HBV-coinfected patients," *Journal of Viral Hepatitis*, vol. 18, no. 1, pp. 61–69, 2011.

[21] R. Huang, N. Jiang, R. Yang et al., "Fibroscan improves the diagnosis sensitivity of liver fibrosis in patients with chronic hepatitis B," *Experimental and Therapeutic Medicine*, vol. 11, no. 5, pp. 1673–1677, 2016.

[22] B. K. Kim, S. U. Kim, H. S. Kim et al., "Prospective validation of Fibrotest in comparison with liver stiffness for predicting liver fibrosis in Asian subjects with chronic hepatitis B," *PLoS ONE*, vol. 7, no. 4, Article ID e35825, 2012.

[23] C. Wang, X. Cheng, C. Meng, and W. Lu, "Diagnostic value of Fibrotest for liver fibrosis in patients with chronic hepatitis," *Chinese Journal of Hepatology*, vol. 23, pp. 738–741, 2015.

[24] X. Cheng, W. Lu, W. Hou, C. Wang, Y. Liu, and J. Wang, "Diagnostic value of FibroTest combined FibroScan for liver fibrosis in patients with chronic hepatitis B," *Journal of Clinical Hepatology*, vol. 30, pp. 424–427, 2014.

[25] D.-R. Dong, M.-N. Hao, C. Li et al., "Acoustic radiation force impulse elastography, FibroScan®, Forns' index and their combination in the assessment of liver fibrosis in patients with chronic hepatitis B, and the impact of inflammatory activity and steatosis on these diagnostic methods," *Molecular Medicine Reports*, vol. 11, no. 6, pp. 4174–4182, 2015.

[26] S. U. Kim, J. K. Kim, Y. N. Park, and K.-H. Han, "Discordance between liver biopsy and fibroscan® in assessing liver fibrosis in chronic hepatitis b: Risk factors and influence of necroinflammation," *PLoS ONE*, vol. 7, no. 2, Article ID e32233, 2012.

[27] D. Liu, Q. Yang, M. Zhang, L. Li, M. Li, and B. Zhao, "Value of Fibroscan in diagnosis of chronic hepatitis B liver fibrosis," *China Practical Medicine*, p. 10, 2015.

[28] Z. Liu, J. Feng, Q. Xiao, L. Ye, X. Wu, and R. Du, "Application of FibroScan for Diagnosis of Liver Fibrosis in Patients with Chronic Hepatitis B," *Chinese General Prac*, vol. 15, pp. 4068–4070, 2012.

[29] Y. Meng, H. Zhang, Z. Yu, H. Liang, and Z. Li, "Value of fibroscan in diagnosis of hepatic fibrosis in patients with chronic hepatitis B infection who had alanine ALT levels lower than 2 times the upper normal limit value," *Chinese J Prac Med*, pp. 43-44, 2016.

[30] H. Qin and H. Yin, "Application of FibroScan combined with APRI for liver fibrosis in patients with chronic hepatitis B," *Anhui Medical Journal*, vol. 36, pp. 552–556, 2015.

[31] Y. S. Seo, M. Y. Kim, S. U. Kim et al., "Accuracy of transient elastography in assessing liver fibrosis in chronic viral hepatitis: A multicentre, retrospective study," *Liver International*, vol. 35, no. 10, pp. 2246–2255, 2015.

[32] C. Wang, J. Wang, B. Jia, C. Li, and C. Liu, "Diagnostic value of FibroScan for liver fibrosis in patients with chronic hepatitis B. Infect Dis Info," *Infectious Disease Information*, pp. 27–226, 2014.

[33] H. Wang, X. Xin, L. Zhang, Q. Ye, and Z. Ye, "Application value analysis of transient elastic wave monitoring in the development of chronic hepatitis," *China Medical Equipment*, pp. 13–61, 2016.

[34] D. Zhang, M. Chen, R. Wang et al., "Comparison of Acoustic Radiation Force Impulse Imaging and Transient Elastography for Non-invasive Assessment of Liver Fibrosis in Patients with Chronic Hepatitis B," *Ultrasound in Medicine & Biology*, vol. 41, no. 1, pp. 7–14, 2015.

[35] J. Zhang, G. Li, S. Ma, and Y. Fang, "Comparative study of shear wave elastography and transient elastography on diagnosing significant liver fibrosis in patients with chronic hepatitis B," *Modern Practical Medicine*, pp. 28–288, 2016.

[36] X. Zhang, W. Lu, and C. Wang, "Diagnostic Value of Fibroscan for Liver Fibrosis in Patients with Chronic Hepatitis B. Tianjin Med," *Tianjin Medical Journal*, pp. 39–236, 2011.

[37] S. Gaia, S. Carenzi, A. L. Barilli et al., "Reliability of transient elastography for the detection of fibrosis in Non-Alcoholic Fatty Liver Disease and chronic viral hepatitis," *Journal of Hepatology*, vol. 54, no. 1, pp. 64–71, 2011.

[38] B. K. Kim, H. S. Kim, J. Y. Park et al., "Prospective validation of ELF test in comparison with fibroscan and fibrotest to predict liver fibrosis in Asian subjects with chronic hepatitis B," *PLoS ONE*, vol. 7, no. 7, Article ID e41964, 2012.

[39] I. Sporea, R. Şirli, A. Deleanu et al., "Liver stiffness measurements in patients with HBV vs HCV chronic hepatitis: A comparative study," *World Journal of Gastroenterology*, vol. 16, no. 38, pp. 4832–4837, 2010.

[40] K. J. M. Stibbe, C. Verveer, J. Francke et al., "Comparison of non-invasive assessment to diagnose liver fibrosis in chronic hepatitis B and C patients," *Scandinavian Journal of Gastroenterology*, vol. 46, no. 7-8, pp. 962–972, 2011.

[41] P. M. Trembling, P. Lampertico, J. Parkes et al., "Performance of Enhanced Liver Fibrosis test and comparison with transient elastography in the identification of liver fibrosis in patients with chronic hepatitis B infection," *Journal of Viral Hepatitis*, vol. 21, no. 6, pp. 430–438, 2014.

[42] M. Viganò, S. Paggi, P. Lampertico et al., "Dual cut-off transient elastography to assess liver fibrosis in chronic hepatitis B: A cohort study with internal validation," *Alimentary Pharmacology & Therapeutics*, vol. 34, no. 3, pp. 353–362, 2011.

[43] X. Cao, Y. Guan, and W. Yu, "Diagnostic study of Fibroscan for liver fibrosis in patients with chronic hepatitis B," *Journal of Tropical Medicine*, pp. 14–779, 2014.

[44] J. Jia, J. Hou, H. Ding et al., "Transient elastography compared to serum markers to predict liver fibrosis in a cohort of Chinese patients with chronic hepatitis B," *Journal of Gastroenterology and Hepatology*, vol. 30, no. 4, pp. 756–762, 2015.

[45] S. U. Kim, J. K. Kim, J. Y. Park et al., "Variability in liver stiffness values from different intercostal spaces," *Liver International*, vol. 29, no. 5, pp. 760–766, 2009.

[46] G. L.-H. Wong, H. L.-Y. Chan, P. C.-L. Choi et al., "Non-invasive algorithm of enhanced liver fibrosis and liver stiffness measurement with transient elastography for advanced liver fibrosis in chronic hepatitis B," *Alimentary Pharmacology & Therapeutics*, vol. 39, no. 2, pp. 197–208, 2014.

[47] G. L.-H. Wong, V. W.-S. Wong, P. C.-L. Choi et al., "Metabolic syndrome increases the risk of liver cirrhosis in chronic hepatitis B," *Gut*, vol. 58, no. 1, pp. 111–117, 2009.

[48] C. R. A. Lesmana, S. Salim, I. Hasan et al., "Diagnostic accuracy of transient elastography (FibroScan) versus the aspartate transaminase to platelet ratio index in assessing liver fibrosis in chronic hepatitis B: the role in primary care setting," *Journal of Clinical Pathology*, vol. 64, no. 10, pp. 916–920, 2011.

[49] A.-C. Cardoso, R. J. Carvalho-Filho, C. Stern et al., "Direct comparison of diagnostic performance of transient elastography in patients with chronic hepatitis B and chronic hepatitis C," *Liver International*, vol. 32, no. 4, pp. 612–621, 2012.

[50] X.-B. Chen, X. Zhu, L.-Y. Chen, E.-Q. Chen, and H. Tang, "Accuracy of FibroScan for the diagnosis of liver fibrosis influenced by serum alanine aminotransferase levels in patients with chronic hepatitis B," *Chinese Journal of Hepatology*, vol. 19, no. 4, pp. 286–290, 2011.

[51] P. Marcellin, M. Ziol, P. Bedossa et al., "Non-invasive assessment of liver fibrosis by stiffness measurement in patients with chronic hepatitis B," *Liver International*, vol. 29, no. 2, pp. 242–247, 2009.

[52] F. Meng, Y. Zheng, Q. Zhang et al., "Noninvasive evaluation of liver fibrosis using real-time tissue elastography and transient elastography (FibroScan)," *Journal of Ultrasound in Medicine* vol. 34, no. 3, pp. 403–410, 2015.

[53] K. Osakabe, N. Ichino, T. Nishikawa et al., "Reduction of liver stiffness by antiviral therapy in chronic hepatitis B," *Journal of Gastroenterology*, vol. 46, no. 11, pp. 1324–1334, 2011.

[54] X. Zhu, L.-C. Wang, E.-Q. Chen et al., "Prospective evaluation of fibroscan for the diagnosis of hepatic fibrosis compared with liver biopsy/AST platelet ratio index and FIB-4 in patients with chronic HBV infection," *Digestive Diseases and Sciences*, vol. 56, no. 9, pp. 2742–2749, 2011.

[55] H. J. Cho, Y. S. Seo, K. G. Lee et al., "Serum aminotransferase levels instead of etiology affects the accuracy of transient elastography in chronic viral hepatitis patients," *Journal of Gastroenterology and Hepatology*, vol. 26, no. 3, pp. 492–500, 2011.

[56] L. Castéra, P.-H. Bernard, B. Le Bail et al., "Transient elastography and biomarkers for liver fibrosis assessment and follow-up of inactive hepatitis B carriers," *Alimentary Pharmacology & Therapeutics*, vol. 33, no. 4, pp. 455–465, 2011.

[57] F. Degos, P. Perez, B. Roche et al., "Diagnostic accuracy of FibroScan and comparison to liver fibrosis biomarkers in chronic viral hepatitis: a multicenter prospective study (the FIBROSTIC Study)," *Journal of Hepatology*, vol. 53, no. 6, pp. 1013–1021, 2010.

[58] J. Cheng, J. Hou, H. Ding et al., "Validation of ten noninvasive diagnostic models for prediction of liver fibrosis in patients with chronic hepatitis B," *PLoS ONE*, vol. 10, no. 12, Article ID e0144425, 2015.

[59] R. Goyal, S. R. Mallick, M. Mahanta et al., "Fibroscan can avoid liver biopsy in Indian patients with chronic hepatitis B," *Journal of Gastroenterology and Hepatology*, vol. 28, no. 11, pp. 1738–1745, 2013.

[60] European Association for the Study of the Liver, "EASL Clinical Practice Guidelines: management of hepatitis C virus infection," *Journal of Hepatology*, vol. 60, no. 2, pp. 392–420, 2014.

[61] X. Qi, F. Liu, Z. Li et al., "Insufficient accuracy of computed tomography-based portal pressure assessment in hepatitis B virus-related cirrhosis: An analysis of data from CHESS-1601 trial," *Journal of Hepatology*, vol. 68, no. 1, pp. 210-211, 2017.

[62] Y. Li, Y.-S. Huang, Z.-Z. Wang et al., "Systematic review with meta-analysis: The diagnostic accuracy of transient elastography for the staging of liver fibrosis in patients with chronic hepatitis B," *Alimentary Pharmacology & Therapeutics*, vol. 43, no. 4, pp. 458–469, 2016.

6

The Effect of Antidepressants on the Course of Inflammatory Bowel Disease

Barry J. Hall,[1] **P. John Hamlin**,[1,2] **David J. Gracie**,[1,2] **and Alexander C. Ford**[1,2]

[1]*Leeds Gastroenterology Institute, St. James's University Hospital, Leeds, UK*
[2]*Leeds Institute of Biomedical and Clinical Sciences, University of Leeds, Leeds, UK*

Correspondence should be addressed to Barry J. Hall; bhall@tcd.ie

Academic Editor: Kevork M. Peltekian

Background and Aims. Mood may have an important role in the natural history of inflammatory bowel disease (IBD). However, the impact of antidepressant use on prognosis is unknown. We aimed to address this in a longitudinal study in a referral population. *Methods.* We collected demographic data, clinical disease activity and mood using validated questionnaires, and antidepressant use at baseline. Longitudinal disease activity was defined by disease flare or need for glucocorticosteroids, escalation of medical therapy, hospitalisation, or intestinal resection. We compared rates of these over a minimum period of 2 years according to antidepressant use at baseline. *Results.* In total, 331 patients provided complete data, of whom 54 (15.8%) were taking an antidepressant at study entry. Older age, female gender, and abnormal mood scores were associated with antidepressant use. During longitudinal follow-up, there was a trend towards lower rates of any of the four endpoints of IBD activity of interest in patients with abnormal anxiety scores at baseline and who were receiving an antidepressant (42.3% versus 64.6%, $P = 0.05$). Based on univariate Cox regression analysis, there was a trend towards lower rates of escalation of medical therapy among patients receiving antidepressants at baseline (hazard ratio (HR) = 0.59; 95% confidence interval (CI) 0.35-1.00, $P = 0.05$). None of the differences observed persisted after multivariate Cox regression. *Conclusions.* Antidepressants may have some beneficial effects on the natural history of IBD, but larger studies with longer follow-up are required. Whether these effects are limited to patients with abnormal mood remains uncertain.

1. Introduction

Crohn's disease (CD) and ulcerative colitis (UC) are chronic inflammatory organic disorders of the gastrointestinal (GI) tract of unknown aetiology, which may arise from dysregulation of both the innate and adaptive immune systems, leading to persistent and damaging inflammation of the intestine. Conventional therapies for inflammatory bowel disease (IBD) include glucocorticosteroids, 5-aminosalicylates, immunosuppressants, and biological therapies [1–7], with the aim of treatment being to induce remission of GI inflammation and prevent future disease relapse.

Patients with IBD appear to be at increased risk of exhibiting mood disorders, such as anxiety or depression, compared with healthy individuals [8–12]. However, whether this is a consequence of, or an etiological factor in, GI inflammation remains uncertain. In people with functional GI disorders, such as irritable bowel syndrome, longitudinal studies suggest that there is an increased likelihood of asymptomatic people who demonstrate anxiety or depression at baseline developing GI symptoms *de novo* [13]. This raises the possibility that coexistent anxiety or depression in patients with IBD, particularly if unrecognised or untreated, may have a deleterious effect on the natural history of IBD.

Evidence to support a role of abnormal mood in subsequent IBD activity comes mainly from animal models. Studies have demonstrated that in mouse models of quiescent colitis, inducing depression leads to reactivation of GI inflammation [14] but that this can be prevented by preadministration of antidepressants [15]. There is also limited evidence in humans to suggest that acute psychological stress induces proinflammatory cytokine production in both the serum and the mucosa of IBD patients [16]. Studies that have examined the effect of psychological comorbidity on the natural history of IBD suggest that patients with coexistent mood disorders have higher rates of disease relapse, escalation of therapy, and IBD-related surgery than patients with IBD without psychological disorders [17–20]. Despite this, the benefit of treatments, such as psychological therapies or antidepressants, which target mood abnormalities in patients with IBD is uncertain. A systematic review and meta-analysis of 14 randomised controlled trials (RCTs) of cognitive behavioural therapy, hypnotherapy, and other psychological interventions failed to demonstrate any effect on subsequent disease activity [21]. However, none of the included trials recruited only patients with psychological comorbidity. Another systematic review examining the effect of antidepressants on the course of IBD identified 15 studies [22], but the majority of these were case series or case reports. There were few longitudinal studies and only one small pilot RCT of fluoxetine in CD [23], which appeared to be of no benefit in terms of maintenance of disease remission.

This is an important issue, as patients with quiescent IBD may be at a lower risk of subsequent relapse of disease activity if coexisting mood disorders are identified and treated. This could lead to a more benign disease course, with fewer episodes of flares of disease activity and reductions in treatment escalation, hospitalisation, or surgery. There is, therefore, a need for epidemiological studies that examine the effects of antidepressants on the course of IBD in a setting that is generalisable to the type of patients with IBD seen in secondary care. We have therefore conducted a longitudinal follow-up study examining these issues in a large number of patients with IBD. Our *a priori* hypothesis was that there would be lower rates of, and longer time of onset to, objective markers of subsequent disease activity among those patients prescribed antidepressants at baseline.

2. Materials and Methods

2.1. Participants and Setting. Individuals recruited into a previous cross-sectional survey were included in this longitudinal follow-up study [24, 25]. All patients had an established radiological, histological, or endoscopic diagnosis of CD or UC and were aged ≥16 years at the time of baseline recruitment. Exclusion criteria were an inability to understand written English, a diagnosis of IBD-unclassified, and anyone with an end ileostomy or colostomy, due to the difficulties in assessing disease activity indices in these patients. Participants were followed up after a minimum period of 2 years had elapsed from initial recruitment. The longitudinal follow-up study was approved by the local research ethics committee in September 2014 (REC ref: 12/YH/0443), and data collection continued until June 2017. Study findings were reported in accordance with the STROBE guidelines for observational studies [26].

2.2. Data Collection and Synthesis. Date of recruitment into the original cross-sectional survey, demographic data, type of IBD, medication use for both IBD and non-IBD-related disease, and data concerning anxiety, depression, somatisation, and quality of life data were recorded at baseline, as described in the original cross-sectional survey [24, 25].

2.2.1. Definition of Disease Activity, Anxiety or Depression, and Somatisation. At baseline assessment, a combination of disease activity indices (the Harvey-Bradshaw index (HBI) for CD [27] and the simple clinical colitis activity index (SCCAI) for UC [28]) were utilised. Clinical remission was defined as a score <5 for both CD and UC, as has been recommended by previous investigators [29, 30].

Anxiety and depression data were collected using the hospital anxiety and depression scale (HADS) [31]. This 14-item questionnaire consists of seven questions screening for the presence of anxiety symptoms and seven for depression symptoms, with a 4-point response for each item, ranging from 0 to 3. The total HADS score ranges from a minimum of 0 to a maximum of 21 for both anxiety and depression. Severity was categorised, according to total HADS score, into normal (total HADS depression or anxiety score 0-7), borderline normal (8-10), and abnormal (≥11) as previously recommended [31].

Somatisation data were collected using the patient health questionnaire-15 (PHQ-15), which is derived from the validated full PHQ [32]. Individuals were asked to rate the severity of 15 predefined symptoms as "not bothered at all" (scored as 0), "bothered a little" (scored as 1), or "bothered a lot" (scored as 2). Therefore the total PHQ-15 score ranges from a minimum of 0 to a maximum of 30. Somatisation severity was categorised, using the total PHQ-15 score, into high (total PHQ-15 ≥15), medium (10-14), low (5-9), and minimal (≤4) levels of somatisation severity, again as previously recommended [32].

2.2.2. Antidepressant Use. Use of antidepressants was captured at the baseline visit. We recorded the regular prescription of any of the following drugs at study entry: selective serotonin reuptake inhibitors (SSRIs) including fluoxetine, fluvoxamine, paroxetine, sertraline, citalopram, escitalopram; tricyclic antidepressants (TCAs) including amitriptyline, nortriptyline, imipramine, clomipramine, desipramine, doxepin, or dosulepin; serotonin and noradrenaline reuptake inhibitors (SNRIs) including venlafaxine and duloxetine; tetracyclic antidepressants including mirtazapine; and atypical antidepressants, such as trazodone.

2.2.3. Longitudinal Objective Assessment of IBD Activity. Objective assessment of disease activity during longitudinal follow-up was made by detailed case note review by a sole investigator (DJG), blinded to the baseline questionnaire data. The case notes of each of the patients included at baseline were assessed for the following four clinical endpoints, with the date of each endpoint recorded, where applicable: documented glucocorticosteroid prescription or a flare of disease activity identified by physician's global assessment; escalation of medical therapy due to uncontrolled disease activity, as judged by a physician's global assessment; hospitalisation secondary to objectively confirmed IBD activity; and intestinal resection. All these decisions were made as per usual care, as this was a noninterventional study conducted in routine clinical practice. Escalation of medical therapy in response to therapeutic drug monitoring, but in the absence of inflammatory activity, was not included as an endpoint, nor was surgical intervention for isolated perianal Crohn's disease.

2.3. Statistical Analysis. Baseline demographic, disease-related, and psychological data for all participants were compared between those taking and not taking antidepressants at study entry. Due to multiple comparisons we considered a 2-tailed P value of <0.01 to be statistically significant for these analyses. Proportions of patients experiencing the occurrence of one, or any, of the four objective markers of IBD activity during longitudinal follow-up were then compared between those patients taking an antidepressant at baseline and those who were not. We planned to perform subgroups analyses according to type of antidepressant used (SSRI, TCA, SNRI, or tetracyclic) as well as presence or absence of anxiety and/or depression at baseline, to assess whether these had any impact on the association between antidepressant use and IBD activity during longitudinal follow-up. We compared proportions in all these analyses using a χ^2 test for categorical variables and an independent samples *t*-test for continuous data.

We then performed univariate Cox regression analysis to examine the effect of antidepressant use on IBD activity during longitudinal follow-up for all patients, and according to presence or absence of anxiety and/or depression at baseline. Independent predictors of the occurrence of any of the objective disease activity outcomes of interest were then determined by performing multivariate Cox regression analysis to control for antidepressant use, as well as all other baseline data. The results of these analyses were expressed as hazard ratios (HR) with 95% confidence intervals (CI). As our hypothesis that there would be lower rates of objective markers of IBD activity among those patients prescribed antidepressants at baseline was defined *a priori*, for these analyses we considered a 2-tailed P value of <0.05 to be statistically significant. All statistical analyses were performed using SPSS for Windows version 22.0 (SPSS Inc., Chicago, IL, USA).

3. Results

In total, 54 (15.8%) of 342 patients were taking an antidepressant at study entry. Of these, 32 (59.3%) were taking an SSRI, 17 (31.5%) a TCA, two (3.7%) an SNRI, two (3.7%) both an SSRI and a TCA, and one (1.9%) trazodone. Older age and female gender were both associated with antidepressant use, and there was a trend towards a higher body mass index (BMI) among those using antidepressants (Table 1). Patients with abnormal HADS anxiety or depression scores and those with high somatisation levels were more likely to be taking an antidepressant at baseline (P < 0.001).

3.1. Effect of Antidepressant Use on Subsequent IBD Activity. Of these 342 patients, 331 (96.8%) provided complete follow-up data for longitudinal IBD activity after case note review and were included in subsequent analyses. In all, 142 (42.9%) of 331 patients had a flare of disease activity or required glucocorticosteroid therapy during the 2-year follow-up period. Furthermore, 137 (41.4%) patients underwent escalation of medical therapy in response to uncontrolled disease activity. In terms of hospitalisation and intestinal resection, 43 (13.0%) and 19 (0.6%) patients experienced these endpoints

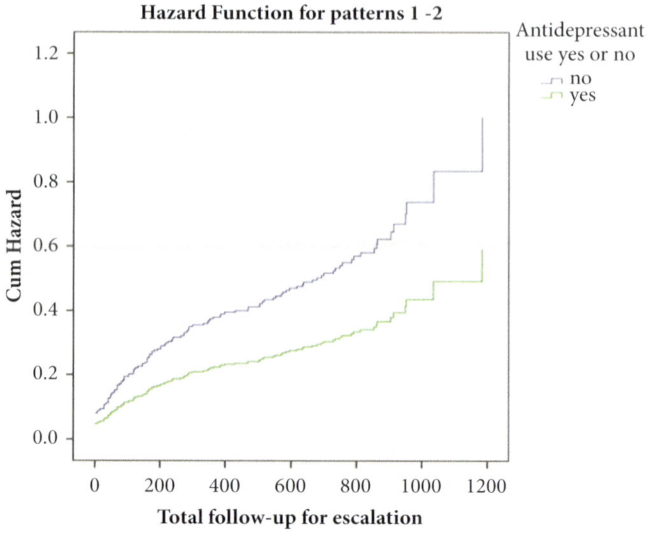

FIGURE 1: Cumulative hazard for escalation of medical therapy in response to uncontrolled IBD between patients receiving or not receiving antidepressants.

of interest, respectively. There were no differences in proportions of patients experiencing a flare of disease activity or glucocorticosteroid use, need for escalation of therapy, hospitalisation, intestinal resection, or any of these endpoints according to use of antidepressants at baseline (Table 2). Limiting our analyses for flare of disease activity or requiring glucocorticosteroid therapy or escalation of medical therapy to only those who were in clinical remission at baseline did not affect our findings—9 (39.1%) of 23 patients receiving antidepressants experienced a flare of disease activity or needed a prescription for glucocorticosteroids versus 49 (32.0%) of 153 not receiving (P = 0.50); 7 (30.4%) of 23 patients receiving antidepressants required escalation of therapy versus 60 (39.2%) of 153 nor receiving (P = 0.42).

Based on univariate Cox regression analysis, there was a trend towards lower rates of escalation of medical therapy among patients receiving antidepressants at baseline, compared with those who were not (HR = 0.59; 95% CI 0.35 to 1.00, P = 0.05) (Table 3, Figure 1), but this was no longer the case based on multivariate Cox regression controlling for all baseline data.

We performed subgroup analyses according to presence or absence of anxiety and/or depression at baseline (Table 2). There was a trend towards lower rates of escalation of therapy among those with either abnormal anxiety or depression scores at baseline and who were receiving an antidepressant, compared with those with either abnormal anxiety or depression scores at baseline but who were not receiving an antidepressant (25.5% versus 46.6%, P = 0.06). There were significantly lower rates of escalation of therapy among patients with abnormal anxiety scores at baseline and who were receiving an antidepressant, compared with those with abnormal anxiety scores at baseline but who were not receiving an antidepressant (23.1% versus 47.7%, P = 0.03). Finally there was a trend towards lower rates of any of the

TABLE 1: Baseline demographic, disease-related, and psychological characteristics of patients with IBD according to use of antidepressants.

	Prescribed Antidepressants at Baseline (n = 54)	Not prescribed Antidepressants at Baseline (n = 288)	P value*
Mean age in years (SD)	47.1 (13.8)	39.6 (16.2)	0.001
Mean duration of follow-up in days (SD) for each endpoint			
Glucocorticosteroid prescription or flare of disease activity	648.3 (409)	502.9 (361.8)	0.02
Escalation of medical therapy in response to uncontrolled disease activity	664.0 (399.1)	531.0 (345.3)	0.03
Hospitalisation due to disease activity (%)	841.4 (284.1)	733.2 (252.1)	0.01
Intestinal resection (%)	861.4 (265.6)	770.7 (218.1)	0.02
Female gender (%)	47 (87.0)	158 (54.9)	<0.001
Caucasian ethnicity (%)	51 (96.2)	267 (93.7)	0.47
Married or co-habiting (%)	27 (50.9)	165 (58.3)	0.32
University/postgraduate (%)	16 (29.6)	102 (36.0)	0.37
Mean BMI (SD)	28.0 (6.2)	25.6 (5.3)	0.01
Tobacco user (%)	14 (25.9)	48 (16.8)	0.11
Alcohol user (%)	31 (57.4)	200 (69.9)	0.07
Crohn's disease (%)	20 (37.0)	118 (41.0)	0.59
5-ASA use (%)	27 (50.0)	124 (43.1)	0.35
Immunosuppressant use (%)	16 (29.6)	117 (40.6)	0.13
Biologic use (%)	6 (11.1)	63 (21.9)	0.07
Glucocorticosteroid use (%)	5 (9.3)	26 (9.0)	0.96
HBI/SCCAI <5 (%)	23 (45.1)	159 (58.7)	0.07
HADS anxiety scores at baseline (%)			
Normal	16 (29.6)	167 (58.6)	
Borderline abnormal	10 (18.5)	10 (18.5)	
Abnormal	28 (51.9)	69 (24.2)	<0.001
HADS depression scores at baseline (%)			
Normal	29 (53.7)	230 (80.1)	
Borderline abnormal	11 (20.4)	35 (12.2)	
Abnormal	14 (25.9)	22 (7.7)	<0.001
PHQ-15 somatisation scores at baseline (%)			
Mild	0 (0)	50 (18.8)	
Low	8 (15.7)	83 (31.2)	
Medium	20 (39.2)	78 (29.3)	
High	23 (45.1)	55 (20.7)	<0.001

*Independent samples t-test for continuous data and $\chi 2$ for comparison of categorical data.

Table 2: Effect of antidepressant use on subsequent development of IBD activity and according to anxiety and depression scores at baseline.

	Antidepressant Use: All Patients			Antidepressant Use: Normal Anxiety and Depression Scores at Baseline			Antidepressant Use: Abnormal Anxiety or Depression Scores at Baseline			Antidepressant Use: Abnormal Anxiety Scores at Baseline			Antidepressant Use: Abnormal Depression Scores at Baseline		
	No	Yes	P value	No	Yes	P value	No	Yes	P value	No	Yes	P value	No	Yes	P value
Glucocorticosteroid prescription or flare of disease activity (%)	121/279 (43.4)	21/52 (40.4)	0.69	82/203 (40.4)	10/25 (40.0)	0.97	38/73 (52.1)	11/27 (40.1)	0.32	35/65 (53.8)	10/26 (38.5)	0.19	9/21 (42.9)	6/14 (42.9)	1.00
Escalation of medical therapy in response to uncontrolled disease activity (%)	120/279 (43.0)	17/52 (32.7)	0.17	85/203 (41.9)	10/25 (40.0)	0.86	34/73 (46.6)	7/27 (25.9)	0.06	31/65 (47.7)	6/26 (23.1)	0.03	8/21 (38.1)	5/14 (35.7)	0.89
Hospitalisation due to disease activity (%)	38/279 (13.6)	5/52 (9.6)	0.43	26/203 (12.8)	4/25 (16.0)	0.66	12/73 (16.4)	1/27 (3.7)	0.09	11/65 (16.9)	1/26 (3.8)	0.10	2/21 (9.5)	0/14 (0)	0.23
Intestinal resection (%)	15/279 (5.4)	4/52 (7.7)	0.51	8/203 (3.9)	3/25 (12.0)	0.08	7/73 (9.6)	1/27 (3.7)	0.34	6/65 (9.2)	1/26 (3.8)	0.38	2/21 (9.5)	0/14 (0)	0.23
Any adverse outcome (%)	148/279 (53.0)	24/52 (46.2)	0.36	102/203 (50.2)	12/25 (48.0)	0.83	45/73 (61.6)	12/27 (44.4)	0.12	42/65 (64.6)	11/26 (42.3)	0.05	10/21 (47.6)	6/14 (42.9)	0.78

TABLE 3: Effect of antidepressant or SSRI use on subsequent IBD activity based on univariate cox regression analysis.

	Glucocorticosteroid prescription or flare of disease activity		Escalation of Medical Therapy in Response to Uncontrolled Disease Activity		Hospitalisation due to Disease Activity		Intestinal resection	
	Hazard ratio (95% CI)	**P value**	**Hazard ratio (95% CI)**	**P value**	**Hazard ratio (95% CI)**	**P value**	**Hazard ratio (95% CI)**	**P value**
Antidepressant use: all patients	0.76 (0.47-1.22)	0.25	0.59 (0.35-1.00)	0.05	0.59 (0.231.50)	0.26	1.15 (0.373.53)	0.81
Antidepressant use: normal anxiety and depression scores at baseline	0.77 (0.38-1.54)	0.77	0.72 (0.36-1.44)	0.35	1.01 (0.352.93)	0.98	2.15 (0.558.50)	0.27
Antidepressant use: abnormal anxiety or depression scores at baseline	0.63 (0.32-1.23)	0.17	0.47 (0.21-1.05)	0.07	0.20 (0.031.57)	0.13	0.37 (0.053.04)	0.36
SSRI use: all patients	0.74 (0.41-1.31)	0.30	0.47 (0.24-0.93)	0.03	0.35 (0.081.46)	0.15	0.86 (0.193.85)	0.84
SSRI use: normal anxiety and depression scores at baseline	0.76 (0.31-1.91)	0.56	0.49 (0.18-1.37)	0.18	0.87 (0.203.75)	0.86	2.39 (0.4712.2)	0.29
SSRI use: abnormal anxiety or depression scores at baseline	0.58 (0.27-1.26)	0.17	0.43 (0.17-1.11)	0.08	0.03 (0.0010.1)	0.24	0.03 (0.0073.9)	0.39

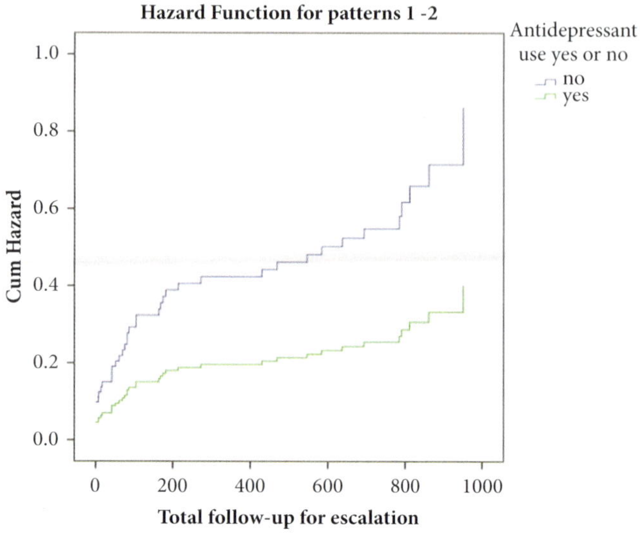

FIGURE 2: Cumulative hazard for escalation of medical therapy in response to uncontrolled IBD between patients with abnormal anxiety or depression scores at baseline receiving or not receiving antidepressants.

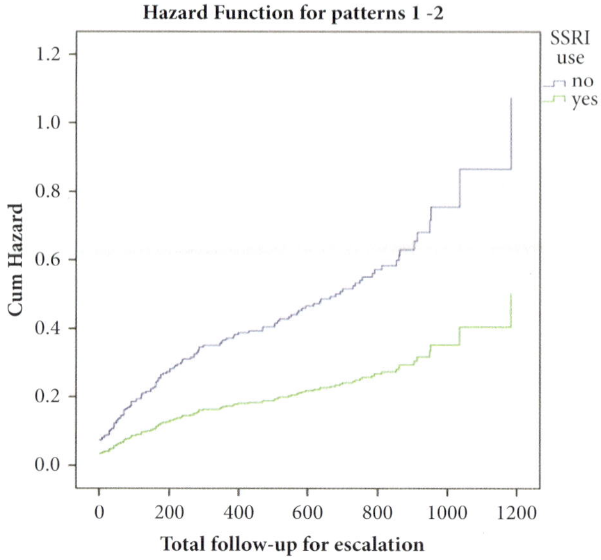

FIGURE 3: Cumulative hazard for escalation of medical therapy in response to uncontrolled IBD between patients receiving or not receiving SSRIs.

four endpoints of IBD activity of interest in patients with abnormal anxiety scores at baseline and who were receiving an antidepressant, compared with those with abnormal anxiety scores at baseline but who were not receiving an antidepressant (42.3% versus 64.6%, P = 0.05). Based on univariate Cox regression analysis, again there was a trend towards lower rates of escalation of medical therapy among patients with either abnormal anxiety or depression scores at baseline who were receiving antidepressants, compared with those with either abnormal anxiety or depression scores at baseline but who were not (HR = 0.47; 95% CI 0.21 to 1.05, P = 0.07) (Table 3) (Figure 2). However, this was no longer the case based on multivariate Cox regression.

3.2. Effect of SSRI Use on Subsequent IBD Activity. In total, 33 (61.1%) of all 54 patients taking an antidepressant at baseline were receiving an SSRI. There were no significant differences in the proportions of patients prescribed an SSRI experiencing one, or any, of the endpoints of interest, compared with those who were not (Table 4).

Based on univariate Cox regression analysis, there was a significantly lower rate of escalation of medical therapy among patients receiving SSRIs at baseline, compared with those who were not (HR = 0.47; 95% CI 0.24 to 0.93, P = 0.03) (Table 3) (Figure 3). This was no longer observed based on multivariate Cox regression.

Due to a reduced number of individuals taking SSRIs we were unable to perform subgroup analyses according to the presence of only abnormal anxiety scores, or only abnormal depression scores, at baseline. In the remaining analyses, there were trends towards higher rates of intestinal resection among patients with normal anxiety and depression scores at baseline who were taking SSRIs (15.4% versus 3.9%, P = 0.06) and lower rates of hospitalisation among patients with either abnormal anxiety or depression scores at baseline receiving SSRIs (0% versus 16.4%, P = 0.05) (Table 4). Based on both univariate (Table 3) and multivariate Cox regression analysis, there were no significant differences in rates of flare or glucocorticoid prescription, escalation of medical therapy, hospitalisation, or intestinal resection among SSRI users according to presence or absence of abnormal anxiety or depression scores at baseline.

4. Discussion

Results from univariate Cox regression analysis in this longitudinal study, adjusted for total duration of follow-up among all individuals, suggest a trend towards lower rates of subsequent escalation of medical therapy among patients with IBD receiving antidepressants at baseline, and this persisted when only those patients with abnormal anxiety or depression scores at study entry were considered in the analysis. Similar findings were observed when only those using SSRIs at baseline were considered in the analysis. However, none of these associations remained statistically significant based on multivariate Cox regression analysis. Our findings, although interesting, should be considered as preliminary only, and larger studies with longer follow-up, or rigorous RCTs, which are powered to examine this issue specifically, will be required before the true effect of antidepressant use on objective disease endpoints in patients with IBD is known.

We obtained longitudinal disease activity outcome data for a cohort of 331 patients with IBD. The observational design and the use of a secondary care population mean that our findings are likely to be generalisable to the majority of patients with IBD seen outside specialist centres. Our use of validated questionnaires to assess for the presence of anxiety [31], depression [31], or somatisation [32] at baseline is a further strength. We controlled for differences in duration

TABLE 4: Effect of SSRI use on subsequent development of IBD activity and according to anxiety and depression scores at baseline.

	SSRI Use: All Patients			SSRI Use: Normal Anxiety and Depression Scores at Baseline			SSRI use: Abnormal Anxiety or Depression Scores at Baseline		
	No	Yes	P Value	No	Yes	P value	No	Yes	P value
Glucocorticosteroid prescription or flare of disease activity (%)	121/279 (43.4)	14/33 (42.4)	0.92	82/203 (40.4)	6/13 (46.2)	0.68	38/73 (52.1)	8/20 (40.0)	0.34
Escalation of medical therapy in response to uncontrolled disease activity (%)	120/279 (43.0)	10/33 (30.3)	0.16	85/203 (41.9)	5/13 (38.5)	0.81	34/73 (46.6)	5/20 (25.0)	0.08
Hospitalisation due to disease activity (%)	38/279 (13.6)	2/33 (6.1)	0.22	26/203 (12.8)	2/13 (15.4)	0.79	12/73 (16.4)	0/20 (0)	0.05
Intestinal resection (%)	15/279 (5.4)	2/33 (6.1)	0.87	8/203 (3.9)	2/13 (15.4)	0.06	7/73 (9.6)	0/20 (0)	0.15
Any adverse outcome (%)	148/279 (53.0)	14/33 (42.4)	0.25	102/203 (50.2)	6/13 (46.2)	0.78	45/73 (61.6)	8/20 (40.0)	0.08

of follow-up between those receiving, or not receiving, antidepressants at baseline and all other baseline data, using multivariate Cox regression. Finally, objective longitudinal disease activity assessment data were collected blinded to baseline disease activity and psychological data, therefore eliminating researcher confirmation bias.

Weaknesses include the sample size and length of follow-up. Based on multivariate Cox regression analysis, there were no statistically significant differences observed in rates of any of the objective markers of disease activity according to antidepressant use at baseline, despite the fact that the absolute proportion of patients reaching these endpoints were generally lower among those taking antidepressants at baseline, particularly among those with abnormal anxiety and/or depression scores at baseline. This suggests that if our sample size had been larger, or the duration of follow-up longer, some of these comparisons may have become statistically significant. Alternatively, there may be a true beneficial effect that was lost when other factors were controlled for in our multivariate analysis. This could be due to either confounding or a loss of time contributed to the analysis from individuals with missing data for these demographic characteristics. Our assessment of psychological well-being was based on questionnaire responses at a single point in time, and our use of HADS scores as a marker of anxiety or depression could be criticised as, although these are widely used, their psychometric properties have been challenged [33]. Although we collected disease activity endpoints based on objectively defined criteria, there is the possibility that some of these endpoints, such as escalation of therapy, were reached based on symptom reporting alone, rather than true inflammatory activity. Due to the low event rate for some of the longitudinal disease activity outcomes, we chose not to present data on IBD patients dichotomised into those with UC and CD, or according to the use of antidepressant subclasses, other than SSRIs. Finally, use of antidepressants at baseline was classified according to a documented current prescription for the drugs of interest, but whether patients were actually adherent to their antidepressant therapy is uncertain. In addition, we did not record the discontinuation or commencement of antidepressant drugs during follow-up and therefore cannot exclude some misclassification of patients.

Due to the chronicity of their disease and the required shifts in coping and self-management skills over time, it is not surprising that patients with IBD are at increased risk of mental health disorders, yet previous studies have demonstrated that these coexistent psychological problems are often undertreated [34]. Undertreatment of mental health disorders can lead to long-term disability and a stigma against seeking treatment [35, 36]. Most IBD specialists have little formal training in the detection and management of such psychological comorbidities. This lack of training, combined with the potential hesitancy of many patients to report psychological symptoms, may influence therapy options. Although our study demonstrated that patients with abnormal anxiety or depression scores and those with high somatisation levels were more likely to be taking an antidepressant at baseline, the prevalence of abnormal anxiety scores, abnormal depression scores, and high somatisation scores in patients not receiving antidepressant therapy was also relatively high at 24.2%, 7.7%, and 20.7%, respectively.

Decreasing potential long-term sequelae by minimising the inflammatory burden in IBD patients is an important treatment strategy. There is some evidence, from studies in both animals and humans with IBD, to suggest that psychological comorbidity can trigger inflammatory activity [14, 16]. Furthermore, patients with IBD are at increased risk of psychological comorbidity, particularly depression and anxiety [37]. Thus, pharmacological therapy for mood disorders may have the potential to alter the natural history of CD and UC. Limited data, to date, have suggested improvements in mood, inflammatory activity, and quality of life with antidepressant therapy [23, 38]. Our own longitudinal follow-up data did not show any statistically significant differences in the proportion of patients experiencing endpoints consistent with inflammatory activity, according to use of antidepressants at baseline. However, the absolute proportions reaching these endpoints were generally lower among those prescribed antidepressants, particularly when only those with abnormal anxiety or depression scores were considered in the analysis.

Mechanisms of any beneficial effect of antidepressant drugs on the course of IBD are uncertain. Some antidepressants, like amitriptyline, appear to have both pain modifying properties [39] and direct effects on proinflammatory cytokines that may arise via actions on the nuclear factor-κB and nitric oxide pathways, which are implicated in the pathogenesis of IBD [40]. The former may explain the trend towards a reduction in escalation of therapy we observed, although given that this was also observed when only patients taking SSRIs, which have less in the way of analgesic effects [39], were considered, this seems unlikely. Therefore, antidepressant therapy may indeed have a beneficial effect on inflammatory activity. However, differentiating the true inflammatory burden in a symptomatic patient with IBD and coexistent mood disorder can be difficult, as the available symptom scoring systems cannot confirm the true origin of symptoms, and patients with IBD with psychological comorbidity may be more likely to report GI symptoms in general [24, 25]. As a result patients with mood disorders and who were on antidepressants in our study may potentially have been less likely to be offered, or indeed accept, a glucocorticosteroid prescription, a step-up in therapy, hospitalisation, or surgery.

In summary, our longitudinal follow-up study demonstrated lower rates of some objective markers of disease activity among patients with IBD receiving antidepressants and SSRIs, at baseline, particularly among those with abnormal anxiety or depression scores at baseline. However, none were statistically significant based on multivariate Cox regression. Further observational studies or RCTs with longer follow-up, which are powered to examine this issue specifically, will be required before the true effect of antidepressant use on disease activity in patients with CD and UC is known.

Abbreviations

BMI: Body mass index
CD: Crohn's disease

CI:	Confidence interval
GI:	Gastrointestinal
HADS:	Hospital anxiety and depression scale
HBI:	Harvey-Bradshaw index
HR:	Hazard ratio
IBD:	Inflammatory bowel disease
PHQ-15:	Patient health questionnaire-15
RCT:	Randomised controlled trial
SCCAI:	Simple clinical colitis activity index
SNRI:	Serotonin and noradrenaline reuptake inhibitor
SSRI:	Selective serotonin reuptake inhibitor
TCA:	Tricyclic antidepressant
UC:	Ulcerative colitis.

Disclosure

David J. Gracie and Alexander C. Ford are joint last authors, and Alexander C. Ford is the guarantor of the article. The study sponsor had no input into the concept, design, analysis, or reporting of the study.

Authors' Contributions

David J. Gracie, Alexander C. Ford, Barry J. Hall, and P. John Hamlin devised the study. David J. Gracie conducted the data collection. Alexander C. Ford, David J. Gracie, and Barry J. Hall analysed and interpreted the data. Barry J. Hall and Alexander C. Ford drafted the manuscript. All authors contributed to and approved the final draft of the manuscript.

Acknowledgments

The authors are thankful for the support provided by the Leeds Teaching Hospitals Charitable Foundation (9R11/14-02) and the unrestricted research funds provided by Tillotts Pharma UK Ltd.

References

[1] S. J. Bickston, B. W. Behm, D. J. Tsoulis et al., "Vedolizumab for induction and maintenance of remission in ulcerative colitis," *Cochrane Database of Systematic Reviews*, vol. 8, 2014.

[2] J. K. MacDonald and J. W. McDonald, "Natalizumab for induction of remission in Crohn's disease," *Cochrane Database of Systematic Reviews*, vol. 1, 2007.

[3] K. J. Khan, M. C. Dubinsky, A. C. Ford, T. A. Ullman, N. J. Talley, and P. Moayyedi, "Efficacy of immunosuppressive therapy for inflammatory bowel disease: a systematic review and meta-analysis," *American Journal of Gastroenterology*, vol. 106, no. 4, pp. 630–642, 2011.

[4] A. C. Ford, J.-P. Achkar, K. J. Khan et al., "Efficacy of 5-aminosalicylates in ulcerative colitis: systematic review and meta-analysis," *American Journal of Gastroenterology*, vol. 106, no. 4, pp. 601–616, 2011.

[5] A. C. Ford, C. N. Bernstein, K. J. Khan et al., "Glucocorticosteroid therapy in inflammatory bowel disease: Systematic review and meta-analysis," *American Journal of Gastroenterology*, vol. 106, no. 4, pp. 590–599, 2011.

[6] A. C. Ford, S. V. Kane, K. J. Khan et al., "Efficacy of 5-aminosalicylates in crohn's disease: systematic review and meta-analysis," *American Journal of Gastroenterology*, vol. 106, no. 4, pp. 617–629, 2011.

[7] A. C. Ford, W. J. Sandborn, K. J. Khan, S. B. Hanauer, N. J. Talley, and P. Moayyedi, "Efficacy of biological therapies in inflammatory bowel disease: systematic review and meta-analysis," *American Journal of Gastroenterology*, vol. 106, no. 4, pp. 644–659, 2011.

[8] A. J. Panara, A. J. Yarur, B. Rieders et al., "The incidence and risk factors for developing depression after being diagnosed with inflammatory bowel disease: A cohort study," *Alimentary Pharmacology & Therapeutics*, vol. 39, no. 8, pp. 802–810, 2014.

[9] L. A. Graff, J. R. Walker, and C. N. Bernstein, "Depression and anxiety in iflammatory bowel disease: a review of comorbidity and management," *Inflammatory Bowel Diseases*, vol. 15, no. 7, pp. 1105–1118, 2009.

[10] E. Fuller-Thomson and J. Sulman, "Depression and inflammatory bowel disease: Findings from two nationally representative Canadian surveys," *Inflammatory Bowel Diseases*, vol. 12, no. 8, pp. 697–707, 2006.

[11] C. Mittermaier, C. Dejaco, T. Waldhoer et al., "Impact of depressive mood on relapse in patients with inflammatory bowel disease: a prospective 18-month follow-up study," *Psychosomatic Medicine*, vol. 66, no. 1, pp. 79–84, 2004.

[12] J. R. Goodhand, M. Wahed, J. E. Mawdsley, A. D. Farmer, Q. Aziz, and D. S. Rampton, "Mood disorders in inflammatory bowel disease: relation to diagnosis, disease activity, perceived stress, and other factors," *Inflammatory Bowel Diseases*, vol. 18, no. 12, pp. 2301–2309, 2012.

[13] N. A. Koloski, M. Jones, J. Kalantar, M. Weltman, J. Zaguirre, and N. J. Talley, "The brain—gut pathway in functional gastrointestinal disorders is bidirectional: a 12-year prospective population-based study," *Gut*, vol. 61, no. 9, pp. 1284–1290, 2012.

[14] J.-E. Ghia, P. Blennerhassett, Y. Deng, E. F. Verdu, W. I. Khan, and S. M. Collins, "Reactivation of Inflammatory bowel disease in a mouse model of depression," *Gastroenterology*, vol. 136, no. 7, pp. 2280–e4, 2009.

[15] J.-E. Ghia, P. Blennerhassett, and S. M. Collins, "Impaired parasympathetic function increases susceptibility to inflammatory bowel disease in a mouse model of depression," *The Journal of Clinical Investigation*, vol. 118, no. 6, pp. 2209–2218, 2008.

[16] J. E. Mawdsley, M. G. Macey, R. M. Feakins, L. Langmead, and D. S. Rampton, "The effect of acute psychologic stress on systemic and rectal mucosal measures of inflammation in ulcerative colitis," *Gastroenterology*, vol. 131, no. 2, pp. 410–419, 2006.

[17] A. N. Ananthakrishnan, V. S. Gainer, R. G. Perez et al., "Psychiatric co-morbidity is associated with increased risk of surgery in Crohn's disease," *Alimentary Pharmacology & Therapeutics*, vol. 37, no. 4, pp. 445–454, 2013.

[18] L. S. Gaines, J. C. Slaughter, S. N. Horst et al., "Association between affective-cognitive symptoms of depression and exacerbation of Crohn's disease," *American Journal of Gastroenterology*, vol. 111, no. 6, pp. 864–870, 2016.

[19] B. Kochar, E. L. Barnes, M. D. Long et al., "Depression is associated with more aggressive inflammatory bowel disease," *American Journal of Gastroenterology*, vol. 113, no. 1, pp. 80–85, 2017.

[20] D. J. Gracie, E. A. Guthrie, P. J. Hamlin, and A. C. Ford, "Bi-directionality of brain–gut interactions in patients with inflammatory bowel disease," *Gastroenterology*, vol. 154, no. 6, pp. 1635–1646.e3, 2018.

[21] D. J. Gracie, A. J. Irvine, R. Sood, A. Mikocka-Walus, P. J. Hamlin, and A. C. Ford, "Effect of psychological therapy on disease activity, psychological comorbidity, and quality of life in inflammatory bowel disease: a systematic review and meta-analysis," *The Lancet Gastroenterology and Hepatology*, vol. 2, no. 3, pp. 189–199, 2017.

[22] B. J. D. Macer, S. L. Prady, and A. Mikocka-Walus, "Antidepressants in inflammatory bowel disease: a systematic review," *Inflammatory Bowel Diseases*, vol. 23, no. 4, pp. 534–550, 2017.

[23] A. Mikocka-Walus, P. A. Hughes, P. Bampton et al., "Fluoxetine for maintenance of remission and to improve quality of life in patients with Crohn's disease: A pilot randomized placebo-controlled trial," *Journal of Crohn's and Colitis*, vol. 11, no. 4, pp. 509–514, 2017.

[24] D. J. Gracie, C. J. M. Williams, R. Sood et al., "Negative effects on psychological health and quality of life of genuine irritable bowel syndrome–type symptoms in patients with inflammatory bowel disease," *Clinical Gastroenterology and Hepatology*, vol. 15, no. 3, pp. 376–384.e5, 2017.

[25] D. J. Gracie, C. J. M. Williams, R. Sood et al., "Poor correlation between clinical disease activity and mucosal inflammation, and the role of psychological comorbidity, in inflammatory bowel disease," *American Journal of Gastroenterology*, vol. 111, no. 4, pp. 541–551, 2016.

[26] E. von Elm, D. G. Altman, M. Egger, S. J. Pocock, P. C. Gøtzsche, and J. P. Vandenbroucke, "The strengthening the reporting of observational studies in epidemiology (STROBE) statement: guidelines for reporting observational studies," *Journal of Clinical Epidemiology*, vol. 61, no. 4, pp. 344–349, 2008.

[27] R. F. Harvey and J. M. Bradshaw, "A simple index of Crohn's-disease activity.," *The Lancet*, vol. 1, no. 8167, p. 514, 1980.

[28] R. S. Walmsley, R. C. S. Ayres, R. E. Pounder, and R. N. Allan, "A simple clinical colitis activity index," *Gut*, vol. 43, no. 1, pp. 29–32, 1998.

[29] S. Vermeire, S. Schreiber, W. J. Sandborn, C. Dubois, and P. Rutgeerts, "Correlation between the Crohn's disease activity and Harvey-Bradshaw indices in assessing Crohn's disease severity," *Clinical Gastroenterology and Hepatology*, vol. 8, no. 4, pp. 357–363, 2010.

[30] S. L. Jowett, C. J. Seal, E. Phillips, W. Gregory, J. R. Barton, and M. R. Welfare, "Defining relapse of ulcerative colitis using a symptom-based activity index," *Scandinavian Journal of Gastroenterology*, vol. 38, no. 2, pp. 164–171, 2003.

[31] A. S. Zigmond and R. P. Snaith, "The hospital anxiety and depression scale," *Acta Psychiatrica Scandinavica*, vol. 67, no. 6, pp. 361–370, 1983.

[32] K. Kroenke, R. L. Spitzer, and J. B. W. Williams, "The PHQ-15: Validity of a new measure for evaluating the severity of somatic symptoms," *Psychosomatic Medicine*, vol. 64, no. 2, pp. 258–266, 2002.

[33] J. C. Coyne and E. van Sonderen, "No further research needed: abandoning the Hospital and Anxiety Depression Scale (HADS)," *Journal of Psychosomatic Research*, vol. 72, no. 3, pp. 173-174, 2012.

[34] I. Marín-Jiménez, M. G. Montoya, A. Panadero et al., "Management of the psychological impact of inflammatory bowel disease: perspective of doctors and patients - The ENMENTE project," *Inflammatory Bowel Diseases*, vol. 23, no. 9, pp. 1492–1498, 2017.

[35] K. A. Collins, H. A. Westra, D. J. A. Dozois, and D. D. Burns, "Gaps in accessing treatment for anxiety and depression: Challenges for the delivery of care," *Clinical Psychology Review*, vol. 24, no. 5, pp. 583–616, 2004.

[36] P. S. Wang, M. Lane, M. Olfson, H. A. Pincus, K. B. Wells, and R. C. Kessler, "Twelve-month use of mental health services in the United States: Results from the National Comorbidity Survey Replication," *Archives of General Psychiatry*, vol. 62, no. 6, pp. 629–640, 2005.

[37] A. Mikocka-Walus, S. R. Knowles, L. Keefer, and L. Graff, "Controversies revisited: a systematic review of the comorbidity of depression and anxiety with inflammatory bowel diseases," *Inflammatory Bowel Diseases*, vol. 22, no. 3, pp. 752–762, 2015.

[38] O. Yanartas, H. T. Kani, E. Bicakci et al., "The effects of psychiatric treatment on depression, anxiety, quality of life, and sexual dysfunction in patients with inflammatory bowel disease," *Neuropsychiatric Disease and Treatment*, vol. 12, pp. 673–683, 2016.

[39] D. A. Drossman, J. Tack, A. C. Ford, E. Szigethy, H. Törnblom, and L. Van Oudenhove, "Neuromodulators for functional gastrointestinal disorders (disorders of gut–brain interaction): a rome foundation working team report," *Gastroenterology*, vol. 154, no. 4, pp. 1140–1171.e1, 2018.

[40] H. R. Rahimi, M. Shiri, and A. Razmi, "Antidepressants can treat inflammatory bowel disease through regulation of the nuclear factor-κB/nitric oxide pathway and inhibition of cytokine production: A hypothesis," *World Journal of Gastrointestinal Pharmacology and Therapeutics*, vol. 3, no. 6, p. 83, 2012.

7

Association between Plasmatic Ceramides Profile and AST/ALT Ratio: C14:0 Ceramide as Predictor of Hepatic Steatosis in Adolescents Independently of Obesity

Jorge Maldonado-Hernández, Gabriela E. Saldaña-Dávila, Mónica I. Piña-Aguero, Benjamín A. Núñez-García, and Mardia G. López-Alarcón

Laboratorio de Espectrometría de Masas, Unidad de Investigación Médica en Nutrición, Hospital de Pediatría, Centro Médico Nacional Siglo XXI, IMSS, Ciudad de México, Mexico

Correspondence should be addressed to Jorge Maldonado-Hernández; jormh@yahoo.com.mx

Academic Editor: Kevork M. Peltekian

Objective. To assess the association between plasma ceramides and hepatic steatosis (HS) in adolescents, independently of obesity. *Materials and Methods*. Ninety-four adolescents from two previous studies conducted and published by our crew were included. Study subjects were stratified in three groups: normal weight ($n = 18$), obesity ($n = 34$), and obesity + HS ($n = 42$). The presence of HS was defined when ALT/AST ratio was <1. Ceramides subspecies (C14:0, C16:0, C18:0, C24:0, and C24:1) were determined by LC/MS. *Results*. All ceramides correlated directly with ALT levels and inversely with ALT/AST ratio; the strongest correlation was observed among C14:0 ceramide ($r = 0.41$ and $r = -0.54$, resp.; $P < 0.001$). Furthermore, significant correlations were observed between cholesterol and all ceramides except for C24:1 ceramide. Interestingly ceramides C14:0, C18:0, and C24:1 correlated directly with both fasting insulin and HOMA-IR index. For assessing HS, a cut-off point of 10.3 nmol/L for C14:0 ceramide reported a sensitivity of 92.7% and a specificity of 73.5% when normal weight and obesity groups ($n = 52$) were compared against obesity + HS group ($n = 42$). Positive and negative predictive values were 77.5% and 90.2%, respectively. *Conclusions*. Plasma ceramides are closely associated with hepatic steatosis in adolescents. C14:0 ceramide could be a novel biomarker of HS independently of obesity.

1. Introduction

Ceramides (Cer) belongs to the sphingolipid family and are formed by a sphingosine and a fatty acid group linked by an amide bond. Typically, the fatty acid moiety is 14 to 26 carbon atoms' chain length, most of them saturated or monounsaturated. Ceramides are produced in the organism by three different pathways: (1) the novo synthesis from palmitate and serine in four sequential reactions in the endoplasmic reticulum, (2) from the hydrolysis of plasma membrane sphingomyelin via sphingomyelinase (SMase), and (3) a salvage pathway from sphingosine that can be recycled back to ceramide [1]. Several isoforms of SMase that can be distinguished by their optima pH, neutral SMase (NSMase), and acid SMase (ASMase) are mostly found in mitochondria and lysosomes, respectively [2].

It has been described that during obesity there is an accumulation of several ceramides species in human tissues as muscle, adipose tissue, liver, and heart. Obesity leads to the activation of inflammatory signals that promote ceramides production [3, 4]. It is well known that TNF-α increases ceramides production via SMase that hydrolyses sphingomyelin, the most abundant sphingolipid specie in cell membranes [5]. Ceramides accumulation has been involved in insulin signaling mechanisms that induce insulin resistance in muscle and adipose tissue [6–8]. In the liver, in addition to glucose impairment metabolism, ceramides have been implicated in the induction of hepatic steatosis [9].

Most of the studies that analyzed the role of ceramides and their relationship with hepatic steatosis (HS) have been conducted in animal models. It has been hypothesized that ceramides could have a role as second messengers in the development and progression of nonalcoholic fatty liver disease (NAFLD) through mechanisms that promote oxidative stress, inflammation, and apoptosis [9, 10]. The liver is an important site of ceramides production due to an increased free fatty acid flux as observed in higher adiposity and inflammation settings. It has been estimated that 80% of plasma ceramides are present in both hepatic lipoproteins: VLDL and LDL [11]. The aspartate aminotransferase (AST)/alanine transaminase (ALT) ratio is a useful screening biomarker of hepatic steatosis. Serum AST and ALT concentrations increase with body weight, although it is more prominent for ALT. Metabolic disturbances as insulin resistance, dyslipidemia, and hyperglycemia are closely related to elevated ALT; a cut-off point of AST/ALT ratio <1 has been defined for hepatic steatosis assessment in obese patients [12].

Global prevalence of NAFLD in children is estimated in 3% and could increase up to 40% in the presence of obesity [13]. Ceramides could play an important role in the pathogenesis of this disease, although clinical studies in pediatric population are limited and the role of ceramides is not well established. The aim of this study was to describe plasma ceramides profile in adolescents with and without hepatic steatosis and evaluate the association between specific ceramides and ALT/AST ratio, independently of obesity as well as assess if any of the analyzed ceramides could be an adequate biomarker to predict hepatic steatosis.

2. Materials and Methods

2.1. Study Population. Clinical data and biological samples of ninety-four adolescents from two previous studies conducted and published by our crew were selected by convenience [14, 15]. Only those subjects who had intact plasma for liver enzymes and ceramides determinations were included. Subjects of both studies were enrolled during 2011 and 2012 in Mexico City, Mexico. Both studies complied with the World Medical Association Declaration of Helsinki regarding ethical conduct of research in human subjects. Protocols were approved by the Ethics Committee of the Mexican Institute of Social Security with register numbers R-2010-3603-35 [14] and R-2010-3603-14 [15], respectively. Informed consent was obtained from the representative of all the study subjects.

2.2. Biochemical Determinations. Peripheral blood samples were obtained after 10–12 hours of overnight-fast in Vacutainer test tubes with and without EDTA. Samples were centrifuged at 3000 rpm during 10 minutes. Plasma and serum were preserved at −70°C until analysis. Concentrations of fasting glucose, triglycerides, HDL, and VLDL were previously determined with commercial kits in an automated spectrophotometer Spin 120 (Spinreact Girona, Spain; coefficients of variation ~3.9%). Fasting insulin was determined by radioimmunoassay kits (Millipore, Billerica, MA) with coefficient of variation (CV) of 7.5%.

AST and ALT concentrations were determined in intact serum samples preserved all the time at −70°C, with enzymatic-colorimetric kits in a Spin 120 spectrophotometer.

2.3. Plasma Ceramides Extraction and Quantification. An adaptation of the method described by Kasumov et al. was performed [16]. All solvents used in the following description were of chromatographic grade. First, 1.4 mL of methanol was added to 200 μL of blood plasma to precipitate the proteins. Then the sample was centrifuged at 3500 rpm for 10 minutes. Once the phases were separated, the supernatant was decanted in a new test tube and 1.2 mL of chloroform was added. Mixture was vortexed for one minute; afterwards 1 mL of water was added and vortexed for another minute. Sample was centrifuged once again at 3500 rpm for 10 minutes. The aqueous phase (upper layer) was discarded and the organic phase (bottom) was evaporated with ultra high purity nitrogen at 40°C. The dried extract was reconstituted with 500 μL of dichloromethane and passed through a Strata® SI-1 Silica column (55 μm, 70 Å, 200 mg/3 mL) (Phenomenex; California, USA) previously washed with 500 μL of dichloromethane. Ceramides were eluted 3 times with 500 μL of dichloromethane/isopropanol solution (70 : 30, v/v). The elution was lead to evaporation with ultra high pure nitrogen. The extract was reconstituted with 200 μL of ethanol and stored at −70°C. Samples were analyzed by LC-MS on a Waters Xevo TQD Acquity UPLC H-Class (Waters; Milford, USA) equipment with a LC Column 50 × 21 mm Kinetex® 2.6 μm C8 100 Å (Phenomenex; California, USA). The column was preheated at 50°C, the flow was established at 0.4 mL/min, and the total run time was of 18 minutes. The aqueous phase (A) was prepared with ultrapure water and formic acid at 0.2%; organic phase (B) was a mixture of acetonitrile and 2-propanol (60 : 40, v/v) and 0.2% of formic acid. Ceramides species were resolved with a gradient starting from 40% mobile phase A and 60% of mobile phase B during 0.2 minutes to 100% phase B over 13.8 minutes at linear gradient and then 100% B for 0.5 min. Mass spectrometer capillary voltage was 3.9 kV, cone voltage 40 V, and the source temperature 150°C.

Ceramide external standards with a d18:1 sphingoid base (C14:0, C16:0, C18:0, C24:0, and C24:1 subspecies; Avanti Polar Lipids, Inc., Alabaster, Alabama, USA) were diluted with 1 mL of $CHCl_3$ in order to obtain a 5 mg/mL concentration. A "Standard Mix" containing the 5 ceramides was prepared at a concentration of 1000 ng/mL (1 μg/mL) of each ceramide, in a total volume of 25 mL in ethanol. Several dilutions were prepared to create a calibration curve with the following concentrations: 1000 ng/mL, 500 ng/mL, 250 ng/mL, 125 ng/mL, 62.5 ng/mL, 31.25 ng/mL, and 7.81 ng/mL. The coefficient of variation for the LC-MS analysis was <6.5%. Ceramides data was converted to nmol/L.

2.4. Statistical Analysis. Data were analyzed using the Statistical Package for the Social Studies (SPSS version 20, SPSS Inc., Chicago, IL, USA). Kolmogorov-Smirnov test was used to assess data distribution. Biochemical results are expressed as median (percentile 25–percentile 75); comparison among study groups was performed with Mann–Whitney *U* test. Plasmatic ceramides concentrations are expressed as mean (confidence interval 95%); comparison between study groups was made by ANOVA test with Tukey post hoc analysis. Correlation between plasmatic ceramides and biochemical features was performed with a Spearman's correlation analysis. A receiver operator characteristic (ROC) curve was constructed

Table 1: Biochemical characteristics of study subjects.

	Normal weight (n = 18)	Obesity (n = 34)	Obesity + HS (n = 42)
Gender (female/male)	8/10	17/17	16/26
Age (years)	14 (12.75–15)	12 (11–13)[a]	13.5 (12–15)[b]
BMI (kg/m^2)	20 (19–20.6)	26.8 (25.1–30.8)[a]	30.1 (27.5–36.1)[b,c]
AST (U/L)	31 (27–38.5)	39 (29.5–47.5)	37.5 (25–56)
ALT (U/L)	19 (16–22.5)	31 (21.5–45.5)[a]	54.5 (33.5–79.5)[b,c]
Ratio (AST/ALT)	1.7 (1.4–1.8)	1.3 (1–1.5)[a]	0.7 (0.6–0.8)[b,c]
Triglycerides (mg/dL)	82 (62.8–98.3)	114 (103.5–218)[a]	135.5 (92–179.3)[b]
Cholesterol (mg/dL)	151.5 (133.5–171)	159 (145.5–187.5)	161 (144.8–185.3)
HDL (mg/dL)	54.5 (48–60)	46 (41–51.5)[a]	47.5 (38–54)
VLDL (mg/dL)	16 (12.5–19.5)	23 (21–44)[a]	29 (18–36)[b]
Fating glucose (mg/dL)	84 (78–86)	87 (81–93.5)	87.5 (82.75–93)[b]
Fasting insulin (μU/mL)	9.6 (7.5–14.7)	18.4 (15.7–22.2)[a]	19 (14.9–25.1)[b]
HOMA-IR	2.03 (1.6–2.9)	4.11 (3.2–4.8)[a]	4.12 (3.2–5.4)[b]

Data are presented as median (percentile 25–percentile 75). Comparison between groups was made with a Mann–Whitney U test. [a]Significant difference ($P < 0.05$) between obesity and normal weight group; [b]between obesity + HS and normal weight group; [c]between obesity + HS and obesity group. HOMA-IR: Homeostasis Model Assessment for Insulin Resistance.

to determine an optimal cut-off point for a specific ceramide to predict hepatic steatosis. Area Under the Curve (AUC) with 95% confidence interval (CI) was obtained; positive and negative predictive values were determined.

3. Results

Ninety-four adolescents were included in the present study; 41 were females (43.6%) and 53 males (56.4%). According to BMI and AST/ALT ratio, subjects were stratified in 3 groups: normal weight group (P15th to P85th of the WHO Child Growth Standards [17] and AST/ALT ratio > 1); obesity group (P > 95th and AST/ALT ratio > 1); and obesity group with hepatic steatosis (P > 95th and AST/ALT ratio < 1). Biochemical characteristics of the subjects are shown in Table 1. Significant differences were found between normal weight group and obesity group in almost all variables except for AST, cholesterol, and fasting glucose levels. A similar behavior was observed when comparing normal weight group and obesity group + HS but, additionally, no significant difference was found in HDL levels. Interestingly, when comparing obesity group and obesity + HS group we just found significant differences in BMI, ALT levels, and AST/ALT ratio.

Plasma ceramides profile stratified by study groups are shown in Figure 1. For C14:0 ceramide (C14:0 Cer) significant differences were observed when comparing normal weight group versus obesity and obesity + HS groups. Likewise, obesity + HS group had significantly higher levels of C14:0 Cer than obesity group. For the other ceramides, significantly higher levels were observed in obesity and obesity + HS groups when comparing to normal weight subjects, although no significance was observed when comparing obesity group versus obesity + HS group.

Spearman's correlation coefficient between specific ceramides and biochemical markers of hepatic function, dyslipidemia, and insulin resistance surrogates are shown in Table 2. All ceramides correlated directly with ALT levels and inversely with AST/ALT ratio; the strongest correlation was observed among C14:0 Cer. Furthermore, significant correlations were observed between cholesterol and all ceramides except for C24:1 subspecies. Interestingly ceramides C14:0, C18:0, and C24:1 correlated directly with both fasting insulin and HOMA-IR index.

Finally, a ROC analysis was performed to determine an optimal cut-off point for a specific ceramide as an adequate biomarker of hepatic steatosis. C14:0 Cer reported the best attributes to predict HS. ROC curve was computed contrasting data from normal weight and obesity groups (n = 52) versus obesity + HS group (n = 42). Figure 2 shows the ROC curve obtained; a cut-off point of 10.3 nmol/L for C14:0 Cer had a sensitivity of 92.7% and a specificity of 73.5% (AUC = 80.4%, $P < 0.001$; 95% CI = 70.2–90.5%). Positive and negative predictive values were 77.5% and 90.2%, respectively.

4. Discussion

The present study demonstrated that hepatic steatosis is closely related to plasmatic ceramides concentration. All the subspecies analyzed correlated inversely with AST/ALT ratio and directly with ALT levels. Although, only C14:0 ceramide was significantly different among the three study groups, no differences were observed in the other analyzed ceramides between obesity group and obesity + HS group. C14:0 ceramide proved to be the better predictor of HS in comparison with the other ceramides analyzed with adequate diagnosis features, independently of obesity. Interestingly, Tomita et al. found similar results to ours for serum-free

TABLE 2: Correlation matrix between different ceramides and biochemical features.

	C14:0 Cer	C16:0 Cer	C18:0 Cer	C24:0 Cer	C24:1 Cer
AST	0.085	0.045	0.12	0.06	0.08
ALT	0.41^{***}	0.21^{**}	0.34^{***}	$0.19^{\$}$	0.3^{**}
AST/ALT ratio	-0.54^{***}	-0.34^{***}	-0.36^{***}	-0.21^{*}	-0.33^{***}
Triglycerides	0.25^{*}	0.12	0.17	0.13	0.17
Cholesterol	0.25^{*}	0.28^{**}	0.28^{**}	0.3^{**}	0.16
HDL	−0.062	−0.11	−0.13	−0.31	-0.31^{**}
VLDL	0.305^{**}	0.16	0.21^{*}	0.15	$0.21^{\$}$
Fasting glucose	0.062	−0.09	−0.02	−0.15	0.01
Fasting insulin	0.21^{*}	$0.19^{\$}$	0.27^{**}	$0.17^{\$}$	0.31^{**}
HOMA-IR	0.21^{*}	0.15	0.23^{*}	0.1	0.25^{*}

Data correspond to Spearman correlation coefficients. ***Significant P values ≤ 0.001; $^{**}P \leq 0.01$; $^{*}P \leq 0.05$. $^{\$}$Statistical trend ($0.05 \geq P < 0.1$).

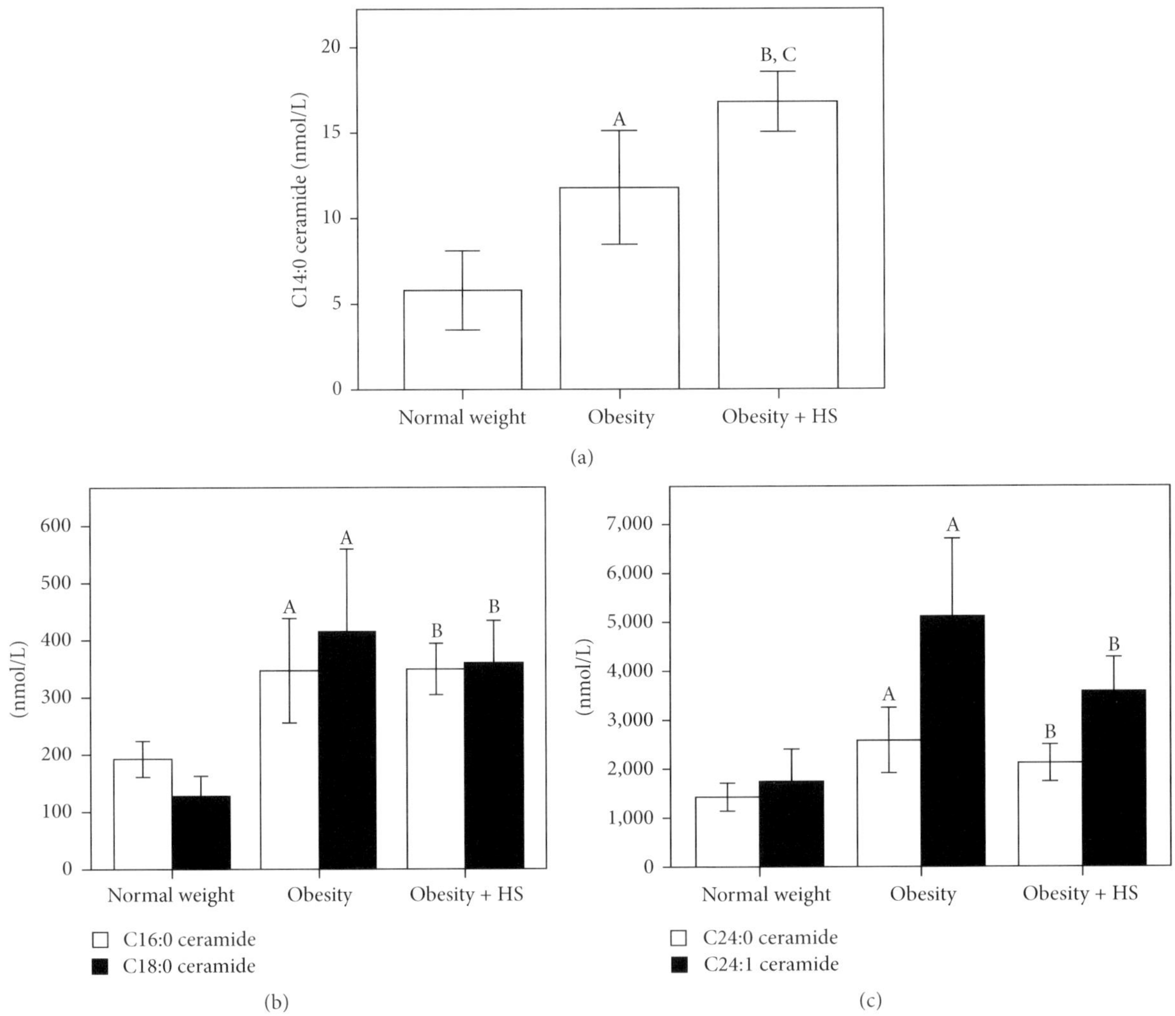

FIGURE 1: Comparison of ceramides subspecies among study groups. ^{A}Significant difference ($P < 0.05$) between obesity and normal weight group; ^{B}between obesity + HS and normal weight group; ^{C}between obesity + HS and obesity group.

myristic acid (C14:0) to predict nonalcoholic steatohepatitis (NASH) with a sensitivity and a specificity of 57.1% and 85%, respectively. Positive and negative predictive values were in turn 93.6% and 34.0% [18]. The C14:0 ceramide analyzed in this study have had enhanced diagnostic attributes than myristic acid, probably because liver is a key site of ceramides production and is therefore a more specific indicator of what happens in liver tissue [9]. Serum-free fatty acids may be reflecting global lipid metabolism that may be influenced by diet, β-oxidation, and lipid mobilization. On the other hand,

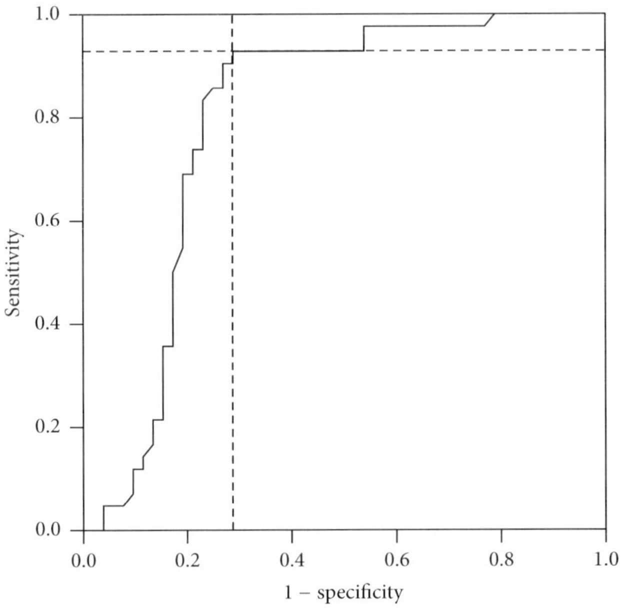

FIGURE 2: Receiver operator characteristic (ROC) curve for C14:0 ceramide. ROC curve was computed contrasting data from normal weight and obesity groups ($n = 52$) versus obesity group with HS ($n = 42$).

a strength of the study of Tomita et al. is that NASH was established by histological assessment in liver biopsy.

In addition to the correlations observed among ALT and the AST/ALT ratio, the examined ceramides also correlated with higher levels of cholesterol (except C24:1 Cer) and C14:0, C18:0, and C24:1 ceramides were directly associated with fasting insulin and HOMA-IR index. Recently, Kasumov et al. found that C14:0 ceramide is related to insulin sensitivity improvement after a 12-week exercise training program. A decrease in plasma levels of C14:0 ceramide was associated with changes in insulin-stimulated glucose disposal ($r = -0.56$; $P < 0.01$) in adult subjects with obesity or type 2 diabetes (T2D). It is well known that ceramides are associated with insulin resistance, although most of the published works have been done in adult population. There are few studies that have described the association between plasma ceramides, insulin resistance, and other metabolic disorders in pediatric population. Lopez et al. found that children and adolescents with T2D have higher concentrations of different subspecies of ceramides in comparison with lean healthy subjects [19].

A limitation of our study could be the use of the AST/ALT ratio as diagnostic criteria to establish the presence of fatty liver in the studied population. The *Ritis* ratio is not the gold standard for hepatic steatosis assessment and there are more precise methods for its diagnosis, such as liver biopsy or imaging studies as ultrasound, tomography, or magnetic resonance [12]. However, these techniques are not available for us and the retrolective character of this study did not allow us to use any of the above methods. It is therefore likely that the presence of fatty liver will become inconsistent particularly in some of the subjects in the groups categorized as "obesity" and "obesity + HS." Regardless, the association found among the subspecies of ceramides and hepatic steatosis markers are independent of this stratification and it might even be more likely that a better delimitation of hepatic steatosis in the study subjects could enhance diagnostic attributes of C14:0 ceramide to predict the disease.

The increase of FFA flux towards the liver tissue observed in states of obesity and inflammation could be increasing the synthesis of ceramides and other lipid species in the liver. Locally, ceramides increase mitochondrial generation of reactive oxygen species that promote apoptosis and hepatic inflammation. The increase of FFA flux ratio overcomes the capacity of the liver to oxidize lipids so its exportation through low density lipoproteins could be a strategy of the liver to decrease the hepatotoxic effect of them. Since liver seems to be a key site for ceramides production, plasma ceramides levels could be a reflection of hepatic disturbances and a new goal for intervention studies to prevent the development of more serious liver diseases.

5. Conclusion

In summary, plasma ceramides are closely associated with hepatic steatosis in adolescents. As far as we know this is the first study to demonstrate that C14:0 ceramide could be a novel biomarker of HS independently of obesity.

Acknowledgments

This study was supported by grants from *Consejo Nacional de Ciencia y Tecnología de México* (CONACYT) with Register no. Salud-2015-2-0261774 and from *Fondo de Investigación en Salud* (FIS/IMSS) with Register no. FIS/IMSS/PROT/G15/1452.

References

[1] H. Aburasayn, R. Al Batran, and J. R. Ussher, "Targeting ceramide metabolism in obesity," *American Journal of Physiology, Endocrinology and Metabolism*, vol. 311, pp. 423–435, 2016.

[2] R. Kolesnick, "The therapeutic potential of modulating the ceramide/sphingomyelin pathway," *Journal of Clinical Investigation*, vol. 110, no. 1, pp. 3–8, 2002.

[3] B. Chaurasia and S. A. Summers, "Ceramides—lipotoxic inducers of metabolic disorders," *Trends in Endocrinology and Metabolism*, vol. 26, no. 10, pp. 538–550, 2015.

[4] W. L. Holland and S. A. Summers, "Sphingolipids, insulin resistance, and metabolic disease: new insights from in vivo manipulation of sphingolipid metabolism," *Endocrine Reviews*, vol. 29, no. 4, pp. 381–402, 2008.

[5] M. Marí and J. C. Fernández-Checa, "Sphingolipid signalling and liver diseases," *Liver International*, vol. 27, no. 4, pp. 440–450, 2007.

[6] F. Amati, J. J. Dubé, E. Alvarez-Carnero et al., "Skeletal muscle triglycerides, diacylglycerols, and ceramides in insulin

resistance: another paradox in endurance-trained athletes?" *Diabetes*, vol. 60, no. 10, pp. 2588–2597, 2011.

[7] J. A. Chavez and S. A. Summers, "A ceramide-centric view of insulin resistance," *Cell Metabolism*, vol. 15, no. 5, pp. 585–594, 2012.

[8] P. J. Larsen and N. Tennagels, "On ceramides, other sphingolipids and impaired glucose homeostasis," *Molecular Metabolism*, vol. 3, no. 3, pp. 252–260, 2014.

[9] M. Pagadala, T. Kasumov, A. J. McCullough, N. N. Zein, and J. P. Kirwan, "Role of ceramides in nonalcoholic fatty liver disease," *Trends in Endocrinology and Metabolism*, vol. 23, no. 8, pp. 365–371, 2012.

[10] M. N. Nikolova-Karakashian and K. A. Rozenova, "Ceramide in stress response," *Advances in Experimental Medicine and Biology*, vol. 688, pp. 86–108, 2010.

[11] S. Lightle, R. Tosheva, A. Lee et al., "Elevation of ceramide in serum lipoproteins during acute phase response in humans and mice: Role of serine-palmitoyl transferase," *Archives of Biochemistry and Biophysics*, vol. 419, no. 2, pp. 120–128, 2003.

[12] M. Botros and K. A. Sikaris, "The de ritis ratio: the test of time," *The Clinical Biochemist Reviews*, vol. 34, pp. 117–130, 2013.

[13] R. Loomba, C. B. Sirlin, J. B. Schwimmer, and J. E. Lavine, "Advances in pediatric nonalcoholic fatty liver disease," *Hepatology*, vol. 50, no. 4, pp. 1282–1293, 2009.

[14] A. Salas-Fernández, J. Maldonado-Hernández, A. Martínez-Basila, G. Martínez-Razo, and F. Jasso-Saavedra, "The 13C-glucose breath test is a valid non-invasive screening tool to identify metabolic syndrome in adolescents," *Clinical Chemistry and Laboratory Medicine*, vol. 53, no. 1, pp. 133–138, 2015.

[15] M. López-Alarcón, O. Perichart-Perera, S. Flores-Huerta et al., "Excessive refined carbohydrates and scarce micronutrients intakes increase inflammatory mediators and insulin resistance in prepubertal and pubertal obese children independently of obesity," *Mediators of Inflammation*, vol. 2014, Article ID 849031, 7 pages, 2014.

[16] T. Kasumov, H. Huang, Y.-M. Chung, R. Zhang, A. J. McCullough, and J. P. Kirwan, "Quantification of ceramide species in biological samples by liquid chromatography electrospray ionization tandem mass spectrometry," *Analytical Biochemistry*, vol. 401, no. 1, pp. 154–161, 2010.

[17] M. de Onis and A. W. Onyango, "WHO child growth standards," *The Lancet*, vol. 371, no. 9608, p. 204, 2008.

[18] K. Tomita, T. Teratani, H. Yokoyama et al., "Plasma free myristic acid proportion is a predictor of nonalcoholic steatohepatitis," *Digestive Diseases and Sciences*, vol. 56, no. 10, pp. 3045–3052, 2011.

[19] X. Lopez, A. B. Goldfine, W. L. Holland, R. Gordillo, and P. E. Scherer, "Plasma ceramides are elevated in female children and adolescents with type 2 diabetes," *Journal of Pediatric Endocrinology and Metabolism*, vol. 26, no. 9-10, pp. 995–998, 2013.

8

Living with Hepatitis C Virus: A Systematic Review and Narrative Synthesis of Qualitative Literature

Laura E. Dowsett,[1,2] Stephanie Coward,[1,2] Diane L. Lorenzetti,[1,2,3] Gail MacKean,[1,2] and Fiona Clement[1,2]

[1] *The Department Community Health Sciences, Teaching, Research and Wellness Building, 3280 Hospital Drive NW, Calgary, AB, Canada T2N 4N1*
[2] *O'Brien Institute for Public Health, Teaching, Research and Wellness Building, 3280 Hospital Drive NW, Calgary, AB, Canada T2N 4N1*
[3] *Institute of Health Economics, 1200, 10405 Jasper Avenue, Edmonton, AB, Canada T5J 3N4*

Correspondence should be addressed to Fiona Clement; fclement@ucalgary.ca

Academic Editor: Aldo J. Montano-Loza

Background and Aims. The lived experience of HCV has not been well documented in the literature. The aim of this systematic review was to understand the experiences of living with Hepatitis C Virus (HCV). *Methods.* Five databases were searched from inception until January 19, 2015. Studies were included if they focused on adults diagnosed with HCV; reported experience living with HCV; and described original research. *Results.* 46 studies were included. Studies found that participants had reduced quality of life due to physical symptoms. Due to physical symptoms and discrimination, many participants switched to part-time work or quit their jobs. Many individuals reported negative experiences with the healthcare system; themes of feeling unsupported, not having adequate information, and not feeling involved in decisions were reported. Stigma significantly impacted those living with HCV. *Conclusions.* Published literature indicates that those with HCV often feel stigmatized and unsupported in their care, relationships, and work environments, while simultaneously coping with physical and psychological symptoms. This synthesis points to areas where greater education, compassion, and patient-centered healthcare could improve the experience of people living with HCV.

1. Background

Chronic Hepatitis C Virus (HCV) is a growing public health concern. HCV is transmitted through exposure to infected blood and cannot be spread through intact skin or mucous membranes [1]. Globally, there are approximately 170 million people diagnosed with chronic HCV [2, 3], with 3 to 4 million new cases per year [2]. It has been estimated that approximately 30% of individuals infected with HCV are unaware that they have the disease [4]. Approximately 350,000 deaths per year are attributed to a HCV related cause [5]. Those most at risk of contracting HCV include the following: those born between 1950 and1970, current or former intravenous drug users (IDUs), children born to HCV positive mothers, people in prison, hemodialysis patients, indigenous peoples, those from high prevalence countries, and recipients of blood, blood products, or organs prior to July 1992 [6–9].

Until recently antiviral medication, specifically pegylated interferon-α (PEG-INF) and ribavirin (RBV), was the current standard therapy for treating HCV [10]. These drugs are associated with severe side-effects (fatigue, headaches, fever, muscle pain, insomnia, nausea, hair loss, anorexia, depression, irritability, and joint pain [11]) and low cure rates of approximately 40–50% for those with Genotype 1 and 80% for those with Genotypes 2 and 4 [12]. The development of direct acting antivirals (DAAs) has changed the treatment landscape. In comparison to PEG-INF or RBV based treatments, DAAs have been found to have higher cure

TABLE 1: Inclusion and exclusion criteria for systematic review of patient experiences with HCV.

Inclusion criteria	Exclusion criteria
(i) Women or men diagnosed with HCV Virus (ii) Report on experience living with HCV from the patients perspective (iii) Original qualitative research (iv) Full-text available (v) Adult participants	(i) Individuals included in the study who do not have Hepatitis C (ii) Patient perspective (iii) Did not report experience living with HCV from the patients perspective (iv) Inclusion of participants under 18 years old (v) Physician accounts of patient experience (vi) Experience of treatment with peg-interferon medication (vii) Abstracts or posters (with no full-text available) (viii) Case studies, reviews, meta-analyses (ix) Quantitative study designs

rates (90–100% viral clearance rates at 12 weeks) and virtually no side-effects [13]. Many consider these new drugs to be curative [14, 15].

Within this new paradigm, countries are reassessing their approach to HCV identification and management. Patient perspectives on living with HCV should be integral to clinical and policy decisions; patients' perspectives on access to treatment, quality of life, burden of illness, impact on productivity, and experiences with healthcare system help create informed evidence-based patient-centered healthcare. However, the lived experience of HCV from the patient perspective has not yet been comprehensively documented. Thus, the objective of this research synthesis was to document the experience of living with HCV from the perspective of those with an HCV diagnosis.

2. Methods

2.1. Data Sources. Using the ENTREQ guidelines for qualitative synthesis [16], a systematic review on patient perspectives of living with HCV was completed. MEDLINE, PubMED, EMBASE, PsychINFO, CINAHL, and SocINDEX were searched from inception until January 19, 2015. A library and information specialist developed the search strategy. Terms capturing the disease (e.g., hepatitis C, hep c, hepatitis c antigens, and hcv) were combined with terms reflecting the patient experience (e.g., attitude, health behaviour, experiences, and quality of life). These results were then focused to include only qualitative studies by using terms such as "qualitative research," "focus groups," and "grounded theory." Terms were searched as both keywords and relevant database-specific subject headings. Results were filtered to exclude non-English results, nonhuman studies, and pediatric studies. No other limitations were used. The detailed search strategy is available in Appendix in Supplementary Material available online at https://doi.org/10.1155/2017/3268650.

2.2. Study Selection. Two trained independent reviewers screened the identified abstracts. Abstracts were assessed for relevance by using the following inclusion criteria: adult (over 18 years of age) women or men diagnosed with HCV; reporting on patient experience living with HCV; and original qualitative research. Abstracts were excluded if they did not meet the above inclusion criteria; or if they did not report findings from the patient perspective; reported only experience with treatment; presented primarily quantitative data; or if all of the participants were coinfected with another disease (i.e., Human Immunodeficiency Virus). Abstracts included by either reviewer proceeded to full-text review.

Studies that were included after the first screen were read in full text by two independent reviewers. Full texts were included if they met all of the inclusion criteria and did not meet any of the exclusion criteria presented in Table 1. Consensus was required for inclusion and disagreement was resolved through discussion or, if required, by consultation with a third reviewer. In order to ensure that all relevant articles were included, systematic reviews were hand-searched.

2.3. Data Extraction and Quality Assessment. Included studies were assessed for quality using the Critical Appraisal Skills Programme (CASP) checklist for qualitative literature [17]. This checklist is comprised of ten questions, each assessing areas of potential bias; for example, was a clear objective stated? Was the recruitment strategy appropriate? Was data analysis rigorous [17]? Each question is answered with "yes," "no," or "can't tell." [17] Studies were not excluded based on quality.

2.4. Analysis. A narrative synthesis approach was used to identify and understand the key findings from the included studies. This approach is commonly used to synthesize heterogeneous literature [18], including qualitative studies. In the first stage of this narrative synthesis, independent reviewers extracted the overarching themes presented by each study in order to identify themes most frequently discussed within the included studies. Any discrepancies in the themes identified by the two reviewers were resolved through consensus. Using these overarching themes as a framework, subthemes and more detailed description were subsequently extracted from each study. Relationships between themes were explored. During data extraction, information, such as journal, study design, participant selection, participant inclusion and exclusion criteria, participant characteristics, and findings, was also extracted in duplicate from each included study.

3. Findings

Seven hundred and ninety-eight abstracts were retrieved (Figure 1). During abstract review, 118 abstracts met the inclusion criteria to continue to full-text review. Hand searching of two systematic reviews [19, 20] identified two additional

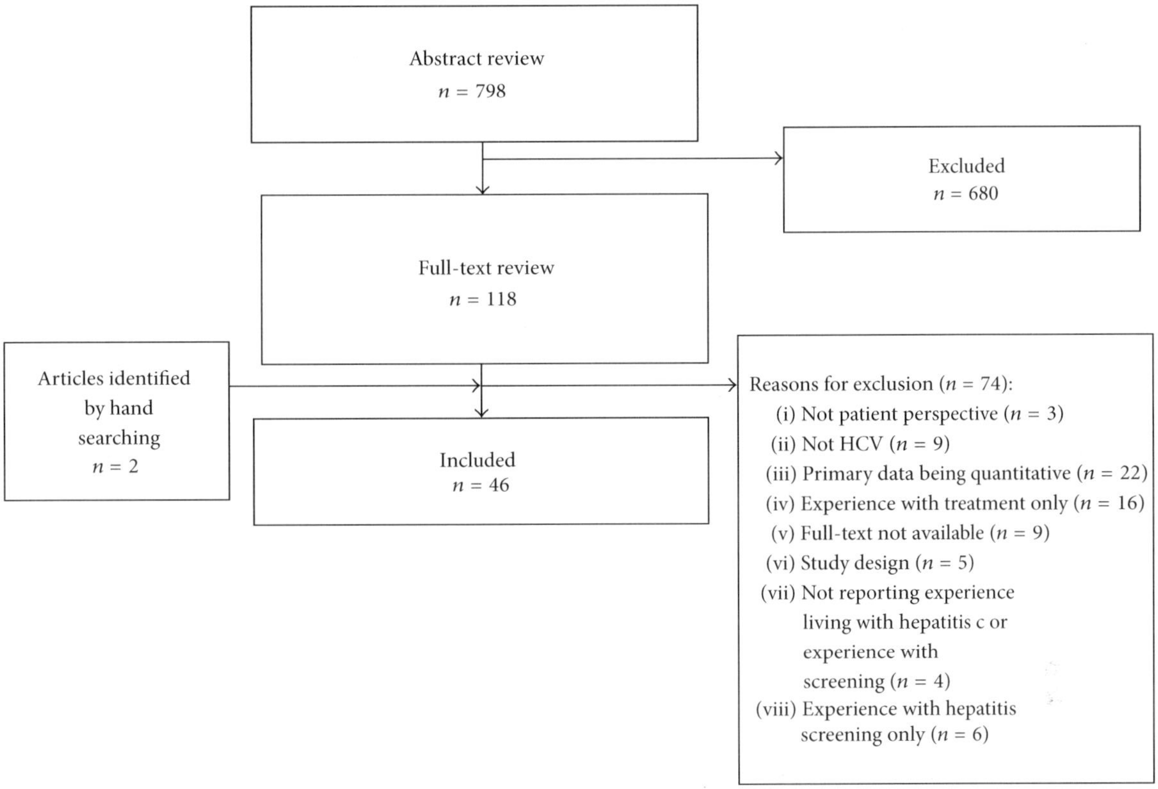

FIGURE 1: Flow chart of included and excluded studies.

studies to include in full-text review, for a total of 120 studies. Seventy-four studies were excluded for the following reasons: no patient perspective ($n = 3$), not HCV ($n = 9$), primarily quantitative data ($n = 22$), only exploring experience with treatment ($n = 16$), only focusing on experiences with HCV screening ($n = 6$), not available in full text ($n = 9$), not a relevant study design ($n = 5$), and not reporting experiences of living with HCV ($n = 4$). Forty-six studies were included in the final data set.

The included studies reported on forty-two populations (total $n = 1619$) (Table 2 and Appendix in Supplementary Material). Some of the included studies assessed the same group of people but reported on different aspects of living with HCV: Olsen et al. [21], Olsen et al. [22], and Olsen et al. [23]; Harris [24] and Harris [25]; and Tompkins et al. [60] and Wright et al. [61]. Thirty-eight studies included participants from a general population [21, 23–59], seven included participants who were IDUs [22, 60–65], and one included participants who received contaminated blood products [66]. The broad themes identified did not differ across these populations, so the findings are described together.

Seventeen studies were conducted in Australia [21–23, 25, 30, 32, 33, 38, 39, 51, 53, 56–59, 64, 65], fifteen in the UK [24, 31, 34, 35, 37, 40, 46, 47, 49, 52, 55, 60, 61, 63, 66], eight in the United States [26, 27, 36, 41, 43, 48, 54, 62], four in Canada [28, 29, 45, 50], and one each from Pakistan [42] and France [44]. The studies were published between 1999 [39] and 2014 [40, 48]. Data in these studies were analyzed using a variety of methods, including thematic and content analysis [21–23, 27, 45, 48, 56, 60, 64], inductive approach [28, 54, 57, 59], grounded theory [30, 32, 35, 46, 63], framework approach [61], phenomenological approach [31, 37, 40, 43, 51, 52, 66], interpretive approach [33, 39], and constant comparative analysis [41, 50]. Various software programs were used by these studies: NVivo [28, 29, 47, 48, 55, 62], atlas.ti [21–23, 26], and QSR∗NUDIST [41].

Broadly, the studies were of high quality; the objectives of studies were clear, as were the findings; the methods of recruitment were reasonable; and the analysis was rigorous. The areas where quality was most lacking, based on the CASP checklist, was Question 6, which asked, has the relationship between researcher and participants been adequately considered? [17] with a focus on researcher bias influencing results (Figure 2). Only four of the included studies reported any information on the relationship between researcher and participant; the remaining 42 studies were unclear. Question 7, which asked "have ethical issues been taken into consideration," was poorly reported, with only 36 out of 46 studies reporting any information on ethical issues or ethics approval.

Initial analysis revealed five overarching themes that were frequently reported by the included studies (Box 1): disruption to daily life, communication, impact of diagnosis, preferences for care, and stigma. The key findings related to each of these five overarching themes are summarized here. The key findings related to each of these five overarching themes are summarized here.

Table 2: Characteristics of included studies.

	Author	Study design	Number of participants included	Themes: Disruption to daily life	Themes: Communication	Themes: Impact of diagnosis	Themes: Preferences for care	Themes: Stigma
General population	Blasiole et al., 2006	Semistructured interview	342			√		√
	Bova et al., 2008	Semistructured interviews	39	√				
	Brunings et al., 2013	Semistructured focus group interviews	44		√		√	
	Butt et al., 2008	Interviews and daily think-aloud recordings	26					√
	Conrad et al., 2006	Semistructured interviews	70	√		√		√
	Dudley et al., 2007	In-depth interviews	8	√				
	Faye and Irurita, 2003	Semistructured interviews	24					√
	Fry and Bates, 2012	Semistructured interviews	15	√	√	√		√
	Glacken et al., 2003	In-depth interviews	28	√				
	Glacken et al., 2001	Descriptive exploratory design	9	√		√		
	Groessl et al., 2008	Semistructured interviews	22	√		√		
	Grundy and Beeching, 2004	Semistructured interviews	8					√
	Harris, 2010	Phenomenological research design	40	√				
	Harris, 2005	Not reported	20			√	√	√
	Harris, 2009	Semistructured interviews	40		√	√		
	Hepworth and Krug, 1999	Semistructured interviews	66		√	√		
	Hill et al., 2015	Unstructured interviews	23	√	√	√	√	√
	Janke et al., 2008	Focus groups	40					√
	Jiwani et al., 2013	Semistructured interviews	10	√		√	√	
	Kinder, 2009	Interviews using open-ended questions	8			√		
	Le Talec, 2013	Semistructured, open-ended interviews	31			√		
	MacNeil, 2012	Semistructured, open-ended interviews	9			√		
	McCreaddie et al., 2011	Semistructured interviews	16	√			√	√
	Moore et al., 2009	Written questionnaire with open ended questions	39		√	√		√
	North et al., 2014	Semistructured focus group interviews	48		√		√	√
	Olsen et al., 2013	Semistructured, open-ended interviews	109			√		
	Olsen et al., 2009	Semistructured, open-ended interviews	109	√				
	Owen, 2008	In-depth, open-ended interviews	6					√
	Paterson et al., 2006	"Think aloud" approach during a face-to-face interview	33		√		√	
	Sgorbini et al., 2009	Semistructured, open-ended interview	5			√	√	√
	Sinclair et al., 2011	Semi-structured open-ended interview	13			√		
	Stewart et al., 2012	Semistructured, open-ended interviews	13		√		√	√
	Stoller et al., 2009	Semi-structured, open-ended interviews	42	√				
	Sutton and Treloar, 2007	Semistructured, open-ended interviews	36			√		√
	Temple-Smith et al., 2004	Open-ended interview	32		√		√	√
	Treloar et al., 2010	Open-ended interview	24		√			
	Treloar and Hopwood, 2008	Open-ended interview	20		√			
	Treloar and Hopwood, 2004	Semistructured, open-ended interviews	19		√			

Table 2: Continued.

	Author	Study design	Number of participants included	Themes: Disruption to daily life	Communication	Impact of diagnosis	Preferences for care	Stigma
Injection drug users	Contreras and Jason, 2013	Semistructured interviews	4	√		√		
	Copeland, 2004	Semistructured interviews, conducted in groups			√			
	Crockett and Gifford, 2004	Semistructured interviews	25	√	√	√	√	√
	Habib and Adorjany, 2003	Self-reported questionnaire with open- and closed-ended questions	274		√		√	√
	Olsen et al., 2012	Semistructured, open-ended interviews	83			√		
	Tompkins et al., 2005	In-depth, open-ended interviews	17		√	√		
	Wright et al., 2005	In-depth interviews	17	√				
Other	Dunne and Quayle, 2001	Semistructured focus groups	32	√		√		

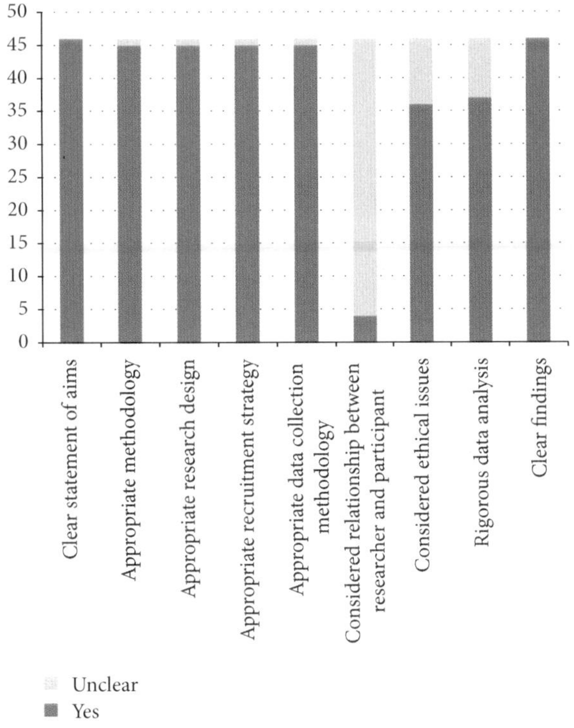

FIGURE 2: CASP Quality Assessment [22].

3.1. Disruption to Daily Life. Broadly, studies reported that participants experienced considerable disruption to daily living, impaired quality of life, and chronic physical and psychological symptoms related to HCV. Study participants reported a variety of physical symptoms, such as fatigue [27, 30, 33–36, 40, 42, 46, 54, 62, 64, 66], weakness [27, 35], nausea [27, 30, 34, 64], pain [27, 34, 36, 42, 64, 66], swelling [27], headaches [30, 64], and sweating [30]. In addition, a number of studies reported participants experiencing psychological symptoms such as depression [27, 30, 66], anxiety or panic attacks [35], and irritability [36, 62]. Other symptoms such as poor memory [30, 35] and inability to concentrate [30, 35, 46] were also reported by participants. Fry and Bates found fatigue and other physical symptoms often made full-time work difficult to maintain; many participants switched to working part-time, quit their job, or changed sectors [33].

For participants who had undergone a liver transplant because of HCV, Dudley et al. found that they suffered from symptoms such as weight loss, lethargy, weakness, and anorexia, to the extent that, within one year of the operation, they wished that they had not received a transplant [31]. However, after one year, none of the participants regretted having the transplant [31]. Participants described that they needed "…deliberate and conscious effort to adapt to living with a transplant." [31] Despite the long-term symptoms, participants also expressed feeling that they had a new and positive outlook on life [31].

Individuals found it difficult to abstain from alcohol or limit consumption of alcohol because their social life was tied to drinking or because they felt alienated from their social network as a nondrinker [24]. When talking about the experience of abstaining from alcohol after HCV diagnosis, patients spoke about not knowing how much alcohol they could safely consume, and receiving mixed messages from healthcare practitioners regarding alcohol consumption [24]. Some participants continued to drink heavily, often justifying their decision as prioritizing pleasure over fear of death [24].

Diagnosis of HCV was found to not significantly impact women's decisions around contraceptives [21]. Women with HCV used a variety of contraceptives or, in some cases, had reasonable justification for not using contraceptives [21]. The type of contraceptive used was dictated by women's own experiences, the experiences of other women, availability, and doctor recommendations [21].

For some, a diagnosis of HCV changes their perceptions towards injection drug use. Some people reported that, after a HCV diagnosis, a fear of transmitting HCV to others led them to develop new strategies to prevent transmission such as covering wounds, using separate injection material, and not allowing anyone to use their personal hygiene items [61]. Some participants, despite knowing that they had HCV, chose not to adopt safe injection practices to reduce transmission to others [61]. Some individuals described using more drugs after diagnosis, due to symptoms related to HCV [61].

3.2. Communication. Poor communication at the time of diagnosis was frequently reported. Both the level of communication and the source of the communication affected patients' perceptions of their diagnosis. One study found that the experience of diagnosis was seen in a more positive light by patients diagnosed by a family doctor or GP than those diagnosed in an organizational setting (i.e., prison and injection drug service) [56]. One participant diagnosed at a detox center said that *"he was sort of cold and…unsympathetic…it was like he does it everyday sort of thing"* and another at a prison was quoted saying that *"there's 750 prisoners. So he goes on and tells people 'Right you've got AIDS, you've got hep C, you've got this, you've got that. Next customer'"* [56]. Participants also voiced that their experience of diagnosis was more distressing when they were not given sufficient information [25, 33, 40] or when they felt that the information was delivered insensitively (e.g., over the phone [25]).

Those with HCV expressed a desire to have involvement in decision-making regarding their care [50], to feel like healthcare practitioners were listening to their concerns [28], to feel cared for [28], and to not be spoken to insensitively [28]. Many patients believed that they were treated insensitively [40, 47, 53, 60], adequate time was not spent with them [64], confusing medical terms were used [64], and healthcare practitioners refused them treatment [47, 65].

Individuals reported that they had been given negligible information about HCV after diagnosis or were poorly informed [25, 40, 48, 59, 64], that they were told different information every visit [39], and that they were not given practical advice [40, 50]. One patient said "a lack of information from health care practitioners resulted in individuals seeking information from other sources" [48, 59]. People generally felt less stressed when more information was given [33]. One participant suggested that an education class would be valuable to those diagnosed with HCV [48]. In only one

Disruption to daily life (n = 17)
"You cannot fight it; it is not a tiredness that you can fight like a normal tiredness. A normal tiredness, you can fight it and get a second wind or if you had a few cups of coffee, it would keep you going. None of this works with this tiredness" [3].
Communication (n = 11)
"There's 750 prisoners. So he goes on and tells people 'Right you've got AIDS, you've got hep C, you've got this, you've got that. Next customer'" [1].
Impact of diagnosis (n = 22)
"My youngest...keeps asking me how old I am because I don't go here, there and everywhere with her. And she says 'How old is that now, does that mean that you are middle aged now?'...And she would say how old is her friend's mum and she is always comparing me with her" [4].
Preferences for care (n = 16)
"There isn't a network, there is just a specialist that sort of looks at one aspect of everything it seems. What I feel like sometimes is that you [health care practitioners] are building or putting together a puzzle without the picture" [2].
Stigma (n = 20)
"The Doctor rang me at home at 11.30pm and said 'you've got Hep C. You're a junkie, aren't you?...' I had never been a drug user, I had never met an intravenous drug user in my life! He said 'you could have only got it if you were a junkie'. So I thought that was just stupid, I dismissed the diagnosis" [5].

Box 1: Themes explored by included studies.

study, by Temple-Smith et al., did participants note that they felt that they had received adequate information [56].

3.3. Impact of Diagnosis. After receiving a positive HCV diagnosis, patients report a range of emotions, including distress (being overwhelmed and frightened and feelings of hopelessness) [25, 33, 34, 36, 39, 44, 51, 60, 62–64, 66]; shame or disgust [36, 39, 40, 44, 60]; denial or doubt [36, 44, 60]; and relief [36, 62, 66]. Studies reported that some patients were shocked or surprised by their HCV diagnosis [23, 25, 33, 34, 36, 40, 43, 44, 51, 52, 60, 63], while others were not surprised or had expected a positive HCV result [23, 33, 36, 38]. Those who were not shocked or surprised at the time of diagnosis were often current IDUs who viewed contracting HCV as inevitable [22, 23, 25, 36, 38], often thinking of HCV as a *"legacy of drug use...the junky flu, that's one of the by-products"* [40]. Some IDUs felt that they had accepted the risk of becoming HCV positive when they began using injection drugs [23, 63], as expressed by one participant *"I guess, after a while I just came to realize that if I'm going to use heroin I'll end up with hep C. It's probably inevitable...hand in hand, you know."* [67] Participants that were former IDUs found that a positive HCV diagnosis was troubling because it forced them to acknowledge their previous drug use [22, 33, 67]; *"I really wanted to put all that behind me...The diagnosis was ten years or whatever after I'd stopped using...I didn't really want to deal with it"* [67].

Other studies reported patients' lack of concern with their HCV diagnosis [22, 25, 33, 40, 55, 63]. This attitude appeared to stem from a variety of sources, including a lack of physical symptoms or physical impact [55] and feeling like they had bigger problems than a HCV diagnosis [22] such as a HIV diagnosis [63]. One individual was quoted as saying *"I wasn't concerned... I've got HIV anyway... just another one to add to the list"* [63].

A diagnosis of HCV impacted individuals' relationships to varying degrees. Some reported that relationships were strengthened due to the diagnosis [33, 36, 42, 52, 60, 62], while others found that HCV negatively impacted relationships [26, 30, 33, 42, 51]. Those who felt that their relationships were strengthened said that they felt more supported and closer to their family after being diagnosed with HCV [33, 36, 42, 52, 60, 62]. Those who experienced a deterioration in their relationships cited irrationality and irritability [26, 42, 51, 62], fatigue [26, 33, 51, 66], physical pain [42, 66], stress and financial burden [26], fear of transmitting HCV to family and children [30, 64], and fear of sexual transmission or pregnancy [22, 42, 47, 64], as the factors contributing to weaker relationships.

Children may be affected by their parents' diagnosis of HCV. Some individuals reported experiencing behavioural problems with their children due to the tension and deterioration of relationships between parents [51]. Some children became confused and frustrated by the symptoms their parents were exhibiting, such as lack of energy and change in their parent's behaviour [66]. One woman expressed this by saying *"my youngest...keeps asking me how old I am because I don't go here, there and everywhere with her. And she says 'How old is that now, does that mean that you are middle aged now?'...And she would say how old is her friend's mum and she is always comparing me with her"* [66].

3.4. Preferences for Care. Many participants cited having a negative relationship with their healthcare providers. Examples of negative relationships included healthcare provider focusing on disease rather than the person [50, 51]; not feeling supported [42, 48, 64]; and being treated like a *"leper"* or feeling unworthy of medical care [46, 53, 56, 64, 65]. One patient was quoted as saying *"you were treated like a leper when you went into the hospital...because I had the hepatitis C, right away they think, drug addict...You know, I'd be stuck in a room and on the front of the door, it'd have 'do not enter, infectious'"* [46].

Participants ideally wanted a health practitioner who was both well-informed and respected confidentiality. In one study, Brunings et al. reported that healthcare practitioners were poorly informed and patients felt that they were educating the doctor [28]. In another study, one patient was concerned because their healthcare practitioner had breached confidentiality [53].

Concerns about continuity of care were discussed in one study [50]. Here, participants felt that their care was fragmented, that specialists assumed that all they had to do was treat the disease and monitor disease progression, and that GPs and specialists worked in silos [50]. A patient was quoted as saying *"there isn't a network, there is just a specialist that sort of looks at one aspect of everything it seems. What I feel like sometimes is that you [health care practitioners] are building or putting together a puzzle without the picture"* [50].

Some study participants also expressed a wish for more holistic care [38, 40, 50, 51]. Participants felt that the medical model of care used by healthcare practitioners did not address all of the issues faced by those with HCV [38, 40, 50, 51].

3.5. Stigma. Many individuals, across these studies, described the stigma associated with HCV. The cause of stigma was consistently found to be based on either an association of HCV with injection drug use or risky behaviours [29, 30, 32, 33, 40, 41, 46, 47, 49, 51, 53, 64] and/or ignorance or misconception about transmission [26, 29, 32, 33, 41, 46–48, 53, 65]. Individuals with HCV reported that misinformation made those around them afraid of touching them [29, 41, 46, 65], and afraid of them using regular utensils and plates (e.g., those with HCV would be offered plastic utensils and paper plates) [30, 41, 46–48]. One individual said *"there's a powerlessness that goes with being represented as, you know, I'm part of the hepatitis C statistics, so when I'm reading misinformation, I feel misrepresented"* [33].

Emotional and action-based responses were reported in the included papers. Emotional responses to stigma included hurt feelings [29, 33], shame [29, 33, 49, 53], embarrassment [29, 47], low self-worth [29], fear [29, 47, 49], anger [29, 33, 49], depression [29], isolation [29], feeling dirty [37, 49, 55, 64], and feeling rejected [49]. Action-based responses to stigma included educating others [29], blaming others [29], and changing relationships [29]. Due to perceived stigma or a fear of stigmatization, those with HCV were often afraid to disclose their HCV status [37, 40, 41, 47, 49, 53, 55, 56, 64, 65], lost friends [26], changed employment to avoid stigmatization [26, 47], and isolated themselves to avoid experiencing stigma [40, 41, 46, 48, 55].

In one study, seven participants reported they had disclosed their status at work; of these, three experienced discrimination (two of whom subsequently quit due to discrimination) [33]. This finding was echoed in studies by Crockett and Gifford who found that physical symptoms and concern about disclosure were the key barriers to stable income [64] and Moore et al. who reported that the stigma of HCV deterred people from disclosing their status [47].

Study participants also reported that they experienced either overt or covert stigmatization or discrimination from healthcare practitioners [29, 38, 40, 46, 47, 53, 65]. One participant expressed that stigmatization from a healthcare professional felt particularly degrading [40]. Often, this type of stigmatization created a barrier to understanding HCV and to seeking help from healthcare professionals [33, 53, 64]. One individual was quoted as saying *"the Doctor rang me at home at 11.30pm and said 'you've got Hep C. You're a junkie, aren't you? I know there's a lot to be ashamed of, but you can tell me'. I had never been a drug user, I had never met an intravenous drug user in my life! He said 'you could have only got it if you were a junkie'. So I thought that was just stupid, I dismissed the diagnosis"* [33].

4. Discussion

A sizeable body of qualitative research was found that explored people's experiences of living with HCV, many of which included people's experiences with the healthcare system. Although the studies included a variety of population groups, common themes emerged which focused on the varying ways in which being diagnosed with and living with HCV affected people's quality of life. Both living with the symptoms of HCV and being diagnosed with HCV contributed to the impact that HCV had on people's lives. For example, the stigma associated with being diagnosed with HCV affected people's careers, relationships, and experiences with the healthcare system, as did the physical and mental health symptoms associated with HCV (e.g., fatigue, weakness, nausea, pain, depression, and anxiety).

Study participants also described having a reduced quality of life due to HCV symptoms, such as fatigue, pain, nausea, and psychological changes. Although often seen as an asymptomatic disease, these studies found that the symptoms of HCV result in considerable disruption to daily living. Three studies investigated the impact of HCV on one's career and found that, due to physical symptoms and discrimination, many participants switched to part-time work, quit their jobs, or changed employment sectors. Additionally, the published literature suggests that, for some, an HCV diagnosis strengthened their personal relationships, while, for others, it weakened relationships; symptoms of HCV (whether physical or emotional) and fear of transmission were the factors most cited for contributing to deteriorating relationships. These findings are important as they underscore that while no clinically relevant symptoms may be present, HCV can still substantially impact a patient's life.

Very few of these study participants with HCV reported positive experiences with the healthcare system. Themes of not feeling supported, stigma, not being given adequate information, and not feeling involved in decision-making were frequent in the literature. Although these represent only a small sample of individuals with HCV who interact with healthcare, these finding were generally consistent across studies, and may help practitioners better recognize the specific needs of patients with HCV. Poor experiences with diagnosis and treatment highlight the need for patient-centered care, with a focus on supporting and educating patients with HCV. For example, offering HCV education sessions to newly diagnosed patients may help patients feel more supported within the healthcare system.

Stigma significantly impacted those with HCV. Two contributing factors to HCV related stigma were consistently identified: fear of transmission and association with injection drug use or risky behaviour. Misinformation appears to be the underlying cause of this stigma. It is likely that education, within the healthcare system, for family and friends of individuals diagnosed with HCV, and public education may reduce the stigma associated with HCV. Knowledge about the causes of HCV, as well as transmission mechanisms and transmission patterns, may reduce the feelings of stigmatization felt by those diagnosed and, in turn, may have positive implications such as more interest in being tested for HCV, increased disclosure, and improved quality of life.

At the time of diagnosis, individuals can experience feelings of distress, shame, unconcern, and relief. While most experience a feeling of shock, those who are current drug users are often not surprised and see diagnosis as inevitable. Awareness of these poor experiences with diagnosis may help illuminate areas where diagnosis communication can be improved; confusion, inadequate information, diagnosis over a phone, and diagnosis in an institutional setting all lead to feelings of dissatisfaction among those with HCV. These findings should be taken into account when considering how, where, and by whom HCV screening should be done.

Two limitations of this synthesis are as follows: non-English language studies were excluded and nearly all of the included studies were conducted in English speaking countries, with a large number being completed in Australia and the UK. Two strengths are as follows: a range of countries and a variety of populations were represented in this synthesis, and there was a lot of consistency across the studies. This means that the themes identified here are likely to be transferable to similar contexts.

Additionally, by its nature, this body of literature is difficult to synthesize; there is significant heterogeneity within the studies that have been included due to the variety of at-risk population categories, the diversity of topics explored in each paper, and the vast number of experiences captured by the included papers. Although organized by theme, this systematic review does not intend to suggest that the experiences across all populations (e.g., injection drug users and general population) are the same. However, remarkable consistency of themes across all studies does suggest that different populations may have similar experiences with HCV.

5. Conclusions

Published literature on experiences of living with HCV indicates that those with HCV often feel stigmatized and unsupported in their care, relationships, and work environments, while simultaneously coping with a variety of physical and psychological symptoms. This synthesis points to several areas where greater education, compassion, and patient-centered healthcare could improve the experience of people living with HCV.

Disclosure

Fiona Clement (Corresponding Author) had full access to all the data in the study and takes responsibility for the integrity of the data and the accuracy of the data analysis. She affirms that it is an honest, accurate, and transparent account of the study being reported; that no important aspects of the study have been omitted; and that any discrepancies from the study as planned have been explained.

Authors' Contributions

Laura E. Dowsett, Stephanie Coward, Diane L. Lorenzetti, and Fiona Clement contributed to design of the study; Laura E. Dowsett and Stephanie Coward assisted in collection of data and management of data; Laura E. Dowsett, Stephanie Coward, and Fiona Clement contributed to analysis of data and interpretation of the data; Laura E. Dowsett and Fiona Clement helped in preparation of manuscript; Laura E. Dowsett, Stephanie Coward, Diane L. Lorenzetti, and Fiona Clement reviewed and approved the manuscript.

References

[1] Ontario Ministry of Health and Long-Term Care, *Assessment Guide for Hepatitis C Risk Factors*, Ontario Ministry of Health and Long-Term Care, 2007, http://www.health.gov.on.ca/english/providers/program/hepc/hepc_pdf/hepc_assess_e.pdf.

[2] K. Mohd Hanafiah, J. Groeger, A. D. Flaxman, and S. T. Wiersma, "Global epidemiology of hepatitis C virus infection: new estimates of age-specific antibody to HCV seroprevalence," *Hepatology*, vol. 57, no. 4, pp. 1333–1342, 2013.

[3] H. B. El-Serag, "Epidemiology of viral hepatitis and hepatocellular carcinoma," *Gastroenterology*, vol. 142, no. 6, pp. 1264–1273.e1, 2012.

[4] M. G. Law, G. J. Dore, N. Bath et al., "Modelling hepatitis C virus incidence, prevalence and long-term sequelae in Australia, 2001," *International Journal of Epidemiology*, vol. 32, no. 5, pp. 717–724, 2003.

[5] F. M. Averhoff, N. Glass, and D. Holtzman, "Global burden of hepatitis C: considerations for healthcare providers in the United States," *Clinical Infectious Diseases*, vol. 55, supplement 1, pp. S10–S15, 2012.

[6] Centers for Disease Control and Prevention, "Hepatitis C FAQS for Health Professionals: Centers for Disease Control and Prevention," 2014, http://www.cdc.gov/hepatitis/hcv/hcvfaq.htm#b7.

[7] B. D. Smith, R. L. Morgan, G. A. Beckett et al., "Recommendations for the identification of chronic hepatitis C virus infection among persons born during 1945-1965," *MMWR Recommendations and Reports: Morbidity and Mortality Weekly Report Recommendations and Reports/Centers for Disease Control*, vol. 61, no. RR-4, pp. 1–32, 2012.

[8] M. M. Denniston, R. M. Klevens, G. M. McQuillan, and R. B. Jiles, "Awareness of infection, knowledge of hepatitis C, and medical follow-up among individuals testing positive for

hepatitis C: national Health and Nutrition Examination Survey 2001–2008," *Hepatology*, vol. 55, no. 6, pp. 1652–1661, 2012.

[9] M. Cornberg, H. A. Razavi, A. Alberti et al., "A systematic review of hepatitis C virus epidemiology in Europe, Canada and Israel," *Liver International*, vol. 31, no. 2, pp. 30–60, 2011.

[10] Public Health Agency of Canada (Center for Communicable Diseases and Infection Control), "Hepatitis C in Canada: 2005–2010 Surveillance Report 2012," March 2015, http://www.catie.ca/sites/default/files/1109-0139-Hep%20C%20Report-EN%20FINAL.pdf.

[11] M. W. Fried, "Side effects of therapy of hepatitis C and their management," *Hepatology*, vol. 36, no. 5I, pp. S237–S244, 2002.

[12] R. P. Myers, A. Ramji, M. Bilodeau, S. Wong, and J. J. Feld, "An update on the management of chronic hepatitis C: consensus guidelines from the Canadian Association for the Study of the Liver," *Canadian Journal of Gastroenterology*, vol. 26, no. 6, pp. 359–375, 2012.

[13] T. Asselah and P. Marcellin, "Interferon free therapy with direct acting antivirals for HCV," *Liver International*, vol. 33, no. 1, pp. 93–104, 2013.

[14] G. J. Dore, G. V. Matthews, and J. Rockstroh, "Future of hepatitis C therapy: development of direct-acting antivirals," *Current Opinion in HIV and AIDS*, vol. 6, no. 6, pp. 508–513, 2011.

[15] V. Soriano, P. Labarga, J. V. Fernández-Montero et al., "The changing face of hepatitis C in the new era of direct-acting antivirals," *Antiviral Research*, vol. 97, no. 1, pp. 36–40, 2013.

[16] A. Tong, K. Flemming, E. McInnes, S. Oliver, and J. Craig, "Enhancing transparency in reporting the synthesis of qualitative research: ENTREQ," *BMC Medical Research Methodology*, vol. 12, article 181, 2012.

[17] Critical Appraisal Skills Programme (CASP), *CASP Checklist for Qualitative Research*, 2013.

[18] J. Popay, H. Roberts, A. Sowden et al., "Guidance on the conduct of narrative synthesis in systematic reviews," *ESRC Methods Programme*, vol. 15, no. 1, pp. 47–71, 2006.

[19] C. Treloar and T. Rhodes, "The lived experience of Hepatitis C and its treatment among injecting drug users: qualitative synthesis," *Qualitative Health Research*, vol. 19, no. 9, pp. 1321–1334, 2009.

[20] L. Jones, A. Atkinson, G. Bates et al., "Views and experiences of hepatitis C testing and diagnosis among people who inject drugs: systematic review of qualitative research," *International Journal of Drug Policy*, vol. 25, no. 2, pp. 204–211, 2014.

[21] A. Olsen, C. Banwell, and P. Dance, "Internal or infernal devices: experiences of contraception among Australian women living with hepatitis C," *Health Care for Women International*, vol. 30, no. 6, pp. 456–474, 2009.

[22] A. Olsen, C. Banwell, P. Dance, and L. Maher, "Positive health beliefs and behaviours in the midst of difficult lives: women who inject drugs," *International Journal of Drug Policy*, vol. 23, no. 4, pp. 312–318, 2012.

[23] A. Olsen, C. Banwell, and P. Dance, "Reinforced biographies among women living with hepatitis C," *Qualitative Health Research*, vol. 23, no. 4, pp. 531–540, 2013.

[24] M. Harris, "Pleasure and guilt: alcohol use and hepatitis C," *Qualitative Health Research*, vol. 20, no. 9, pp. 1262–1271, 2010.

[25] M. Harris, "Troubling biographical disruption: narratives of unconcern about hepatitis C diagnosis," *Sociology of Health and Illness*, vol. 31, no. 7, pp. 1028–1042, 2009.

[26] J. A. Blasiole, L. Shinkunas, D. R. LaBrecque, R. M. Arnold, and S. L. Zickmund, "Mental and physical symptoms associated with lower social support for patients with hepatitis C," *World Journal of Gastroenterology*, vol. 12, no. 29, pp. 4665–4672, 2006.

[27] C. Bova, C. Jaffarian, P. Himlan, L. Mangini, and L. Ogawa, "The symptom experience of HIV/HCV-coinfected adults," *Journal of the Association of Nurses in AIDS Care*, vol. 19, no. 3, pp. 170–180, 2008.

[28] P. Brunings, S. Klar, G. Butt, M. D. Nijkamp, and J. A. Buxton, ""It's a big part of our lives": a qualitative study defining quality of hepatitis C care from the patient's perspective," *Gastroenterology Nursing*, vol. 36, no. 4, pp. 249–257, 2013.

[29] G. Butt, B. L. Paterson, and L. K. McGuinness, "Living with the stigma of hepatitis C," *Western Journal of Nursing Research*, vol. 30, no. 2, pp. 204–221, 2008.

[30] S. Conrad, L. E. Garrett, W. G. E. Cooksley, M. P. Dunne, and G. A. Macdonald, "Living with chronic hepatitis C means "you just haven't got a normal life any more"," *Chronic Illness*, vol. 2, no. 2, pp. 121–131, 2006.

[31] T. Dudley, D. Chaplin, C. Clifford, and D. J. Mutimer, "Quality of life after liver transplantation for hepatitis C infection," *Quality of Life Research*, vol. 16, no. 8, pp. 1299–1308, 2007.

[32] B. Faye and V. F. Irurita, "Balancing perspective: the response to feelings of being condemned with the hepatitis C virus," *Journal of Substance Use*, vol. 8, no. 2, pp. 92–103, 2003.

[33] M. Fry and G. Bates, "The tasks of self-managing hepatitis C: the significance of disclosure," *Psychology and Health*, vol. 27, no. 4, pp. 460–474, 2012.

[34] M. Glacken, G. Kernohan, and V. Coates, "Diagnosed with Hepatitis C: a descriptive exploratory study," *International Journal of Nursing Studies*, vol. 38, no. 1, pp. 107–116, 2001.

[35] M. Glacken, V. Coates, G. Kernohan, and J. Hegarty, "The experience of fatigue for people living with hepatitis C," *Journal of Clinical Nursing*, vol. 12, no. 2, pp. 244–252, 2003.

[36] E. J. Groessl, K. R. Weingart, R. M. Kaplan, J. A. Clark, A. L. Gifford, and S. B. Ho, "Living with hepatitis C: qualitative interviews with hepatitis C-infected veterans," *Journal of General Internal Medicine*, vol. 23, no. 12, pp. 1959–1965, 2008.

[37] G. Grundy and N. Beeching, "Understanding social stigma in women with hepatitis C.," *Nursing Standard*, vol. 19, no. 4, pp. 35–39, 2004.

[38] M. Harris, "Living with hepatitis C: the medical encounter," *New Zealand Sociology*, vol. 20, no. 1, pp. 4–19, 2005.

[39] J. Hepworth and G. J. Krug, "Hepatitis C. A socio-cultural perspective on the effects of a new virus on a community's health," *Journal of Health Psychology*, vol. 4, no. 2, pp. 237–246, 1999.

[40] R. Hill, M. Pfeil, J. Moore, and B. Richardson, "Living with hepatitis C: a phenomenological study," *Journal of Clinical Nursing*, vol. 24, no. 3-4, pp. 428–438, 2015.

[41] E. A. Janke, S. McGraw, G. Garcia-Tsao, and L. Fraenkel, "Psychosocial issues in hepatitis C: a qualitative analysis," *Psychosomatics*, vol. 49, no. 6, pp. 494–501, 2008.

[42] N. S. Jiwani, R. B. Gul, A. Ali, M. Salih, and M. Hanzala, "Experiences and perceptions of patients living with hepatitis C in Karachi, Pakistan," *Journal of Transcultural Nursing*, vol. 24, no. 3, pp. 297–304, 2013.

[43] M. Kinder, "The lived experience of treatment for Hepatitis C," *Gastroenterology Nursing*, vol. 32, no. 6, pp. 401–408, 2009.

[44] J.-Y. Le Talec, "When 'raw sex' turns to a 'raw deal' ... taking the opportunity to think about sex? Interviews with HIV-positive gay men diagnosed with acute hepatitis C," *Culture, Health and Sexuality*, vol. 15, no. 10, pp. 1133–1147, 2013.

[45] J. M. MacNeil, "The complexity of living with hepatitis C: a Newman perspective," *Nursing Science Quarterly*, vol. 25, no. 3, pp. 261–266, 2012.

[46] M. McCreaddie, I. Lyons, D. Horsburgh, M. Miller, and J. Frew, "The isolating and insulating effects of hepatitis C: a substantive grounded theory," *Gastroenterology Nursing*, vol. 34, no. 1, pp. 49–59, 2011.

[47] G. A. Moore, D. A. Hawley, and P. Bradley, "Hepatitis C: experiencing stigma," *Gastroenterology Nursing*, vol. 32, no. 2, pp. 94–104, 2009.

[48] C. S. North, R. Devereaux, D. E. Pollio, B. A. Hong, and M. K. Jain, "Patient perspectives on hepatitis C and its treatment," *European Journal of Gastroenterology and Hepatology*, vol. 26, no. 1, pp. 74–81, 2014.

[49] G. Owen, "An 'elephant in the room'? Stigma and hepatitis C transmission among HIV-positive 'serosorting' gay men," *Culture, Health and Sexuality*, vol. 10, no. 6, pp. 601–610, 2008.

[50] B. L. Paterson, G. Butt, L. McGuinness, and B. Moffat, "The construction of hepatitis C as a chronic illness," *Clinical Nursing Research*, vol. 15, no. 3, pp. 209–224, 2006.

[51] M. Sgorbini, L. O'Brien, and D. Jackson, "Living with hepatitis C and treatment: the personal experiences of patients," *Journal of Clinical Nursing*, vol. 18, no. 16, pp. 2282–2291, 2009.

[52] M. Sinclair, S. Mcpherson, R. Bor, and L. Orban, "Another dragon in the kitchen: psychological experiences of hepatitis C treatment among HIV-hepatitis C co-infected gay men," *Counselling and Psychotherapy Research*, vol. 11, no. 3, pp. 228–236, 2011.

[53] B. J. Stewart, A. A. Mikocka-Walus, H. Harley, and J. M. Andrews, "Help-seeking and coping with the psychosocial burden of chronic hepatitis C: a qualitative study of patient, hepatologist, and counsellor perspectives," *International Journal of Nursing Studies*, vol. 49, no. 5, pp. 560–569, 2012.

[54] E. P. Stoller, N. J. Webster, C. E. Blixen et al., "Lay management of chronic disease: a qualitative study of living with hepatitis C infection," *American Journal of Health Behavior*, vol. 33, no. 4, pp. 376–390, 2009.

[55] R. Sutton and C. Treloar, "Chronic illness experiences, clinical markers and living with hepatitis C," *Journal of Health Psychology*, vol. 12, no. 2, pp. 330–340, 2007.

[56] M. Temple-Smith, S. Gifford, and M. Stoov Eacute, "The lived experience of men and women with hepatitis C: implications for support needs and health information," *Australian Health Review*, vol. 27, no. 2, pp. 46–56, 2004.

[57] C. Treloar and M. Hopwood, "Infection control in the context of hepatitis C disclosure: implications for education of healthcare professionals," *Education for Health*, vol. 17, no. 2, pp. 183–191, 2004.

[58] C. Treloar and M. Hopwood, "'Look, I'm fit, I'm positive and I'll be all right, thank you very much': coping with hepatitis C treatment and unrealistic optimism," *Psychology, Health and Medicine*, vol. 13, no. 3, pp. 360–366, 2008.

[59] C. Treloar, J. Newland, M. Harris, R. Deacon, and L. Maher, "A diagnosis of hepatitis C: insights from a study on patients' experiences," *Australian Family Physician*, vol. 39, no. 8, pp. 589–592, 2010.

[60] C. N. E. Tompkins, N. M. J. Wright, and L. Jones, "Impact of a positive hepatitis C diagnosis on homeless injecting drug users: a qualitative study," *British Journal of General Practice*, vol. 55, no. 513, pp. 263–268, 2005.

[61] N. M. J. Wright, C. N. E. Tompkins, and L. Jones, "Exploring risk perception and behaviour of homeless injecting drug users diagnosed with hepatitis C," *Health and Social Care in the Community*, vol. 13, no. 1, pp. 75–83, 2005.

[62] R. Contreras and L. A. Jason, "Experiences of Oxford house residents living with the Hepatitis C virus," *Frontiers in Psychological and Behavioral Science*, vol. 2, no. 2, pp. 57–63, 2013.

[63] L. Copeland, "The drug user's identity and how it relates to being hepatitis C antibody positive: a qualitative study," *Drugs: Education, Prevention and Policy*, vol. 11, no. 2, pp. 129–147, 2004.

[64] B. Crockett and S. M. Gifford, ""Eyes wide shut" narratives of women living with hepatitis C in Australia," *Women and Health*, vol. 39, no. 4, pp. 117–137, 2004.

[65] S. E. Habib and L. V. Adorjany, "Hepatitis C and injecting drug use: the realities of stigmatisation and discrimination," *Health Education Journal*, vol. 62, no. 3, pp. 256–265, 2003.

[66] E. A. Dunne and E. Quayle, "The impact of Iatrogenically acquired hepatitis C infection on the well-being and relationships of a group of Irish women," *Journal of Health Psychology*, vol. 6, no. 6, pp. 679–692, 2001.

[67] A. Olsen, M. Temple-Smith, and C. Banwell, "Consideration of gender in diagnosis and management of blood-borne viruses: the case of hepatitis C," *Australian Journal of Primary Health*, vol. 19, no. 2, pp. 124–129, 2013.

9

Predictive Role of Interleukin-18 in Liver Steatosis in Obese Children

Marta Flisiak-Jackiewicz,[1] **Anna Bobrus-Chociej,**[1]
Eugeniusz Tarasów,[2] **Małgorzata Wojtkowska,**[3] **Irena Białokoz-Kalinowska,**[4]
and Dariusz Marek Lebensztejn[1]

[1]*Department of Pediatrics, Gastroenterology and Allergology, Medical University of Białystok, Białystok, Poland*
[2]*Department of Radiology, Medical University of Białystok, Białystok, Poland*
[3]*Department of Radiology, University Children Hospital, Białystok, Poland*
[4]*Łomża State University of Applied Sciences, Łomża, Poland*

Correspondence should be addressed to Marta Flisiak-Jackiewicz; m_flisiak@op.pl

Academic Editor: Peter Jarčuška

Introduction. Interleukin-18 (IL-18) is a proinflammatory cytokine associated with metabolic syndrome (MS). Nonalcoholic fatty liver disease (NAFLD) can be recognized as a feature of MS. *Material and Methods*. Serum IL-18 concentration was evaluated in serum of 108 obese children, determined with ELISA, and referred to degree of liver steatosis in USG or total intrahepatic lipid content assessed by magnetic resonance proton spectroscopy (^{1}HMRS). *Results*. Fatty liver was confirmed in 89 children with USG and in 72 with ^{1}HMRS. IL-18 concentration demonstrated significantly higher values in patients than in controls. Significant correlations between IL-18 and ALT, GGT, triglycerides, hsCRP, and the degree of liver steatosis were demonstrated. NAFLD children had significantly higher level of IL-18, ALT, GGT, HOMA-IR, waist circumference, and total lipids content in ^{1}HMRS than other obese children. IL-18 level was also significantly higher in obese children with advanced liver steatosis. Measurement of serum IL-18 showed ability to differentiate children with fatty liver from those without steatosis. *Conclusion*. Elevated serum IL-18 concentration and its correlation with hepatocyte injury, systemic inflammation, and degree of liver steatosis support role in NAFLD pathomechanism. IL-18 can be considered to play a role in predicting advanced liver steatosis and fatty liver in obese children.

1. Introduction

Nonalcoholic fatty liver disease (NAFLD) nowadays becomes a leading cause of liver pathology and may be present in 20–30% of general population. Rising prevalence of NAFLD is also observed among children and adolescents, which is closely related to obesity epidemic worldwide [1, 2]. The histological spectrum of NAFLD ranges from simple steatosis to nonalcoholic steatohepatitis (NASH), where steatosis coexists with hepatic inflammation that can be accompanied by fibrosis. Long lasting NASH may progress to severe liver damage and can result in cirrhosis or even hepatocellular carcinoma [3, 4]. Development of NAFLD is strongly associated with visceral obesity and other components of the metabolic syndrome (MS) including dyslipidemia and insulin resistance (IR); that is why NAFLD is regarded as a hepatic manifestation of MS [5, 6]. The pathogenesis of this clinical condition has not been fully understood but usually is explained by a "two-hit" hypothesis [7, 8]. In this mechanism the first "hit" is associated with excess accumulation of lipids in the liver. The second "hit" can lead to progression to NASH through increase of oxidative stress, lipid peroxidation, imbalance of adipokines level, or release of toxic products. Recent studies have revealed more possible factors involved in the development and progression of NAFLD, such as dysregulated intestinal microbiota, mitochondrial dysfunction, abnormalities of iron metabolism, or increased fructose consumption [9–15]. Moreover there are growing evidences showing that NAFLD, as well as IR, is strongly related to low-grade systemic inflammation and probably therefore some mediators are released from obese fat tissue and additionally promoting hepatic and systemic inflammation [16–21]. For this reason we have focused on investigation of proinflammatory cytokine interleukin-18 (IL-18) and its possible association with the development and the potential progression of NAFLD through stimulation of hepatic inflammation and fibrosis. However the most recent studies demonstrate differences between pediatric and adult NAFLD in terms of prevalence, histology, diagnosis, and management [22].

IL-18 plays a crucial role in the inflammatory cascade. This molecule is a member of the IL-1 family of cytokines and it was initially described as an interferon-γ- (IFN-gamma-) inducing factor. IL-18 is secreted in many different cell types, including macrophages, endothelial cells, vascular smooth muscle cells, dendritic cells, Kupffer cells, and adipocytes [23, 24]. It is primarily synthesized as a precursor protein, pro-IL-18, which requires activation by caspase-1 cleavage into bioactive mature form. IL-18 is inactivated by specific binding protein, which results from a negative feedback mechanism in response to increased IL-18 production, protecting cells from accelerated proinflammatory activity [25, 26]. Previously published studies demonstrated elevated circulating levels of IL-18 in adult patients with metabolic syndrome and its components. There are several reports suggesting its usefulness as a marker of insulin resistance in type 2 diabetes and predictor of cardiovascular disease development [27–30]. Furthermore there is some evidence that plasma levels of IL-18 are elevated in adults with chronic liver disease and correlate with severity of the disease [31–33].

These findings were demonstrated in adults and led us to investigate whether there is an association between serum IL-18 concentration and NAFLD in obese children. Moreover we analyzed effect of steatosis degree on serum IL-18 levels to establish its possible predictive role for the disease progression in comparison to several other markers of hepatic injury, metabolic dysfunction, and systemic inflammation.

2. Materials and Methods

2.1. Patients. This study comprised a group of 108 consecutive obese children (84 boys and 24 girls) aged 7–17 years (mean age 12,8 years) admitted to our department because of suspected liver disease based on hepatomegaly and/or elevated alanine aminotransferase (ALT) activity and/or fatty liver features on ultrasound (USG) examination. Informed consent was obtained from all patients' parents. The protocol was approved by the local bioethics committee. Viral infection due to hepatitis C virus (negative testing for anti-HCV) and hepatitis B virus (negative testing for HBsAg), autoimmune hepatitis, selected metabolic liver diseases (Wilson disease, alpha-1-antitrypsin deficiency, and cystic fibrosis), and drug-induced liver injury (DILI) were excluded in all children. Moreover, children with diabetes (elevated fasting plasma glucose) and those having infectious diseases on admission (white blood cell (WBC) count less than 3500 cells/μl or more than 10 500 cells/μl; C-reactive protein (CRP) more than 5 mg/L; body temperature more than 38°C) were excluded from this study.

All participants underwent a detailed medical history and physical examination with anthropometric measurements, including weight, height, body mass index (BMI), and waist circumference. BMI was calculated by dividing weight in kilograms by the square of height in meters (kg/m2). Obesity was defined as a BMI over the 95th percentile based on age and gender [34]. The diagnosis of NAFLD was established in children with both elevated serum ALT activity and liver steatosis on ultrasound examination. Liver steatosis was diagnosed with positive imaging results. Patients were divided into two groups: with NAFLD ($n = 39$) and obese without NAFLD ($n = 69$) that did not fulfil criteria of NAFLD diagnosis. All patients with elevated ALT had steatosis, but there were 50 patients with steatosis and normal ALT.

Age matched control group comprised of 15 nonobese children without any somatic organ pathology was recruited at the time of the study and blood samples were collected as a part of their routine checkup to obtain normal values of IL-18.

2.2. Laboratory Measurements. In all patients routine biochemical measurements were performed, including alanine aminotransferase (ALT), aspartate aminotransferase (AST), gamma glutamyltransferase (GGT), bilirubin, total cholesterol, high-density lipoprotein (HDL-C) and low-density lipoprotein (LDL-C) cholesterol, triglycerides (TG), uric acid, ferritin, glucose, and insulin, by using the enzymatic colorimetric method at laboratory department of our hospital. In all patients alpha-1-antitrypsin (A1AT) level and in 45 patients high-sensitive C-reactive protein (hsCRP) level were determined by a nephelometric method with a DADE Behring Nephelometer Analyzer (Germany).

Insulin resistance (IR) was calculated by homeostasis model assessment of insulin resistance (HOMA-IR) using the following formula: HOMA-IR = fasting insulin (μU/ml) × fasting plasma glucose (mmol/L)/22.5 [35].

Serum IL-18 levels were determined by an enzyme-linked immunosorbent assay (Human IL-18 ELISA Kit, Medical & Biological Laboratories Co., Ltd., Nagoya, Japan). Samples were centrifuged and frozen in −80°C until further analysis. The minimum detection limit for IL-18 was 12.5 pg/ml. The intra- and interassay CVs of IL-18 ranged from 4.9 to 10.8% and 5.2 to 10.1%, respectively. The assays were conducted according to the manufacturer's instructions.

2.3. Liver Examination. Liver ultrasound examination was performed with Voluson E8 instrument (General Electric, USA), equipped with convex sonde 3–5 MHz. The degree of liver steatosis was graded using a four-grade scale (0–3) according to Saverymuttu et al. [36]. Advanced liver steatosis was defined as a score > 1. Steatosis grade was assessed by the same radiologist without knowledge of the patients' data. Proton magnetic resonance spectroscopy (^{1}HMRS) was performed with a 1.5 T scanner (Picker Eclipse) and with PRESS sequencing. Total intrahepatic lipid content was assessed in relative units (r.u.) in comparison to unsuppressed water signal. Voxel's size 3 × 3 × 3 cm (27 cm3) was localized in the right liver lobe to avoid vessels and bile ducts [37].

Table 1: Analyzed parameters in all obese patients included in the study.

Parameters	NAFLD median; Q1–Q3 ($n = 39$)	Non-NAFLD median; Q1–Q3 ($n = 69$)	p
Gender, M/F	33/6	51/18	NS
IL-18 (pg/ml)	335; 257–493	299; 219–383	0.034
BMI (kg/m^2)	29; 27–34	27; 25–31	0.007
Waist (cm)	100; 94–108	93; 86–103	0.008
ALT (IU/l)	64; 50–101	26; 19–33	0.000
AST (IU/l)	39; 32–52	25; 21–30	0.000
GGT (IU/l)	30; 23–45	18; 14–23	0.000
Bilirubin (mg/dl)	0.6; 0.5–0.9	0.6; 0.45–0.7	NS
Total cholesterol (mg/dl)	177; 153–216	174; 145–190	NS
HDL-C (mg/dl)	44; 39–51	46; 38–54	NS
LDL-C (mg/dl)	97; 79–143	99; 78–116	NS
TG (mg/dl)	132; 85–173	108; 85–142	NS
Glucose (mg/dl)	93; 85–99	91; 86–96	NS
Insulin (μIU/ml)	18; 14–22	15; 11–18	0.011
HOMA-IR	4.2; 3.2–5.8	3.2; 2.1–4	0.005
Uric acid (mg/dl)	6.5; 5.5–7.4	5.7; 4.8–6.6	0.023
hsCRP (mg/l)	0.9; 0.7–1.8	1.3; 0.6–2	NS
Ferritin (ng/ml)	61; 50–105	52; 34–65	0.005
A1AT (g/l)	1.3; 1.2–1.5	1.4; 1.2–1.5	NS
USG grade of steatosis	2; 1–3	1; 0-1	0.000
^{1}HMRS (r.u.)	163; 106–210	80; 40–148	0.000

2.4. Statistical Analysis. Results are reported as median, 25–75 quartiles. The statistical analysis was evaluated using the Mann–Whitney two-sample test for nonparametric data. The relationship between serum IL-18 concentration and variables was analyzed by the Spearman rank-correlation test for nonparametric data. Statistical significance level was set at $p < 0.05$. Logistic regression analysis was performed using IBM SPSS Statistics 20.0. The receiver operating characteristics (ROC) analysis was used to calculate the power of IL-18 to detect liver steatosis on ^{1}HMRS. The comparison of the area under curve (AUC) was performed using a two-tailed p-test, which compares the AUC to the diagonal line of no information (AUC 0.5).

To perform combined ROC analysis of multiple parameters, linear combination of logistic regressions was carried out to detect children with liver steatosis in ^{1}HMRS.

3. Results

Eighty-nine children (82,5%) had liver steatosis in ultrasound examination and 72 (78,2%) in ^{1}HMRS with concordance rate of 100%. Moreover thirty-nine had also an elevated serum ALT activity (NAFLD patients).

Median IL-18 concentration measured in all obese patients (309; 237–410 pg/mL) was significantly ($p = 0.038$) higher than in controls (242; 197–318 pg/mL). As demonstrated in Table 1 median IL-18 level was significantly higher in NAFLD patients than in other obese children ($p = 0.034$). Moreover, patients with NAFLD showed significantly higher values of ALT, AST, and GGT activities, insulin, HOMA-IR, uric acid, ferritin, BMI, waist circumferences, degree of liver steatosis (USG), and total amount of lipids in ^{1}HMRS compared to children without NAFLD (Table 1).

Significant positive correlations of IL-18 with ALT ($r = 0.2$, $p = 0.036$), AST ($r = 0.21$, $p = 0.032$), GGT ($r = 0.23$, $p = 0.016$), TG ($r = 0.21$, $p = 0.027$), hsCRP ($r = 0.36$, $p = 0.014$), and the degree of liver steatosis (USG) ($r = 0.2$, $p = 0.044$) were found (Table 2). Patients with steatosis in USG and elevated ALT demonstrated significantly higher IL-18 activity than those with steatosis but normal ALT (310 versus 339 pg/mL; $p = 0.044$). However it was not a case in patients with steatosis diagnosed using ^{1}HMRS (341 versus 349 pg/mL; p-0.064).

Among 108 obese children included in the study, 19 had no steatosis in USG (grade 0), 47 (44%) demonstrated moderate steatosis (grade 1), and 42 (39%) had advanced liver steatosis defined as grade 2 or 3 (Table 3). The concentration of IL-18 was significantly higher in obese children with advanced liver steatosis compared to children without steatosis ($p = 0.027$) (Figure 1).

As shown in Table 4 children with liver steatosis measured with ^{1}HMRS had significantly higher levels of IL-18, ALT, AST, GGT, TG, and intensity of liver steatosis in USG examination than those without liver steatosis in ^{1}HMRS.

TABLE 2: Correlation (Spearman) between IL-18 serum concentrations and selected parameters.

	r	p
ALT	0.20	**0.036**
AST	0.21	**0.032**
GGT	0.23	**0.016**
Bilirubin	−0.13	0.185
Total cholesterol	−0.02	0.811
HDL-C	−0.08	0.399
LDL-C	−0.02	0.841
TG	0.21	**0.027**
Glucose	0.11	0.253
Insulin	0.07	0.462
HOMA - IR	0.08	0.396
Uric acid	−0.04	0.704
hsCRP	0.36	**0.014**
Ferritin	0.05	0.599
A1AT	−0.05	0.588
USG grade of steatosis	0.19	**0.044**
1HMRS	0.12	0.252
BMI	−0.12	0.219
Waist	−0.29	**0.009**

In the logistic regression analysis IL-18 (OR-1.006, 95% CI for OR—1.001–1.010, and $p = 0.018$) and triglycerides (OR-1.015, 95% CI for OR—1.003–1.028, and $p = 0.012$) were the only measures useful in the differentiation of obese patients with liver steatosis confirmed using ^{1}HMRS. This finding was confirmed in ROC analysis, which demonstrated a cut-off of IL-18 concentration on the level of 326.8 pg/ml as effective (AUC = 0.68; $p = 0.006$) for differentiation between children with or without fatty liver in ^{1}HMRS (Table 5). Sensitivity was 60% and specificity 75%, whereas negative and positive predictive values were 34% and 90%, respectively (Figure 2(a)). ROC curves for ALT, AST, GGT, and TG demonstrate similar pattern to IL-18 (Figures 2(b), 2(c), 2(d), and 2(e)) as well as AUC values (Table 5). Combined ROC analysis of all five parameters was carried out to find out possible superior measure for steatosis corresponding to intrahepatic lipid content evaluated with ^{1}HMRS. ROC analysis of combined parameters demonstrated superior AUC of 0.7826 ($p < 0.0001$), sensitivity 61%, specificity 85%, and negative or positive predictive value of 38% and 94%, respectively. However the ROC of the combined logistic regression model did not demonstrate statistical significance compared to individual AUC (Figure 2(f), Table 5).

4. Discussion

Early diagnosis of NAFLD in obese children is important for possible prediction of further metabolic disorders, which was supported in our study through significantly higher insulin concentration and HOMA-IR values related to insulin resistance. In this group of obese children with diagnosed NAFLD, we demonstrated significantly higher IL-18 serum concentration compared to both healthy controls and non-NAFLD obese children. This is in line with results from the study of Vecchiet at al. [33] who demonstrated higher IL-18 in NAFLD adult patients compared to controls but lower IL-18 than in patients with chronic hepatitis C, indicating possible role of hepatic inflammation in addition to steatosis regarding IL-18 production. The significant positive correlations between serum IL-18 and ALT and other indices of hepatocytes injury as well as hsCRP shown in our study support this hypothesis. However, we were not able to demonstrate significant elevation of hsCRP in any group, because its measurement was carried out in limited number of patients.

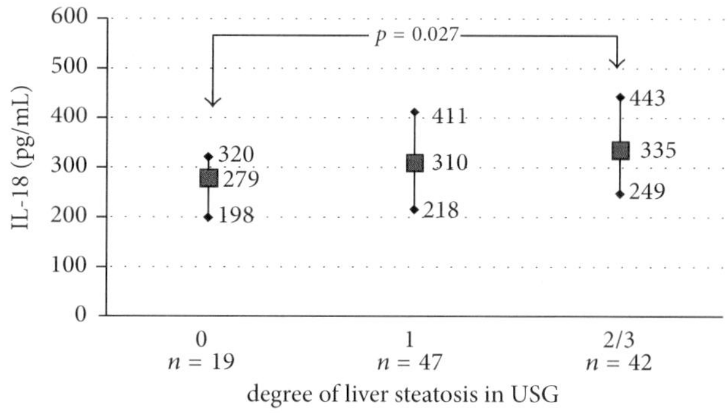

FIGURE 1: Median (min., max.) of IL-18 serum concentration depending on degree of liver steatosis in USG.

Contrary results with no effect on IL-18 in the absence of metabolic risk factors were demonstrated by Tapan et al. [38], but the study was conducted in male adults with NASH. IL-18 is a proinflammatory cytokine that can be produced by adipocytes, but also macrophages and Kupffer and endothelial cells [23, 24]. Therefore serum IL-18 production can be released as a result of inflammatory activity related to numerous concomitant health conditions, which obviously are much more frequent in adults than in children. Since children are less likely to have concomitant proinflammatory conditions than adults, measurement of IL-18 concentration can be useful for NAFLD diagnosis in children. In this study we were able to demonstrate significant increase of IL-18 serum concentrations with degree of liver steatosis measured using USG. To support results obtained with USG we applied ^{1}HMRS. Obtained results demonstrated that hepatopathic children with liver steatosis measured with ^{1}HMRS have significantly higher levels of serum IL-18 as well as steatosis score of 2 or 3 in USG than those without liver steatosis in ^{1}HMRS. IL-18 serum level above 326.8 pg/mL was finally demonstrated with ROC analysis as an optimal border for differentiation of NAFLD in children. Interestingly elevated IL-18 was accompanied by higher activities of hepatocyte injury enzymes in more advanced steatosis irrespective of diagnostic method with USG or ^{1}HMRS. On the other hand there was no effect of steatosis degree on cholesterol and glucose levels, but possible future metabolic problems in children with more advanced steatosis were indicated by significantly higher triglycerides level and insulin resistance.

TABLE 3: Comparison of obese children without liver steatosis ($n = 19$) and with advanced liver steatosis ($n = 42$) evaluated in USG according to Saverymuttu et al.

Parameters	No liver steatosis USG grade 0 median; Q1–Q3 ($n = 19$)	Advanced liver steatosis USG grade 2-3 median; Q1–Q3 ($n = 42$)	p
Gender, M/F	12/7	36/6	NS
IL-18 (pg/ml)	279; 198–320	335; 249–443	0.027
BMI (kg/m^2)	27; 25–30	28; 27–33	NS
Waist (cm)	90; 83–98	99; 93–107	0.014
ALT (IU/l)	20; 16–31	48; 36–77	0.000
AST (IU/l)	23; 20–29	32; 26–45	0.000
GGT (IU/l)	18; 13–23	27; 21–35	0.000
Bilirubin (mg/dl)	0.6; 0.5–0.7	0.6; 0.4–0.85	NS
Total cholesterol (mg/dl)	164; 137–182	170; 153–191	NS
HDL-C (mg/dl)	47; 39–56	42; 37–50	NS
LDL-C (mg/dl)	92; 73–111	96; 79–121	NS
TG (mg/dl)	86; 65–116	120; 88–167	0.004
Glucose (mg/dl)	90; 83–96	95; 90–99	NS
Insulin (μIU/ml)	14; 8–17	17; 12–21	NS
HOMA-IR	3.2; 1.9–3.7	3.9; 3–5.4	0.020
Uric acid (mg/dl)	5.9; 4.8–7	6.7; 5.6–7.3	NS
hsCRP (mg/l)	1.1; 0.7–2.2	1.1; 0.5–1.7	NS
Ferritin (ng/ml)	54; 29–66	58; 46–85	NS
A1AT (g/l)	1.4; 1.2–1.6	1.3; 1.2–1.4	NS
^{1}HMRS (r.u.)	38; 17–61	172; 123–216	0.000

TABLE 4: Comparison of obese children with ($n = 72$) and without ($n = 20$) liver steatosis diagnosed with measurement of intrahepatic lipid content using ^{1}HMRS.

Parameters	No liver steatosis in ^{1}HMRS median; Q1–Q3 ($n = 20$)	Liver steatosis in ^{1}HMRS median; Q1–Q3 ($n = 72$)	p
Gender, M/F	12/8	58/14	NS
IL-18 (pg/ml)	275; 205–340	342; 249–455	0.014
BMI (kg/m^2)	29; 27–32	28; 26–32	NS
Waist (cm)	96; 88–104	94; 90–105	NS
ALT (IU/l)	25; 16–45	37; 26–63	0.022
AST (IU/l)	24; 21–33	30; 25–39	0.013
GGT (IU/l)	17; 12–23	23; 18–31	0.016
Bilirubin (mg/dl)	0.7; 0.5–1.2	0.6; 0.4–0.8	NS
Total cholesterol (mg/dl)	172; 142–182	176; 150–192	NS
HDL-C (mg/dl)	50; 42–52	46; 39–55	NS
LDL-C (mg/dl)	92; 78–114	97; 78–121	NS
TG (mg/dl)	90; 61–120	115; 88–164	0.008
Glucose (mg/dl)	90; 85–95	92; 85–96	NS
Insulin (μIU/ml)	14; 8–18	15; 12–20	NS
HOMA-IR	3; 1.9–4	3.6; 2.8–4.6	NS
Uric acid (mg/dl)	5.7; 4.8–7	6; 5–6.8	NS
hsCRP (mg/l)	1; 0.7–2	1.3; 0.6–1.9	NS
Ferritin (ng/ml)	55; 29–73	57; 45–86	NS
A1AT (g/l)	1.4; 1.2–1.6	1.3; 1.2–1.5	NS
USG grade of steatosis	0.5; 0-1	1.5; 1-2	0.000

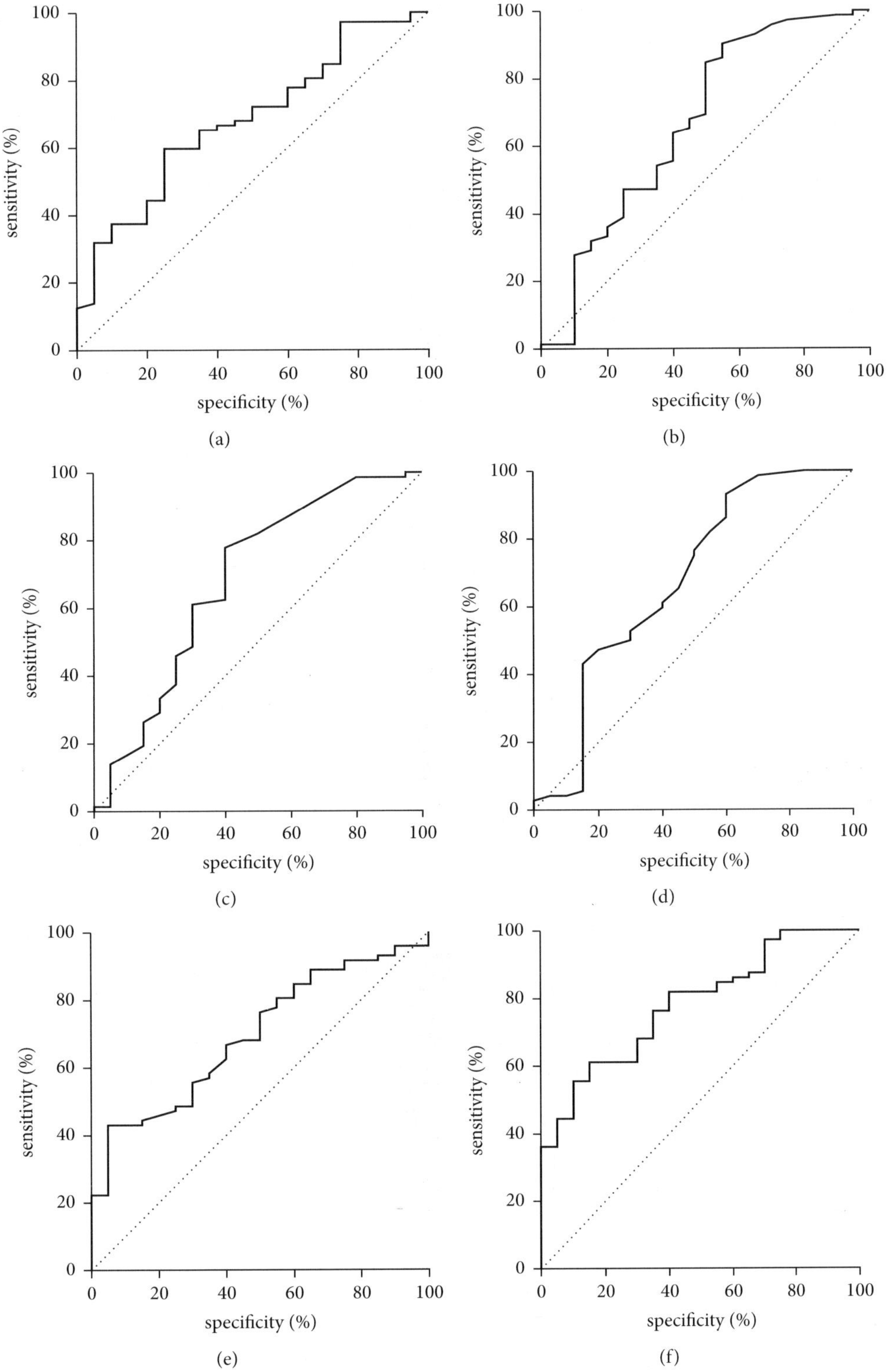

FIGURE 2: ROC curve for ability of IL-18 (a), ALT (b), AST (c), GGT (d), TG (e), and their combination (f) to detect children with liver steatosis in ^{1}HMRS.

TABLE 5: Analysis of AUC for IL-18, ALT, AST, GGT, and TG and their combination to detect children with liver steatosis in ^{1}HMRS.

Parameters	AUC	SE	95% CI (AUC)	p (AUC = 0,5)	p (AUC individual versus combined)
IL-18	0,6802	0,0653	(0,552–0,808)	0,0058	0,263
ALT	0,6681	0,0787	(0,514–0,822)	0,0327	0,253
AST	0,6830	0,0769	(0,532–0,834)	0,0173	0,279
GGT	0,6767	0,0792	(0,521–0,832)	0,0257	0,324
TG	0,6944	0,0614	(0,574–0,815)	0,0015	0,316
Combined	0,7826	0,0532	(0,678–0,887)	<0,0001	-

The studies on adults population have suggested that iron overload plays a significant role in pathogenesis of NAFLD and progression from simple steatosis to nonalcoholic steatohepatitis (NASH) through increasing oxidative stress and altering insulin signaling and lipid metabolism [13]. Since serum ferritin level is related to liver iron storage in NAFLD [39], we included measurement of ferritin in our study. Kowdley at al. [40] demonstrated recently elevated serum ferritin as an independent predictor of advanced hepatic fibrosis among adult patients with NAFLD. Our data confirmed possibility of similar effect in younger population, because of significantly higher ferritin serum concentration among obese NAFLD children. However, in contrast to IL-18 increase of ferritin serum level was not related to liver steatosis, which is contrary to data from adult population that showed predictive role of high serum ferritin as a risk factor for steatosis [41]. Based on these data we can conclude that serum ferritin is related mostly to inflammatory activity in NAFLD patients [42]. However according to results from our study and some literature data, this component of the disease can also be measured using hsCRP [43]. In contrast, elevated IL-18 can reflect degree of steatosis in addition to inflammation and therefore can be recognized as more representative for complexity of NAFLD pathogenesis.

This is a first study in obese children population investigating serum IL-18 concentration. Studies carried out in children may be more reliable compared to those in adults, because of infrequent confounding factors and less advanced disease. Large sample size of obese children is a main strength of our study. Additional value of our study was inclusion of new sensitive imaging technique to assess liver steatosis, such as proton magnetic resonance spectroscopy (^{1}HMRS), providing an opportunity of precise data interpretation [44]. However there are some potential limitations of the study. First of all, we did not perform histological examination to confirm diagnosis in the studied group. According to the ESPGHAN Hepatology Committee guidelines liver biopsy is preferred but imperfect gold standard, because as an invasive procedure it has important limitations in children, including risk of complications, cost, and possible sampling error [45]. Therefore, according to accepted recommendations liver biopsy should be performed only in children in very specific cases of NAFLD suspicion, such as suspected advanced disease, to exclude coexisting diseases, in patients below 10 years of age with elevated ALT activity and before therapeutic intervention [46]. Children included in our study did not meet these criteria; therefore we did not perform a liver biopsy. We still need to validate reliable, noninvasive tests that could be useful to evaluate children with suspected NAFLD and determine disease progression. Another limitation of our study was selection bias, because examined patients were recruited from a tertiary center, which is focused on pediatric hepatology. Therefore children with suspected liver disease were initially referred to the center and then included in the study group.

In conclusion, the study demonstrated association between NAFLD and IL-18 serum concentration in children. Based on this finding we can consider IL-18 as a useful novel noninvasive biomarker for differential diagnosis between obese children with and without NAFLD and prediction of possible metabolic disorders development.

Abbreviations

ALT:	Alanine aminotransferase
A1AT:	Alpha-1-antitrypsin
AUC:	Area under curve
AST:	Aspartate aminotransferase
BMI:	Body mass index
CRP:	C-reactive protein
DILI:	Drug-induced liver injury
GGT:	Gamma glutamyltransferase
HBV:	Hepatitis B virus
HCV:	Hepatitis C virus
HDL:	High-density lipoprotein
hsCRP:	High-sensitive C-reactive protein
HOMA-IR:	Homeostasis model assessment of insulin resistance
IR:	Insulin resistance
IFN-gamma:	Interferon-γ
IL-18:	Interleukin-18
LDL:	Low-density lipoprotein
MS:	Metabolic syndrome
NAFLD:	Nonalcoholic fatty liver disease
NASH:	Nonalcoholic steatohepatitis
^{1}HMRS:	Proton magnetic resonance spectroscopy
ROS:	Reactive oxygen species
ROC:	Receiver operating characteristics
TG:	Triglycerides
USG:	Ultrasonography
WBC:	White blood cell.

Ethical Approval

The study was approved by the bioethics committee of the Medical University of Białystok. All procedures performed in studies involving human participants were in accordance with the ethical standards of the institutional and/or national research committee and with the 1964 Helsinki declaration and its later amendments or comparable ethical standards.

Acknowledgments

The study was financially supported by Grants from Medical University of Białystok, Poland, nos. 143-43618L and 153-43771L.

References

[1] A. Alisi, G. Carpino, and V. Nobili, "Paediatric nonalcoholic fatty liver disease," *Current Opinion in Gastroenterology*, vol. 29, no. 3, pp. 279–284, 2013.

[2] C. Della Corte, A. Alisi, A. Saccari, R. De Vito, A. Vania, and V. Nobili, "Nonalcoholic fatty liver in children and adolescents: An overview," *Journal of Adolescent Health*, vol. 51, no. 4, pp. 305–312, 2012.

[3] M. Masarone, A. Federico, L. Abenavoli, C. Loguercio, and M. Persico, "Non alcoholic fatty liver: epidemiology and natural history," *Reviews on Recent Clinical Trials*, vol. 9, no. 3, pp. 126–133, 2014.

[4] E. M. Brunt, "Histopathology of nonalcoholic fatty liver disease," *World Journal of Gastroenterology*, vol. 16, no. 42, pp. 5286–5296, 2010.

[5] V. Nobili, G. Bedogni, R. Berni Canani et al., "The potential role of fatty liver in paediatric metabolic syndrome: a distinct phenotype with high metabolic risk?" *Pediatric Obesity*, vol. 7, no. 6, pp. e75–e80, 2012.

[6] J. B. Moore, "Non-alcoholic fatty liver disease: the hepatic consequence of obesity and the metabolic syndrome," *Proceedings of the Nutrition Society*, vol. 69, pp. 211–220, 2010.

[7] Z. Tariq, C. J. Green, and L. Hodson, "Are oxidative stress mechanisms the common denominator in the progression from hepatic steatosis towards non-alcoholic steatohepatitis (NASH)?" *Liver International*, vol. 34, no. 7, pp. e180–e190, 2014.

[8] M. Basaranoglu, G. Basaranoglu, and H. Sentürk, "From fatty liver to fibrosis: a tale of 'second hit'," *World Journal of Gastroenterology*, vol. 19, no. 8, pp. 1158–1165, 2013.

[9] D. Festi, R. Schiumerini, L. H. Eusebi, G. Marasco, M. Taddia, and A. Colecchia, "Gut microbiota and metabolic syndrome," *World Journal of Gastroenterology*, vol. 20, no. 43, pp. 16079–16094, 2014.

[10] S. Ferolla, G. Armiliato, C. Couto, and T. Ferrari, "The role of intestinal bacteria overgrowth in obesity-related nonalcoholic fatty liver disease," *Nutrients*, vol. 6, no. 12, pp. 5583–5599, 2014.

[11] J. M. Lotowska, M. E. Sobaniec-Lotowska, S. B. Bockowska, and D. M. Lebensztejn, "Pediatric non-alcoholic steatohepatitis: The first report on the ultrastructure of hepatocyte mitochondria," *World Journal of Gastroenterology*, vol. 20, no. 15, pp. 4335–4340, 2014.

[12] R. S. Rector, J. P. Thyfault, G. M. Uptergrove et al., "Mitochondrial dysfunction precedes insulin resistance and hepatic steatosis and contributes to the natural history of non-alcoholic fatty liver disease in an obese rodent model," *Journal of Hepatology*, vol. 52, no. 5, pp. 727–736, 2010.

[13] J. E. Nelson, H. Klintworth, and K. V. Kowdley, "Iron metabolism in Nonalcoholic Fatty Liver Disease," *Current Fungal Infection Reports*, vol. 14, no. 1, pp. 8–16, 2012.

[14] F. Demircioğlu, G. Görünmez, E. Dağıstan et al., "Serum hepcidin levels and iron metabolism in obese children with and without fatty liver: case-control study," *European Journal of Pediatrics*, vol. 173, no. 7, pp. 947–951, 2014.

[15] M. F. Abdelmalek, A. Suzuki, C. Guy et al., "Increased fructose consumption is associated with fibrosis severity in patients with nonalcoholic fatty liver disease," *Hepatology*, vol. 51, no. 6, pp. 1961–1971, 2010.

[16] H. Xu, G. T. Barnes, Q. Yang et al., "Chronic inflammation in fat plays a crucial role in the development of obesity-related insulin resistance," *The Journal of Clinical Investigation*, vol. 112, no. 12, pp. 1821–1830, 2003.

[17] H. Tilg and A. R. Moschen, "Evolution of inflammation in nonalcoholic fatty liver disease: the multiple parallel hits hypothesis," *Hepatology*, vol. 52, no. 5, pp. 1836–1846, 2010.

[18] R. De Vito, A. Alisi, A. Masotti, S. Ceccarelli, N. Panera, A. Citti et al., "Markers of activated inflammatory cells correlate with severity of liver damage in children with nonalcoholic fatty liver disease," *International Journal of Molecular Medicine*, vol. 30, pp. 49–56, 2012.

[19] M. Asrih and F. R. Jornayvaz, "Inflammation as a potential link between nonalcoholic fatty liver disease and insulin resistance," *Journal of Endocrinology*, vol. 218, no. 3, pp. R25–R36, 2013.

[20] S. Stojsavljevic, M. Gomerčić Palčić, L. Virović Jukić, L. Smirčić Duvnjak, and M. Duvnjak, "Adipokines and proinflammatory cytokines, the key mediators in the pathogenesis of nonalcoholic fatty liver disease," *World Journal of Gastroenterology*, vol. 20, no. 48, pp. 18070–18091, 2014.

[21] H. Tilg, "The role of cytokines in non-alcoholic fatty liver disease," *Digestive Diseases*, vol. 28, no. 1, pp. 179–185, 2010.

[22] M. Crespo, S. Lappe, A. E. Feldstein, and N. Alkhouri, "Similarities and differences between pediatric and adult nonalcoholic fatty liver disease," *Metabolism - Clinical and Experimental*, vol. 65, no. 8, pp. 1161–1171, 2016.

[23] C. A. Dinarello, "Interleukin-18 and the pathogenesis of inflammatory diseases," *Seminars in Nephrology*, vol. 27, no. 1, pp. 98–114, 2007.

[24] T. Skurk, H. Kolb, S. Müller-Scholze, K. Röhrig, H. Hauner, and C. Herder, "The proatherogenic cytokine interleukin-18 is secreted by human adipocytes," *European Journal of Endocrinology*, vol. 152, no. 6, pp. 863–868, 2005.

[25] J. A. Gracie, S. E. Robertson, and I. B. McInnes, "Interleukin-18," *Journal of Leukocyte Biology*, vol. 73, no. 2, pp. 213–224, 2003.

[26] C. A. Dinarello, D. Novick, S. Kim, and G. Kaplanski, "Interleukin-18 and IL-18 binding protein," *Frontiers in Immunology*, vol. 4, Article ID Article 289, 2013.

[27] M. Trøseid, I. Seljeflot, and H. Arnesen, "The role of interleukin-18 in the metabolic syndrome," *Cardiovascular Diabetology*, vol. 9, article no. 11, 2010.

[28] G. P. Van Guilder, G. L. Hoetzer, J. J. Greiner, B. L. Stauffer, and C. A. DeSouza, "Influence of metabolic syndrome on biomarkers of oxidative stress and inflammation in obese adults," *Obesity*, vol. 14, no. 12, pp. 2127–2131, 2006.

[29] C. P. Fischer, L. B. Perstrup, A. Berntsen, P. Eskildsen, and B.

K. Pedersen, "Elevated plasma interleukin-18 is a marker of insulin-resistance in type 2 diabetic and non-diabetic humans," *Clinical Immunology*, vol. 117, no. 2, pp. 152–160, 2005.

[30] M. Trøseid, I. Seljeflot, E. M. Hjerkinn, and H. Arnesen, "Interleukin-18 is a strong predictor of cardiovascular events in elderly men with the metabolic syndrome synergistic effect of inflammation and hyperglycemia," *Diabetes Care*, vol. 32, no. 3, pp. 486–492, 2009.

[31] O. Ludwiczek, A. Kaser, D. Novick et al., "Plasma levels of interleukin-18 and interleukin-18 binding protein are elevated in patients with chronic liver disease," *Journal of Clinical Immunology*, vol. 22, no. 6, pp. 331–337, 2002.

[32] A. López-Bermejo, M. Bosch, M. Recasens et al., "Potential role of interleukin-18 in liver disease associated with insulin resistance," *Obesity Research*, vol. 13, no. 11, pp. 1925–1931, 2005.

[33] J. Vecchiet, K. Falasca, P. Cacciatore et al., "Association between plasma interleukin-18 levels and liver injury in chronic hepatitis C virus infection and non-alcoholic fatty liver disease," *Annals of Clinical & Laboratory Science*, vol. 35, no. 4, pp. 415–422, 2005.

[34] J. J. Reilly, "Diagnostic accuracy of the BMI for age in paediatrics," *International Journal of Obesity*, vol. 30, no. 4, pp. 595–597, 2006.

[35] D. R. Matthews, J. P. Hosker, A. S. Rudenski, B. A. Naylor, D. F. Treacher, and R. C. Turner, "Homeostasis model assessment: insulin resistance and β-cell function from fasting plasma glucose and insulin concentrations in man," *Diabetologia*, vol. 28, no. 7, pp. 412–419, 1985.

[36] S. H. Saverymuttu, A. E. A. Joseph, and J. D. Maxwell, "Ultrasound scanning in the detection of hepatic fibrosis and steatosis," *British Medical Journal*, vol. 292, no. 6512, pp. 13–15, 1986.

[37] E. Tarasów, L. Siergiejczyk, A. Panasiuk et al., "MR proton spectroscopy in liver examinations of healthy individuals in vivo," *Medical Science Monitor*, vol. 8, no. 2, pp. MT36–MT40, 2002.

[38] S. Tapan, T. Dogru, M. Kara et al., "Circulating levels of interleukin-18 in patients with non-alcoholic fatty liver disease," *Scandinavian Journal of Clinical & Laboratory Investigation*, vol. 70, no. 6, pp. 399–403, 2010.

[39] M. D. Beaton, S. Chakrabarti, and P. C. Adams, "Inflammation is not the cause of an elevated serum Ferritin in non-alcoholic fatty liver disease," *Annals of Hepatology*, vol. 13, no. 3, pp. 353–356, 2014.

[40] K. V. Kowdley, P. Belt, L. A. Wilson et al., "Serum ferritin is an independent predictor of histologic severity and advanced fibrosis in patients with nonalcoholic fatty liver disease," *Hepatology*, vol. 55, no. 1, pp. 77–85, 2012.

[41] A. Licata, M. E. Nebbia, G. Cabibbo et al., "Hyperferritinemia is a risk factor for steatosis in chronic liver disease," *World Journal of Gastroenterology*, vol. 15, no. 17, pp. 2132–2138, 2009.

[42] J. H. Na, S. W. Park, Y. Kang, H. Koh, and S. Kim, "The clinical significance of serum ferritin in pediatric non-alcoholic fatty liver disease," *Pediatric Gastroenterology, Hepatology and Nutrition*, vol. 17, no. 4, pp. 248–256, 2014.

[43] K. Kitsios, M. Papadopoulou, K. Kosta, N. Kadoglou, M. Papagianni, and K. Tsiroukidou, "High-sensitivity C-reactive protein levels and metabolic disorders in obese and overweight children and adolescents," *Journal of Clinical Research in Pediatric Endocrinology*, vol. 5, no. 1, pp. 44–49, 2013.

[44] N. F. Schwenzer, F. Springer, C. Schraml, N. Stefan, J. Machann, and F. Schick, "Non-invasive assessment and quantification of liver steatosis by ultrasound, computed tomography and magnetic resonance," *Journal of Hepatology*, vol. 51, no. 3, pp. 433–445, 2009.

[45] P. Vajro, S. Lenta, P. Socha et al., "Diagnosis of nonalcoholic fatty liver disease in children and adolescents: position paper of the ESPGHAN hepatology committee," *Journal of Pediatric Gastroenterology and Nutrition*, vol. 54, no. 5, pp. 700–713, 2012.

[46] E. A. Roberts, "Pediatric nonalcoholic fatty liver disease (NAFLD): A "growing" problem?" *Journal of Hepatology*, vol. 46, no. 6, pp. 1133–1142, 2007.

10

Macroscopic Portal Vein Thrombosis in HCC Patients

Hikmet Akkiz,[1] Brian I. Carr,[2] Sedef Kuran,[1] Ümit Karaoğullarından,[1] Oguz Üsküdar,[1] Salih Tokmak,[1] Burcu Arslan,[1] Figen Doran,[1] Hüseyin Tugsan Balli,[1] Abdulalh Ülkü,[1] Tolga Atılgan Akçam,[1] Halil İbrahim Bahçeci,[3] Kamil Yalçın Polat,[4] Necati Örmeci,[5] Halis Şimşek,[6] Abdullah Sonsuz,[7] Ali Demir,[8] Engin Altıntaş,[9] Mehmet Demir,[10] Kendal Yalçın,[11] Nazım Ekinci,[11] Ayşegül Harmancı Özakyol,[12] Mehmet Yücesoy,[13] Ahmet Uygun,[14] Vito Guerra,[15] Anıl Delik,[1] Yaman Tokat,[16] Sezai Yilmaz,[17] Ahmet Bektaş,[18] and Murat Kılıç[19]

[1] *Çukurova University Gastroenterology Department, Adana, Turkey*
[2] *İzmir Biomedicine and Genome Institute, Dokuz Eylül University, İzmir, Turkey*
[3] *Fırat University, Turkey*
[4] *İstanbul Memorial Hospital, Turkey*
[5] *Ankara University, Turkey*
[6] *Hacettepe University, Turkey*
[7] *İstanbul Cerrahpaşa University, Turkey*
[8] *Konya Necmettin Erbakan University, Turkey*
[9] *Mersin University, Turkey*
[10] *Hatay Mustafa Kemal University, Turkey*
[11] *Dicle University, Turkey*
[12] *Eskişehir Osmangazi University, Turkey*
[13] *Erciyes University, Turkey*
[14] *Haydarpaşa Sultan Abdülhamid Eğitim Araştırma Hospital, Turkey*
[15] *Trials Centre, National Institute for Digestive Diseases, IRCCS "Saverio de Bellis", Castellana, Bari, Italy*
[16] *Florence Nightingale Hospital, İstanbul, Turkey*
[17] *İnonu University, Malatya, Turkey*
[18] *Ondokuz Mayıs University, Turkey*
[19] *Izmir Kent Hospital, Turkey*

Correspondence should be addressed to Brian I. Carr; brianicarr@hotmail.com

Academic Editor: Pascal Lapierre

Macroscopic portal vein invasion (PVT) by hepatocellular carcinoma (HCC) in the liver is one of the most important negative prognostic factors for HCC patients. The characteristics of a large cohort of such patients were examined. We found that the percent of patients with PVT significantly increased with increasing maximum tumor diameter (MTD), from 13.7% with tumors of MTD <5cm to 56.4% with tumors of MTD >10cm. There were similar numbers of HCC patients with very large tumors with and without PVT. Thus, MTD alone was insufficient to explain the presence of PVT, as were high AFP levels, since less than 50% of high AFP patients had PVT. However, the percent of patients with PVT was also found to significantly increase with increasing blood alpha-fetoprotein (AFP) levels and tumor multifocality. A logistic regression model that included these 3 factors together showed an odds ratio of 17.9 for the combination of MTD>5.0cm plus tumor multifocality plus elevated AFP, compared to low levels of these 3 parameters. The presence or absence of macroscopic PVT may therefore represent different HCC aggressiveness phenotypes, as judged by a significant increase in tumor multifocality and AFP levels in the PVT positive patients. Factors in addition to MTD and AFP must also contribute to PVT development.

1. Introduction

The prognosis of patients with hepatocellular carcinoma (HCC) depends upon both tumor factors and liver factors [1]. The tumor factors include the maximum tumor diameter (MTD), number of tumors, presence of macroscopic (clinically evident) portal vein thrombosis (PVT), and blood levels of alpha-fetoprotein (AFP). The presence of PVT may be the most important tumor factor, as it reflects tumor aggressiveness (migration, invasion, and potential for metastasis), limits the options for curative resection or transplantation, and can also worsen residual liver function. It is thought that up to 45% of HCC patients have some form of macroscopic PVT [2–5] and may be gross or macroscopic as shown on CT or MRI scan or microscopic as evidenced only on pathology. It is poorly understood, with few biological models and little understanding of its causes. However, predisposing factors include increased MTD, with increased levels of the HCC plasma tumor markers des-gamma carboxyprothrombin (DCP) and AFP, decreased serum albumin, and elevated platelet counts [6–11]. The current study in a large HCC cohort confirms the increased percent of PVT with increasing MTD, as well as with increasing multifocality and AFP. Furthermore, we found that PVT occurred in 13.7% of small HCCs <5cm, but in 56.4% of large HCCs >10cm.

2. Methods

2.1. Patient Data. We analyzed a database of 1773 prospectively accrued HCC patients who had full baseline tumor parameter data, including CT scan information on HCC size, number of tumor nodules, and presence or absence of PVT and plasma AFP levels; complete blood count; routine blood liver function tests (total bilirubin, GGTP, ALKP, albumin, and transaminases); and patient demographics. Diagnosis was made either via tumor biopsy or according to international guidelines. Of these patients, 1029 had low AFP levels (≤100 IU/ml) and are the subject of this study. Database management conformed to legislation on privacy and this study conforms to the ethical guidelines of the Declaration of Helsinki and approval for this retrospective study on deidentified HCC patients was obtained by the Institutional Review Board.

2.2. Statistical Analysis. Mean and SD for continuous variables and relative frequency for categorical variables were used as indices of centrality and dispersion of the distribution. For categorical variables, the Chi-square and z test for proportions were used. The Wilcoxon rank-sum (Mann–Whitney) test was to test the difference between two categories and the Kruskal-Wallis rank test to test the difference among categories.

Logistic regression model was to evaluate the associations between PVT (No/Yes) on single variables examined.

Final multiple linear or logistic regression models were obtained with the backward stepwise method and the variables that showed associations with $p<0.10$ were left in the models.

When testing the null hypothesis of no association, the probability level of α error, two tailed, was 0.05. All the statistical computations were made using STATA 12.1 Statistical Software (StataCorp), 2014, release 12 (College Station, TX).

3. Results

3.1. PVT in Tumor Size (MTD) Groups. Patients were initially analyzed according to PVT status in different tumor size (MTD) groups (Table 1). There was a large percent increase in PVT positive patients with increase in MTD, 13.7% for small tumors, 33.9% for intermediate tumors, and 56.4% for very large tumors. For small and intermediate size tumor patients, there were more Child-Pugh score A patients without PVT. However, the prevalence of cirrhosis was not different across MTD groups, nor were there differences in total serum bilirubin values. Albumin values were lower in the patients with PVT, but significant only for the small tumor groups. Patients with PVT had a small but significant increase in MTD, in the small and intermediate size tumor groups compared to patients without PVT. However, the AFP levels were significantly higher in the PVT positive patients, for all 3 tumor size groups, as was tumor multifocality. Thus, on the whole, patients with PVT had larger and more multifocal tumors with higher AFP values, yet similar bilirubin levels, across the tumor size groups.

3.2. PVT-Associated Parameters. The parameters that were associated with presence of PVT were next examined. A logistic regression model of PVT showed significance for several single parameters as continuous variables (Table 2(A)), but when all parameters were considered together, there was significance in the final model (Table 2(B)) for tumor multifocality, MTD, AFP, ALKP, and albumin. Two of these parameters versus PVT values are shown graphically in Figure 1, which shows significant increases in percent PVT, in relation to increase of both MTD and AFP. However, even in the highest AFP categories, less than r50% of patients had PVT (Figure 2).

A logistic regression model of PVT was then performed for the variables of MTD (large or small), AFP (high or low), and tumor multifocality versus unifocality, considered singularly (Table 3(A)) or together (Table 3(B)), as these were the 3 parameters with highest odds ratio (OR) in Table 2. High ORs were found for the high values of each of the 3 parameters, whether considered singularly or together. However, when we combined all 3 parameters of MTD >5cm plus tumor multifocality plus AFP >100 IU/ml, an OR of 17.9 was obtained (Table 3(C)).

4. Discussion

Clinical macroscopic PVT is typically diagnosed as obstruction and expansion of the portal vein on CT or MRI scan [12–14] or by contrast-enhanced ultrasonography [15]. It is associated with several serum changes, such as the des-gamma-carboxy-prothrombin/vitamin K pathway [16–23] and is a well-recognized predictor of poor survival in

Table 1: Comparisons amongst HCC patients between portal vein thrombosis groups, in single MTD categories.

Parameter*	MTD<5.0 (cm)			5.0≤MTD≤10.0 (cm)			MTD>10.0 (cm)		
	PVT(No) (n=701)	PVT(Yes) (n=112) (13.7%)	p^{ψ}	PVT(No) (n=388)	PVT(Yes) (n=199) (33.9%)	p^{ψ}	PVT(No) (n=84)	PVT(Yes) (n=109) (56.4%)	p^{ψ}
Sex (M) (%)	145 (79.32)	88 (78.57)	0.86^	319 (82.22)	164 (82.41)	0.95^	72 (85.71)	96 (88.07)	0.63^
Age (yr)	61.55±11.04	61.59±11.53	0.98	63.86±10.95	61.24±11.88	0.005	63.89±12.52	60.69±13.68	0.08
Cigarettes smoke (%)	159 (44.04)	32 (42.11)	0.76^	129 (60.85)	79 (56.03)	0.37^	26 (55.32)	32 (57.14)	0.85^
Alcohol (%)	63 (17.65)	8 (11.11)	0.17^	27 (13.85)	25 (18.12)	0.29^	7 (20.00)	7 (12.07)	0.30^
Child-Pugh (B&C)			0.01 ^			<0.001^			0.47 ^
A	217 (39.19)	18 (22.22)		138 (44.23)	44 (26.04)		26 (35.14)	23 (26.44)	
B	212 (38.27)	41 (50.62)		118 (37.82)	70 (41.42)		28 (37.84)	39 (44.83)	
C	125 (22.56)	22 (27.16)		56 (17.95)	55 (32.54)		20 (27.03)	25 (28.74)	
Cirrhosis (%)	542 (79.47)	88 (87.13)	0.07 ^	301 (77.98)	168 (85.71)	0.03^	62 (73.81)	81 (77.88)	0.51 ^
Albumin (g/dL)	3.15±0.76	2.95±0.76	0.02	3.11±0.75	2.97±0.71	0.07	3.04±0.74	3.00±0.63	0.60
GGTP (U/L)	148.07±186.14	143.42±134.30	0.41	147.47±153.36	210.61±206.48	0.0003	186.06±153.04	213.74±175.12	0.34
AST (U/L)	118.06±226.07	102.20±92.59	0.86	100.88±121.40	114.37±105.87	0.02	146.35±425.67	114.46±112.63	0.07
ALKP (U/L)	190.97±216.09	191.34±168.76	0.40	193.97±139.92	279.19±313.31	0.02	232.77±149.04	268.86±241.38	0.96
Bilirubin (mg/dL)	2.41±3.45	2.52±3.41	0.67	2.27±3.67	3.60±5.44	0.009	1.96±3.06	2.58±3.61	0.22
Platelet counts ($10^3/\mu L$)	139.16±85.58	141.80±90.29	0.92	161.86±89.36	180.04±108.38	0.10	226.94±141.19	227.79±127.74	0.63
AFP (IU/mL)	1774.84±13163.19	2722.60±8062.90	<0.0001	3504.43±18586.15	10976.9±54278.4	0.0007	9395.0±29325.7	18393.3±55766.2	0.02
MTD (cm)	2.91±1.01	3.13±0.94	0.03	7.00±1.73	7.47±1.66	0.0004	14.29±3.56	14.24±3.17	0.91
Nodules number (%)			0.002 ^			<0.001^			<0.001^
Unifocal	507 (72.53)	62 (57.94)		271 (70.76)	98 (50.52)		67 (79.76)	55 (55.00)	
Multifocality (≥2)	192 (27.47)	45 (42.06)		112 (29.24)	96 (49.48)		17 (20.24)	45 (45.00)	

* All values: means ± standard deviation as continuous; Frequencies and percentage (%) as categorical.
$^{\psi}$ Wilcoxon rank-sum (Mann–Whitney) test; ^ Chi-square test.
GGTP, gamma glutamyl transpeptidase; ALKP, alkaline phosphatase; AFP, alpha-fetoprotein; MTD, maximum tumor diameter; PVT, portal vein thrombosis.

TABLE 2: Logistic regression model of PVT *(No/Yes)*, on single variables **(A)**. Final multiple logistic regression model in stepwise method of PVT *(No/Yes)*, on all variables included together in the model **(B)**. All models in total cohort.

Parameter *	OR	se(OR)	p-value	95% C.I.
(A)				
Platelet counts ($10^3/\mu L$)	1.002	0.001	0.003	1.001 to 1.004
Hemoglobin (g/dL)	0.899	0.034	0.005	0.835 to 0.969
GGTP (U/L)	1.001	0.0004	0.006	1.0003 to 1.0021
ALKP (U/L)	1.001	0.0004	0.002	1.0004 to 1.0019
Total Bilirubin (mg/dL)	1.042	0.021	0.04	1.002 to 1.084
Albumin (g/dL)	0.711	0.080	0.002	0.571 to 0.887
AFP (IU/mL)				
≤100 *[Ref. category]*	1			
>100	2.091	0.354	<0.001	1.500 to 2.913
MTD (cm)	1.178	0.027	<0.001	1.127 to 1.231
Tumor Nodule #	1.714	0.284	0.001	1.238 to 2.372
Cirrhosis (yes)	1.388	0.303	0.13	0.905 to 2.130
(B)				
ALKP (U/L)	1.001	0.0004	0.02	1.0001 to 1.0017
Albumin (g/dL)	0.758	0.093	0.02	0.595 to 0.965
AFP (IU/mL)				
≤100 *[Ref. category]*	1			
>100	1.632	0.297	0.007	1.143 to 2.331
MTD (cm)	1.166	0.027	<0.001	1.114 to 1.219
Tumor Nodule #	1.558	0.281	0.01	1.094 to 2.219

* All variables included in the model were considered as continuous, except the AFP which was considered as categorical.
OR, odds ratio; se(OR), standard error of odds ratio; GGTP, gamma glutamyl transpeptidase; ALKP, alkaline phosphatase; AFP, alpha-fetoprotein; MTD, maximum tumor diameter; PVT, portal vein thrombosis.

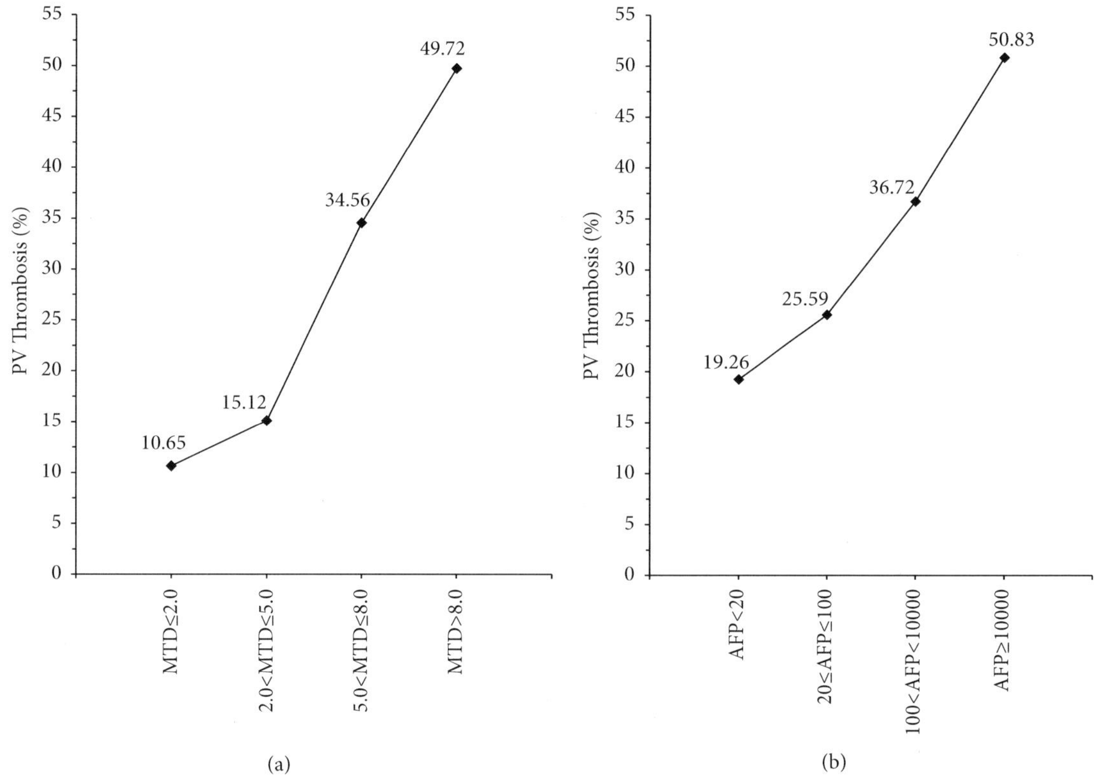

FIGURE 1: Percentage of patients with PV Thrombosis in **(a)** MTD (cm) categories, in total cohort ($p < 0.0001^*$)$^;$ **(b)** AFP (IU/mL) categories ($p < 0.0001^*$)$^;$ * Chi-square test for trend; PVT, portal vein thrombosis; MTD, maximum tumor dimension; AFP, alpha-fetoprotein.

TABLE 3: Logistic regression model of PVT (*No/Yes*), on single variables (**A**), all as categories. Final multiple logistic regression model in stepwise method of PVT (*No/Yes*), on all variables as categories, included together in the model (**B**). Combination of MTD (<5.0/≥5.0), focality (Unifocality/Multifocality), and AFP (≤100/>100) (**C**).

Parameter	OR	se(OR)	p-value	95% C.I.
(A)				
MTD (cm)				
<5.0 *[Ref. category]*	1			
≥5.0	3.97	0.53	<0.001	3.05 to 5.17
Tumor Nodule #				
Unifocality (n=1) *[Ref. category]*	1			
Multifocality (n≥2)	2.43	0.31	<0.001	1.90 to 3.11
AFP (IU/mL)				
≤100 *[Ref. category]*	1			
>100	2.55	0.32	<0.001	2.00 to 3.25
(B)				
MTD (cm)				
<5.0 *[Ref. category]*	1			
≥5.0	3.49	0.48	<0.001	2.66 to 4.57
Tumor Nodule #				
Unifocality (n=1) *[Ref. category]*	1			
Multifocality (n≥2)	2.22	0.29	<0.001	1.71 to 2.88
AFP (IU/mL)				
≤100 *[Ref. category]*	1			
>100	2.05	0.27	<0.001	1.58 to 2.65
(C)				
Combination of: MTD, Focality, and AFP				
MTD<5.0 & Unifocality & AFP≤100 *[Ref. category]*	1			
MTD<5.0 & Unifocality & AFP>100	2.80	0.82	<0.001	1.57 to 4.99
MTD<5.0 & Multifocality & AFP≤100	2.17	0.71	0.02	1.15 to 4.11
MTD<5.0 & Multifocality & AFP>100	6.93	2.31	<0.001	3.60 to 13.31
MTD≥5.0 & Unifocality & AFP≤100	4.68	1.20	<0.001	2.83 to 7.73
MTD≥5.0 & Unifocality & AFP>100	7.48	1.92	<0.001	4.52 to 12.38
MTD≥5.0 & Multifocality & AFP≤100	9.50	2.76	<0.001	5.37 to 16.80
MTD≥5.0 & Multifocality & AFP>100	17.94	4.80	<0.001	10.62 to 30.30

OR, odds ratio; se(OR), standard error of odds ratio; PVT, portal vein thrombosis; MTD, maximum tumor diameter; AFP, alpha-fetoprotein.

HCC patients [1, 5–7, 24–26]. It is typically diagnosed radiologically [13–15] and although pathological confirmation often requires examination of resected or transplantation specimens, percutaneous biopsy material can also be used [27, 28]. Despite this, some factors have been associated with discriminate better survival among patients with PVT. These include serum albumin levels [9], C-reactive protein [11], and AFP levels [29] and some subsets of patients have been identified as having better prognosis [24, 25, 30, 31]. The causes of increased death in HCC patients with PVT include worsened residual liver function and the presence of tumor cells in the vein as a pathway to systemic spread of tumor and distant metastasis.

The mechanisms involved in the pathogenesis of PVT include disruption of the tumor matrix, migration and invasion of the tumor cells, systemic inflammation [32], and DCP [16–19]. AFP levels are typically elevated in HCC patients with PVT, but whether they are cause or consequence is unclear.

Treatment of HCC patients with PVT is controversial [5] with more than usual complications and some limited survival benefit [33, 34]. Recently, radioembolization has emerged as a safer therapy [35, 36], but its effects on survival have yet to be proved. However, some evidence suggests that chemoembolization may also be useful in the presence of PVT [37, 38]. Furthermore, Sorafenib has been found to be a safe treatment in this setting [39] and may be as effective as radioembolization. In additional, multiple different radiation modalities have been evaluated in the presence of PVT, with few differences between them [40].

A major finding in this analysis was the increase in % of patients with PVT as MTD increased (Tables 1, 2, and 3, Figure 1). We considered 2 possible explanations for this. One is that the same factors that induce tumor growth, such as stem cells or growth factors, also enhance tumor invasion and thus MTD. Alternatively, there might be some change in HCC biology beyond a certain size that is associated with more

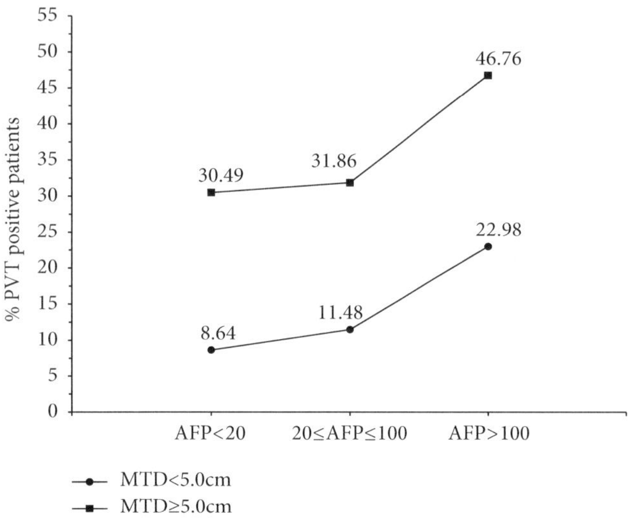

FIGURE 2: Percentage of patients with PVT in MTD (cm) categories: MTD<5.0cm ($p < 0.0001^*$) and MTD≥5.0cm ($p < 0.0001^*$). * Chi-square test for trend; PVT, portal vein thrombosis; MTD, maximum tumor dimension (cm); AFP, alpha-fetoprotein (IU/mL).

aggressive features. Table 1 shows that the proportion of very large MTD tumors with and without PVT is similar. Furthermore, within this category, average MTD is almost identical. This suggests that it is not tumor size per se. Perhaps there are 2 different growth pathways, one associated with PVT and the other not. This could explain why large tumors are well represented in the PVT positive and negative groups (Table 1). The same Table 1 also shows that both tumor multifocality and average AFP values are always significantly higher in every MTD category that has PVT patients compared to each PVT negative category, suggesting that the tumors are more aggressive in the PVT patients, whether they are larger or not. However, even in the highest AFP groups, less than 50% of the patients were PVT positive, as shown in Figure 2. Other reports have found elevated bilirubin levels in PVT patients, but our data do not really show this. Thus, the patients with PVT in this cohort have aggressive HCCs which did not destroy sufficient liver parenchyma to cause liver failure. PVT is generally classified as macroscopic or microscopic [5]. The current study was based on clinical/nonsurgical evidence (macroscopic) for PVT. Thus, a proportion of our patients classed as PVT negative macroscopically could still be PVT positive microscopically. It has also been reported that PVT seems to occur at a very early stage of HCC evolution [41]. These findings support the idea of 2 possible HCC developmental pathways, namely, HCCs with and without macroscopic PVT. Factors other than MTD and AFP must also be involved in the development of PVT.

Abbreviations

HCC: Hepatocellular carcinoma
PVT: Portal vein thrombosis
AFP: Alpha-fetoprotein
GGTP: Gamma glutamyl transpeptidase
ALKP: Alkaline phosphatase
AST: Aspartate aminotransferase
Alb: Albumin
MTD: Maximum tumor diameter
CRP: C-reactive protein
CT: Computerized axial tomography
MRI: Magnetic resonance imaging.

Authors' Contributions

Hikmet Akkiz and Brian I. Carr contributed equally.

Acknowledgments

This work is supported in part by NIH Grant CA 82723 (Brian I. Carr)

References

[1] B. I. Carr, P. Pancoska, and R. A. Branch, "Tumor and liver determinants of prognosis in unresectable hepatocellular carcinoma: a large case cohort study," *Hepatology International*, vol. 4, no. 1, pp. 396–405, 2010.

[2] M. Schöniger-Hekele, C. Müller, M. Kutilek, C. Oesterreicher et al., "Hepatocellular carcinoma in Central Europe: prognostic features and survival," *Gut*, vol. 48, pp. 103–109, 2001.

[3] M. Pirisi, C. Avellini, C. Fabris et al., "Portal vein thrombosis in hepatocellular carcinoma: Age and sex distribution in an autopsy study," *Journal of Cancer Research and Clinical Oncology*, vol. 124, no. 7, pp. 397–400, 1998.

[4] S. Roayaie, I. N. Blume, S. N. Thung et al., "A system of classifying microvascular invasion to predict outcome after resection in patients with hepatocellular carcinoma," *Gastroenterology*, vol. 137, no. 3, pp. 850–855, 2009.

[5] M. Quirk, Y. H. Kim, S. Saab, and E. W. Lee, "Management of hepatocellular carcinoma with portal vein thrombosis," *World Journal of Gastroenterology*, vol. 21, no. 12, pp. 3462–3471, 2015.

[6] S. Hagiwara, M. Kudo, T. Kawasaki et al., "Prognostic factors for portal venous invasion in patients with hepatocellular carcinoma," *Journal of Gastroenterology*, vol. 41, no. 12, pp. 1214–1219, 2006.

[7] M. Gotoh, "Prediction of invasive activities in hepatocellular carcinomas with special reference to alpha-fetoprotein and des-gamma-carboxyprothrombin," *Japanese Journal of Clinical Oncology*, vol. 33, no. 10, pp. 522–526, 2003.

[8] Y. Koike, Y. Shiratori, S. Sato et al., "Des-gamma-carboxy prothrombin as a useful predisposing factor for the development of portal venous invasion in patients with hepatocellular carcinoma: a prospective analysis of 227 patients," *Cancer*, vol. 91, pp. 561–569, 2001.

[9] B. I. Carr and V. Guerra, "Serum Albumin Levels in Relation to Tumor Parameters in Hepatocellular Carcinoma Patients," *The International Journal of Biological Markers*, vol. 32, no. 4, pp. 391–396, 2017.

[10] A. Kinoshita, H. Onoda, K. Takano et al., "Pretreatment serum C-reactive protein level predicts poor prognosis in patients with hepatocellular carcinoma," *Medical Oncology*, vol. 29, no. 4, pp. 2800–2808, 2012.

[11] J. M. Kim, C. H. D. Kwon, J.-W. Joh et al., "C-reactive protein may be a prognostic factor in hepatocellular carcinoma with malignant portal vein invasion," *World Journal of Surgical Oncology*, vol. 11, article no. 92, 2013.

[12] C. R. Taylor, "Computed tomography in the evaluation of the portal venous system," *Journal of Clinical Gastroenterology*, vol. 14, no. 2, pp. 167–172, 1992.

[13] M. E. Tublin, G. D. Dodd 3rd, and R. L. Baron, "Benign and malignant portal vein thrombosis: differentiation by CT characteristics," *American Journal of Roentgenology*, vol. 168, no. 3, pp. 719–723, 1997.

[14] S. Rossi, G. Ghittoni, V. Ravetta et al., "Contrast-enhanced ultrasonography and spiral computed tomography in the detection and characterization of portal vein thrombosis complicating hepatocellular carcinoma," *European Radiology*, vol. 18, no. 8, pp. 1749–1756, 2008.

[15] L. Tarantino, P. Ambrosino, and M. N. D. Di Minno, "Contrast-enhanced ultrasound in differentiating malignant from benign portal vein thrombosis in hepatocellular carcinoma," *World Journal of Gastroenterology*, vol. 21, no. 32, pp. 9457–9460, 2015.

[16] M. Suzuki, H. Shiraha, T. Fujikawa et al., "Des-γ-carboxy prothrombin is a potential autologous growth factor for hepatocellular carcinoma," *The Journal of Biological Chemistry*, vol. 280, no. 8, pp. 6409–6415, 2005.

[17] Y. Zhang, J. Chu, S. Cui, Z. Song, and X. Qu, "Des-gamma-carboxy prothrombin (DCP) as a potential autologous growth factor for the development of hepatocellular carcinoma," *Cellular Physiology and Biochemistry*, vol. 34, no. 3, pp. 903–915, 2014.

[18] P. Yue, Z.-H. Gao, X. Xue et al., "Des-γ-carboxyl prothrombin induces matrix metalloproteinase activity in hepatocellular carcinoma cells by involving the ERK1/2 MAPK signalling pathway," *European Journal of Cancer*, vol. 47, no. 7, pp. 1115–1124, 2011.

[19] T. Suehiro, T. Matsumata, H. Itasaka, A. Taketomi, K. Yamamoto, and K. Sugimachi, "Des-gamma-carboxy prothrombin and proliferative activity of hepatocellular carcinoma," *Surgery*, vol. 117, no. 6, pp. 682–691, 1995.

[20] M. Ma, X.-J. Qu, G.-Y. Mu et al., "Vitamin K2 inhibits the growth of hepatocellular carcinoma via decrease of des-gamma-carboxy prothrombin," *Chemotherapy*, vol. 55, pp. 28–35, 2009.

[21] M. Otsuka, N. Kato, R.-X. Shao et al., "Vitamin K2 inhibits the growth and invasiveness of hepatocellular carcinoma cells via protein kinase A activation," *Hepatology*, vol. 40, no. 1, pp. 243–251, 2004.

[22] B. I. Carr, Z. Wang, M. Wang, and G. Wei, "Differential effects of vitamin K1 on AFP and DCP levels in patients with unresectable HCC and in HCC cell lines," *Digestive Diseases and Sciences*, vol. 56, no. 6, pp. 1876–1883, 2011.

[23] Z. Wang, M. Wang, F. Finn, and B. I. Carr, "The growth inhibitory effects of vitamins K and their actions on gene expression," *Hepatology*, vol. 22, no. 3, pp. 876–882, 1995.

[24] J. Bruix, A. Cheng, G. Meinhardt, K. Nakajima, Y. De Sanctis, and J. Llovet, "Prognostic factors and predictors of sorafenib benefit in patients with hepatocellular carcinoma: Analysis of two phase III studies," *Journal of Hepatology*, vol. 67, no. 5, pp. 999–1008, 2017.

[25] A. A. Mokdad, A. G. Singal, J. A. Marrero, H. Zhu, and A. C. Yopp, "Vascular Invasion and Metastasis is Predictive of Outcome in Barcelona Clinic Liver Cancer Stage C Hepatocellular Carcinoma," *Journal of the National Comprehensive Cancer Network*, vol. 15, no. 2, pp. 197–204, 2017.

[26] The Cancer of the Liver Italian Program (CLIP) Investigators, "Prospective validation of the CLIP score: a new prognostic system for patients with cirrhosis and hepatocellular carcinoma," *Hepatology*, vol. 31, pp. 840–845, 2000.

[27] Dodd GD 3rd and B. I. Carr, "Percutaneous biopsy of portal vein thrombus: A new staging technique for hepatocellular carcinoma," *American Journal of Roentgenology*, vol. 161, pp. 229–233, 1993.

[28] I. De Sio, L. Castellano, M. Calandra, M. Romano, M. Persico, and C. Del Vecchio-blanco, "Ultrasound guided fine needle aspiration biopsy of portal vein thrombosis in liver cirrhosis: results in 15 patients," *Journal of Gastroenterology and Hepatology*, vol. 10, pp. 662–665, 1995.

[29] B. I. Carr and V. Guerra, "Low Alpha-Fetoprotein Levels Are Associated with Improved Survival in Hepatocellular Carcinoma Patients with Portal Vein Thrombosis," *Digestive Diseases and Sciences*, vol. 61, pp. 937–947, 2016.

[30] K.-W. Lee, S.-W. Suh, Y. Choi et al., "Macrovascular invasion is not an absolute contraindication for living donor liver transplantation," *Liver Transplantation*, vol. 23, no. 1, pp. 19–27, 2017.

[31] S. H. Kang, D. Y. Kim, S. M. Jeon et al., "Clinical characteristics and prognosis of hepatocellular carcinoma with different sets of serum AFP and PIVKA-II levels," *European Journal of Gastroenterology & Hepatology*, vol. 24, no. 7, pp. 849–856, 2012.

[32] X. Li, Z.-H. Chen, Y.-F. Xing et al., "Platelet-to-lymphocyte ratio acts as a prognostic factor for patients with advanced hepatocellular carcinoma," *Tumor Biology*, vol. 36, no. 4, pp. 2263–2269, 2015.

[33] Y. Yamamoto, H. Ikoma, R. Morimura, K. Shoda et al., "Post-hepatectomy survival in advanced hepatocellular carcinoma with portal vein tumor thrombosis," *World Journal of Gastroenterology*, vol. 21, no. 1, pp. 246–253, 2015.

[34] Y. P. Le Treut, J. Hardwigsen, P. Ananian et al., "Resection of Hepatocellular Carcinoma with Tumor Thrombus in the Major Vasculature. A European Case-Control Series," *Journal of Gastrointestinal Surgery*, vol. 10, no. 6, pp. 855–862, 2006.

[35] L. M. Kulik, B. I. Carr, M. F. Mulcahy, and R. J. Lewandowski, "Safety and efficacy of 90Y radiotherapy for hepatocellular carcinoma with and without portal vein thrombosis," *Hepatology*, vol. 47, pp. 71–81, 2008.

[36] W.-Y. Lau, B. Sangro, P.-J. Chen et al., "Treatment for hepatocellular carcinoma with portal vein tumor thrombosis: the emerging role for radioembolization using yttrium-90," *Oncology*, vol. 84, no. 5, pp. 311–318, 2013.

[37] B. I. Carr, W. Irish, and M. P. Federle, "Chemoembolization for unresectable hepatocellular carcinoma in patients with or without portal vein thrombosis," *Hepato-Gastroenterology*, vol. 57, no. 104, pp. 1375–1381, 2010.

[38] J. Y. Cheong, K. M. Lee, S. W. Cho et al., "Survival benefits of intra-arterial infusion chemotherapy in patients with advanced hepatocellular carcinoma with portal vein tumor thrombosis," *Hepatology Research*, vol. 32, no. 2, pp. 127–133, 2005.

[39] J. Edeline, L. Crouzet, B. Campillo-Gimenez et al., "Selective internal radiation therapy compared with sorafenib for hepatocellular carcinoma with portal vein thrombosis," *European Journal of Nuclear Medicine and Molecular Imaging*, vol. 43, no. 4, pp. 635–643, 2016.

[40] C. H. Rim, C. Y. Kim, D. S. Yang, and W. S. Yoon, "Comparison of radiation therapy modalities for hepatocellular carcinoma with portal vein thrombosis: A meta-analysis and systematic review," *Radiotherapy & Oncology*, vol. 17, pp. 32730–32735, Dec, 2017.

[41] Y. Zhong, M. Deng, and R. Xu, "Reappraisal of evidence of microscopic portal vein involvement by hepatocellular carcinoma cells with stratification of tumor size," *World Journal of Surgery*, vol. 39, no. 5, pp. 1142–1149, 2015.

11

Comparison of Fecal Calprotectin Methods for Predicting Relapse of Pediatric Inflammatory Bowel Disease

Saranya Kittanakom,[1,2] Md. Sharif Shajib,[1,3] Kristine Garvie,[4] Joceline Turner,[4] Dan Brooks,[4] Sufian Odeh,[5] Robert Issenman,[3,5] V. Tony Chetty,[1,4] Joseph Macri,[1,4] and Waliul I. Khan[1,3,4]

[1]*Department of Pathology & Molecular Medicine, McMaster University, Hamilton, ON, Canada L8S 4K1*
[2]*Pathology and Laboratory Medicine, Schulich School of Medicine & Dentistry, Western University, London, ON, Canada*
[3]*Farncombe Family Digestive Health Research Institute, Hamilton, ON, Canada*
[4]*Hamilton Regional Laboratory Medicine Program, Hamilton Health Sciences, Hamilton, ON, Canada*
[5]*Division of Pediatric Gastroenterology, McMaster University, Hamilton, ON, Canada*

Correspondence should be addressed to Waliul I. Khan; khanwal@mcmaster.ca

Academic Editor: Michael Beyak

Background. Pediatric inflammatory bowel disease (IBD) is on the rise worldwide. Endoscopies are necessary for IBD assessment but are invasive, expensive, and inconvenient. Recently, fecal calprotectin (FCal) was proposed as a noninvasive and specific marker of gut inflammation. We evaluated the analytical performance of three FCal assays and their clinical performance in predicting relapse in pediatric IBD. *Methods.* This study used 40 pediatric IBD and 40 random non-IBD patients' fecal samples. Two automated ELISAs (Bühlmann and PhiCal® Calprotectin-EIA) and an EliA (Phadia 250 EliA-Calprotectin) were used to evaluate the analytical performance. The clinical performance was assessed by PhiCal Calprotectin-EIA, EliA-Calprotectin, and Bühlmann immunochromatographic point-of-care test (POCT). *Results.* All assays displayed acceptable analytical performance below and above the medical decision cut-off [imprecision (CV < 10% intra-assay; <15% interassay); linearity (overall mean % deviation < 16.5%)]. The agreement with PhiCal Calprotectin-EIA was 100% and 78.6% for Bühlmann (95% CI, 87.5–100; Kappa: 1) and EliA-Calprotectin (95% CI, 60.5–89.8; Kappa: 0.32), respectively, and 63.6% between Bühlmann and EliA-Calprotectin (95% CI, 46.6–77.8; Kappa: 0.16). All assays evaluated had similar clinical performance [AUC: 0.84 (EliA-Calprotectin); 0.83 (POCT and PhiCal Calprotectin-EIA)]. *Conclusion.* FCal levels determined using the same method and assay together with clinical history would be a noninvasive and useful tool in monitoring pediatric IBD.

1. Introduction

Inflammatory bowel disease (IBD) encompasses two chronic, relapsing, life-long gastrointestinal (GI) inflammatory conditions, Crohn's disease (CD) and ulcerative colitis (UC). In 2012, it was reported that Canada has one of the highest prevalence rates and the highest incidence rate for IBD in the world [1]. Currently, the prevalence of IBD in Canada is approximately 0.7%, meaning one in every 150 Canadians has IBD [1]. The age of onset for IBD is early adulthood, but the disease may occur at any age. Canada also has one of the highest rates of childhood-onset IBD in the world [1]. The severity of IBD can significantly impact the quality of life, especially in children. They sometimes develop negative emotions and poor self-esteem resulting in troubled behavior and depression [2]. Therefore, detection and monitoring are very important in the clinical management of IBD. Timely diagnosis is particularly crucial for children, as IBD may affect their growth and sexual development [3]. However, month-long delays in diagnosis are quite common. Diagnostic criteria in IBD include nonspecific signs and symptoms such as chronic diarrhea, blood in the stool, abdominal pains, and weight loss. Several blood tests can help in the diagnosis of IBD, such as C-reactive protein (CRP), Erythrocyte Sediment Rate (ESR), *Saccharomyces cerevisiae* antibodies (ASCA), and perinuclear anti-neutrophilic cytoplasmic antibodies (p-ANCA), but none can definitively diagnose IBD. Endoscopy with biopsies is the gold standard for assessing intestinal inflammation in IBD. Endoscopy is an expensive and invasive procedure that requires a skilled operator. Furthermore, the preparatory regimen can be uncomfortable for patients. These limitations of endoscopy prevent the frequent assessment of disease activity in IBD patients.

In recent years, fecal calprotectin (FCal) has become a popular diagnostic tool in assessing IBD activity. Numerous studies have shown that the calprotectin levels detected in stool correlate well with histopathological and endoscopic findings of IBD activity [4, 5]. Calprotectin is an abundant calcium-binding protein found predominantly in neutrophils. Functions of calprotectin include inhibiting zinc-dependent enzymes by competing for zinc, potential biostatic activity against microbes through chelation of zinc ions, inducing apoptosis in malignant cells, and regulating the inflammatory process [6, 7]. The increase in FCal levels can be detected, following inflammatory damage of the intestinal mucosa and an influx of neutrophils into the intestinal lumen [8]. Calprotectin is stable in stool for up to a week at room temperature [9]. This remarkable property of FCal allows for sample collection at home by the patient and delivery to a laboratory within a few days for analysis.

FCal is a useful tool for determining the cause of abdominal discomfort, whether it is organic or functional when it is difficult to discern from symptoms or by clinical examination. An additional utility of FCal is that changes in FCal levels are a good indicator of mucosal healing. Therefore, FCal levels might be worth monitoring in patients with IBD under therapy, as well as to predict the risk of recurrence of disease prior to clinical relapse [10–16]. Calprotectin extracted from stool can be quantified using enzyme-linked immunosorbent assays (ELISAs) with the manufacturer-recommended cut-off values. This may help facilitate the diagnostic processes and may be an efficient method of monitoring IBD therapy.

A cut-off value of 50 μg/g of FCal has been established for adults as well as children over the age 4 years and is used by most of the commercial ELISA kits [17]. In adults, the cut-off value of 50 μg/g was found to have a 95% sensitivity and 91% specificity in differentiating IBD from healthy controls and was identified as the optimal cut-off value for detecting endoscopically active IBD [18, 19]. Children under the age of 4 tend to have higher levels of FCal, which stabilizes with age and is not gender-specific. One study recently reported three cut-off levels based on the 97.5% percentiles of FCal in different age groups, which were 538 μg/g (1 < 6 months), 214 μg/g (6 months < 3 years), and 75 μg/g (3 < 4 years) [20].

In pediatric IBD, FCal has an excellent sensitivity for monitoring disease activity and the response to treatment [21]. Determination of FCal levels is more convenient than having repeated endoscopies. To our knowledge, this is the first Canadian study to evaluate and compare the performance of three FCal assays from different manufacturers, which is necessary given that the results of these assays may play an important role in shaping clinical decisions in pediatric IBD management. We also assessed the clinical performance of a point-of-care test (POCT) by utilizing samples from pediatric IBD patients.

2. Methods

2.1. Study Design. This retrospective study was approved by Hamilton Integrated Research Ethics Board (HiREB).

2.2. Participants. All stool samples were collected from consenting pediatric participants, which includes any participants up to their 18th birthday. A total of forty anonymous stool samples were randomly selected and obtained from the microbiology laboratory of Hamilton Regional Laboratory Medicine Program (HRLMP) and were used as non-IBD controls. These samples were stored at 4°C and FCal extractions were performed within 48 hours of obtaining the samples.

Eighty-nine of 125 patients attending the pediatric IBD clinic at McMaster Children's Hospital were approached and invited to participate in the study from January 2013 to July 2013, and samples were obtained from forty of the patients approached via convenience sampling. The participants had previously been diagnosed with IBD and had recently developed symptoms suggestive of relapse. The exclusion criteria for IBD patients included (1) any positive results from stool culture, ova, and parasites or *Clostridium difficile* tests, (2) inability to provide informed consent, (3) presence of serious life threatening comorbidities, (4) colectomy, (5) toxic megacolon, and (6) acute gastrointestinal bleeding. The diagnosis was made by a pediatric gastroenterologist who was unaware of FCal levels measured. The Pediatric Crohn's Disease Activity Index (PCDAI) and Pediatric Ulcerative Colitis Activity Index (PUCAI) disease activity indices were obtained prospectively for all patients with CD and UC at the time of each visit and were available for comparison [22, 23]. It is important to note here that all PCDAI scores reported exclude the height item [24]. During the colonoscopy, two biopsy specimens were obtained from the ileum and each segment of the colon in all patients. The endoscopic impression of disease activity was noted as normal or as inflamed with disease location and histological assessment by the pathologist based on standard criteria [25] was relied upon to reduce interrater variability and to assess deep tissue healing (reference standard). For patients with IBD, stool samples were collected at least 2 weeks prior to bowel preparation for a colonoscopy and neither the endoscopist nor the pathologist was made aware of the FCal levels determined.

2.3. Test Methods

2.3.1. Fecal Calprotectin Extraction. For all assays evaluated, FCal extractions were performed within 48 hours of sample collection using the Smart Prep Extraction device from Roche Diagnostics according to respective manufacturer's instructions. Following homogenization, the extracts were centrifuged at 3000 ×g for 5 minutes; thereafter, supernatants were collected and stored at −20°C until assay. The laboratory technologist was unaware of the patient history and performed all analyses according to the manufacturer's instructions.

2.3.2. Measurement of Fecal Calprotectin. Two conventional ELISA methods and a fluorescence-immunoassay (EliA) test system were used for measuring FCal levels. All three immunoassays evaluated in this study are based on the same principle of two-site sandwich technique, in which monoclonal capture antibodies highly specific to the calprotectin heterodimeric and polymeric complex are coated on the microtiter plate. For the conventional ELISAs the Bühlmann Calprotectin ELISA, extended range (30–1,800 μg/g; ALPCO, Cat# 01-EK-CAL) and the PhiCal Calprotectin-EIA (Nova Century, Cat# K6927) kits were used. For the fluorescence-immunoassay method, we used the Phadia 250 EliA-Calprotectin, where ImmunoCAP 250 was the instrument (Somagen). All assays were performed according to the respective manufacturer's instructions.

Additionally, we measured FCal levels in pediatric IBD patient samples using the immunochromatographic Bühlmann point-of-care test (POCT), for which the extended range cartridge of Bühlmann POCT (30–1800 μg/g; ALPCO, Cat# 01-LF-CHR25) was used according to manufacturer's instructions. Briefly, the aforementioned FCal extracts were further diluted to 1 : 150 in the extraction buffer and 80 μl of the diluted samples was applied to the rapid test cartridges. Following 15 minutes of incubation at room temperature, the FCal levels were quantified using the Quantum Blue® Lateral Flow Reader (ALPCO Cat# 02-BI-POCTR-ABS).

(a) Imprecision. The repeatability and between-run variability of the FCal kits were assessed following Clinical and Laboratory Standards Institute (CLSI) EP05. The within-run imprecision and the between-run imprecision were evaluated ($n = 20$) at two levels of FCal. Three FCal extracts from low (non-IBD patient samples) and three from high (IBD patient samples) pools were selected for the purposes of these experiments; we additionally used controls supplied by the manufacturers. These samples were tested 20 times and the within-run imprecision was calculated. The between-run imprecision was determined by testing the samples twice a day for 10 days.

(b) Reproducibility around (below and above) the Cut-Off. To verify the repeatability of the FCal test results, especially around the medical decision cut-off established by the manufacturers, where FCal level below 50 μg/g is considered negative and above 100 μg/g is positive in IBD, we used the adopted cut-off suggested by the manufactures. These adopted values are FCal levels 20% lower than the medical decision cut-off point of a negative test (40 μg/g) and 20% higher than positive test (120 μg/g). Here, the pooled samples were prepared from 3 different extracts that reported FCal concentrations above (120 μg/g) or below (40 μg/g) the cut-off. Each pooled sample was tested 10 times to assess the reproducibility.

(c) Linearity. To assess the linearity over the analytical measuring range of the calprotectin assays, two fecal extract pools, low and high, were prepared from the samples based on the CLSI EP06A guidelines. The low calprotectin pool was prepared from 3 non-IBD patient samples and the high calprotectin pool was prepared from three IBD patient samples. Both pools were subjected to seven serial dilutions (e.g., pool 1 = 58, pool 2 = 335, pool 3 = 609, pool 4 = 885, pool 5 = 1161, pool 6 = 1435, and pool 7 = 1712 μg/g) and were tested in triplicate. Mean percentage differences were calculated to represent the average percentage deviation between the expected and observed calprotectin concentrations across the seven dilutions of each extract using the EP Evaluator®.

(d) Agreement between Assays. To assess the agreement among the three assays using medical decision cut-off of below 50 μg/g for FCal levels as negative, 50–100 μg/g as grey zone, and above 100 μg/g as positive for IBD, the forty IBD patient stool samples were evaluated.

(e) Predicting Relapse in Pediatric IBD. To assess the clinical cut-off of IBD relapse, FCal levels were measured using enzyme-linked immunoassays, the PhiCal Calprotectin-EIA, and the EliA assay (EliA-Calprotectin on ImmunoCAP 250), as well as using the immunochromatographic Bühlmann POCT (research study only) within 48 hours of obtaining the stool samples. As mentioned earlier, the stool sample was collected at least 2 weeks before the colonoscopy. Following the colonoscopy, the pediatric gastroenterologists' endoscopic impression of normal (negative) or inflamed (positive) bowel was made available to us.

2.4. Analysis. All FCal levels measured are represented as microgram of calprotectin detected per gram of fecal matter (μg/g). The sample size of the study was determined based on CLSI EP9-A2 guidelines [26]. Only available data were included as part of the analysis and all statistical analyses and graphics were examined using Analyse-it® version 2.22 (Analyse-it Software Ltd., Leeds, UK) and EP Evaluator (EE) (Data Innovations, LLC, USA). The agreement between the different extraction devices, linearity, precision, and the correlation between three assays was assessed using a Bland-Altman plot, a nonparametric Passing-Bablok regression analysis, and spearman rank correlation, respectively. Indeterminate FCal values were not considered when comparing agreement between assays. The receiver operating characteristic (ROC) analyses were performed to evaluate the optimal cut-offs and to determine the FCal cut-off in evaluating IBD relapse in our study population.

3. Results

3.1. Characterization of IBD Patients and Non-IBD Patient Samples. A total of 40 pediatric IBD patients were enrolled in this study and their demographic information is presented in Table 1. The maximal extents of CD for three of the 22 patients were colonic. 11 patients with CD presented with ileocolonic disease and one patient from this group had concomitant upper GI tract involvement. Eight others had their disease restricted to the ileum, but one presented with concomitant perianal disease. In addition to that, 14 of the 22 patients with

TABLE 1: Pediatric IBD patient demographic information.

	Crohn's disease	Ulcerative colitis
Number of participants	22	18
Mean age (range) in years	14.6 (11–17)	14.1 (11–17)
% female	45.5	33.3
Mean disease duration (range) in years	2.8 (0.33–7)	2.3 (0.66–9)

TABLE 2: Studied imprecision.

Manufacturer	Within run ($n = 20$)				Between run ($n = 20$)	
	Mean	SD	95% CI	% CV	Mean	% CV
Bühlmann						
Low sample	58	4.7	3.6–7.1	8.1	38	9.1
High sample	396	15.1	11.3–22.1	3.8	408	12.4
PhiCal						
Low sample	43	3.3	2.3–5.9	7.6	50	6.9
High sample	147	6.7	4.6–12.2	4.5	160	8.4
EliA						
Low sample	64	2.5	1.8–4.2	3.9	42	7.5
High sample	342	15.6	11.9–22.8	4.6	640	6.5

TABLE 3: The linearity of dilution.

Manufacturer	Slope	Intercept	Overall mean % deviation
Bühlmann	0.87 (0.85 to 0.89)	4.1 (−2.6 to 10.9)	9.9
PhiCal	1.24 (1.16 to 1.31)	−1.8 (−9.4 to 5.6)	16.5
EliA	1.11 (1.07 to 1.16)	−1.3 (−4.9 to 2.2)	11.1

CD had a PCDAI score of less than 7.5 and 8 had scores higher than or equal to 7.5. Sixteen out of the 18 patients with UC had extensive UC and two had ulcerative proctitis. Furthermore, 14 of the 18 UC patients enrolled had a PUCAI less than 10 and the remaining 4 were equal to or greater than 10. Endoscopic description of IBD appearance correlated with the histological assessment of biopsy specimens obtained during colonoscopy. All 40 anonymous non-IBD pediatric patient samples obtained through HRLMP microbiology laboratory tested negative for *C. difficile*.

3.2. Imprecision. The imprecision levels for both low and high pools were adequate and acceptable for all three platforms (overall CV < 10% for intra-assay and <15% for interassay). Among the three assays, the PhiCal Calprotectin-EIA exhibited the best intrabatch precision in which the CV at low FCal level of 43 μg/g is 7.6% and the CV at high FCal level of 147 μg/g is 4.5% and interbatch imprecision of 6.9% at 50 μg/g and 8.4% at 160 μg/g (Table 2).

3.3. Reproducibility above and below the Medical Decision Cut-Off. Using adopted cut-offs suggested by the manufacturers, we found that of the 2 automated ELISA platforms evaluated, Bühlmann and PhiCal Calprotectin-EIA, the latter exhibited overall good calprotectin reproducibility with the CV of 8% (at 40 μg/g) and 4.5% (at 120 μg/g) compared to the Bühlmann (18.7% and 13.4%, resp.) automated immunoassay.

3.4. Linearity. In the linearity study, the observed FCal concentrations were plotted versus the expected values and the relationship was assessed using linear regression analysis (Table 3). It is noted that the analytical measuring range of FCal was stated to be up to 1,800 μg/g by Bühlmann Calprotectin ELISA, up to 1970 μg/g by PhiCal Calprotectin-EIA, and up to 3,000 μg/g by EliA-Calprotectin. There were mean percentage deviations observed at the high concentration of FCal. Three methods were linear for the concentrations tested, which included the medical decision limit.

3.5. Method Comparison. To evaluate variability among the three assays, FCal of 40 stool samples was determined. The descriptive comparative plot (Figure 1(a)) represents overall higher FCal values from EliA-Calprotectin assay (mean value of 765.6 μg/g) compared to the other two assays (mean FCal of 222.5 μg/g for Bühlmann Calprotectin ELISA and 247.2 μg/g, for PhiCal Calprotectin-EIA). The Passing-Bablok analysis showed the same finding of positive bias in the EliA-Calprotectin assay compared to Bühlmann Calprotectin ELISA and PhiCal Calprotectin-EIA (Table 4 and Figure 1(b)), especially at the higher end of the measuring

TABLE 4: Summary of assay performance (Passing-Bablok).

Bühlmann				
PhiCal	30	1.3 (1.1 to 1.4)	−4.4 (−16.0 to 8.1)	0.94 (0.87 to 0.97)
EliA	30	5.0 (4.4 to 5.6)	−56.0 (−108.3 to −4.0)	0.94 (0.88 to 0.97)
PhiCal				
EliA	33	3.8 (3.5 to 4.1)	−21.0 (−44.3 to −0.4)	0.93 (0.87 to 0.97)

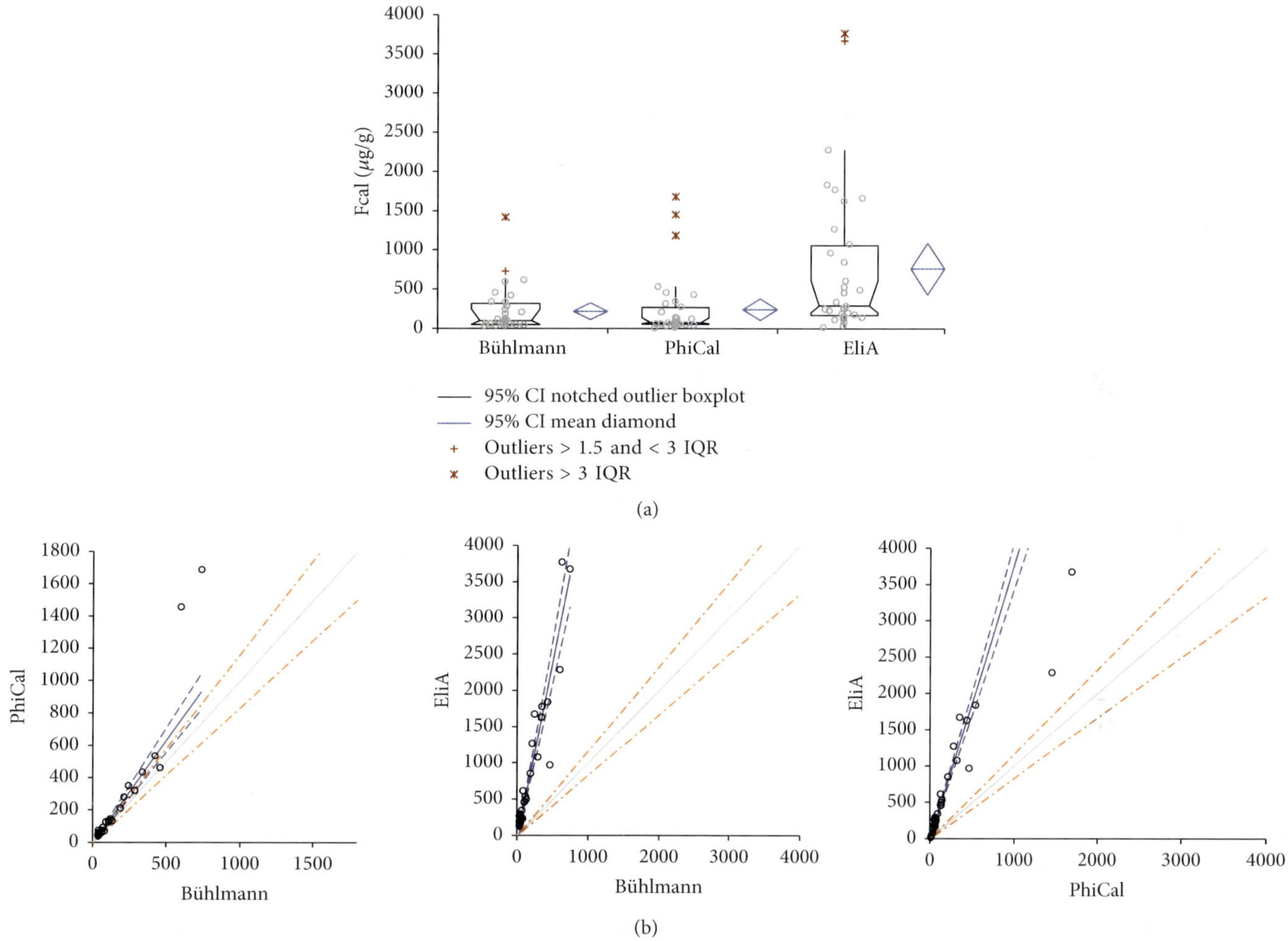

FIGURE 1: *Method comparison between three assays.* Direct comparison between the Bühlmann Calprotectin ELISA (n = 32; mean = 225.2; 95% CI = 119.9–330.4; SE = 51.62; SD = 292.01), PhiCal Calprotectin-EIA (n = 35; mean = 247.2; 95% CI = 110.0–384.4; SE = 67.516; SD = 399.432), and Phadia 250 EliA-Calprotectin (n = 35; mean = 765.6; 95% CI = 438.3–1092.8; SE = 161.04; SD = 952.70) using (a) descriptive comparative plot and (b) Passing-Bablok regression analysis.

range (>1,000 μg/g). A good correlation between assays (R > 0.9) revealed both proportional and consistent differences; this is summarized in Table 4.

3.6. Agreement between Assays. The method comparison study exhibits the disagreement of the quantitative FCal results (Table 5). Bühlmann and PhiCal revealed very high overall agreement (100%, 95% CI, and 87.5 to 100.0%) with an excellent Cohen's Kappa coefficient. However, this agreement is not considering the discordant data in the grey zone in which six negative results and one grey zone measured by Bühlmann Calprotectin ELISA were grey zones and positive results by PhiCal Calprotectin-EIA, respectively. Bühlmann Calprotectin ELISA and EliA-Calprotectin demonstrated the least overall agreement and Kappa's coefficient. These findings implied that there is a significant difference between these two assays. PhiCal Calprotectin-EIA and EliA-Calprotectin, however, exhibited a moderate overall agreement with weak Kappa's coefficient of 0.32 (95% CI, 0.10–0.80). It is noted that the negative agreement between

TABLE 5: Agreement between assays.

Comparison	*N*	Cohen's Kappa	Positive agreement	Negative agreement	Overall agreement
Bühlmann					
PhiCal	27	1 (1 to 1)	100%	100%	100.0% (87.5 to 100.0%)
EliA	33	0.16 (0 to 0.54)	100%	14%	63.6% (46.6 to 77.8%)
PhiCal					
EliA	28	0.32 (0 to 0.80)	100%	25%	78.6% (60.5 to 89.8%)

TABLE 6: Clinical performance of FCal.

Platform	AUC	95% CI	Cut-off (μg/g)	Sensitivity (%)	Specificity (%)	Positive predictive value (%)	Negative predictive value (%)
PhiCal	0.83	0.71 to 0.96	400	100.0 (69.2–100.0)	75.9 (56.5–89.7)	58.8 (32.9–81.6)	100.0 (84.6–100.0)
EliA	0.86	0.74 to 0.98	800	100.0 (69.2–100.0)	72.4 (52.8–87.3)	55.6 (30.8–78.5)	100.0 (83.9–100.0)
Bühlmann (POCT)	0.83	0.70 to 0.96	500	100.0 (69.2–100.0)	72.4 (52.8–87.3)	55.6 (30.8–78.5)	100.0 (83.9–100.0)

EliA-Calprotectin assay and either Bühlmann Calprotectin ELISA or PhiCal Calprotectin-EIA was found, indicating higher FCal results from EliA-Calprotectin (positive bias).

3.7. FCal in Predicting Relapse in Pediatric IBD. Our data suggests that all three FCal assays have an overall equal area under the curve (AUC) of 0.83 (95% CI 0.71–0.96) (Figure 2 and Table 6). The ROC curve showed that a cut-off of 400 μg/g represents the highest sensitivity at 100% (95% CI: 69.2%–100.0%) and specificity at 75.9% (95% CI: 56.5%–89.7%) for PhiCal Calprotectin-EIA. Consistent with the method comparison data, EliA-Calprotectin revealed the highest cut-off (800 μg/g) to use in monitoring disease activity compared to the other two assays (400 μg/g by PhiCal Calprotectin-EIA and 500 μg/g by Bühlmann POCT) with a 100.0% sensitivity (95% CI: 69.2%–100.0%) and 72.4% specificity (95% CI: 52.8%–87.3%) (Table 6).

The cut-offs for each assay (400 μg/g by PhiCal Calprotectin-EIA, 500 μg/g by Bühlmann POCT, and 800 μg/g by EliA-Calprotectin) were then applied to evaluate the relapse of IBD; and, at each cut-off value, IBD disease activity displayed a positive correlation with FCal levels. The Bühlmann POCT and PhiCal Calprotectin-EIA discriminated well between active and inactive IBD (Figure 3). Once again higher FCal values were reported by EliA-Calprotectin in comparison with the aforementioned two tests (Figure 3). However, this cut-off correlated with previous publications [5, 27–29]. All three assays exhibited 100% negative predictive value (95% CI ranging between 83.9% and 100.0%) and about 55.6% positive predictive value (95% CI ranging between 30.8% and 81.6%), highlighting the ability of FCal in determining relapse in this pediatric IBD population (Table 6).

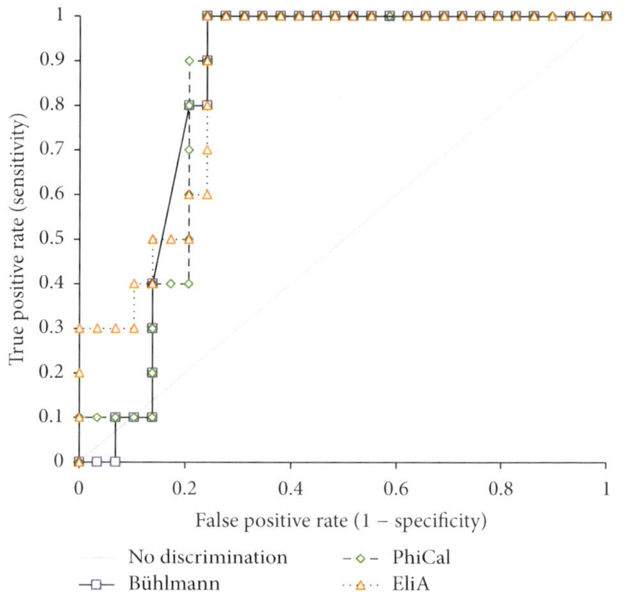

FIGURE 2: *Receiver operating characteristic (ROC) curve of fecal calprotectin (FCal).* ROC of FCal comparing Bühlmann Calprotectin ELISA, PhiCal Calprotectin-EIA, and Phadia 250 EliA-Calprotectin with colonoscopy in 40 pediatric fecal samples. The solid line indicates values that have no discrimination. The performance of a test that exhibits the highest sensitivity and specificity shows an optimum cut-off value to evaluate the relapse of IBD.

4. Discussion

The establishment of noninvasive biomarkers is of growing interest in clinical practice, as they facilitate the objective evaluation of the disease activity and serve as a prognostic indicator of treatment outcome. Determination of FCal levels is considered to be a reliable marker of inflammatory activity in the GI tract. FCal can be used to differentiate between IBD and functional diseases like irritable bowel syndrome (IBS) [30]. In addition, it is useful in monitoring the effectiveness of IBD treatment and in detecting IBD relapses. In this study, we

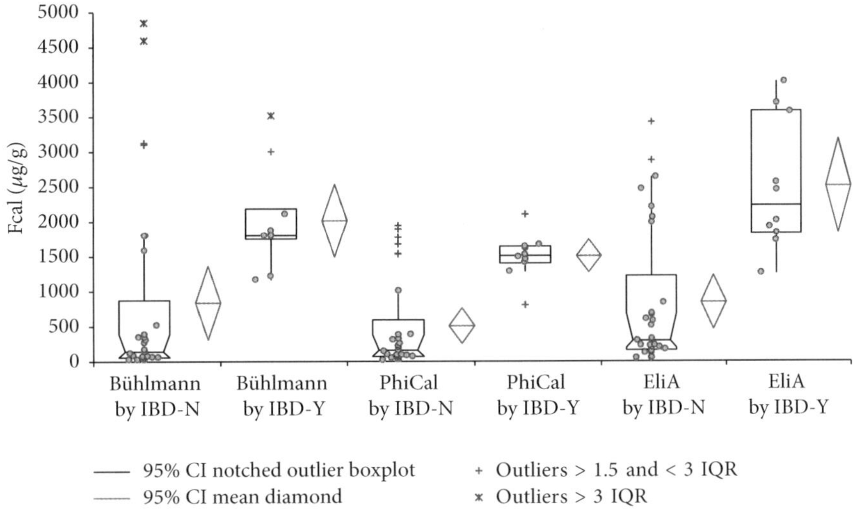

FIGURE 3: *FCal in predicting relapse in pediatric IBD patients.* FCal levels were assessed in 40 pediatric patients with IBD to evaluate the capacity of FCal to determine relapse. FCal levels (μg/g) were analyzed using Bühlmann Calprotectin POCT, PhiCal Calprotectin-EIA, and Phadia 250 EliA-Calprotectin with positive (Y) or negative (N) colonoscopy of active IBD.

compared three immunoassay based FCal detection methods with a view to implement an effective and reliable procedure for the FCal test in a clinical laboratory setting.

Keeping in mind the crucial preanalytical aspects, such as stool sampling technique and transportation and storage of stool and reagents as stated by UK NEQAS external quality assurance program, herein, the performance of three immunoassays was validated and evaluated. One of the limitations of this study is the lack of a true-negative population, such as IBD patients who are not symptomatic and/or have no disease at endoscopy. We found that the PhiCal Calprotectin-EIA demonstrated the best intra- and interbatch performance. Our findings are in opposition to the findings of Whitehead et al. [31], where the authors reported that the Bühlmann Calprotectin ELISA exhibited the better interbatch assay precision. The imprecision of the three assays was comparable, but method comparisons have shown a proportional bias between assays. The linearity, however, was not as the manufacturers had stated which was demonstrated by the drift at high FCal concentrations. This drift was not reported by the previous publication [31] and this may be due to the preanalytical issues in sample extraction or analytical considerations due to the nonstandardized FCal testing. To that end, we performed several extractions with the Thermo Fisher FCal extraction device in addition to the Roche Diagnostics device (data not shown); and our findings are in line with the findings of Whitehead et al. [31] and Oyaerta et al. [32]. Both of these studies reported that the Thermo Fisher extraction devices underestimate FCal concentrations, particularly with fluid samples, as they are not as well captured by the grooves on the dosing tips as stool samples that keep their shape. It was additionally reported that FCal extracts from this device yield higher values when measured using the EliA method. We made similar observations; however, the Thermo Fisher extraction kit may be a good alternative to the Smart Prep by Roche Diagnostics due to its ease of use.

Bühlmann Calprotectin ELISA and PhiCal Calprotectin-EIA have the closest relationship for cross-kit variation study and, EliA-Calprotectin showed the highest FCal read-out with very good precision (imprecision studies), supporting the findings of a previous publication [31]. Moreover, the quantitative agreement between three assays suggested that the differences between Bühlmann Calprotectin ELISA and EliA-Calprotectin could be due to the different antibodies used, which may recognize different epitopes of the heteroduplex of calprotectin. Our findings demonstrate that the FCal levels measured by different assays are not interchangeable and laboratories should state the methods used.

The medical decision cut-off of FCal has been proposed by many studies [18, 30, 31, 33, 34] with an overall good sensitivity and specificity in differentiating IBD from other forms of inflammation. The clinical usefulness of calprotectin and cut-off values has been intensively studied, including, in the diagnosis and differential diagnosis of IBD, disease activity monitoring, disease course, and effect of treatment [35, 36]. Chung-Faye et al. [37] and Carroccio et al. [38] used significantly different cut-offs of 25 μg/g and 170 μg/g in their studies, respectively. In IBD relapse prediction, the study by Tibble et al. [39] had applied FCal > 50 μg/g in adults patients, whereas Walkiewicz et al. used the cut-off as high as >400 μg/g of FCal in pediatric IBD population [28]. Though many studies have suggested different cut-off values, which take into account the type of assay used and the population that the tests were applied to, Waugh et al.'s suggestion of using a cut-off value of 50 μg/g FCal is reasonably sensitive and specific [30]. A greater accuracy was found when using an FCal cut-off value of 100 μg/g instead of 50 μg/g in the diagnosis of IBD [40]. Using a cut-off of 250 μg/g, the sensitivity and specificity of detecting disease activity were found to be 90% and 75%, respectively, for one study [35] and 80% and 82%, respectively, in other similar studies [40, 41]. In addition to that, an accuracy of 88% and 74% with a cut-off value of 250 μg/g in detecting disease activity of UC and CD, respectively, was reported [42]. Based on our results of the ROC curve, the optimal FCal cut-off point to differentiate active from inactive IBD in pediatric patients was 400, 500, and 800 μg/g measured by PhiCal Calprotectin-EIA, Bühlmann POCT, and EliA-Calprotectin, respectively, and this is in agreement with previous studies [5]. With the above-selected cut-off in predicting relapse, the sensitivity of 100% and specificity of 75.9% were achieved. Our data also showed a 100% negative predictive value for all assays evaluated, which emphasizes the potential usefulness of FCal in eliminating unnecessary endoscopic evaluations of patients with negative FCal results. It is noted that the optimal medical decision cut-off point for monitoring and predicting the recurrence of pediatric IBD is not yet clear, but significantly higher values have been reported [5]. However, FCal levels > 500 μg/g have been proposed as the cut-off point for adult IBD patients as it correlates well with disease activity. This emphasizes the need for standardization of FCal assays, as well as a well-defined cut-off point for its clinical utility, especially FCal levels ranging within 51–99 μg/g (the grey zone) to abolish the interpretive ambiguity.

The other important factors which are preanalytical, such as sample collection, disease activity, treatment, and specific method used, as well as FCal stability, consistency of sample analyzed (firm or loose stool), sample storage, and the freeze-thaw cycle of the sample, may considerably influence the FCal level measured. Therefore, the medical decision cut-off should be established by taking these factors into account. Dhaliwal et al. reported that FCal levels decrease significantly when the extract is stored at room temperature, whereas extracts stored at −20°C remain stable for up to two and a half months [40].

In our study, the Bühlmann POCT showed as good and comparable sensitivity as the automated platforms, PhiCal Calprotectin-EIA and EliA-Calprotectin. The introduction of the automated platform in our facility led to flexibility reduced cost and improved quality of service. Given the good performance characteristics of the automated platforms, they can be used as the first screening tool in patients with suspected IBD but with a different cut-off point in mind. Our findings are in agreement with others [43] and demonstrate that determination of FCal levels may be useful in avoiding the unnecessary, undesirable, and invasive procedure such as endoscopy and/or selecting the best treatment plan especially for children with IBD. FCal testing has the potential to become a clinically relevant tool in determining whether patients have IBD and even predicting relapse in IBD patients, in consideration with the limitations of assay/platform as well as their differences. Regardless of the grey zone and differing cut-off values reported, the clinical interpretation of FCal results should be made with caution depending on the assay used. Therefore, we highly recommended the use of the same test by the same manufacturer during follow-ups or monitoring of the treatment.

Disclosure

Saranya Kittanakom and Md. Sharif Shajib are co-first authors.

Acknowledgments

The authors thank Ms. Celynne Grewe of Hamilton Regional Laboratory Medicine Program, Hamilton Health Sciences, for her technical assistance.

References

[1] A. Rocchi, E. I. Benchimol, C. N. Bernstein et al., "Inflammatory bowel disease: a Canadian burden of illness review," *Canadian Journal of Gastroenterology*, vol. 26, no. 11, pp. 811–817, 2012.

[2] E. M. Szigethy, A. O. Youk, D. Benhayon et al., "Depression subtypes in pediatric inflammatory bowel disease," *Journal of Pediatric Gastroenterology and Nutrition*, vol. 58, no. 5, pp. 574–581, 2014.

[3] R. B. Canani, L. T. de Horatio, G. Terrin et al., "Combined use of noninvasive tests is useful in the initial diagnostic approach to a child with suspected inflammatory bowel disease," *Journal of Pediatric Gastroenterology & Nutrition*, vol. 42, no. 1, pp. 9–15, 2006.

[4] D. Desai, W. A. Faubion, and W. J. Sandborn, "Review article: biological activity markers in inflammatory bowel disease," *Alimentary Pharmacology and Therapeutics*, vol. 25, no. 3, pp. 247–255, 2007.

[5] I. D. Kostakis, K. G. Cholidou, A. G. Vaiopoulos, I. S. Vlachos, D. Perrea, and G. Vaos, "Fecal calprotectin in pediatric inflammatory bowel disease: a systematic review," *Digestive Diseases and Sciences*, vol. 58, no. 2, pp. 309–319, 2013.

[6] I. Dale, M. K. Fagerhol, and I. Naesgaard, "Purification and partial characterization of a highly immunogenic human leukocyte protein, the L1 antigen," *European Journal of Biochemistry*, vol. 134, no. 1, pp. 1–6, 1983.

[7] R. Mao, Y.-L. Xiao, X. Gao et al., "Fecal calprotectin in predicting relapse of inflammatory bowel diseases: a meta-analysis of prospective studies," *Inflammatory Bowel Diseases*, vol. 18, no. 10, pp. 1894–1899, 2012.

[8] M. Erbayrak, C. Turkay, E. Eraslan, H. Cetinkaya, B. Kasapoglu, and M. Bektas, "The role of fecal calprotectin in investigating inflammatory bowel diseases," *Clinics*, vol. 64, no. 5, pp. 421–425, 2009.

[9] A. G. Røseth, M. K. Fagerhol, E. Aadland, and H. Schjønsby, "Assessment of the neutrophil dominating protein calprotectin in feces. A methodologic study," *Scandinavian Journal of Gastroenterology*, vol. 27, no. 9, pp. 793–798, 1992.

[10] G. Vaos, I. D. Kostakis, N. Zavras, and A. Chatzemichael, "The role of calprotectin in pediatric disease," *BioMed Research International*, vol. 2013, Article ID 542363, 8 pages, 2013.

[11] A. D. Sutherland, R. B. Gearry, and F. A. Frizelle, "Review of fecal biomarkers in inflammatory bowel disease," *Diseases of the Colon and Rectum*, vol. 51, no. 8, pp. 1283–1291, 2008.

[12] K. L. Kolho, D. Turner, G. Veereman-Wauters et al., "Rapid test for fecal calprotectin levels in children with Crohn disease," *Journal of Pediatric Gastroenterology and Nutrition*, vol. 55, no. 4, pp. 436–439, 2012.

[13] U. L. Fagerberg, L. Lööf, J. Lindholm, L.-O. Hansson, and Y. Finkel, "Fecal calprotectin: a quantitative marker of colonic inflammation in children with inflammatory bowel disease," *Journal of Pediatric Gastroenterology & Nutrition*, vol. 45, no. 4, pp. 414–420, 2007.

[14] A. Diamanti, F. Colistro, M. S. Basso et al., "Clinical role of calprotectin assay in determining histological relapses in children affected by inflammatory bowel diseases," *Inflammatory Bowel Diseases*, vol. 14, no. 9, pp. 1229–1235, 2008.

[15] J. Däbritz, J. Musci, and D. Foell, "Diagnostic utility of faecal biomarkers in patients with irritable bowel syndrome," *World Journal of Gastroenterology*, vol. 20, no. 2, pp. 363–375, 2014.

[16] R. Caccaro, R. D'Incà, S. Pathak, and G. C. Sturniolo, "Clinical utility of calprotectin and lactoferrin in patients with inflammatory bowel disease: is there something new from the literature?" *Expert Review of Clinical Immunology*, vol. 8, no. 6, pp. 579–585, 2012.

[17] J. P. Gisbert and A. G. McNicholl, "Questions and answers on the role of faecal calprotectin as a biological marker in inflammatory bowel disease," *Digestive and Liver Disease*, vol. 41, no. 1, pp. 56–66, 2009.

[18] A. C. Von Roon, L. Karamountzos, S. Purkayastha et al., "Diagnostic precision of fecal calprotectin for inflammatory bowel disease and colorectal malignancy," *American Journal of Gastroenterology*, vol. 102, no. 4, pp. 803–813, 2007.

[19] U. Menon, A. Ryan, J. Kalsi et al., "Risk algorithm using serial biomarker measurements doubles the number of screen-detected cancers compared with a single-threshold rule in the United Kingdom Collaborative Trial of Ovarian Cancer Screening," *Journal of Clinical Oncology*, vol. 33, no. 18, pp. 2062–2071, 2015.

[20] T. Oord and N. Hornung, "Fecal calprotectin in healthy children," *Scandinavian Journal of Clinical and Laboratory Investigation*, vol. 74, no. 3, pp. 254–258, 2014.

[21] T. Sipponen and K.-L. Kolho, "Fecal calprotectin in diagnosis and clinical assessment of inflammatory bowel disease," *Scandinavian Journal of Gastroenterology*, vol. 50, no. 1, pp. 74–80, 2014.

[22] J. S. Hyams, G. D. Ferry, F. S. Mandel et al., "Development and validation of a pediatric crohn's disease activity index," *Journal of Pediatric Gastroenterology and Nutrition*, vol. 12, no. 4, pp. 439–447, 1991.

[23] D. Turner, D. Mack, N. Leleiko et al., "Severe pediatric ulcerative colitis: a prospective multicenter study of outcomes and predictors of response," *Gastroenterology*, vol. 138, no. 7, pp. 2282–2291, 2010.

[24] D. Turner, A. M. Griffiths, T. D. Walters et al., "Appraisal of the pediatric Crohn's disease activity index on four prospectively collected datasets: recommended cutoff values and clinimetric properties," *The American Journal of Gastroenterology*, vol. 105, no. 9, pp. 2085–2092, 2010.

[25] F. Magro, C. Langner, A. Driessen et al., "European consensus on the histopathology of inflammatory bowel disease," *Journal of Crohn's and Colitis*, vol. 7, no. 10, pp. 827–851, 2013.

[26] *Method Comparison and Bias Estimation Using Patient Samples; Approved Guideline*, vol. 22, no. 19 of *CLSI Document EP9-A2*, CLSI, Wayne, Pa, USA, 2nd edition, 2002.

[27] A. Hämäläinen, T. Sipponen, and K.-L. Kolho, "Serum infliximab concentrations in pediatric inflammatory bowel disease," *Scandinavian Journal of Gastroenterology*, vol. 48, no. 1, pp. 35–41, 2013.

[28] D. Walkiewicz, S. L. Werlin, D. Fish, M. Scanlon, P. Hanaway, and S. Kugathasan, "Fecal calprotectin is useful in predicting disease relapse in pediatric inflammatory bowel disease," *Inflammatory Bowel Diseases*, vol. 14, no. 5, pp. 669–673, 2008.

[29] P. F. Van Rheenen, "Role of fecal calprotectin testing to predict relapse in teenagers with inflammatory bowel disease who report full disease control," *Inflammatory Bowel Diseases*, vol. 18, no. 11, pp. 2018–2025, 2012.

[30] N. Waugh, E. Cummins, P. Royle et al., "Faecal calprotectin testing for differentiating amongst inflammatory and non-inflammatory bowel diseases: systematic review and economic evaluation," *Health Technology Assessment*, vol. 17, no. 55, pp. 1–211, 2013.

[31] S. J. Whitehead, J. French, M. J. Brookes, C. Ford, and R. Gama, "Between-assay variability of faecal calprotectin enzyme-linked immunosorbent assay kits," *Annals of Clinical Biochemistry*, vol. 50, no. 1, pp. 53–61, 2013.

[32] M. Oyaerta, C. Trouvéa, F. Baert, D. De Smet, M. Langlois, and H. Vanpoucke, "Comparison of two immunoassays for measurement of faecal calprotectin in detection of inflammatory bowel disease: (pre)-analytical and diagnostic performance characteristics," *Clinical Chemistry and Laboratory Medicine*, vol. 52, no. 3, pp. 391–397, 2014.

[33] A. M. Schoepfer, M. Trummler, P. Seeholzer, B. Seibold-Schmid, and F. Seibold, "Discriminating IBD from IBS: comparison of the test performance of fecal markers, blood leukocytes, CRP, and IBD antibodies," *Inflammatory Bowel Diseases*, vol. 14, no. 1, pp. 32–39, 2008.

[34] M. D. Jensen, J. Kjeldsen, and T. Nathan, "Fecal calprotectin is equally sensitive in Crohn's disease affecting the small bowel and colon," *Scandinavian Journal of Gastroenterology*, vol. 46, no. 6, pp. 694–700, 2011.

[35] F. Costa, M. G. Mumolo, L. Ceccarelli et al., "Calprotectin is a stronger predictive marker of relapse in ulcerative colitis than in Crohn's disease," *Gut*, vol. 54, no. 3, pp. 364–368, 2005.

[36] L. A. Smith and D. R. Gaya, "Utility of faecal calprotectin analysis in adult inflammatory bowel disease," *World Journal of Gastroenterology*, vol. 18, no. 46, pp. 6782–6789, 2012.

[37] G. Chung-Faye, B. Hayee, S. Maestranzi, N. Donaldson, I. Forgacs, and R. Sherwood, "Fecal M2-pyruvate kinase (M2-PK): a novel marker of intestinal inflammation," *Inflammatory Bowel Diseases*, vol. 13, no. 11, pp. 1374–1378, 2007.

[38] A. Carroccio, G. Iacono, M. Cottone et al., "Diagnostic accuracy of fecal calprotectin assay in distinguishing organic causes of chronic diarrhea from irritable bowel syndrome: a prospective study in adults and children," *Clinical Chemistry*, vol. 49, no. 6, part 1, pp. 861–867, 2003.

[39] J. Tibble, K. Teahon, B. Thjodleifsson et al., "A simple method for assessing intestinal inflammation in Crohn's disease," *Gut*, vol. 47, no. 4, pp. 506–513, 2000.

[40] A. Dhaliwal, Z. Zeino, C. Tomkins et al., "Utility of faecal calprotectin in inflammatory bowel disease (IBD): what cut-offs should we apply?" *Frontline Gastroenterology*, vol. 6, no. 1, pp. 14–19, 2015.

[41] J.-F. Lin, J.-M. Chen, J.-H. Zuo et al., "Meta-analysis: fecal calprotectin for assessment of inflammatory bowel disease activity," *Inflammatory Bowel Diseases*, vol. 20, no. 8, pp. 1407–1415, 2014.

[42] S. Nancey, G. Boschetti, D. Moussata et al., "Neopterin is a novel reliable fecal marker as accurate as calprotectin for predicting endoscopic disease activity in patients with inflammatory bowel diseases," *Inflammatory Bowel Diseases*, vol. 19, no. 4, pp. 1043–1052, 2013.

[43] Z. Yang, N. Clark, and K. T. Park, "Effectiveness and cost-effectiveness of measuring fecal calprotectin in diagnosis of inflammatory bowel disease in adults and children," *Clinical Gastroenterology and Hepatology*, vol. 12, no. 2, pp. 253–262, 2014.

12

Long-Term Management of Recurrent Cholecystitis after Initial Conservative Treatment: Endoscopic Transpapillary Gallbladder Stenting

Hideki Kamada,[1] Hideki Kobara,[1] Naohito Uchida,[1] Kiyohito Kato,[1] Takayuki Fujimori,[1] Kiyoyuki Kobayashi,[1] Takuma Yamashita,[1] Masahiro Ono,[1] Yuichi Aritomo,[1] Kunihiko Tsutsui,[1] Keiichi Okano,[2] Yasuyuki Suzuki,[2] and Tsutomu Masaki[1]

[1]*Department of Gastroenterology and Neurology, Faculty of Medicine, Kagawa University, Kagawa, Japan*
[2]*Department of Gastroenterological Surgery, Faculty of Medicine, Kagawa University, Kagawa, Japan*

Correspondence should be addressed to Hideki Kamada; kamacho@med.kagawa-u.ac.jp

Academic Editor: Michael Beyak

Background. Endoscopic transpapillary gallbladder stenting (ETGBS) is an effective procedure for treating high-risk patients with acute cholecystitis and severe comorbidities. However, the efficacy of ETGBS for recurrent cholecystitis (RC) remains unclear. This study aimed to explore its efficacy in patients with RC for whom cholecystectomy is contraindicated because of its high surgical risk. *Methods.* Data on 19 high-risk patients who had undergone ETGBS for RC after initial conservative therapy in our institution between June 2006 and May 2012 were retrospectively examined. The primary outcome was the clinical success rate, which was defined as no recurrences of acute cholecystitis after ETGBS until death or the end of the follow-up period. Secondary outcomes were technical success rate and adverse events (AEs). *Results.* The clinical success rate of ETGBS was 100%, the technical success rate 94.7%, and AE rate 5%: one patient developed procedure-related mild acute pancreatitis. The clinical courses of all patients were as follows: four died of nonbiliary disease, and the remaining 15 were subsequently treated conservatively. The median duration of follow-up was 14.95 months (range 3–42 months). *Conclusions.* ETGBS is an effective alternative for managing RC in high-risk patients with severe comorbidities.

1. Introduction

Laparoscopic cholecystectomy is currently the standard treatment for patients with early stage acute cholecystitis [1, 2]. Cholecystectomy is a commonly performed and safe procedure; however, invasive surgery is sometimes contraindicated in high-risk patients with complex comorbidities such as severe coagulopathy or poor performance status [3]. Moreover, although percutaneous transhepatic gallbladder aspiration/drainage (PTGBA/D) is considered a temporary therapy aimed at decompressing the gallbladder, the percutaneous transhepatic approach is controversial in patients at high risk of intra-abdominal bleeding or of removing their drainage tubes themselves [4–7]. Thus, endoscopic transpapillary gallbladder drainage (ETGBD) has recently been proposed as an alternative procedure for high-risk patients with acute cholecystitis [8–12]. ETGBD generally involves endoscopic nasotranspapillary gallbladder drainage and endoscopic transpapillary gallbladder stenting (ETGBS) without risks of tube self-withdrawal. In particular, ETGBS has been adopted as the initial approach in high-risk patients with acute cholecystitis or in patients with end-stage liver disease related to advanced cancer or those awaiting liver transplantation [13–19]. However, ETGBS has a mild risk of related pancreatitis due to the transpapillary approach, and conservative therapy may sometimes be curative for acute cholecystitis without the need for additional therapy. Accordingly, ETGBS may be a suitable option for recurrent cholecystitis (RC) after conservative treatment with antibiotics or PTGBA/D. Few studies have reported the long-term clinical outcomes of ETGBS for the prevention of RC. Hence, this retrospective study aimed to assess the clinical efficacy and long-term outcomes of ETGBS after initial conventional therapy in surgically high-risk patients with RC.

2. Methods

2.1. Patients. This retrospective study was conducted at a single center, Kagawa University Hospital. Data on 19 high-risk patients who had undergone ETGBS for RC after initial conservative therapy in our institution between June 2006 and May 2012 were retrospectively examined. Patient characteristics, including age, comorbidities (benign and malignant), physical status, presence of dementia, severity of cholecystitis, and therapy prior to ETGBS, were collected. The inclusion criteria were high-risk patients with RC within 2 months after conservative treatment with antibiotics or PTGBA/D for first episodes of acute cholecystitis for whom cholecystectomy was contraindicated because of its high surgical risk. High-risk patients with acute cholecystitis were defined as follows: (1) patients with increased postoperative morbidity and mortality, such as those with cirrhosis, cerebral disease, cardiopulmonary disease, malignancy, or other significant medical illnesses; (2) those with severe coagulopathy or thrombocytopenia; (3) patients with anatomically inaccessible gallbladder or other anatomic abnormalities; (4) those with a large amount of ascites, which is a known contraindication to percutaneous therapy.

ETGBS was performed with the aim of permanently managing RC. Scheduled stent exchanges were not performed in this study; however, patients were prospectively followed for stent exchange at the discretion of the endoscopist, surgical intervention, or death.

Acute cholecystitis was diagnosed based on (1) presence of symptoms, (2) abnormalities of relevant laboratory data (white blood cell count and C-reactive protein), and (3) a thickened gallbladder wall, pericholecystic fluid, and a distended gallbladder shown by imaging studies (transabdominal ultrasonography and computed tomography). The severity of acute RC was graded according to the Tokyo Guidelines (TG) grading system [20]. American Society of Anesthesiologists (ASA) scores were used to denote the patients' preoperative physical health status. All patients with acute or RC had been treated under fasting with antibiotics and intravenous administration of lactated Ringer's solution.

This study was approved by the Clinical Ethics Committee of Kagawa University Hospital. All patients had provided written informed consent to undergo the ETGBS procedures.

2.2. ETGBS Procedure. ETGBS was performed as previously described [12] and as shown in Figure 1. All patients were placed in a prone position before undergoing endoscopic retrograde cholangiopancreatography (ERCP) with side-viewing endoscopes (TJF240 or TJF260V; Olympus, Tokyo, Japan) after sedation with intravenous midazolam (0.05 mg/kg). Selective bile duct cannulation was achieved by advancing an ERCP catheter (MTW, Düsseldorf, Germany) over a 0.025- or 0.032-inch hydrophilic guidewire (e.g., Radifocus; Terumo, Tokyo, Japan) into the cystic duct and gallbladder. After the catheter had been inserted over the guide wire into the fundus of the gallbladder (Figure 2(a)), a stiff guide wire was substituted for the hydrophilic guidewire (VisiGlide; Olympus, Tokyo, Japan, or Hydra Jagwire; Boston Scientific Japan, Tokyo, Japan). A 7F, 10 to 15 cm long, double-pigtail polyethylene stent (Olympus, Tokyo, Japan) was then deployed (Figure 2(b)), crossing the ampulla with the proximal and distal pigtails in the gallbladder and duodenum, respectively. The length of the stent was determined by pulling the guide wire out of the gallbladder to the ampulla and measuring that distance.

2.3. Outcome Measures. The primary outcome was clinical success rate. Secondary outcomes were the rates of technical success and procedure-related adverse events (AEs). Clinical success was defined as no recurrences of acute cholecystitis after ETGBS until death or the end of the follow-up period. Technical success was defined as successful placement of a double-pigtail stent in the gallbladder. Procedure-related AEs were graded according to the American Society for Gastrointestinal Endoscopy lexicon's grading system [24].

3. Results

Data of 19 consecutive patients (10 men, 9 women; median age of 84 years; range 60–93 years) were examined. Detailed patient characteristics are summarized in Table 1. All included patients had severe comorbidities, 15 (78.9%) of them having severe dementia. ASA scores were used to assess the patients' preoperative physical status: 15 patients (78.9%) were classified as having Class 4 status, three (15.8%) Class 3, and one (5.3%) Class 2, contraindicating cholecystectomy. The severity of acute cholecystitis according to TG13 grades was as follows: four patients (21.1%) were classified as having Grade I acute cholecystitis and 15 patients (78.9%) as having Grade II. Prior to ETGBS, 12 patients had received conservative therapy with antibiotics and seven had undergone PTGBA/D. Outcomes are shown in Table 2. ETGBS was technically successful in 18 (94.7%) of the 19 patients. ETGBS failed in one patient, after which PTGBD was performed. Endoscopic sphincterotomy (EST) was performed to remove common bile duct stones in three patients. The clinical success rate was 100% in the 18 patients for whom ETGBS had been successful. Although no severe procedure-related AEs occurred, one patient developed mild acute pancreatitis; thus the AE rate was 5.3%. The clinical courses of all patients were as follows. Four patients died of nonbiliary diseases, namely, malignant lymphoma (3 months after ETGBS), chronic respiratory failure (9 months after ETGBS), aspiration pneumonitis (17 months after ETGBS), and cerebral infarction (42 months after ETGBS). The remaining 15 patients, including the one in whom ETGBS was unsuccessful, were thereafter managed conservatively. Figure 3 is a flow diagram showing the patients' clinical courses. The median duration of follow-up was 14.95 months (range 3–42 months). Although spontaneous distal migration of the stent occurred in one patient 23 months after ETGBS, no patients who had undergone ETGBS required stent removal or exchange during follow-up. None of the included patients received oral antibiotics and biliary

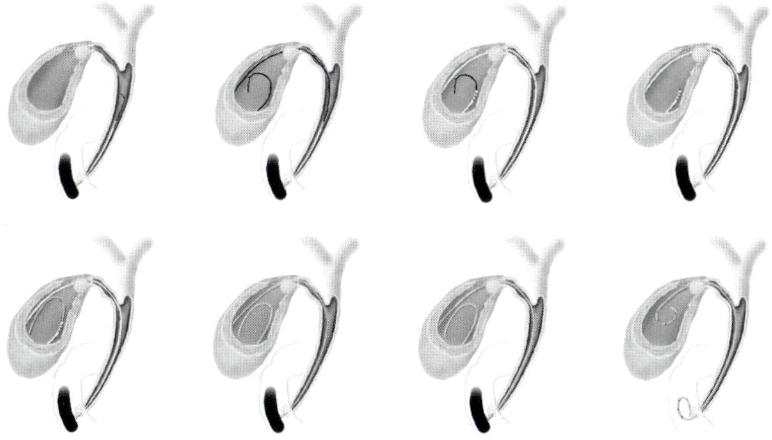

FIGURE 1: Depiction of the procedure for endoscopic stenting of the common bile duct and gallbladder. A catheter is inserted deep into the bile duct and a guidewire advanced into the cystic duct and gallbladder. The catheter is inserted over the guidewire up to the fundus of the gallbladder. A double-pigtail polyethylene stent is then inserted.

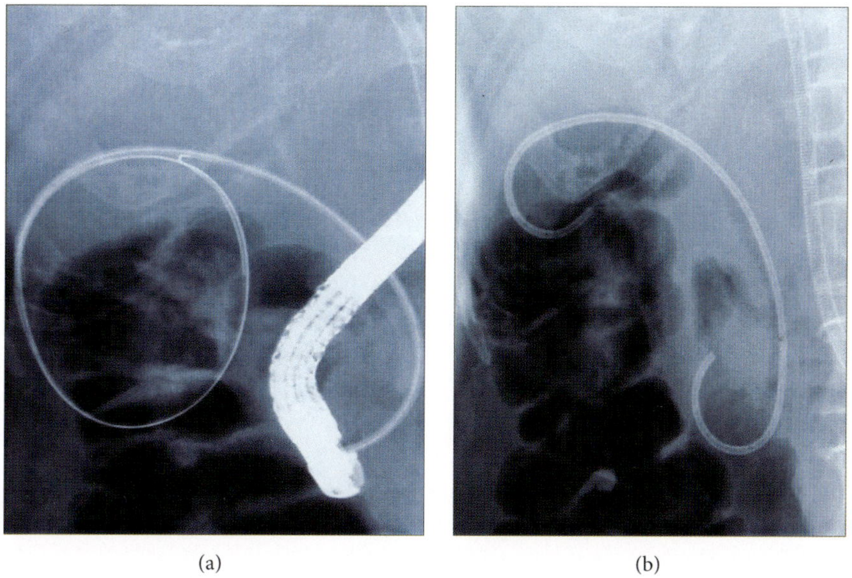

FIGURE 2: (a) Fluoroscopic image of a guidewire coiled in the gallbladder. (b) Fluoroscopic image of a stent extending from the duodenum into the gallbladder.

medicines such as ursodeoxycholic acid during follow-up after recovering from acute cholecystitis.

4. Discussion

ETGBS is considered an effective treatment option for acute cholecystitis in poor surgical candidates with severe comorbidities. However, there are few published data on long-term outcomes in terms of symptomatic cholelithiasis in such patients. Because advanced skills are required to perform ETGBS and there is a risk of procedure-related severe pancreatitis because of the transpapillary approach, conventional measures such as conservative therapy or PTGBA/D are generally selected as the initial approach for managing acute cholecystitis. Thus, in the present study, ETGBS was performed for RC occurring after such initial therapies rather than for the first episode of acute cholecystitis. This is the first study demonstrating that ETGBS is a reasonable option for long-term management of RC after initial conventional therapy.

Cholecystectomy is the mainstay of management of acute cholecystitis [1, 2]. However, the mortality rate of emergency cholecystectomy (approximately 30%) is still unsatisfactory in high-risk patients with severe comorbidities such as liver cirrhosis, serious cardiopulmonary disease, or significant medical illness [21]. Therefore, such patients may be treated with conservative therapy with antibiotics or PTGBA/D as a temporary means of decompressing the gallbladder.

Table 1: Patient characteristics.

Characteristics	Value
Number of patients, *n*	19
Sex, male/female, *n*.	10/9
Age, median (range), yr	84 (60–93)
Comorbidities, *n*	
Benign	
Poor cerebral condition	8
Poor cardiovascular condition	2
Poor cerebral and cardiovascular condition	2
Poor pulmonary function	1
Ulcerative colitis	1
Bedridden due to gonarthrosis	1
Multiorgan failure	1
Malignant	
Bile duct cancer	1
Gastric cancer	1
Lymphoma	1
ASA class	
I	0
II	1
III	3
IV	15
Dementia	
YES	15
NO	4
Severity grading per Tokyo guidelines 2013	
I	4
II	15
First therapy prior to ETGBS	
Conservative with antibiotics	12
PTGBA/D	7

F, female; M, male.

Reported technical success rates for PTGBA and PTGBD range between 82%–97% and 97%–100%, respectively [4–7]. However, PTGBA/D procedures are sometimes contraindicated by factors such as severe coagulopathy, severe thrombocytopenia, anatomically inaccessible lesions, or the presence of ascites [7]. Recently, ETGBD has been reported as an alternative to percutaneous gallbladder drainage for managing acute cholecystitis in such patients. Since Kozarek introduced endoscopic transpapillary cannulation of the gallbladder in 1984 [25], several endoscopists, including our senior colleagues [12], have developed ETGBD techniques for treating acute cholecystitis. However, ETGBD has the limitation that older persons with dementia are at risk of removing their drainage tubes themselves and these tubes cannot be implanted in the gallbladder long term. Thus, ETGBD is best considered a temporary and bridge therapy to surgery. Consequently, there is a need for an effective long-term therapeutic strategy for managing acute cholecystitis in high-risk patients who are poor candidates for emergency cholecystectomy. Recently, several authors have reported that ETGBS is an effective long-term option for managing acute cholecystitis in high-risk patients [17, 21, 22]. Previously reported outcomes of ETGBS are shown in Table 3 [8, 13–17, 21–23]. The mean overall clinical success rate was 92.6% (range 64%–100%) (216 cases), including our results. Although there are few studies on long-term clinical courses, our data on patients undergoing ETGBS demonstrate excellent long-term outcomes with a clinical success rate of 100% in 19 patients in whom the procedure was technically successful. None of our patients required stent removal or exchange, likely because stents have the following favorable effects. First, stents prevent impaction or migration of gallstones into the cystic duct. Second, even occluded stents may still provide drainage of the gallbladder because bile may flow around them. Third, bile flow may improve because the cystic duct is straightened by the placement of the stent. However, more studies are needed to clarify the reasons for the excellent patency results.

The reported technical success rate of ETGBS ranges from 79.3% to 100%, as shown in Table 3. In our study, the technical success rate of ETGBS (94.7%) was similar to that in previous studies. One limitation of ETGBD/S is that it can be technically difficult to perform in some patients, considerable skill being required to pass the guidewire through the cystic duct. Several factors can contribute to failure, namely, severe inflammatory or malignant strictures, obstruction of the neck of the gallbladder by impacted stones, tortuosity of the duct, and cystic duct outlet not visible on the cholangiogram. These high rates of technical success may be attributable to the level of skills gained by performing many of these procedures.

As shown in Table 3, the mean overall rate of AEs was 2.5% in 216 cases; there were no serious AEs. In our series, there was only one case of postprocedure mild pancreatitis. However, although ETGBS is thus relatively safe, a careful approach is needed to prevent post-ERCP. Moreover, great care should be taken to avoid perforation of the cystic duct or gallbladder. Pannala et al. reported that biliary perforation occurred in 2% of patients who underwent this procedure [26]. Other AEs, including migration of the stent and cholangitis, have been reported. In 20 patients with long-term follow-up (median 606.5 days) after ETGBS, Lee et al. [21] reported that spontaneous distal migration occurred in two patients 7 months after ETGBS with EST and that one patient who had undergone ETGBS without EST developed cholangitis with choledocholithiasis 19 months after the procedure. In our study, spontaneous distal migration of a stent occurred in one patient 23 months after ETGBS without EST; there were no complications and no additional interventions were required.

Jang et al. recently reported that endoscopic ultrasound-guided transmural gallbladder drainage (EUS-GBD) is comparable with PTGBD for nonsurgical patients with comorbidities in terms of technical feasibility, efficacy, and safety [27]. In contrast, the consensus report of Tokyo Guidelines 13 reported that EUS-GBD results in a relatively high incidental rate of AEs of 11%–33% [28]. Because severe and uncontrolled

TABLE 2: Outcomes of endoscopic transpapillary gallbladder stenting (n = 19).

Primary outcome	Clinical success rate, % (n)	100 (18/18)
Secondary outcomes	Technical success rate, % (n)	94.7 (18/19)
	Procedure-related adverse events rate, % (n)	5.3 (1/19)[#]

[#]Mild acute pancreatitis.

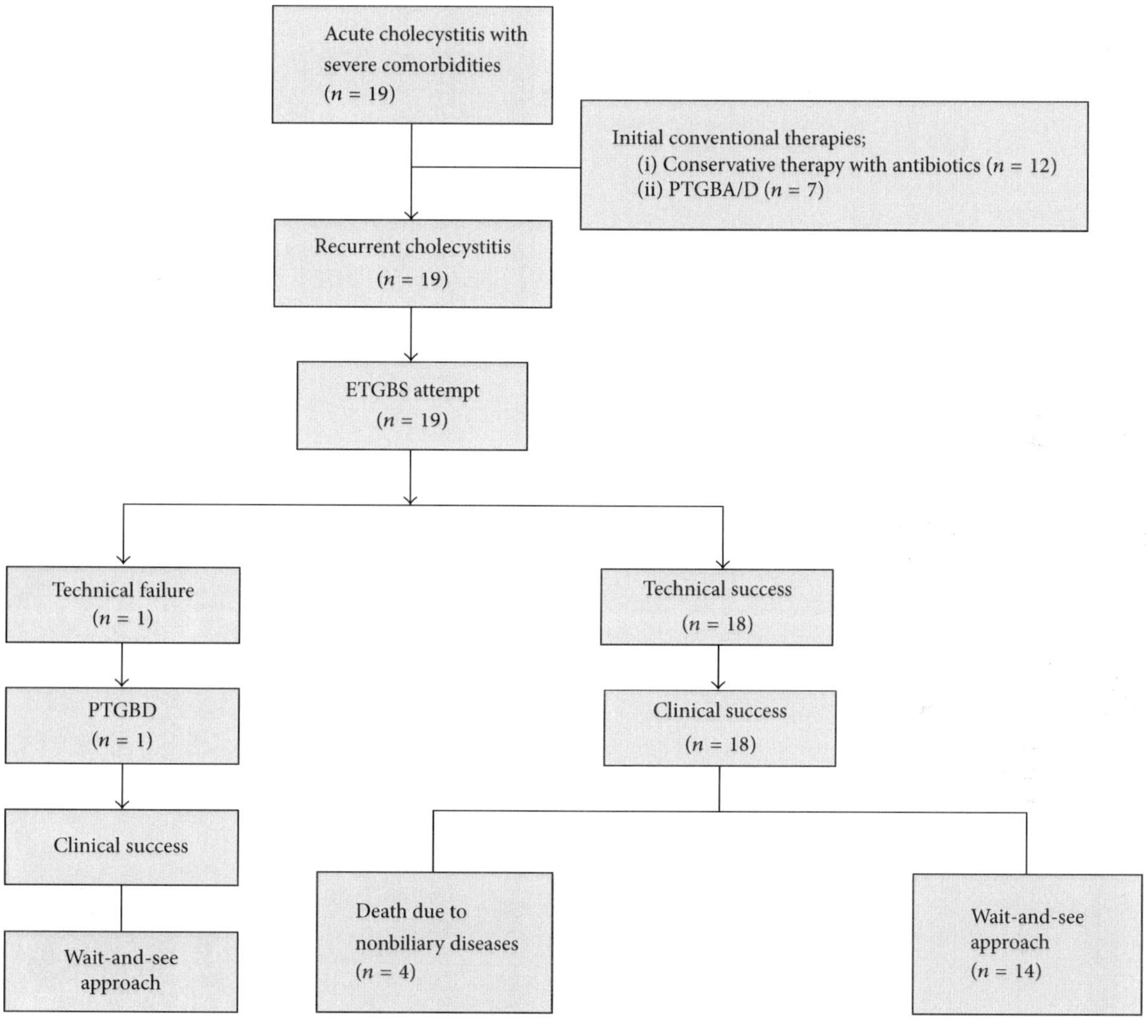

FIGURE 3: Flow diagram of patient's clinical courses.

complications such as bile leakage, stent migration into the gallbladder or intra-abdominal space, deviation of the stent from the gallbladder, puncture-induced hemorrhage, and perforation of the peritoneum are expected, EUS-GBD has not yet been established as a standard therapy for gallbladder drainage. Further research is needed to determine whether EUS-GBD or ETGBS is superior.

Finally, first-line therapy for acute cholecystitis in high-risk patients should be discussed to establish a therapeutic strategy. Performing ETGBS requires advanced skills and has the potential risk of procedure-related severe pancreatitis because of the transpapillary approach. Regarding the rate of recurrence of acute cholecystitis, Ha et al. reported that 1-year and 3-year recurrence rates of in-patients who did not undergo subsequent cholecystectomies were 35% and 46% [29], respectively. Schmidt et al. reported a recurrence rate of 24% [30]. In other words, conservative approaches are appropriate for 50%–70% of all patients treated for acute cholecystitis. Therefore, we recommend conventional therapies such as conservative treatment or PTGBA/D for the initial approach to acute cholecystitis. After such initial therapy, ETGBS should be considered for long-term management when RC occurs. However, no data are available on how long stents remain patent or when and whether stent removal and exchange are necessary. A large study is needed to resolve these issues.

TABLE 3: Published outcomes of endoscopic transpapillary gallbladder stenting.

Author (year) [Ref.]	Type of study	Number of cases	Technical success rate (%)	Clinical success rate (%)	Rate of adverse events (%)	Follow-up, months	Number of relapses
Tamada et al. (1991) [8]	R	14	100	64	0	2	0
Kalloo et al. (1994) [13]	R	4	100	100	0	11–17	0
Gaglio et al. (1996) [14]	R	3	100	100	0	4–6	2
Shrestha and Lasch (2001) [15]	R	13	100	100	0	1–36	1
Conway et al. (2005) [16]	R	29	89.7	97	0	9.4	2
Schlenker et al. (2006) [17]	R	23	100	78.3	0	2–54	3
Lee et al. (2011) [21]	P	29	79.3	100	17.2	20	2
Maekawa et al. (2013) [22]	R	46	80.4	96.8	0	1–60	1
Itoi et al. (2015) [23]	P	36	86.1	90.3	2.7	1	0
Our study	R	19	94.7	100	5.3	3–42	0
Total		216	93.6	92.6	2.5		

P, prospective; R, retrospective.

In conclusion, ETGBS may be an effective and reasonable option for long-term management of recurrent cholecystitis after initial conventional therapies in high-risk patients who are poor candidates for cholecystectomy.

References

[1] R. Shrestha, T. E. Trouillot, and G. T. Everson, "Endoscopic stenting of the gallbladder for symptomatic gallbladder disease in patients with end-stage liver disease awaiting orthotopic liver transplantation," *Liver Transplantation and Surgery*, vol. 5, no. 4, pp. 275–281, 1999.

[2] H. Lau, C. Y. Lo, N. G. Patil, and W. K. Yuen, "Early versus delayed-interval laparoscopic cholecystectomy for acute cholecystitis: a metaanalysis," *Surgical Endoscopy*, vol. 20, no. 1, pp. 82–87, 2006.

[3] A. Puggioni and L. L. Wong, "A metaanalysis of laparoscopic cholecystectomy in patients with cirrhosis," *Journal of the American College of Surgeons*, vol. 197, no. 6, pp. 921–926, 2003.

[4] E. J. Patterson, R. F. McLoughlin, J. R. Mathieson, P. L. Cooperberg, and J. K. MacFarlane, "An alternative approach to acute cholecystitis. Percutaneous cholecystostomy and interval laparoscopic cholecystectomy," *Surgical Endoscopy*, vol. 10, no. 12, pp. 1185–1188, 1996.

[5] S. Chopra, G. D. Dodd III, A. L. Mumbower et al., "Treatment of acute cholecystitis in non-critically III patients at high surgical risk: Comparison of clinical outcomes after gallbladder aspiration and after percutaneous cholecystostomy," *American Journal of Roentgenology*, vol. 176, no. 4, pp. 1025–1031, 2001.

[6] K. Ito, N. Fujita, Y. Noda et al., "Percutaneous cholecystostomy versus gallbladder aspiration for acute cholecystitis: A prospective randomized controlled trial," *American Journal of Roentgenology*, vol. 183, no. 1, pp. 193–196, 2004.

[7] T. Itoi, A. Sofuni, F. Itokawa et al., "Endoscopic transpapillary gallbladder drainage in patients with acute cholecystitis in whom percutaneous transhepatic approach is contraindicated or anatomically impossible (with video)," *Gastrointestinal Endoscopy*, vol. 68, no. 3, pp. 455–460, 2008.

[8] K. Tamada, H. Seki, K. Sato et al., "Efficacy of endoscopic retrograde cholecystoendoprosthesis (ERCCE) for cholecystitis," *Endoscopy*, vol. 23, no. 1, pp. 2-3, 1991.

[9] F. C. Johlin Jr. and G. A. Neil, "Drainage of the gallbladder in patients with acute acalculous cholecystitis by transpapillary endoscopic cholecystotomy," *Gastrointestinal Endoscopy*, vol. 39, no. 5, pp. 645–651, 1993.

[10] C. Feretis, N. Apostolidis, E. Mallas, A. Manouras, and J. Papadimitriou, "Endoscopic drainage of acute obstructive cholecystitis in patients with increased operative risk," *Endoscopy*, vol. 25, no. 6, pp. 392–395, 1993.

[11] T. H. Baron, M. B. Farnell, and A. J. LeRoy, "Endoscopic transpapillary gallbladder drainage for closure of calculous gallbladder perforation and cholecystoduodenal fistula," *Gastrointestinal Endoscopy*, vol. 56, no. 5, pp. 753–755, 2002.

[12] T. Nakatsu, "Endoscopie transpapillary gallbladder drainage (ETGBD) for the treatment of acute cholecystitis," *Journal of Hepato-Biliary-Pancreatic Sciences*, vol. 4, no. 1, pp. 31–35, 1997.

[13] A. N. Kalloo, P. J. Thuluvath, and P. J. Pasricha, "Treatment of high-risk patients with symptomatic cholelithiasis by endoscopic gallbladder stenting," *Gastrointestinal Endoscopy*, vol. 40, no. 5, pp. 608–610, 1994.

[14] P. J. Gaglio, B. Buniak, and C. B. Leevy, "Primary endoscopic retrograde cholecystoendroprosthesis: A nonsurgical modality for symptomatic cholelithiasis in cirrhotic patients," *Gastrointestinal Endoscopy*, vol. 44, no. 3, pp. 339–342, 1996.

[15] R. Shrestha and H. Lasch, "Endoscopic therapy for biliary tract disease before orthotopic liver transplantation," *Gastrointestinal Endoscopy Clinics of North America*, vol. 11, pp. 45–64, 2001.

[16] J. D. Conway, M. W. Russo, and R. Shrestha, "Endoscopic stent insertion into the gallbladder for symptomatic gallbladder disease in patients with end-stage liver disease," *Gastrointestinal Endoscopy*, vol. 61, no. 1, pp. 32–36, 2005.

[17] C. Schlenker, J. F. Trotter, R. J. Shah et al., "Endoscopic gallbladder stent placement for treatment of symptomatic cholelithiasis in patients with end-stage liver disease," *American Journal of Gastroenterology*, vol. 101, no. 2, pp. 278–283, 2006.

[18] D. W. Kjaer, A. Kruse, and P. Funch-Jensen, "Endoscopic gallbladder drainage of patients with acute cholecystitis," *Endoscopy*, vol. 39, no. 4, pp. 304–308, 2007.

[19] M. Mutignani, F. Iacopini, V. Perri et al., "Endoscopic gallbladder drainage for acute cholecystitis: Technical and clinical results," *Endoscopy*, vol. 41, no. 6, pp. 539–546, 2009.

[20] M. Yokoe, T. Takada, T.-L. Hwang et al., "Validation of TG13 severity grading in acute cholecystitis: Japan-Taiwan collaborative study for acute cholecystitis," *Journal of Hepato-Biliary-Pancreatic Sciences*, vol. 24, no. 6, pp. 338–345, 2017.

[21] T. H. Lee, D. H. Park, S. S. Lee et al., "Outcomes of endoscopic transpapillary gallbladder stenting for symptomatic gallbladder diseases: A multicenter prospective follow-up study," *Endoscopy*, vol. 43, no. 8, pp. 702–708, 2011.

[22] S. Maekawa, R. Nomura, T. Murase, Y. Ann, M. Oeholm, and M. Harada, "Endoscopic gallbladder stenting for acute cholecystitis: A retrospective study of 46 elderly patients aged 65 years or older," *BMC Gastroenterology*, vol. 13, no. 1, article no. 65, 2013.

[23] T. Itoi, H. Kawakami, A. Katanuma et al., "Endoscopic nasogallbladder tube or stent placement in acute cholecystitis: A preliminary prospective randomized trial in Japan (with videos)," *Gastrointestinal Endoscopy*, vol. 81, no. 1, pp. 111–118, 2015.

[24] P. B. Cotton, G. M. Eisen, L. Aabakken et al., "A lexicon for endoscopic adverse events: report of an ASGE workshop," *Gastrointestinal Endoscopy*, vol. 71, no. 3, pp. 446–454, 2010.

[25] R. A. Kozarek, "Selective cannulation of the cystic duct at time of ERCP," *Journal of Clinical Gastroenterology*, vol. 6, no. 1, pp. 37–40, 1984.

[26] R. Pannala, B. T. Petersen, C. J. Gostout, M. D. Topazian, M. J. Levy, and T. H. Baron, "Endoscopic transpapillary gallbladder drainage: 10-year single center experience," *Minerva Gastroenterol Dietol*, vol. 54, pp. 107–113, 2008.

[27] J. W. Jang, S. S. Lee, T. J. Song et al., "Endoscopic ultrasound-guided transmural and percutaneous transhepatic gallbladder drainage are comparable for acute cholecystitis," *Gastroenterology*, vol. 142, no. 4, pp. 805–811, 2012.

[28] T. Tsuyuguchi, T. Itoi, T. Takada et al., "TG13 indications and techniques for gallbladder drainage in acute cholecystitis (with videos)," *Journal of Hepato-Biliary-Pancreatic Sciences*, vol. 20, no. 1, pp. 81–88, 2013.

[29] J. P. Ha, K. K. Tsui, C. N. Tang, W. T. Siu, K. H. Fung, and M. K. Li, "Cholecystectomy or not after percutaneous cholecystostomy for acute calculous cholecystitis in high-risk patients," *Hepatogastroenterology*, vol. 55, pp. 1497–1502, 2008.

[30] M. Schmidt, K. Sondenaa, M. Vetrhus, T. Berhane, and G. E. Eide, "Long-term follow-up of a randomized controlled trial of observation versus surgery for acute cholecystitis: Non-operative management is an option in some patients," *Scandinavian Journal of Gastroenterology*, vol. 46, no. 10, pp. 1257–1262, 2011.

13

Efficacy and Safety of Single-Session Endoscopic Stone Removal for Acute Cholangitis Associated with Choledocholithiasis

Junya Sato,[1] Kazunari Nakahara,[1] Ryo Morita,[1] Nozomi Morita,[1] Keigo Suetani,[1] Yosuke Michikawa,[1] Shinjiro Kobayashi,[2] and Fumio Itoh[1]

[1] *Department of Gastroenterology and Hepatology, St. Marianna University School of Medicine, 2-16-1 Sugao, Miyamae-ku, Kawasaki 216-8511, Japan*

[2] *Department of Gastroenterological and General Surgery, St. Marianna University School of Medicine, 2-16-1 Sugao, Miyamae-ku, Kawasaki 216-8511, Japan*

Correspondence should be addressed to Kazunari Nakahara; nakahara@marianna-u.ac.jp

Academic Editor: Yousuke Nakai

Background/Aims. In early endoscopic retrograde cholangiopancreatography (ERCP) for acute cholangitis due to choledocholithiasis, it is unclear that single-session stone removal can be safely performed. We examined the efficacy and safety of early single-session stone removal for mild-to-moderate acute cholangitis associated with choledocholithiasis. *Methods.* Among patients with mild-to-moderate acute cholangitis associated with choledocholithiasis who underwent early ERCP (n = 167), we retrospectively compared the removal group (patients who underwent single-session stone removal; n = 78) with the drainage group (patients who underwent biliary drainage alone; n = 89) and examined the effectiveness and safety of single-session stone removal by early ERCP. *Results.* The patients in the removal group had significantly fewer and smaller stones compared with those in the drainage group. The single-session complete stone removal rate was 85.9% in the removal group. The complication rate in early ERCP was 11.5% in the removal group and 10.1% in the drainage group, with no significant difference (P = 0.963). On comparing patients who underwent early endoscopic sphincterotomy (EST) with those who underwent elective EST after cholangitis had improved, the post-EST bleeding rates were 6.8% and 2.7%, respectively, with no significant difference (P = 0.600). The mean duration of hospitalization was 11.9 days for the removal group and 19.9 days for the drainage group, indicating a shorter stay for the removal group (P < 0.001). In multiple linear regression analysis, stone removal in early ERCP, number of stones, and C-reactive protein level were significant predictors of hospitalization period. *Conclusions.* Single-session stone removal for mild-to-moderate acute cholangitis can be safely performed. It is useful from the perspective of shorter hospital stay.

1. Introduction

According to the Tokyo Guidelines 2013 (TG13) for acute cholangitis, endoscopic transpapillary drainage is the most recommended for acute cholangitis [1, 2]. It is recommended that the timing to perform biliary drainage should be determined in accordance with the severity of acute cholangitis [3–5], with urgent drainage indicated for severe cases and early drainage for moderate cases; biliary drainage is needed when initial treatment such as antibiotic treatment is ineffective for mild cases. Moreover, when performing early endoscopic retrograde cholangiopancreatography (ERCP) for acute cholangitis associated with choledocholithiasis, if the cholangitis is severe, it is recommended to perform biliary drainage alone [3]; however, in moderate-to-mild cases, there is insufficient evidence regarding whether or not single-session stone removal can be safely performed.

Some previous reports indicate that endoscopic sphincterotomy (EST) for patients with acute cholangitis has a risk of bleeding [6, 7] and that acute cholangitis in itself is a risk factor for post-EST bleeding [8]. Furthermore, in acute cholangitis, stone removal may carry the risk of exacerbating cholangitis. On the other hand, if the acute cholangitis is mild-to-moderate, when performing early ERCP, it has been reported that EST does not increase the bleeding rate and that it shortens the length of hospital stay [9]. In a single-arm prospective study, it was reported that, in the absence of coagulopathy, single-session stone removal by EST for mild-to-moderate acute cholangitis is effective and can be safely performed [10]. In another report [11] comparing the therapeutic outcomes of single-session stone removal with elective stone removal after drainage for acute cholangitis, there was no difference in the rates of cholangitis improvement and procedural complications. However, the report [11] had limitations such as a small number of cases and a low single-session stone removal rate of 30.5%.

In the present study, we retrospectively examined patients who underwent early ERCP for mild-to-moderate acute cholangitis associated with choledocholithiasis and compared the therapeutic outcomes and safety of single-session stone removal with biliary drainage alone.

2. Materials and Methods

2.1. Patients. During the period from January 2011 to March 2017, 212 consecutive patients with mild-to-moderate acute cholangitis associated with choledocholithiasis underwent early ERCP at the Department of Gastroenterology and Hepatology of St. Marianna University School of Medicine. Early ERCP was defined as ERCP performed within 24 h of diagnosis. Among these patients, 14 who underwent postoperative reconstruction other than the Billroth I reconstruction, 21 with concurrent gallstone pancreatitis, and 10 with concurrent cholecystitis were excluded; thus, a total of 167 patients were included in the study. Six of 167 patients were enrolled twice because of recurrence of choledocholithiasis and cholangitis during the study period. For those six patients, the time to recurrence was 13.2±7.5 months (mean±standard deviation), and complete stone removal was confirmed by cholangiography using a balloon catheter at the initial ERCP.

In early ERCP, stone removal was attempted in a single session for 78 patients (removal group) and biliary drainage alone was performed in 89 patients (drainage group). Six patients registered twice were enrolled in 7 in the removal group and 5 in the drainage group. The decision to perform single-session stone removal or drainage alone was made at the discretion of the endoscopist; however, patients receiving antithrombotic therapy for native papilla underwent drainage alone. We discontinued any kind of antithrombotic drugs in principle and EST was performed after the appropriate discontinuation period for each drug. For the patients who had difficulty in discontinuation of antithrombotic drugs, heparin was substituted. All ERCPs were performed under the supervision of an expert with experience in over 500 ERCP procedures. In our institution, biliary cannulation is first attempted using the conventional contrast cannulation (CC). However, in case where biliary cannulation is difficult to perform by CC but in which a guidewire can be placed in the pancreatic duct, the pancreatic duct guidewire placement method (P-GW) is employed as the second choice. Then, we usually place a pancreatic stent for the prevention of pancreatitis over the guidewire used in the P-GW. The high-frequency device used in EST was 120-Watt Endocut mode Effect 3 (ICC 200; ERBE Corp., Tuebingen, Germany) or ESG-100 in 50-Watt pulse cut slow mode (Olympus Corp., Tokyo, Japan). Endoscopic papillary large balloon dilatation (EPLBD) was defined as papillary dilatation performed using a balloon of ≥12-mm diameter, and endoscopic papillary balloon dilatation (EPBD) was defined as papillary dilatation performed using a balloon of ≤10-mm diameter. EPLBD was performed for the papilla after performing EST or with a history of EST. Endoscopic nasobiliary drainage (ENBD) was performed using a 6-Fr catheter, and endoscopic biliary drainage (EBD) was performed using a 7-Fr stent. Complete stone removal confirmation was performed by cholangiography using balloon catheter. The contrast was injected from the proximal side hole of the balloon catheter after performing procedure for papilla such as EST. All patients were given antibiotics, with the type of antibiotic and administration period determined at the discretion of the attending physician. With the aim of preventing post-ERCP pancreatitis, on the day of the ERCP procedure, all patients were given 600 mg/day of gabexate mesilate. Furthermore, all patients underwent blood tests 3 h after the procedure and on the following day. Thereafter, blood and imaging tests were performed as required at the discretion of the attending physician to ascertain the patient's condition.

2.2. Measurements. In this study, the primary outcome was to evaluate the safety of early stone removal for mild-to-moderate acute cholangitis associated with choledocholithiasis, and the secondary outcome was to evaluate the clinical benefit of early single-session stone removal.

We retrospectively compared the patient characteristics, the details of ERCP procedure, the procedural duration, total number of ERCP sessions, stone removal rate, cholangitis improvement rate, period from early ERCP to the second ERCP for stone removal, length of hospital stay, and procedural complications in patients in the removal group (n = 78) with those in the drainage group (n=89). Furthermore, procedural complications were compared between patients who underwent EST in early ERCP and those who underwent EST in elective ERCP following improvement in cholangitis in the drainage group. Moreover, stepwise multiple linear regression analysis was performed to evaluate the factors related to hospitalization period.

Improvement of cholangitis was defined as a body temperature <37°C maintained for >24h and normalization of white blood cell count in blood test. On the other hand, worsening of cholangitis was defined as that blood test values and/or clinical symptoms such as fever or abdominal pain showed an exacerbation tendency. The diagnosis of procedural complications included pancreatitis, perforation, and cholangitis based on the consensus guidelines by Cotton et al. [12]. Post-EST bleeding was defined as requiring endoscopic hemostasis. However, simple hemostasis with coagulation using EST knife immediately after EST was excluded.

The present study was performed with the approval of the ethical review board of our hospital (approval number: 3667). Informed consent about present study participation was officially announced on a web page.

Table 1: Patient characteristics.

	Removal group (n=78)	Drainage group (n=89)	*P* value
Age (mean±SD)	71.1±16.1	77.3±9.9	0.002
Sex (Male/Female)	41/37	52/37	0.447
Performance status (0-2/3-4)	66/12	72/17	0.527
Severity of cholangitis (Moderate/Mild)	37/41	39/50	0.640
Blood test values			
WBC (/μl) (mean±SD)	10661±4280	10903±4320	0.717
CRP (mg/dl) (mean±SD)	6.26±5.55	6.09±6.09	0.851
T-Bil (mg/dl) (mean±SD)	3.80±2.71	3.30±2.42	0.213
Number of stones (mean±SD)	2.33±2.29	3.37±3.47	0.002
Diameter of stones (mm)(mean±SD)	8.55±4.80	12.24±6.36	<0.001
Post-endoscopic sphincterotomy (n (%))	19 (24.4)	23 (25.8)	0.825
Parapapillary diverticulum (n (%))	44 (56.4)	52 (58.4)	0.793
Antithrombotic drug (n (%))	6 (7.7)	59 (66.3)	<0.001

SD: standard deviation, WBC: white blood cell count, CRP: C-reactive protein, and T-Bil: total bilirubin.

Table 2: Procedures of early endoscopic retrograde cholangiopancreatography.

Endoscopic procedures (n (%))	Removal group (n=78)	Drainage group (n=89)	*P* value
Techniques for successful biliary cannulation			
CC	69 (88.5)	77 (86.5)	0.705
P-GW	7 (9.0)	12 (13.5)	0.360
Pre-cut	2 (2.6)	0 (0)	0.420
Endoscopic sphincterotomy	58 (74.4)	11 (12.4)	<0.001
Endoscopic papillary balloon dilatation	9 (11.5)	0 (0)	0.003
Endoscopic papillary large balloon dilatation	8 (10.3)	0 (0)	0.006
Intraductal ultrasonography	8 (10.3)	1 (1.1)	0.024
Endoscopic mechanical lithotripsy	10 (12.8)	–	–
Basket catheter	42 (53.8)	–	–
Balloon catheter	49 (62.8)	–	–
Endoscopic nasobiliary drainage	9 (11.5)	16 (18.0)	0.245
Endoscopic biliary stenting	8 (10.3)	74 (83.1)	<0.001
Incidental pancreatography	30 (38.5)	33 (37.1)	0.854
Pancreatic stenting to prevent pancreatitis	6 (7.7)	12 (13.5)	0.229

CC: conventional contrast cannulation, P-GW: pancreatic duct guidewire placement method.

2.3. Statistical Analysis. Chi-square test, Fisher's exact test, and Welch's t-test were used for statistical analysis where appropriate. Stepwise multiple linear regression analysis with a forward approach using cutoff value of 0.05 was performed to identify independent predictors of hospitalization period. A P value of <0.05 was regarded as significant. Statistical analysis was performed with StatMate IV (ATMS Co., Ltd., Tokyo, Japan) and SPSS (version 19; SPSS, Chicago, IL, USA).

3. Results

3.1. Patient Characteristics. Patient characteristics are shown in Table 1. There was no difference in terms of gender, performance status (PS), severity of cholangitis, proportion of post-EST papilla, and presence or absence of parapapillary diverticulum between the removal and drainage groups; however, the patients in the removal group were significantly younger and had fewer and smaller stones compared with those in the drainage group. Moreover, the drainage group included many patients who were taking antithrombotic agents.

3.2. Procedures. The details of the early ERCP procedure are shown in Table 2. Biliary cannulation was achieved in all 167 patients. Techniques for successful biliary cannulation included CC in 69 patient, P-GW in 7, and Pre-cut in 2 in the removal group and CC in 77 and P-GW in 12 in the drainage group. There was no difference in the technique of successful biliary cannulation between the two groups. The procedures for papilla included EST in 58 patients, EPBD in 9, and EPLBD in 8 in the removal group and EST in 11 in the drainage group. EST, EPBD, EPLBD, and intraductal ultrasonography were more frequently performed in the removal group, whereas endoscopic biliary stenting (EBS) was more frequently performed in the drainage group. There

Table 3: Comparison of the treatment results between the removal and drainage groups.

	Removal group (n=78)	Drainage group (n=89)	*P* value
Procedure time of early ERCP (min)(mean±SD)	38.8±18.6	27.0±15.2	0.036
Number of ERCP administrations (mean±SD)	1.2±0.50	2.2±0.8	<0.001
Complete stone removal ratio in early ERCP (n (%))	67 (85.9)	–	–
Final complete stone removal ratio (n (%))	78 (100)	84 (94.4)	0.095
Improvement rate of cholangitis after early ERCP (n (%))	78 (100)	89 (100)	–
Final improvement rate of cholangitis (n (%))	78 (100)	89 (100)	–
Period to second ERCP for stone removal (day)(mean±SD)	7.8±3.9	9.8±4.7	0.068
Hospitalization period (day)(mean±SD)	11.9±7.16	19.9±8.69	<0.001

ERCP: endoscopic retrograde cholangiopancreatography, SD: standard deviation.

Table 4: Comparison of adverse events in early ERCP between the removal and drainage groups.

	Removal group (n=78)	Drainage group (n=89)	*P* value
Adverse events ratio (n (%))	9 (11.5)	9 (10.1)	0.963
Pancreatitis	2 (2.6)	1 (1.1)	0.484
Post-EST bleeding	4 (5.1)	1 (1.1)	0.259
Post-EPLBD bleeding	1 (1.3)	0 (0)	0.947
Perforation	0 (0)	0 (0)	–
Worsening cholangitis	0 (0)	0 (0)	–
Acute cholecystitis	0 (0)	0 (0)	–
Mallory-Weiss syndrome	1 (1.3)	1 (1.1)	0.536
ENBD self-removal	1 (1.3)	3 (3.4)	0.709
Stent migration	0 (0)	3 (3.4)	0.292

EST: endoscopic sphincterotomy, EPLBD: endoscopic papillary large balloon dilatation, and ENBD: endoscopic nasobiliary drainage.

was no difference in the proportion of pancreatic stenting between the two groups (P = 0.229).

In 84 out of the 89 patients in the drainage group, elective stone removal was performed after cholangitis had improved. The procedures for papilla involved EST in 37 patients, EPBD in 13, EPLBD in 26, and pre-cutting in 1. Furthermore, five patients had concurrent malignant tumors or severe illness and were thus discharged after undergoing EBD alone without stone removal.

3.3. Therapeutic Outcomes. The therapeutic outcomes are shown in Table 3. The procedural duration for early ERCP was 38.8 min in the removal group and 27.0 min in the drainage group, which was significantly shorter (P = 0.036); however, the total number of ERCP sessions was 1.2 in the removal group and 2.2 in the drainage group, indicating that significantly fewer sessions were performed for the removal group (P < 0.001). The single-session complete stone removal rate in early ERCP was 85.9% for the removal group. The overall complete stone removal rate was 100% for the removal group and 94.4% for the drainage group, with no significant difference observed (P = 0.095). The improvement rate in acute cholangitis following early ERCP and the overall improvement rate in acute cholangitis were 100% for both groups. The mean period from early ERCP to second ERCP for stone removal was 7.8 days for the removal group and 9.8 days for drainage group with no statistical difference (P = 0.068). The mean length of hospital stay was 11.9 days for the removal group and 19.9 days for the drainage group, indicating a significantly shorter stay for the removal group (P < 0.001).

3.4. Procedural Complications. The procedural complications in early ERCP are shown in Table 4. The overall procedural complication rate was 11.5% for the removal group and 10.1% for the drainage group, with no significant difference observed between the two groups (P = 0.963). In the removal group, pancreatitis occurred in 2.6%, post-EST bleeding in 5.1%, post-EPLBD bleeding in 1.3%, Mallory–Weiss syndrome in 1.3%, and ENBD self-removal in 1.3%, whereas in the drainage group, pancreatitis occurred in 1.1%, post-EST bleeding in 1.1%, Mallory–Weiss syndrome in 1.1%, ENBD self-removal in 3.4%, and stent migration in 3.4%; no difference was observed between the two groups. Furthermore, perforation, worsening of cholangitis, and acute cholecystitis were not observed in either group, and there were no fatalities. In patients who underwent early EST, including those in the removal and drainage groups, the post-EST bleeding rate was 6.8% (5/69), including 6.9% (4/58) in the removal group and 9.1% (1/11) in the drainage group, with no significant difference observed (P = 0.706). Moreover, upon comparing early EST (n = 69) with elective EST after cholangitis had improved (n = 37), the post-EST bleeding rates were 6.8% (5/69) and 2.7% (1/37), respectively, with no significant difference observed (P = 0.600) (Table 5). In all patients with post-EST bleeding and post-EPLBD

TABLE 5: Comparison of adverse events between early and elective endoscopic sphincterotomy.

	Early EST (n=69)	Elective EST (n=37)	*P* value
Adverse events ratio (n (%))	7 (10.1)	1 (2.7)	0.319
Pancreatitis	2 (2.9)	0 (0)	0.767
Post-EST bleeding	5 (6.8)	1 (2.7)	0.600
Perforation	0 (0)	0 (0)	–
Worsening cholangitis	0 (0)	0 (0)	–
Acute cholecystitis	0 (0)	0 (0)	–

EST: endoscopic sphincterotomy.

TABLE 6: Stepwise multiple linear regression analysis for variables associated with hospitalization period.

Variables	B	SE	β	T value	P value
Stone removal in early ERCP	7.467	1.223	0.418	6.107	< 0.001
Number of stones	0.568	0.203	0.192	2.792	0.006
CRP level	0.250	0.104	0.163	2.412	0.017

B: partial regression coefficient, SE: standard error, β: standardized partial regression coefficient, ERCP: endoscopic retrograde cholangiopancreatography, and CRP: C-reactive protein.

bleeding, hemostasis was achieved by endoscopic hemostasis (injection of hypertonic saline-epinephrine: 4, compression using balloon catheter for stone removal or EPBD: 3, and clipping: 1), and all other complications were improved with conservative treatment.

3.5. Predictors of Hospitalization Period. Stepwise multiple linear regression was calculated to predict hospitalization period. Independent variables included age, sex, PS, severity of cholangitis, white blood cell count (WBC), C-reactive protein (CRP) level, total bilirubin (T-Bil) level, number of stones, diameter of stones, naïve papilla, use of antithrombotic drug, procedure for naïve papilla in early ERCP, stone removal in early ERCP, development of adverse event, development of pancreatitis, and development of bleeding. A significant regression equation was found ($F(3, 163) = 18.973$, $p < 0.001$, with an R^2 of 0.259). Participants' predicted hospitalization period is equal to 9.008 + 0.250 (CRP level) + 0.568 (number of stones) + 7.467 (stone removal in early ERCP), where CRP level is measured in mg/dl, and stone removal in early ERCP is coded as 1 = without, 0 = with. Participants' hospitalization period increased 7.467 days in without stone removal in early ERCP, 0.568 days for each number of stones, and 0.250 days for each mg/dl of CRP level. As a result, stone removal in early ERCP, number of stones, and CRP level were significant predictors of hospitalization period (Table 6).

4. Discussion

In this study, we evaluated the safety and clinical benefit of single-session stone removal for mild-to-moderate acute cholangitis associated with choledocholithiasis. As a result, regarding safety, there was no difference in the incidence of adverse events such as cholangitis exacerbation or post-EST bleeding between single-session stone removal and only drainage; that is, it was considered that the single-session stone removal could be performed with the same safety level as only drainage. Regarding clinical benefit, single-session stone removal contributed to a significant shortening of the hospitalization period. Furthermore, a multiple linear regression analysis revealed that the factor most related to the hospitalization period was stone removal in early ERCP. Therefore, in this study, we found that single-session stone removal for mild-to-moderate acute cholangitis can be performed safely, moreover, with the perspective of shorter length of hospital stay.

As for EST in the presence of acute cholangitis, Sugiyama et al. [6] retrospectively compared the presence or absence of EST prior to ENBD for acute cholangitis and found that, in patients without EST, the overall complication rate was 2% and the bleeding rate was 0%, whereas in those with EST, the overall complication rate was 11% and the bleeding rate was 4%, which were significantly higher ($P < 0.05$). However, in the report, among patients who underwent EST, 19% had severe cholangitis and 8% had coagulopathy. In addition, two among the three patients with bleeding had coagulopathy. Hui et al. [7] retrospectively compared the presence or absence of EST prior to EBS for acute cholangitis associated with choledocholithiasis. The overall complication rate was 2.7% and the bleeding rate was 0% in patients without EST, whereas the overall complication rate was 10.8% and the bleeding rate was 8.1% in patients with EST, indicating higher rates in those who underwent EST. However, in the report by Hui et al. [7], all patients had severe cholangitis or acute suppurative cholangitis. Therefore, for patients with severe acute cholangitis, EST may increase the risk of bleeding.

On the other hand, Ueki et al. [9] retrospectively compared single-session EST against elective EST prior to EBD for moderate acute cholangitis associated with choledocholithiasis and reported that the rate of bleeding was 13% in single-session EST and 5% in elective EST, with no significant difference observed ($P = 0.127$). In addition, Eto et al. [10]

reported that the rate of post-EST bleeding of single stage EST for mild-to-moderate cholangitis was 4% (2/5), and Ito et al. [11] reported that the rate of post-EST bleeding of immediate EST for acute suppurative cholangitis was 0% (0/59). Therefore, these reports concluded that the risk of post-EST bleeding is not high in patients with mild-to-moderate cholangitis. In the present study, the post-EST bleeding rate among patients with EST was 6.8% (removal group: 6.9%, drainage group: 9.1%), which was comparable to that in previously reported results, and on comparing early EST with elective EST after cholangitis had improved, there was no difference in procedural complications including bleeding; thus, it was suggested that, in mild-to-moderate cholangitis, EST can be performed with equal safety similar to that performed in patients without cholangitis.

With regard to single-session stone removal, Jang et al. [13] retrospectively compared urgent and elective single-session stone removal for mild-to-moderate acute cholangitis and demonstrated that there was no significant difference in clinical success rate and intervention-related complications. Furthermore, the urgent group has a shorter length of hospital stay ($P < 0.001$). Moreover, Eto et al. [10] conducted a prospective single-arm study of single-session stone removal for 50 patients with mild-to-moderate acute cholangitis associated with choledocholithiasis and reported that, within 4 days of the procedure, the improvement rate of acute cholangitis was 90%, the overall procedural complication rate was 10%, and the bleeding rate was 4%; thus, in the absence of coagulopathy and oral antithrombotic therapy, they found that single-session stone removal by EST was useful. In the present study, we observed no cases of cholangitis exacerbation following single-session stone removal, with an improvement observed in cholangitis in all cases. Therefore, if the acute cholangitis is mild-to-moderate, then we consider that single-session stone removal does not carry a high risk of cholangitis exacerbation. Furthermore, other procedural complication rate, such as pancreatitis, was comparable in patients who underwent drainage alone; thus, single-session stone removal by EST can be safely performed.

Same as present study, Ito et al. [11] compared the therapeutic results of single-session stone removal for acute cholangitis associated with choledocholithiasis with those of elective stone removal following drainage and reported that there was no difference in the cholangitis improvement rate and procedural complication rate. However, it cannot be ruled out that the results were affected by the fact that the sample size for elective stone removal following drainage was small at 28 patients and that the single-session complete stone removal rate was low at 30.5%. The present study included more patients (removal group: 78 patients, drainage group: 89 patients), and the single-session complete stone removal rate was high at 85.9%. However, consequently, there was no difference in the cholangitis improvement rate and procedural complication rate, which is consistent with the findings by Ito et al. Therefore, even if stone removal was performed with a high complete stone removal rate, it could be safely performed without exacerbation of cholangitis. Furthermore, in the report by Ito et al., there was no statistically significant difference in the length of hospital stay between the single-session stone removal group (n=59) and the group that underwent elective stone removal after drainage (n=28) (P=0.09). However, when limited to the patients with successful complete stone removal in the single-session stone removal group (n=18), the hospitalization period was significantly shorter than the elective EST group (P=0.02). In the present study, the removal group had a significantly shorter length of hospital stay and we consider that the high complete stone removal rate in the removal group could have contributed to shorter length of hospital stay. Since stone removal in early ERCP was identified as a factor most related to hospitalization period in multiple linear regression analysis, high complete stone removal rate may contribute to shortening of hospitalization period. Besides, the number of stones and CRP level are also identified as a factor related to hospitalization period; therefore, requiring multiple ERCP sessions for many stones or severe inflammation may have affected the prolonged hospitalization.

Limitations of the present study are that it was a retrospective study and that there may have been a selection bias in the drainage group comprising patients receiving oral antithrombotic therapy, patients with many stones, and patients with large stone. Therefore, further prospective comparative studies of patients with consistent backgrounds are needed.

5. Conclusions

In the present study, we found that, in patients with mild-to-moderate acute cholangitis associated with choledocholithiasis, without receiving oral antithrombotic therapy, single-session stone removal can be performed with the same safety level as that for elective stone removal after drainage, moreover, with the perspective of shorter length of hospital stay.

Acknowledgments

The authors are grateful to Dr. T Ueno from Unit of Medical Statistics, Faculty of Medical Education and Culture, St. Marianna University School of Medicine for constructive advice on statistical analysis. They also thank Crimson Interactive Pvt Ltd. for their assistance in manuscript translation and editing.

References

[1] T. Takada, S. M. Strasberg, J. S. Solomkin et al., "TG13: updated Tokyo Guidelines for the management of acute cholangitis and cholecystitis," *Journal of Hepato-Biliary-Pancreatic Surgery*, vol. 20, pp. 1–7, 2013.

[2] T. Itoi, T. Tsuyuguchi, T. Takada et al., "TG13 indications and techniques for biliary drainage in acute cholangitis (with videos)," *Journal of Hepato-Biliary-Pancreatic Sciences*, vol. 20, no. 1, pp. 71–80, 2013.

[3] F. Miura, T. Takada, S. M. Strasberg et al., "TG flowchart for the management of acute cholangitis and cholecystitis," *Journal of Hepato-Biliary-Pancreatic Surgery*, vol. 20, pp. 47–54.

[4] S. Kiriyama, T. Takada, S. M. Strasberg et al., "New diagnostic criteria and severity assessment of acute cholangitis in revised Tokyo Guidelines," *Journal of Hepato-Biliary-Pancreatic Surgery*, vol. 19, pp. 548–556, 2012.

[5] M. A. Khashab, A. Tariq, U. Tariq et al., "Delayed and Unsuccessful Endoscopic Retrograde Cholangiopancreatography Are Associated With Worse Outcomes in Patients With Acute Cholangitis," *Clinical Gastroenterology and Hepatology*, vol. 10, no. 10, pp. 1157–1161, 2012.

[6] M. Sugiyama and Y. Atomi, "The benefits of endoscopic nasobiliary drainage without sphincterotomy for acute cholangitis," *American Journal of Gastroenterology*, vol. 93, no. 11, pp. 2065–2068, 1998.

[7] C.-K. Hui, K.-C. Lai, M.-F. Yuen et al., "Does the addition of endoscopic sphincterotomy to stent insertion improve drainage of the bile duct in acute suppurative cholangitis?" *Gastrointestinal Endoscopy*, vol. 58, no. 4, pp. 500–504, 2003.

[8] M. L. Freeman, D. B. Nelson, S. Sherman et al., "Complications of endoscopic biliary sphincterotomy," *The New England Journal of Medicine*, vol. 335, no. 13, pp. 909–918, 1996.

[9] T. Ueki, K. Otani, N. Fujimura et al., "Comparison between emergency and elective endoscopic sphincterotomy in patients with acute cholangitis due to choledocholithiasis: Is emergency endoscopic sphincterotomy safe?" *Journal of Gastroenterology*, vol. 44, no. 10, pp. 1080–1088, 2009.

[10] K. Eto, H. Kawakami, S. Haba et al., "Single-stage endoscopic treatment for mild to moderate acute cholangitis associated with choledocholithiasis: a multicenter, non-randomized, open-label and exploratory clinical trial," *Journal of Hepato-Biliary-Pancreatic Sciences*, vol. 22, no. 12, pp. 825–830, 2015.

[11] T. Ito, J. K. Sai, H. Okubo et al., "Safety of immediate endoscopic sphincterotomy in acute suppurative cholangitis caused by choledocholithiasis," *World Journal of Gastrointestinal Endoscopy*, vol. 8, no. 3, p. 180, 2016.

[12] P. B. Cotton, G. Lehman, J. Vennes et al., "Endoscopic sphincterotomy complications and their management: an attempt at consensus," *Gastrointestinal Endoscopy*, vol. 37, no. 3, pp. 383–393, 1991.

[13] S. E. Jang, S. W. Park, B. S. Lee et al., "Management for CBD stone-related mild to moderate acute cholangitis: Urgent versus elective ERCP," *Digestive Diseases and Sciences*, vol. 58, no. 7, pp. 2082–2087, 2013.

14

Increased Duodenal Iron Absorption through Upregulation of Ferroportin 1 due to the Decrement in Serum Hepcidin in Patients with Chronic Hepatitis C

Masanori Sato,[1] Koji Miyanishi,[1] Shingo Tanaka,[1] Akira Sakurada,[1] Hiroki Sakamoto,[1] Yutaka Kawano,[1] Kohichi Takada,[1] Masayoshi Kobune,[2] and Junji Kato[1]

[1] *Department of Medical Oncology, Sapporo Medical University School of Medicine, South-1, West-16, Chuo-Ku, Sapporo 060-8543, Japan*
[2] *Department of Medical Hematology, Sapporo Medical University School of Medicine, South-1, West-16, Chuo-Ku, Sapporo 060-8543, Japan*

Correspondence should be addressed to Koji Miyanishi; miyako@sapmed.ac.jp and Masayoshi Kobune; mkobune@sapmed.ac.jp

Academic Editor: Alessandro Granito

Hepatic iron accumulation is generally increased in the chronic hepatitis C (CHC) liver; however, the precise mechanism of such accumulation remains unclear. We evaluated iron absorption from the gastrointestinal tract of patients with CHC and control participants. We measured the expression of a panel of molecules associated with duodenal iron absorption and serum hepcidin levels to determine the mechanism of iron accumulation in the CHC liver. We enrolled 24 patients with CHC and 9 patients with chronic gastritis without *Helicobacter pylori* infection or an iron metabolism disorder as control participants. An oral iron absorption test (OIAT) was administered which involved a dosage of 100 mg of sodium ferrous citrate. Serum level of hepcidin-25 was measured by liquid chromatography-tandem mass spectrometry. Ferroportin 1 (FPN) mRNA was measured by RT-PCR and FPN protein was analyzed by western blot. Samples were obtained from duodenum biopsy tissue from each CHC patient and control participant. Caco-2/TC7 cells were incubated in Costar transwells (0.4 μm pores). The OIAT showed significantly greater iron absorption in CHC patients than control participants. Serum hepcidin-25 in the CHC group was significantly lower than in the control group. Compared with control participants, duodenal FPN mRNA expression in CHC patients was significantly upregulated. The FPN mRNA levels and protein levels increased significantly in Caco-2/TC7 cell monolayers cultured in transwells with hepcidin. Lower serum hepcidin-25 levels might upregulate not only FPN protein expression but also mRNA expression in the duodenum and cause iron accumulation in patients with CHC.

1. Introduction

Hepatic iron overload has long been known to develop in patients with chronic hepatitis C (CHC) [1]. We previously revealed that excess free iron in hepatocytes promotes not only the production of reactive oxygen species (ROS) causing damage to hepatocytes and hepatic fibrosis but also increases the level of 8-hydroxy-2′-deoxyguanosine (8-OH-dG), a mutagenic base, in the liver, resulting in the development of hepatocellular carcinoma (HCC). In addition, we found that iron reduction therapy in combination with phlebotomy and a low iron diet improved hepatitis and hepatic fibrosis while normalizing the elevated 8-OH-dG level [2]. We also found that long-term iron depletion significantly reduced the incidence of HCC in patients with CHC (F2/F3 grade) [3]. However, the precise mechanisms involved in iron overload remain to be clarified.

The body's iron supply is obtained largely by iron absorption from the intestine and reabsorption from hemoglobin in the reticuloendothelial system [4]. Intestinal iron absorption is mainly from the duodenum. Two iron transport proteins, divalent metal transporter 1 (DMT1) and ferroportin 1 (FPN), are expressed in duodenal enterocytes [4, 5]. Hepcidin is a 2.7 kDa peptide consisting of 25 amino acids that is produced mainly in hepatocytes and acts as a major regulator of iron homeostasis [6]. Hepcidin affects macrophages, Hela cells, or human embryonic kidney cells, so that they regulate iron efflux and storage and the duodenum so that it inhibits iron absorption [7–9]. Although several reports have shown decreased expression of hepcidin in CHC patients [10, 11], no reported study has investigated the dynamics of iron absorption in patients with nonalcoholic steatohepatitis.

In the current study, we aimed to investigate the mechanism of hepatic iron overload in CHC patients. For this purpose we measured the expression of a panel of molecules in association with iron absorption in the duodenum and serum hepcidin levels.

2. Materials and Methods

2.1. Patients and Tissue Samples. Duodenum tissue samples were obtained from 24 CHC cases between February 2008 and January 2016. In addition, biopsied duodenum tissue samples were examined from 9 control participants with chronic gastritis who did not have *Helicobacter pylori* infection or an iron metabolism disorder. The ethical committee for human genome/gene analysis research of our hospital approved this study. All participants provided written informed consent at the time of tissue sampling to take part in this study after receiving a detailed explanation of the procedures involved according to the Declaration of Helsinki.

2.2. Criteria for Definition of CHC. CHC was defined according to an ALT value ≥30 U/L and HCV RNA positivity by polymerase chain reaction (PCR). Patients younger than 18 years and those with hepatitis B surface antigen (HBs Ag) positivity, previous IFN treatment, serum HCV RNA negativity, and history of heavy alcohol abuse were excluded from this study.

2.3. Laboratory Tests. Laboratory tests were done at the same time as tissue sampling. Venous blood samples were taken in the morning after a 12-h overnight fast. Complete blood cell counts, determinations of serum iron, ferritin, total iron-binding capacity, and %transferrin saturation (Tf sat), and biochemical examinations, including that for serum ALT, were performed using automated procedures in the clinical laboratories of Sapporo Medical University Hospital (Sapporo, Japan).

2.4. Oral Iron Absorption Test. Iron absorption from the gastrointestinal (GI) tract was measured using the oral iron absorption test (OIAT) established in our laboratory as described previously [12, 13]. In brief, at 9 a.m. after an overnight fast a blood sample was taken to measure serum iron and total iron-binding capacity (TIBC). Subsequently, the participant ingested 100 mg of iron in the form of two tablets of sodium ferrous citrate (SFC). Blood samples for measurement of iron parameters were taken after 15, 30, 60, and 120 min. Participants were not permitted to eat during the test.

2.5. Serum Hepcidin-25 Concentration. Serum concentration of hepcidin-25 was measured by liquid chromatography-tandem mass spectrometry (LC-MS/MS) as described previously [13, 14]. The assay was performed by Medical Care Proteomics Biotechnology Co., Ltd. (Kanazawa, Japan).

2.6. Quantitative Real-Time Reverse-Transcriptase Polymerase Chain Reaction. We followed the methods of our previous report [13]. Assay numbers for the endogenous control (18S ribosomal RNA [rRNA]) and target genes were as follows: Hs00167206 m1 (DMT1) and Hs00205888 m1 (FPN). Total RNAs were extracted from cultured cells using RNeasy Mini Kits (QIAGEN, Valecia, CA, USA) according to the manufacturer's protocol. cDNA was prepared using the Super Script VILO kit (Invitrogen, Carlsbad, CA, USA). The cDNA was added to the TaqMan Universal PCR Master Mix (Applied Biosystems, Tokyo, Japan). Each mixture was transferred to a 96-well optical tray. Target mRNAs were reverse transcribed at 60°C for 30 min, followed by a PCR cycle with a melting step for 20 s at 94°C and annealing for 1 min at 60°C for a total of 40 cycles using the ABI PRISM 7300 Sequence Detection System (Applied Biosystems). The parameter Ct was defined as the fractional cycle number at which the fluorescence generated by cleavage of the probe passes a fixed threshold above baseline. The standard curve was constructed with 10-fold serial dilutions of total RNA from Caco-2/TC7 cell monolayers (calibrator) and composed of 4 points (200, 20, 2, and 0.2 ng of total RNA). The target RNA and relative messages to the calibrator, termed [Target]c and [18S rRNA] c, respectively, in unknown samples were quantified by measuring Ct and using a standard curve to determine the starting target message quantity. The final relative mRNA expression level was expressed as follows: relative target mRNA level = [Target] c/[18S rRNA] c. We performed duplicate measurements for each data point. Each RT-PCR run included 5 points on the standard curve, a no-template control, the calibrator total RNA, and 36 unknown total RNAs. All of the samples with a coefficient of variation for relative messages to the calibrator data >10% were retested as previously reported [13, 15].

2.7. Western Blot Experiments. Proteins were extracted from cultured Caco-2/TC7 cell monolayers using RIPA buffer (150 mmol/L NaCl, 1% Nonidet P-40, 0.5% deoxycholate, 0.1% sodium dodecyl sulfate, 50 mmol/L Tris HCl pH 8.0, 0.2 mmol/L phenylmethylsulfonyl fluoride, 1 μg/mL pepstatin, 0.5 μg/mL leupeptin), and 50 μg of total protein was used for immunoblotting. Blots were incubated with 1 μg/mL anti-DMT1 antibody or FPN antibody for 24 h at 4°C. For western blots, the specific antibodies used were: DMT1 catalog #ab55735 from abcam Cambridge, MA; and FPN #LS-B1836 from Lifespan Bioscience, Seattle, WA.

2.8. Cell Cultures. Caco-2/TC7 cells were obtained from American Type Culture Collection (ATCC; Manassas, VA, USA). To achieve a fully differentiated monolayer, cells were grown in Dulbecco's modified Eagle's medium (DMEM) containing 10% fetal bovine serum (FBS) on Costar transwell

TABLE 1: Baseline characteristics of study participants.

Characteristic	Control group	CHC group	P values
Number of patients	9	24	
Gender, M/F	4/5	11/13	0.9431
Age, y	61 (46-74)	59 (22-73)	0.5709
Body mass index, kg/m2	21.6 (19.0-25.5)	23.3 (16.3-32.5)	0.0688
AST, IU/L	18 (13-32)	56 (28-303)	0.0002
ALT, IU/L	20 (17-30)	71 (35-501)	0.0108
GGT, IU/L	32 (11-64)	52 (10-260)	0.0881
Hb, g/dL	14.8 (11.4-16.2)	13.4 (11.6-16.3)	0.6900
Platelet count, x104/μL	221 (182-265)	176 (57-308)	0.0596
Serum Fe, μg/dL	68 (55-99)	106 (44-234)	0.0038
Serum ferritin, μg/dL	75.0 (25.0-115.0)	184 (12.4-1550)	0.0084
Tf saturation, %	23.8 (19.0-31.8)	41.0 (20.8-63.9)	0.0103
Total cholesterol, mg/dL	201 (140-258)	180 (90-257)	0.1455
Triglyceride, mg/dL	120 (77-235)	118 (64-359)	0.7772

membrane inserts with 0.4 μm pores (Corning, St. Louis, MO, USA) for 21 days. At the 22nd day of culture, serum-free DMEM was added to the upper well and DMEM containing 2% FBS was added to the lower well after which the cells were cultured for 48 h. At the 24th day of culture, DMEM containing 2% FBS was added to the upper well and the cells were treated with DMEM containing 10% FBS either with or without human 25-amino acid synthetic hepcidin for 48 h. We followed the methods of our previous report [13].

2.9. Immunohistochemistry. Biopsy tissues were fixed in 10% buffered formaldehyde. After overnight fixation, they were embedded in paraffin wax and 4-mm thick sections were cut. All immunohistochemical staining was carried out on a Leica Bond-Max autostainer (Leica Biosystems, Nussloch, Gmbh, Germany) according to the manufacturer's protocol, with appropriate positive and negative controls. Sections were baked at 60°C for 60 min in a dehydration oven, then dewaxed in Bond Dewax solution, and rehydrated in Bond Wash solution (Leica Microsystems). Antigen retrieval was carried out at pH 6 with Novocastra Epitope Retrieval solution (Leica Bioosystems) for 20 min at 100°C. Slides were then incubated for 15 min at room temperature with ferroportin antibody (HPA065634 dilution 1 : 150; Atlas Antibodies Stockholm, Sweden).

The staining intensity of FPN in the duodenum biopsy tissues was evaluated by the immunohistochemical score. The method was described previously [16, 17].

2.10. Statistical Analysis. Statistical evaluation was performed with GraphPad Prism (GraphPad Inc, La Jolla, CA, USA). Quantitative values are expressed as means ± standard deviation (SD) or median (range). Each data set was first evaluated for normality of distribution by the Kolmogorov-Smirnov's test to decide whether a nonparametric rank-based analysis or a parametric analysis should be used. Two groups were compared using Fisher's exact test for categorical data and either the Wilcoxon-Mann-Whitney U test or the one-way analysis of variance (ANOVA) for quantitative data. Spearman's rank correlation was used to quantify the association between continuous or ordered categorical variables. Comparison of chronologic changes in parameters in the OIAT was done by repeated-measures ANOVA. Comparison of changes in the starting target message quantity in qRT-PCR was made using the Jonckheere-Terpstra test.

3. Results

3.1. Characteristics of the CHC Group and Control Group. The levels of AST, ALT, serum iron, serum ferritin, and TF sat in the CHC group at diagnosis were significantly higher than those in the control group. There were no between-group differences in gender or hemoglobin, body mass index, and total cholesterol and triglyceride levels (Table 1).

3.2. Oral Iron Absorption Test. To investigate the mechanism of hepatic iron overload in CHC patients, we performed the OIAT to evaluate iron absorption from the intestine. Compared with the control group, iron absorption was significantly increased from the GI tract in the CHC group (Figure 1(a); $P < 0.001$). Also, Tf sat was significantly increased in the CHC group compared with the control group (Figure 1(b); $P < 0.001$). Despite the increased Tf sat levels before the administration of SFC, iron absorption was upregulated in CHC patients.

3.3. Serum Hepcidin-25 Concentrations. We measured serum hepcidin-25 using LC-MS/MS. The normal range of serum hepcidin-25 using LC-MS/MS analysis was reported to be 10-34 ng/mL [18]. The median serum hepcidin-25 level in the CHC group was 7.2 ng/mL (range, 0-27.3) and was 23.3 ng/mL (range, 3.9-47.3) in the control group, with the CHC group having a significantly lower value (Figure 2; P = 0.0002). Serum hepcidin-25 level was significantly correlated with OIAT s-Fe 120 min (ρ = -0.438 and p = 0.0196).

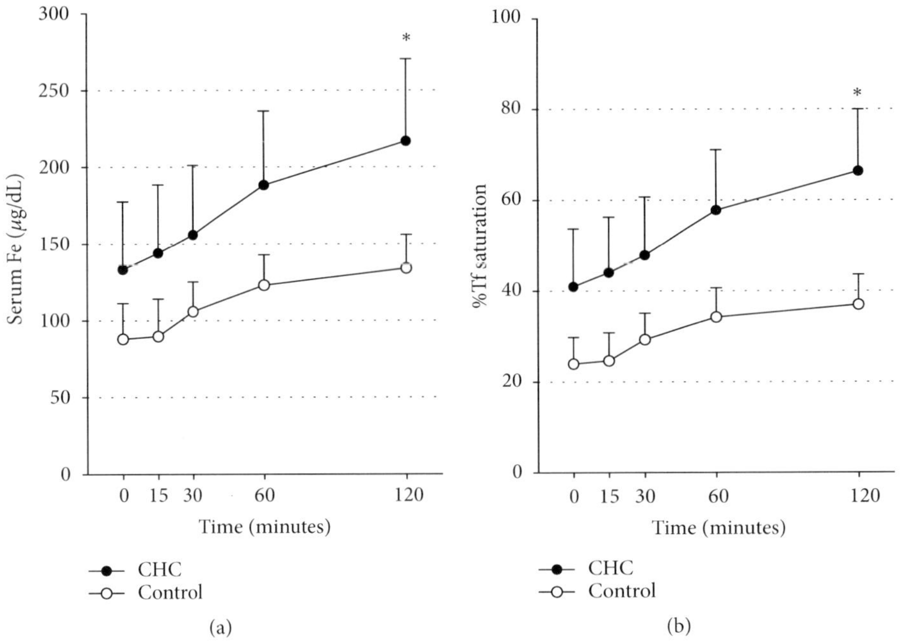

FIGURE 1: Serial changes in sFe (a) and Tf sat (b) after administration of sodium ferrous citrate. Closed circles indicate patients with CHC; open circles indicate controls. Compared to the control group, sFe and Tf sat were significantly increased in the patients with CHC (repeated-measures ANOVA. $^{*}P < 0.001$). These data show that iron absorption from the GI tract was significantly increased in the CHC patients.

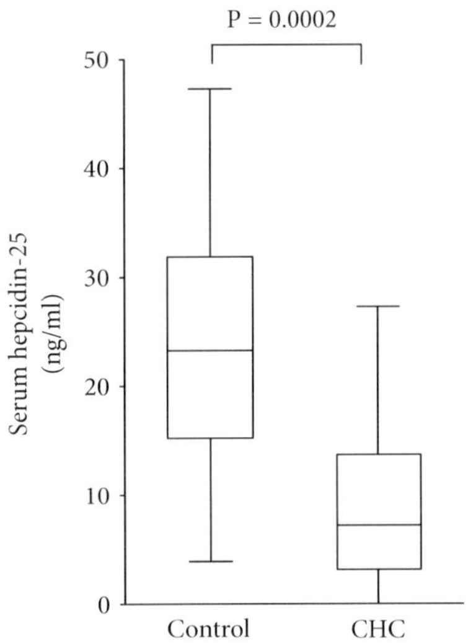

FIGURE 2: Serum hepcidin-25 levels were measured by LC-MS/MS. Median serum hepcidin-25 levels of control participants and CHC patients were 23.3 ng/mL (range, 3.9-47.3) and 7.2 ng/mL (range, 0-27.3). Serum hepcidin-25 levels in patients with CHC were significantly lower than in the control group ($P = 0.0002$; Wilcoxon-Mann-Whitney U test). Bottom and top edges of the boxes are the 25th and 75th percentiles, respectively. Median values are shown by a line within the box.

3.4. mRNA Expression of FPN and DMT1 in the Duodenum. To investigate the mechanism of iron absorption from the intestine, we utilized Taqman real-time RT-PCR to evaluate the mRNA expression of molecules related to iron absorption in biopsy specimens from the duodenum. Median FPN mRNA level in patients with CHC was 36.8 (range, 12.9-104.0) and that in control participants was 19.5 (range, 13.1-30.8); values were significantly higher in CHC patients than in control participants (Figure 3(a); P = 0.0091). On the other hand, the median DMT1 mRNA level in the CHC group was 4.5 (range, 2.23-12.0) and 3.99 (range, 3.08-6.52) in the control group, with no significant between-group difference (Figure 3(b); P = 0.8369). These findings suggested that decreased serum hepcidin-25 levels and the resultant upregulated expression of FPN in the duodenum could promote iron absorption from the intestine, thereby causing hepatic iron overload in CHC patients.

3.5. Immunohistochemical Detection of FPN in Duodenum Biopsy Tissues. To evaluate protein expression of FPN in the duodenum, we performed immunohistochemical detection in biopsy specimens from the duodenum using an anti-SLC40A1 antibody. In comparison with the control group, high FPN expression was observed in the duodenum specimens from CHC patients (Figures 4(a), 4(b), 4(c), and 4(d)). FPN expression was determined by scoring the intensity of immunohistochemical staining and comparing the results between the two groups. The immunohistochemical score for the CHC group was higher than for the control group (Figure 4(e); P < 0.0001).

Thus, these investigations using clinical specimens clearly showed increased iron absorption from the intestine in CHC patients compared with the control participants. These findings suggested that decreased serum hepcidin-25 values and increased FPN expression at both mRNA and protein levels could contribute to the mechanism of the increased iron absorption in CHC patients.

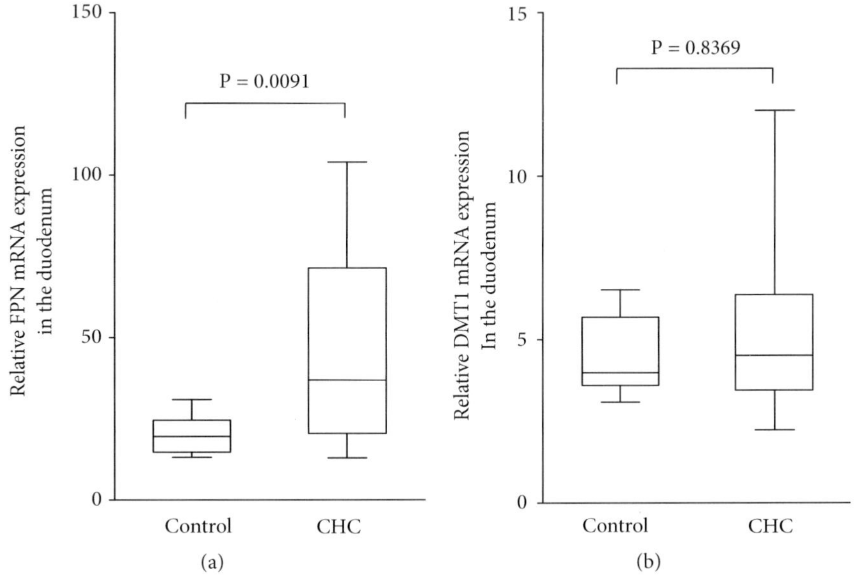

FIGURE 3: FPN and DMT1 mRNA expression in the duodenum. Relative mRNA expression levels of FPN (a) and DMT1 (b) in the duodenum were measured by Taqman real-time PCR. FPN mRNA in the CHC group was significantly upregulated compared with control participants ($P = 0.0091$; Wilcoxon-Mann-Whitney U test). Relative mRNA expression levels of DMT1 were measured by Taqman real-time PCR (b). There was no significant between-group difference ($P = 0.8369$; Wilcoxon-Mann-Whitney U test).

3.6. Induction of FPN in Caco-2/TC7 Cell Monolayers Cultured with Hepcidin. Although it was reported that hepcidin negatively regulates FPN at the protein level in reticuloendothelial cells [7], no study has directly addressed the interaction between hepcidin and FPN in the duodenal epithelium. We therefore examined the effects of hepcidin on the expression of two iron transport proteins *in vitro*. Caco-2/TC7 cells were cultured in a monolayer with or without hepcidin, and the difference in FPN and DMT1 expression was then investigated. The medium contained hepcidin at 5 different concentrations, from 6.25 to 100 nM. Relative FPN mRNA expression in Caco-2/TC7 cell monolayers was 20.46 (16.76-26.14) with no hepcidin, 18.40 (15.26-23.62) with hepcidin at 6.25 nM, 16.70 (13.39-19.73) at 12.5 nM, 15.23 (11.33-17.74) at 25 nM, 13.16 (10.90-15.78) at 50 nM, and 12.94 (9.95-13.85) at 100 nM. Thus, in Caco-2/TC7 cell monolayers, the FPN mRNA expression was significantly decreased as concentrations of hepcidin were increased in a dose-dependent manner (Figure 5(a); $P < 0.001$). On the other hand, relative DMT1 mRNA expression in Caco-2/TC7 cell monolayers was 40.51 (11.60-137.7) with no hepcidin, 39.49 (8.42-90.68) with hepcidin at 6.25 nM, 36.49 (16.12-209.8) at 12.5 nM, 31.48 (12.03-91.78) at 25 nM, 24.90 (9.32-161.0) at 50 nM, and 12.94 (9.95-13.85) at 100 nM, showing no significant differences according to hepcidin concentrations (Online Supplemental Figure S1; $P = 0.561$). Western blot assay was performed to measure expression levels of FPN and DMT1 in Caco-2/TC7 cell monolayers and revealed that FPN expression was increased in accordance with concentrations of hepcidin (Figure 5(b)). There was no correlation between DMT1 expression and hepcidin concentration (Online Supplemental Figure S2).

3.7. Immunohistochemical Detection of FPN in Caco-2/TC7 Cell Monolayers. We also examined changes in FPN expression in Caco-2/TC7 cell monolayers using an immunohistochemical assay. This assay showed that FPN was strongly expressed in Caco-2/TC7 cell monolayers cultured in the medium without hepcidin, but that heptidin decreased FPN expression in a dose-dependent manner (Figure 6).

4. Discussion

Excess iron generates ROS including H_20_2 by the Fenton reaction [4, 19], and oxidative stress is associated with hepatic fibrosis and carcinogenesis [2, 3, 19, 20]. Although hepatic iron overload in CHC patients has been described [21–26], the mechanism of such iron accumulation remains unknown. Possible causes include increased iron absorption from the intestine, increased iron uptake by the liver, and decreased iron release from the liver. To clarify the mechanism of iron overload in the CHC liver, we first examined the dynamics of intestinal iron absorption using the OIAT and found that iron absorption was significantly enhanced in the CHC group compared with the control group. Since iron absorption was enhanced in CHC patients despite the increased Tf sat levels before the OIAT, one possible reason for iron overload could be a breakdown in the negative feedback system that normally suppresses iron absorption in response to systemic iron overload.

Hepcidin was originally isolated from human serum and urine as a peptide with anti-bacterial activity [27–29]. Hepcidin is a hormone produced only in hepatocytes and is involved in iron release by reticuloendothelial macrophages and iron absorption from the intestinal epithelium [8, 30].

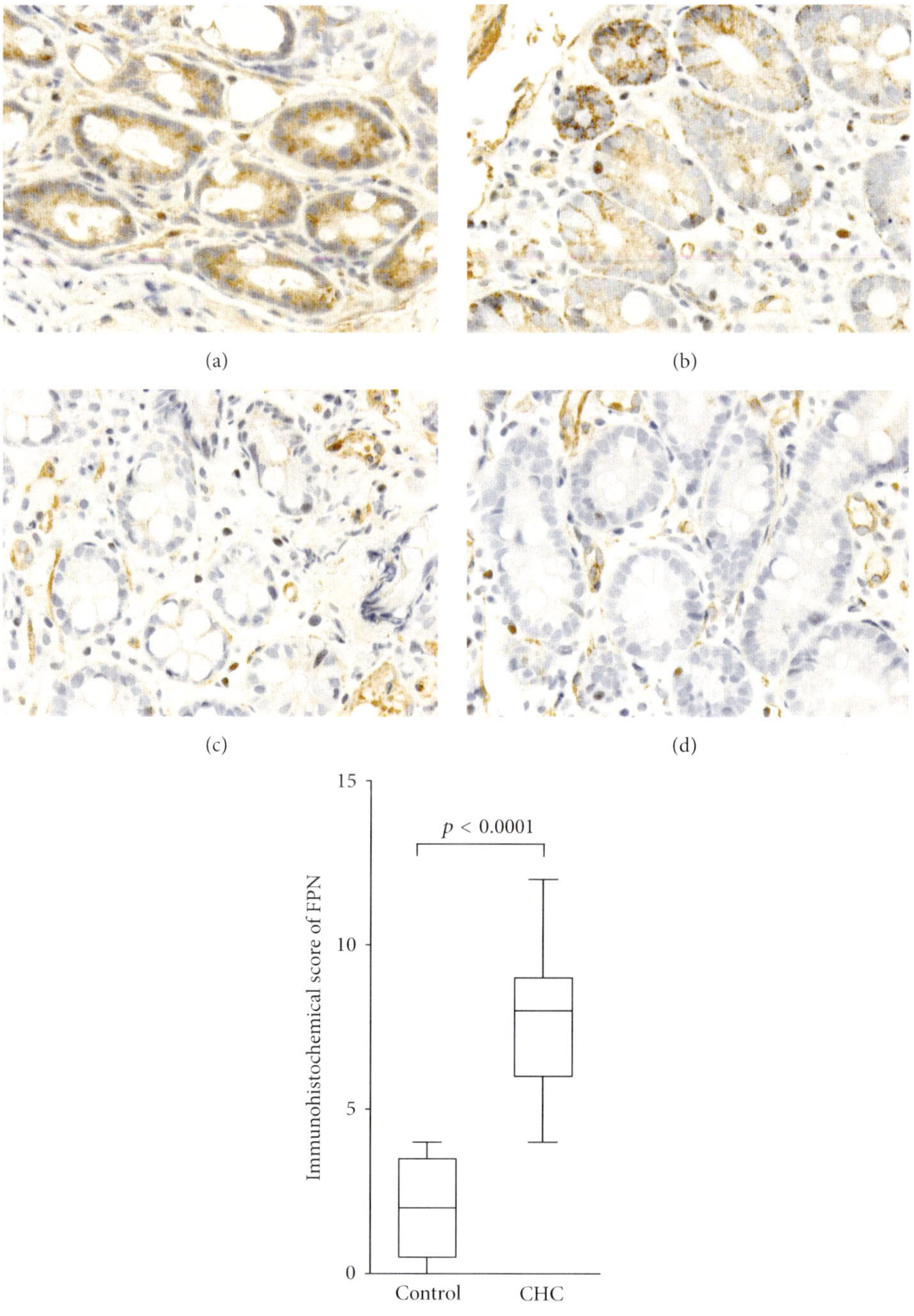

FIGURE 4: Immunohistochemical analysis of FPN in duodenum biopsy tissues from patients with CHC (a, b) and those of control participants (c, d). FPN expression was higher in the CHC group than in the control group. The immunohistochemical score was significantly higher in CHC patients compared with control participants (e).

Regarding hepcidin expression in CHC patients, the hepcidin mRNA/serum ferritin ratio was shown to be decreased in liver biopsy samples [10, 11] and it was suggested that the decreased DNA-binding ability of C/EBPα or HDAC activation by HCV-derived ROS may be responsible for the decreased hepcidin levels in CHC patients [31, 32].

In the present study, we measured serum hepcidin-25 concentrations by LC-MS/MS and found lower concentrations of hepcidin-25 in CHC patients than in the control participants. Though hepcidin is known to inhibit extracellular iron transport by inducing FPN internalization or degradation in Hela cells [7], it remains unclear how hepcidin acts in enterocyte. Our results suggest that there may be tissue-specific differences. We examined mRNA expression levels of molecules related to iron absorption in the duodenum, including FPN and DMT1. Whereas the DMT1 mRNA expression level did not differ between the control and CHC groups, FPN mRNA expression was higher in the CHC group.

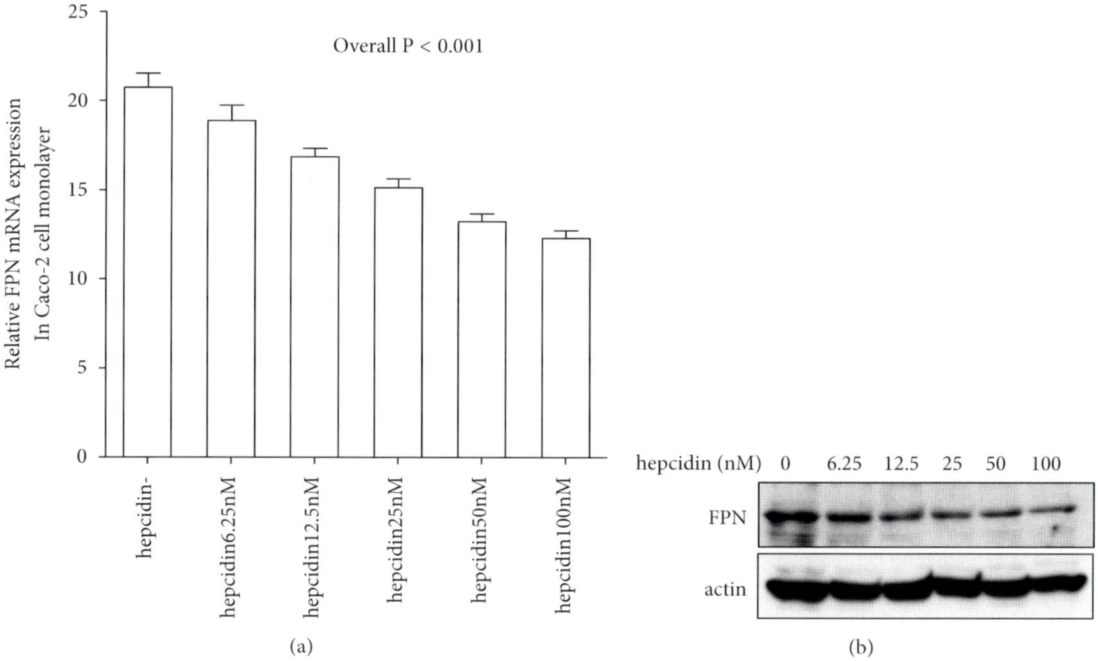

Figure 5: FPN expression in Caco-2/TC7 cell monolayers. FPN mRNA expression levels in Caco-2/TC7 cell monolayers cultured with or without hepcidin were measured by Taqman real-time PCR (a). FPN mRNA levels in Caco-2/TC7 cell monolayers were downregulated dependent on hepcidin concentration ($P < 0.0001$; Jonckheere–Terpstra test). FPN protein expression was analyzed by western blot (b). FPN protein in Caco-2/TC7 cell monolayers was downregulated dependently on hepcidin concentration.

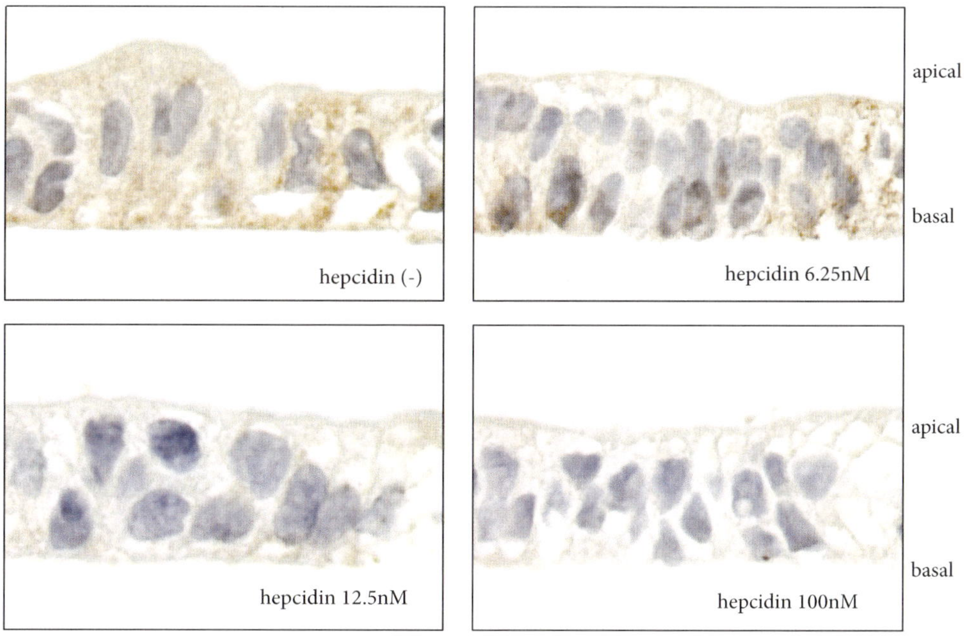

Figure 6: Immunohistochemical detection of FPN in Caco-2/TC7 cell monolayers was cultured with or without hepcidin (0-100 nM). FPN expression in Caco-2/TC7 cell monolayers was downregulated dependently on hepcidin concentration.

Similarly, immunohistochemical staining showed increased expression of FPN protein in the duodenum of CHC patients. Thus, it was suggested that hepcidin might regulate FPN expression not only at the protein level but also at the mRNA level in duodenal epithelial cells. We therefore investigated the effects of hepcidin on FPN and DMT1 in a model of duodenal epithelium in which Caco-2/TC7 cells were cultured in transwells as a monolayer for slightly longer than 3 weeks. In this model, DMT1 mRNA expression did not change in response to different concentrations of hepcidin, but FPN mRNA expression decreased by hepcidin in a dose-dependent manner. Based on these findings, one possible mechanism for the iron overload in CHC patients could be associated with enhanced intestinal iron absorption as a result of increased FPN expression in the duodenal mucosa due to decreased serum hepcidin. It should be supported by significant correlation between serum hepcidin-25 and OIAT s-Fe 120 min.

Increased expression of FPN in the duodenum also has been reported in FL-N/35 transgenic mice, a persistent infection model of HCV [31]. In the present study, we found that FPN mRNA expression was suppressed by hepcidin. FPN mRNA expression was reported to be upregulated by Nrf2 in macrophages [5, 33, 34] or by HIF2α, which binds to the HIF response elements in enterocytes [35]. However, the association of these molecules with hepcidin was not investigated in our present study and further investigation is needed to clarify the mechanism by which hepcidin suppresses FPN mRNA expression.

In conclusion, our present results showed that the serum hepcidin-25 concentration was decreased in CHC patients, which could enhance iron absorption by increasing the expression of FPN in the duodenum. Results of our *in vitro* assays suggested that hepcidin inhibits mRNA expression of FPN in duodenal epithelial cells. Although currently phlebotomy is used to treat iron overload in patients who have persistent HCV infection, our findings raise the possibility of the development of new drugs based on this mechanism. Furthermore, it was reported that, despite an increasing rate of SVR by direct acting antivirals, hepatic fibrosis is exacerbated in a subset (12%) of patients who achieve SVR [36] and that HCC develops continuously even after achieving SVR [37–39]. Therefore, further investigation of the involvement of abnormal iron absorption in these patients and a preventive strategy based on its underlying mechanism could lead to the establishment of a method to prevent cancer in patients with HCC in the future.

Ethical Approval

Ethics approval was obtained from the ethical committee for human genome/gene analysis research of the Sapporo Medical University.

Disclosure

The authors presented an earlier version of this study as another abstract [40].

Acknowledgments

Financial support was in part from grants received from the JSPS KAKENHI (20590787).

References

[1] F. Farinati, R. Cardin, N. De Maria et al., "Iron storage, lipid peroxidation and glutathione turnover in chronic anti-HCV positive hepatitis," *Journal of Hepatology*, vol. 22, no. 4, pp. 449–456, 1995.

[2] J. Kato, T. Nakamura, G. Kuroiwa et al., "Normalization of elevated hepatic 8-hydroxy-2′-deoxyguanosine levels in chronic hepatitis C patients by phlebotomy and low iron diet," *Cancer Research*, vol. 61, no. 24, pp. 8697–8702, 2001.

[3] J. Kato, K. Miyanishi, M. Kobune et al., "Long-term phlebotomy with low-iron diet therapy lowers risk of development of hepatocellular carcinoma from chronic hepatitis C," *Journal of Gastroenterology*, vol. 42, no. 10, pp. 830–836, 2007.

[4] K. Pantopoulos, S. K. Porwal, A. Tartakoff, and L. Devireddy, "Mechanisms of mammalian iron homeostasis," *Biochemistry*, vol. 51, no. 29, pp. 5705–5724, 2012.

[5] H. Drakesmith, E. Nemeth, and T. Ganz, "Ironing out Ferroportin," *Cell Metabolism*, vol. 22, no. 5, pp. 777–787, 2015.

[6] T. Ganz, "Systemic iron homeostasis," *Physiological Reviews*, vol. 93, no. 4, pp. 1721–1741, 2013.

[7] E. Nemeth, M. S. Tuttle, J. Powelson et al., "Hepcidin regulates cellular iron efflux by binding to ferroportin and inducing its internalization," *Science*, vol. 306, no. 5704, pp. 2090–2093, 2004.

[8] T. Ganz and E. Nemeth, "Hepcidin and iron homeostasis," *Biochimica et Biophysica Acta*, vol. 1823, no. 9, pp. 1434–1443, 2012.

[9] G. Rishi, D. F. Wallace, and V. N. Subramaniam, "Hepcidin: regulation of the master iron regulator," *Bioscience Reports*, vol. 35, no. 3, Article ID e00192, 2015.

[10] N. Fujita, R. Sugimoto, M. Takeo, N. Urawa, R. Mifuji, H. Tanaka et al., "Hepcidin expression in the liver: relatively low level in patients with chronic hepatitis C," *Molecular Medicine*, vol. 13, pp. 97–104, 2007.

[11] K. Sikorska, T. Romanowski, P. Stalke, E. I. Swieszewska, and K. P. Bielawski, "Association of hepcidin mRNA expression with hepatocyte iron accumulation and effects of antiviral therapy in chronic hepatitis C infection," *Hepatitis Monthly*, vol. 14, no. 11, 2014.

[12] M. Kobune, K. Miyanishi, K. Takada et al., "Establishment of a simple test for iron absorption from the gastrointestinal tract," *International Journal of Hematology*, vol. 93, no. 6, pp. 715–719, 2011.

[13] T. Hoki, K. Miyanishi, S. Tanaka et al., "Increased duodenal iron absorption through up-regulation of divalent metal transporter 1 from enhancement of iron regulatory protein 1 activity in patients with nonalcoholic steatohepatitis," *Hepatology*, vol. 62, no. 3, pp. 751–761, 2015.

[14] N. Tomosugi, H. Kawabata, R. Wakatabe et al., "Detection of serum hepcidin in renal failure and inflammation by using ProteinChip System," *Blood*, vol. 108, no. 4, pp. 1381–1387, 2006.

[15] K. Miyanishi, T. Takayama, M. Ohi et al., "Glutathione S-transferase-π overexpression is closely associated with K-ras mutation during human colon carcinogenesis," *Gastroenterology*, vol. 121, no. 4, pp. 865–874, 2001.

[16] R. A. Soslow, A. J. Dannenberg, D. Rush et al., "COX-2 is expressed in human pulmonary, colonic, and mammary tumors," *Cancer*, vol. 89, no. 12, pp. 2637–2645, 2000.

[17] A. Yang, J. Zhao, M. Lu et al., "Expression of hepcidin and ferroportin in the placenta, and ferritin and transferrin receptor

1 levels in maternal and umbilical cord blood in pregnant women with and without gestational diabetes," *International Journal of Environmental Research and Public Health*, vol. 13, pp. 766–774, 2016.

[18] H. Kijima, T. Sawada, N. Tomosugi, and K. Kubota, "Expression of hepcidin mRNA is uniformly suppressed in hepatocellular carcinoma," *BMC Cancer*, vol. 8, 2008.

[19] A. V. Ivanov, B. Bartosch, O. A. Smirnova, M. G. Isaguliants, and S. N. Kochetkov, "HCV and oxidative stress in the liver," *Viruses*, vol. 5, no. 2, pp. 439–469, 2013.

[20] C. Hézode, C. Cazeneuve, O. Coué et al., "Liver iron accumulation in patients with chronic active hepatitis C: Prevalence and role of hemochromatosis gene mutations and relationship with hepatic histological lesions," *Journal of Hepatology*, vol. 31, no. 6, pp. 979–984, 1999.

[21] H. Hofer, C. Österreicher, W. Jessner et al., "Hepatic iron concentration does not predict response to standard and pegylated-IFN/ribavirin therapy in patients with chronic hepatitis C," *Journal of Hepatology*, vol. 40, no. 6, pp. 1018–1022, 2004.

[22] S. J. Rulyak, S. C. Eng, K. Patel, J. G. McHutchison, S. C. Gordon, and K. V. Kowdley, "Relationships between hepatic iron content and virologic response in chronic hepatitis C patients treated with interferon and ribavirin," *American Journal of Gastroenterology*, vol. 100, no. 2, pp. 332–337, 2005.

[23] K. Hino, S. Nishina, and Y. Hara, "Iron metabolic disorder in chronic hepatitis C: mechanisms and relevance to hepatocarcinogenesis," *Journal of Gastroenterology and Hepatology*, vol. 28, no. 4, pp. 93–98, 2013.

[24] R. J. Fontana, J. Israel, P. LeClair et al., "Iron reduction before and during interferon therapy of chronic hepatitis C: results of a multicenter, randomized, controlled trial," *Hepatology*, vol. 31, no. 3, pp. 730–736, 2000.

[25] F. Kageyama, Y. Kobayashi, T. Kawasaki, S. Toyokuni, K. Uchida, and H. Nakamura, "Successful interferon therapy reverses enhanced hepatic iron accumulation and lipid peroxidation in chronic hepatitis C," *American Journal of Gastroenterology*, vol. 95, no. 4, pp. 1041–1050, 2000.

[26] A. L. Barton, B. F. Banner, E. E. Cable, and H. L. Bonkovsky, "Distribution of iron in the liver predicts the response of chronic hepatitis C infection to interferon therapy," *American Journal of Clinical Pathology*, vol. 103, no. 4, pp. 419–424, 1995.

[27] A. Krause, S. Neitz, H.-J. Mägert et al., "LEAP-1, a novel highly disulfide-bonded human peptide, exhibits antimicrobial activity," *FEBS Letters*, vol. 480, no. 2-3, pp. 147–150, 2000.

[28] C. Pigeon, G. Ilyin, B. Courselaud et al., "A new mouse liver-specific gene, encoding a protein homologous to human antimicrobial peptide hepcidin, is overexpressed during iron overload," *The Journal of Biological Chemistry*, vol. 276, no. 11, pp. 7811–7819, 2001.

[29] C. H. Park, E. V. Valore, A. J. Waring, and T. Ganz, "Hepcidin, a urinary antimicrobial peptide synthesized in the liver," *The Journal of Biological Chemistry*, vol. 276, no. 11, pp. 7806–7810, 2001.

[30] T. Ganz, "Hepcidin, a key regulator of iron metabolism and mediator of anemia of inflammation," *Blood*, vol. 102, no. 3, pp. 783–788, 2003.

[31] K. Miura, K. Taura, Y. Kodama, B. Schnabl, and D. A. Brenner, "Hepatitis C virus-induced oxidative stress suppresses hepcidin expression through increased histone deacetylase activity," *Hepatology*, vol. 48, no. 5, pp. 1420–1429, 2008.

[32] S. Nishina, K. Hino, M. Korenaga et al., "Hepatitis C virus-induced reactive oxygen species raise hepatic iron level in mice by reducing hepcidin transcription," *Gastroenterology*, vol. 134, no. 1, pp. 226–238, 2008.

[33] C. Delaby, N. Pilard, H. Puy, and F. Canonne-Hergaux, "Sequential regulation of ferroportin expression after erythrophagocytosis in murine macrophages: Early mRNA induction by haem, followed by iron-dependent protein expression," *Biochemical Journal*, vol. 411, no. 1, pp. 123–131, 2008.

[34] N. Harada, M. Kanayama, A. Maruyama et al., "Nrf2 regulates ferroportin 1-mediated iron efflux and counteracts lipopolysaccharide-induced ferroportin 1 mRNA suppression in macrophages," *Archives of Biochemistry and Biophysics*, vol. 508, no. 1, pp. 101–109, 2011.

[35] M. Taylor, A. Qu, E. R. Anderson et al., "Hypoxia-inducible factor-2α mediates the adaptive increase of intestinal ferroportin during iron deficiency in mice," *Gastroenterology*, vol. 140, no. 7, pp. 2044–2055, 2011.

[36] Y. A. Lee and S. L. Friedman, "Reversal, maintenance or progression: What happens to the liver after a virologic cure of hepatitis C?" *Antiviral Research*, vol. 107, no. 1, pp. 23–30, 2014.

[37] N. Yamashita, A. Ohho, A. Yamasaki, M. Kurokawa, K. Kotoh, and E. Kajiwara, "Hepatocarcinogenesis in chronic hepatitis C patients achieving a sustained virological response to interferon: significance of lifelong periodic cancer screening for improving outcomes," *Journal of Gastroenterology*, vol. 49, no. 11, pp. 1504–1513, 2014.

[38] Q.-L. Zeng, B. Li, X.-X. Zhang et al., "Clinical model for predicting hepatocellular carcinomas in patients with post-sustained virologic responses of chronic hepatitis C: A case control study," *Gut and Liver*, vol. 10, no. 6, 2016.

[39] H. B. El-Serag, F. Kanwal, P. Richardson, and J. Kramer, "Risk of hepatocellular carcinoma after sustained virological response in Veterans with hepatitis C virus infection," *Hepatology*, vol. 64, no. 1, pp. 130–137, 2016.

[40] K. Miyanishi, M. Sato, S. Tanaka, H. Sakamoto, Y. Kawano, M. Kobune et al., "Increased duodenal iron absorption through upregulation of ferroportin 1 due to decrement of serum hepcidin in patients with chronic hepatitis C," *Hepatology*, vol. 64, p. 736A, 2016.

15

Clinical and Pathological Characteristics of Autoimmune Hepatitis with Acute Presentation

Yi Shen,[1] Changli Lu,[2] Ruoting Men,[1] Jianping Liu,[2] Tinghong Ye,[1] and Li Yang[1]

[1]*Department of Gastroenterology & Hepatology, West China Hospital, Sichuan University, Chengdu, Sichuan 610041, China*
[2]*Department of Pathology, West China Hospital, Sichuan University, Chengdu, Sichuan 610041, China*

Correspondence should be addressed to Li Yang; yangli_hx@scu.edu.cn

Academic Editor: Hong Shen

Aim. To study the differences between acute presentation-autoimmune hepatitis (A-AIH) and chronic autoimmune hepatitis (C-AIH). *Methods.* Through long-term follow-up, 80 patients were included in our study by using the revised international autoimmune hepatitis group (IAIHG) score and were divided into acute and chronic groups for comparison. *Results.* No significant difference was found in the gender, age, IAIHG score (pretreatment/posttreatment), definite diagnosis rate, extrahepatic autoimmune disease, onset time, or treatment before biopsy between the acute and chronic groups. In terms of clinical symptoms, A-AIH patients were more prone to jaundice, anorexia, yellow urine, and detesting oil than C-AIH patients, but melena only occurred in chronic group ($P < 0.05$). The acute group exhibited more severe injury upon histological evaluation, with lobular inflammation and bile duct injury, especially central necrosis of the lobule, more pronounced in this group ($P < 0.05$). *Conclusion.* A-AIH had manifestations of acute hepatitis and presented cholestasis. Serum indicators could preliminarily distinguish A-AIH and C-AIH. Histologically, the primary manifestation of A-AIH was lobular inflammation, which was usually accompanied by lobular central necrosis. For the diagnosis of A-AIH, more attention should be paid to long-term follow-up. This study was registered at ClinicalTrials.gov (identifier: NCT02994537).

1. Introduction

Typical autoimmune hepatitis (AIH) is a chronic and non-specific inflammatory disease that is primarily characterized by the presence of autoantibodies, elevated alanine aminotransferase (ALT), aspartate transaminase (AST), and immunoglobulin G (IgG) levels, interface inflammation, lymphoplasmacytic infiltration, and hepatocyte rosetting [1–3]. The common criterion for diagnosing AIH is the international autoimmune hepatitis group (IAIHG) score, but acute presentation-AIH (A-AIH) probably lacks the typical presentations described in this score. Moreover, prominent lobular inflammation and sometimes even obvious central necrosis of the lobule may be present [4–7], which restricts the use of the IAIHG score for A-AIH. Various studies have reported different definitions of A-AIH. Most of these studies have divided the disease into acute-onset AIH, acute exacerbation of chronic AIH (C-AIH), and acute-severe AIH [4, 8–12]. In clinical works, 25%–40% of AIH cases are the acute form [1, 4, 13, 14], so an early and accurate diagnosis of A-AIH to improve the prognosis is an important research goal. Therefore, our study included patients with suspected AIH. Ultimately, 80 patients were included in our study after long-term follow-up. And the patients were divided into acute and chronic groups according to their serum examination results. Then, we analysed the differences between A-AIH and C-AIH. Based on these results, physicians may be able to more easily distinguish A-AIH to improve early diagnoses and increase the timeliness of treatment.

2. Materials and Methods

2.1. Inclusion Criteria. This study enrolled patients who visited the West China Hospital of Sichuan University from October 2013 to November 2016 with suspected AIH. Through long-term follow-up [the median follow-up time for all patients was 14 (11.00, 20.25) months], we ultimately included 80 patients with a probable and definitive diagnosis

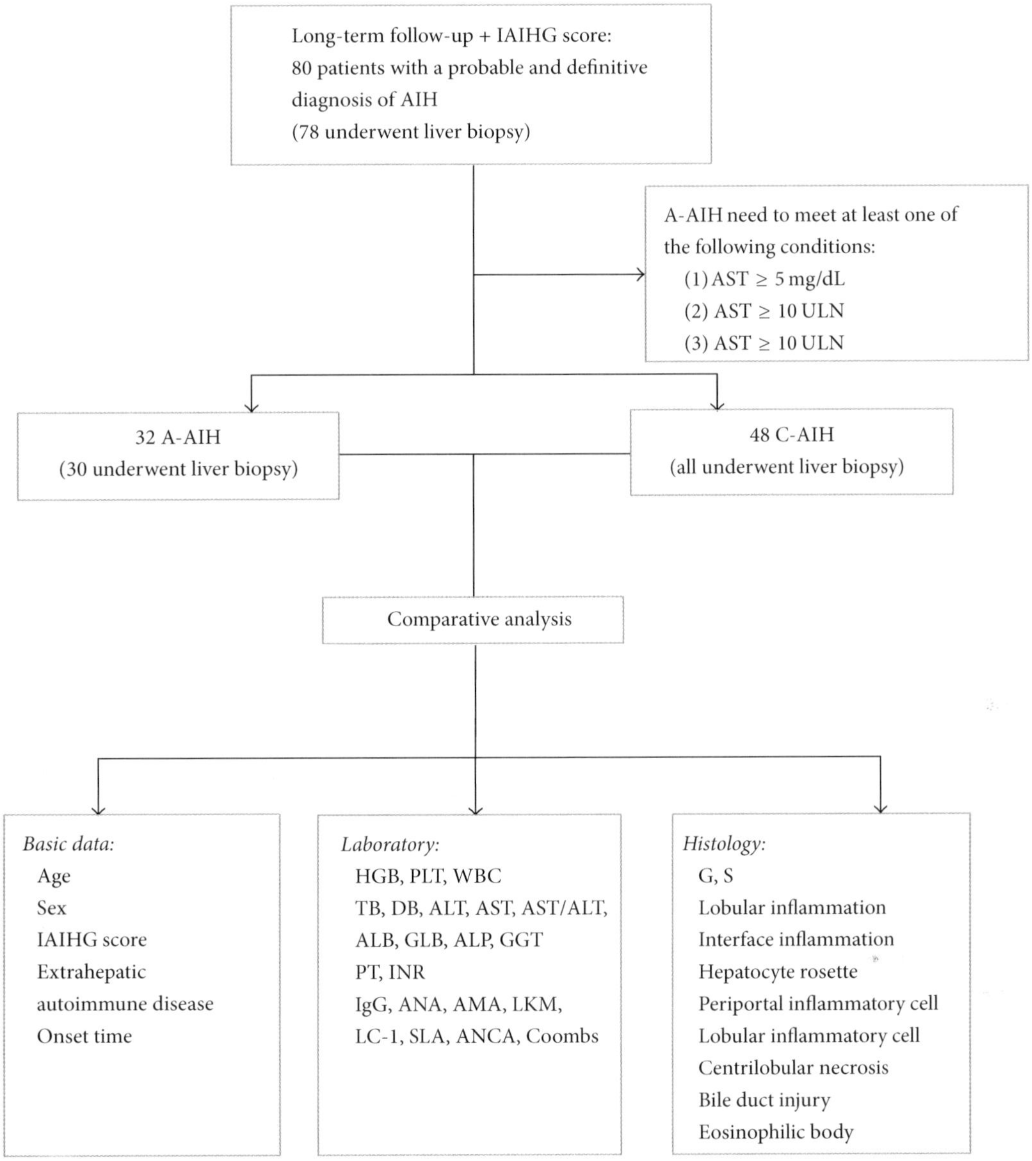

FIGURE 1: Flow chart. The figure shows the entire process and the contents of the study. IAIHG: international autoimmune hepatitis group; AIH: autoimmune hepatitis; A-AIH: acute presentation-autoimmune hepatitis; TB: total bilirubin; ALT: alanine aminotransferase; AST: aspartate transaminase; C-AIH: chronic autoimmune hepatitis; HGB: haemoglobin; PLT: platelet; WBC: white blood cell; DB: direct bilirubin; ALB: albumin; GLB: globulin; ALP: alkaline phosphatase; GGT: gamma-glutamyl transferase; PT: prothrombin time; INR: international normalized ratio; IgG: immunoglobulin G; ANA: anti-nuclear antibody; AMA: anti-mitochondrial antibody; LKM: liver kidney microsomal; LC: liver cytosol; SLA: soluble liver antigen; ANCA: anti-neutrophil cytoplasmic antibody; Coombs: Coombs test; G: inflammation grade; S: fibrosis stage.

of AIH based on the 1999 revised IAIHG score (a score ≥10 indicates probable AIH before treatment and a score ≥16 indicates definite AIH before treatment) [15, 16]. Of these patients, 78 patients underwent a liver biopsy as a diagnostic examination, but 2 patients refused to do it. Then, the 80 patients were divided into the A-AIH group and the C-AIH group. For inclusion in the A-AIH group, the patient needed to meet at least one of the following conditions: (1) total bilirubin (TB) ≥ 5 mg/dL, (2) ALT ≥ X10 upper limits of normal (ULN), or (3) AST ≥ X10 ULN. [8–12, 17]. The onset time was defined as the time from the first instance of liver dysfunction to the time of liver biopsy (or the time of admission for patients who did not have a liver biopsy) [4]. Patient information was acquired from the West China Hospital electronic medical record system and by telephone (see Figure 1).

2.2. Laboratory Examination. Fasting blood samples were collected from the patients, and routine blood, biochemical, and coagulation function examinations were implemented within 3 days before or after the liver biopsy (or implemented at the time of admission). Other blood test results acquired within 1 month before or after the biopsy were considered acceptable [4]. The laboratory indices included the white blood cell (WBC) and platelet (PLT) counts, haemoglobin (HGB), TB, direct bilirubin (DB), ALT, AST, AST/ALT, albumin (ALB), and globulin (GLB) levels, prothrombin time (PT), international normalized ratio (INR), IgG concentration, the anti-nuclear (ANA), anti-mitochondrial (AMA), anti-liver kidney microsomal (LKM), anti-liver cytosol (LC), anti-soluble liver antigen (SLA), and anti-neutrophil cytoplasmic (ANCA) antibodies, and the Coombs test (Coombs). The laboratory tests were performed by the Department of Laboratory Medicine of West China Hospital, which was certified by the College of American Pathologists (CAP).

2.3. Pathological Examination. Liver samples were acquired by ultrasound-guided percutaneous needle biopsy of the liver. The tissues were fixed in 10% formaldehyde (Kelong, China), embedded in paraffin, and used for haematoxylin and eosin (H&E) staining, immunohistochemical staining for CK7 (ZSGB-BIO, China) and CD138 (Maxim, China), and Masson trichrome staining to examine the histological characteristics. Finally, two pathologists (CL and JL) from the Pathology Department of West China Hospital (certified by CAP) interpreted the samples. The Scheuer score system was used to classify the inflammation grade (G0–4) and fibrosis stage (S0–4) of the liver tissues [7, 18]. The pathologists assigned 0 to 4 points for different levels of pathological presentations as follows [4]: (1) lobular inflammation (0–4: no inflammation, piecemeal necrosis, fusion necrosis, multiacinar necrosis, and massive necrosis); (2) interface inflammation (0–3: no, mild, moderate, and severe); (3) hepatocyte rosetting (0 and 1: no and yes); (4) cellular infiltration of the portal area: (0–2: no, few, and many); (5) bile duct injury (0–2: no, bile duct proliferation or vacuolar degeneration, and bile duct deficiency); (6) centrilobular inflammation or necrosis (0 and 1: no and yes); (7) cellular infiltration of the lobule (0–2: no, few, and many); and (8) eosinophilic bodies (0 and 1: no and yes).

2.4. Statistical Analysis. Continuous variables that conformed to the normal distribution were expressed by mean ± SD, while continuous variables which did not conform to the normal distribution were expressed using the median and interquartile range. Categorical variables were expressed as numbers (percentages) (see Tables 1–5). Differences between groups were compared using Student's t-test, the Mann–Whitney U test, and the Chi-square test ($P < 0.05$ was considered significant). Receiver operating characteristic (ROC) curves were used to acquire the cut-off values of valuable parameters. All statistical tests were performed using SPSS version 18.0 (SPSS, Chicago, IL, USA).

3. Results

3.1. Basic Information. Eighty patients were included, of which 32 (40%) patients had A-AIH and 48 (60%) patients had C-AIH. Thirteen (16.25%) were males, and 67 (83.75%) were females, with a male-to-female ratio of 1:5.2. No significant difference was found in the gender, age, IAIHG score (pretreatment/posttreatment), definite diagnosis rate, extrahepatic autoimmune disease status, or the composition of treatment and the time of treatment before biopsy (P = 0.458, P = 0.471, P = 0.696/0.727, P = 0.923, P = 0.732, P = 0.078, and P = 0.805, resp.) between the patients with acute-presentation and chronic AIH. The onset time of the A-AIH patients was 6.5 (1.19, 27) months, whereas the onset time of the C-AIH patients was 16 (2.5, 54) months (P = 0.054) (see Tables 1 and 4). The common clinical symptoms were shown in Table 5. Jaundice, fatigue, and anorexia were the three most common symptoms in all patients. A-AIH patients were more prone to jaundice, anorexia, yellow urine, and detesting oil than C-AIH patients ($P < 0.001$, $P < 0.001$, $P = 0.004$, and $P = 0.009$, resp.), but melena only occurred in chronic group ($P = 0.038$). Other less common symptoms include itching, diarrhea, vomiting, heart fatigue, and shortness of breath.

Table 1: Comparison of basic pieces of information between A-AIH and C-AIH patients.

	Acute n = 32 (40.0%)	Chronic n = 48 (60.0%)	P
Gender (M : F)	1:7	1:4.3	0.458
Age (years)	52 ± 12	54 ± 13	0.471
Pretreatment IAIHG score	13 (12, 17)	14 (12, 16)	0.696
Posttreatment IAIHG score	14 (13, 20)	15 (12, 18)	0.727
Definite diagnosis (%)	11 (34.4%)	16 (33.3%)	0.923
Extrahepatic autoimmune disease	7 (21.9%)	9 (18.8%)	0.732
Onset time (months)	6.5 (1.19, 27)	16 (2.5, 54)	0.054

3.2. Laboratory Examination. The HGB, PLT, WBC, AST/ALT, AMA, LKM, LC-1, SLA, ANCA, and Coombs test results showed no significant differences between the two groups. Bilirubin: TB and DB were higher in the acute group ($P < 0.001$ and $P < 0.001$, resp.). Liver enzymes: ALT and AST were higher in the acute group ($P < 0.001$ and $P < 0.001$, resp.), and ALP and GGT were higher than in the chronic group ($P < 0.001$ and $P = 0.003$, resp.). ALB was higher in the chronic group ($P < 0.001$), whereas GLB was higher in the acute group ($P = 0.001$). Moreover, the cut-off value of ALB deduced by ROC curve was 36.9 g/L (see Figure 3). Regarding coagulation function, the PT was longer ($P < 0.001$) and the INR was greater ($P < 0.001$) in the acute group. IgG was higher in the acute group ($P < 0.001$). In the acute group, 28 (87.5%) patients had an ANA titre greater than or equal to 1:100 (1:100 was equivalent to the international general 1:40 titre in this study [8]) compared with only 26 (55.3%) patients in the chronic group, and the positive rate of ANA was significantly different between the two groups ($P = 0.003$) (see Table 2).

3.3. Histological Examination. A-AIH was primarily performed as acute hepatitis in histology. No significant difference in the fibrosis stage (S) was found between the acute

TABLE 2: Comparison of laboratory data between A-AIH and C-AIH patients.

	Acute $n = 32$ (40.0%)	Chronic $n = 48$ (60.0%)	P
HGB (g/L)	116 ± 21	118 ± 26	0.687
PLT (10^9 /L)	112 (76, 169)	121 (76, 160)	0.757
WBC (10^9 /L)	5.24 (3.51, 6.43)	4.50 (3.72, 5.69)	0.556
TB (μmol/L)	93 (48.1, 198.9)	17.8 (13.5, 24.3)	<0.001[a]
DB (μmol/L)	83.2 (30.3, 157.4)	6.7 (4.7, 11.3)	<0.001[a]
ALT (IU/L)	330 (149, 452)	42 (22, 97)	<0.001[a]
AST (IU/L)	394 (208, 557)	45 (34, 87)	<0.001[a]
AST/ALT	1.21 (0.98, 1.74)	1.13 (0.94, 1.65)	0.694
ALB (g/L)	34.3 ± 5.4	40.1 ± 5.8	<0.001[a]
GLB (g/L)	42.7 (35.8, 47)	35.8 (31.4, 41.3)	0.001[a]
ALP (IU/L)	144 (125, 173)	98 (80, 146)	<0.001[a]
GGT (IU/L)	128 (63, 225)	58 (27, 110)	0.003[a]
PT (s)	14.7 (13.2, 16.3)	12.8 (11.9, 13.4)	<0.001[a]
INR	1.27 (1.12, 1.39)	1.09 (1.01, 1.13)	<0.001[a]
IgG (g/L)	30.8 (21.5, 33.2)	19.3 (16, 24.7)	<0.001[a]
ANA			
<1:100	4 (12.5%)	21 (44.7%)	0.003[a]
≥1:100	28 (87.5%)	26 (55.3%)	
AMA			
−	27 (84.4%)	43 (97.7%)	0.322
+	5 (15.6%)	1 (2.3%)	
LKM			
−	32 (100%)	43 (97.7%)	1.000
+	0	1 (2.3%)	
LC-1			
−	32 (100%)	43 (97.7%)	
+	0	0	1.000
±	0	1 (2.3%)	
SLA			
−	31 (96.9%)	41 (93.2%)	1.000
+	1 (3.1%)	3 (6.8%)	
ANCA			
−	14 (77.8%)	19 (79.2%)	
+	2 (11.1%)	0	0.178
±	2 (11.1%)	5 (20.8%)	
Coombs			
−	6 (42.9%)	14 (66.7%)	
+	8 (57.1%)	6 (28.5%)	0.091
±	0	1 (4.8%)	

[a]$P < 0.05$. AIH: autoimmune hepatitis; IAIHG: international autoimmune hepatitis group; HGB: haemoglobin; PLT: platelet; WBC: white blood cell; TB: total bilirubin; DB: direct bilirubin; ALT: alanine aminotransferase; AST: aspartate transaminase; ALB: albumin; GLB: globulin; ALP: alkaline phosphatase; GGT: gamma-glutamyl transferase; PT: prothrombin time; INR: international normalized ratio; IgG: immunoglobulin G; ANA: antinuclear antibody; AMA: anti-mitochondrial antibody; LKM: liver kidney microsomal; LC: liver cytosol; SLA: soluble liver antigen; ANCA: anti-neutrophil cytoplasmic antibody; Coombs: Coombs test.

and chronic groups. Conversely, the inflammation grade (G) ($P < 0.001$), lobulitis ($P = 0.001$), interface inflammation ($P = 0.001$), rosettes ($P < 0.001$), periportal lymphocytes ($P < 0.001$), plasma cells ($P < 0.001$), neutrophils ($P = 0.001$), monocytes ($P < 0.001$), eosinophils ($P = 0.002$), bile duct injury ($P < 0.001$), centrilobular necrosis ($P = 0.005$), lobular neutrophils ($P < 0.001$), monocytes ($P < 0.001$), eosinophils ($P = 0.002$), and eosinophilic bodies ($P = 0.05$) were all significantly different between the acute and chronic groups (see Table 3 and Figure 2). In the acute group, the patients with onset time less than 3 months and $S < 3$ were defined as acute-onset AIH, while the rest of the patients were acute exacerbation of chronic AIH (there were 2 patients who had no liver biopsy so they could not be included). After comparison, we found that PLT [206 (165, 276), 106 (70, 161), $P = 0.018$], interface inflammation [no or mild: 100%, 16%, $P = 0.001$], periportal eosinocyte (100%, 48%, $P = 0.035$), and centrilobular necrosis (80%, 24%, $P = 0.031$) between the acute-onset and acute-on-chronic groups were statistically different.

4. Discussion

A-AIH can quickly lead to liver decompensation if the diagnosis and treatment are not timely. And A-AIH can be easily confused with other liver dysfunction diseases, leading to misdiagnoses and delayed treatment. Moreover, A-AIH does not usually exhibit the clinical characteristics of typical chronic AIH, which complicates a diagnosis based solely on the existing diagnostic criteria. Therefore, understanding the haematological and histological characteristics of A-AIH is necessary to ensure early diagnosis and treatment.

Previous reports differ in their descriptions of the onset age of A-AIH [10, 13, 19, 20]. In our study, no significant difference was found in the mean age between the two groups; therefore, determining the age of onset of A-AIH requires further study. Moreover, no significant difference was observed in extrahepatic autoimmune disease between the two groups. The two groups of patients (57.1% of A-AIH patients and 44.4% of C-AIH patients) with extrahepatic autoimmune diseases (A-AIH: 4 thyroid disease, 1 systemic lupus erythematosus, and 2 Sjogren's syndrome; C-AIH: 4 thyroid disease, 2 Sjogren's syndrome, 1 Sjogren's syndrome and dermatomyositis, 1 rheumatoid arthritis, and 1 vitiligo) were mainly diagnosed with thyroid disease. The study of Miyake et al. showed that A-AIH concurrent with thyroid disease was often seen in Caucasians, but the inverse was observed in Japanese [10]. Therefore, determining whether autoimmune thyroid disease and A-AIH have the same genetic susceptibility and whether extrahepatic autoimmune diseases in A-AIH patients have ethnic differences requires a larger sample or an international multicentre study for clarification. The onset time of A-AIH has been reported to be 1–3 months in various studies [4, 11]. In our study, no difference was found in the onset time between the two groups ($P = 0.054$). However, the median onset time was significantly lower in the acute group than in the chronic group [6.5 (1.19, 27) and 16 (2.5, 54) months, resp.], possibly because the acute group included patients with acute-onset

TABLE 3: Comparison of histological features between A-AIH and C-AIH patients.

	Acute $n = 30$	Chronic $n = 48$	P
G			
0	0	1 (2.1%)	
1	1 (3.3%)	12 (25.0%)	
2	2 (6.7%)	17 (35.4%)	<0.001[a]
3	21 (70.0%)	18 (37.5%)	
4	6 (20.0%)	0	
S			
0	0	2 (4.2%)	
1	10 (33.3%)	20 (41.7%)	
2	3 (10.0%)	10 (20.8%)	0.135
3	7 (23.3%)	4 (8.3%)	
4	10 (33.3%)	12 (25.0%)	
Lobular inflammation			
0	0	2 (4.2%)	
1	17 (56.7%)	40 (80.3%)	0.002[a]
2	6 (20.0%)	2 (4.2%)	
3	7 (23.3%)	4 (8.3%)	
Interface inflammation			
0	4 (13.3%)	13 (27.1%)	
1	5 (16.7%)	21 (43.8%)	0.001[a]
2	14 (46.7%)	11 (22.9%)	
3	7 (23.3%)	3 (6.3%)	
Hepatocyte rosettes			
No	2 (6.7%)	21 (43.8%)	<0.001[a]
Yes	28 (93.3%)	27 (56.3%)	
Periportal lymphocyte			
0	0	0	
1	1 (3.3%)	19 (39.6%)	<0.001[a]
2	29 (96.7%)	29 (60.4%)	
Periportal plasmocyte			
0	1 (3.3%)	17 (35.4%)	
1	15 (50.0%)	27 (56.3%)	<0.001[a]
2	14 (46.7%)	4 (8.3%)	
Periportal neutrophils			
0	8 (26.7%)	28 (58.3%)	
1	12 (40.0%)	16 (33.3%)	0.002[a]
2	10 (33.3%)	4 (8.3%)	
Periportal monocyte			
0	0	0	
1	1 (3.3%)	19 (39.6%)	<0.001[a]
2	29 (96.7%)	29 (60.4%)	
Periportal eosinocyte			
0	13 (43.3%)	36 (75.0%)	
1	17 (56.7%)	12 (25.0%)	0.005[a]
2	0	0	

Table 3: Continued.

	Acute $n = 30$	Chronic $n = 48$	P
Bile duct injury			
0	5 (16.7%)	31 (64.6%)	
1	21 (70.0%)	17 (35.4%)	<0.001[a]
2	4 (13.3%)	0	
Centrilobular necrosis			
No	20 (66.7%)	44 (91.7%)	0.005[a]
Yes	10 (33.3%)	4 (8.3%)	
Lobular neutrophils			
0	8 (26.7%)	40 (83.3%)	
1	10 (33.3%)	5 (10.4%)	<0.001[a]
2	12 (40.0%)	3 (6.3%)	
Lobular monocyte			
0	8 (26.7%)	39 (81.3%)	
1	11 (36.7%)	7 (14.6%)	<0.001[a]
2	11 (36.7%)	2 (4.2%)	
Lobular eosinocyte			
0	19 (63.3%)	44 (91.7%)	
1	10 (33.3%)	4 (8.3%)	0.002[a]
2	1 (3.3%)	0	
Eosinophilic body			
No	22 (73.3%)	44 (91.7%)	0.05
Yes	8 (26.7%)	4 (8.3%)	

[a] $P < 0.05$.

Table 4: Comparison of treatments between A-AIH and C-AIH before liver biopsy.

	Acute $n = 32$ (40.0%)	Chronic $n = 48$ (60.0%)	P
No treatment	1 (3.1%)	6 (12.5%)	
General treatment	21 (65.6%)	31 (64.6%)	
General treatment + immunosuppressants	1 (3.1%)	5 (10.4%)	0.078
General treatment + UDCA	8 (25%)	3 (6.3%)	
General treatment + immunosuppressants + UDCA	1 (3.1%)	3 (6.3%)	
Time of treatment (months)	2 (0.50, 12)	1 (0.33, 12)	0.805

AIH and acute exacerbation of C-AIH. The results might have been different if we enlarged the sample and divided the A-AIH patients into acute-onset AIH and acute exacerbation of C-AIH groups for separate analyses.

In this study, we only used serum indicators to judge A-AIH without distinguishing acute and chronic histological characteristics; therefore, a portion of the A-AIH patients corresponded to acute exacerbation of C-AIH. However, Abe et al. divided acute and chronic AIH patients using histological characteristics and found that the A-AIH patients also met our blood conditions for A-AIH [9]. This finding indirectly explains the reliability of using blood indicators to distinguish between acute-presentation and chronic AIH. Acute-severe AIH showed markedly abnormal coagulation, and many studies defined AIH with an INR > 1.5 as acute-severe AIH [8, 21–23]. In this study, 6 patients (18.75%) in the acute group but only 1 patient (2.08%) in the chronic group ($P = 0.015$) had an INR > 1.5. Additionally, ALB was lower in the acute group in our study, which also indicated worse A-AIH conditions. Severe AIH patients exhibit severe destruction of the liver tissue, which directly hampers the production of ALB in the liver and explains the difference in ALB between the two groups. Kessler et al. suggested that ALB might play a role in the acute phase response; thus, hypoproteinaemia was a suitable indicator of A-AIH [4]. In our study, the GLB and IgG levels were higher in the acute group than in the chronic group, which was different from the results of many other studies [6, 9, 10, 13, 19]. However,

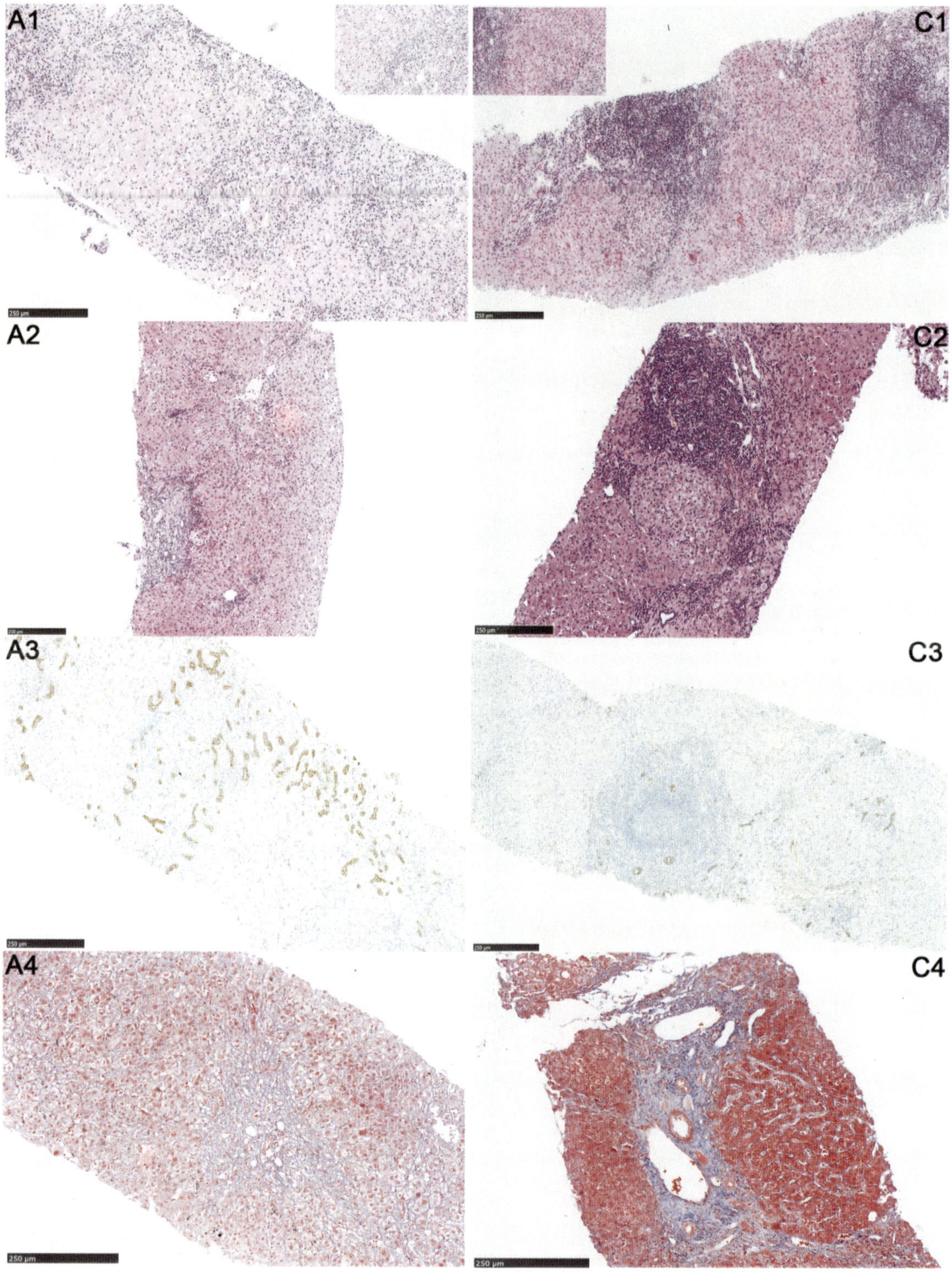

FIGURE 2: Histological features of A-AIH and C-AIH. A-AIH (A1–4) and C-AIH (C1–4): A1, C1: A1 shows multiacinar and centrilobular necrosis in A-AIH, which is uncommon in C-AIH (H&E, ×200, small pictures emphasized the typical areas in the big pictures); A2, C2: the main manifestation of A-AIH is cellular swelling, ballooning change, and lobular inflammation accompanied by mild interface inflammation; however, C-AIH often has moderate-to-severe interface inflammation caused by lymphoplasmacytic infiltration (H&E ×200); A3, C3: CK7 staining showing regeneration of cholangiocytes due to the multiacinar necrosis of hepatocyte in A-AIH. However, bile duct regeneration was less likely to be found in C-AIH (CK7, ×200); A4, C4: blue staining shows fibrosis in the portal area; fibrous septa were found in the chronic group but not the acute group (Masson trichrome staining, ×200).

TABLE 5: Comparison of symptoms between A-AIH and C-AIH.

	Acute $n = 32$ (40.0%)	Chronic $n = 48$ (60.0%)	P
Jaundice	21 (65.6%)	12 (25.0%)	<0.001[a]
Fatigue	14 (43.8%)	18 (37.5%)	0.576
Anorexia	18 (56.3%)	8 (16.7%)	<0.001[a]
Ventosity	10 (31.3%)	13 (27.1%)	0.687
Ascites	9 (28.1%)	13 (27.1%)	0.919
Yellow urine	14 (43.8%)	7 (14.6%)	0.004[a]
Detesting oil	12 (37.5%)	6 (12.5%)	0.009[a]
Abdominal pain	4 (12.5%)	10 (20.8%)	0.337
Nausea	6 (18.8%)	5 (10.4%)	0.333
Weight loss	6 (18.8%)	4 (8.3%)	0.187
Dizziness	2 (6.3%)	8 (16.7%)	0.301
Lower limb swelling	2 (6.3%)	6 (12.5%)	0.466
Arthralgia	1 (3.1%)	6 (12.5%)	0.233
Melena	0	7 (14.6%)	0.038[a]
Hematemesis	0	5 (10.4%)	0.08

[a] $P < 0.05$.

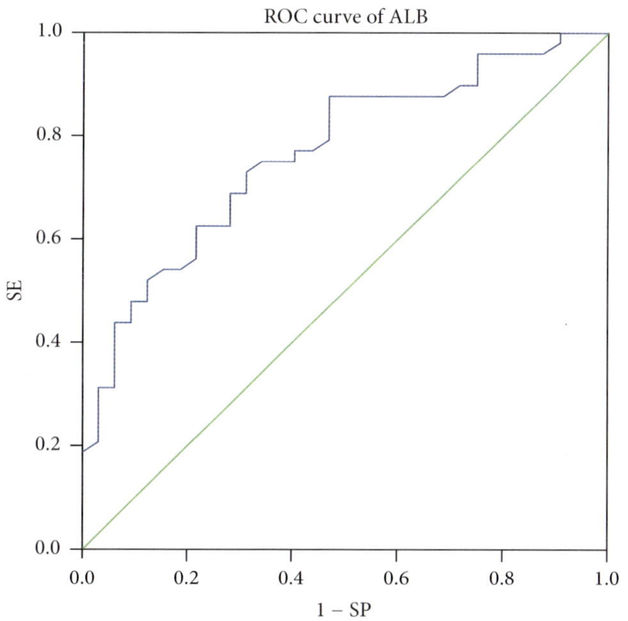

FIGURE 3: ROC curve of ALB. The area under the receiver operating characteristic (ROC) curve was 0.765 for ALB, 95% confidence interval (CI) was 0.662–0.869, and rates for sensitivity and specificity were 72.9% and 68.7%, respectively.

those studies did not include acute exacerbation of C-AIH in their A-AIH groups. Moreover, IgG is not an acute phase protein, and thus A-AIH patients may not have enough time to generate a significant amount of IgG [19, 21]. Miyake et al. showed that A-AIH displayed an IgG concentration <2000 mg/dL; therefore, using the revised IAIHG score to determine A-AIH may correspond to a decreased score and lead to a decreased definite diagnosis of AIH [10]. This finding suggests that the scope of the revised IAIHG score should be reconsidered. In this study, 15 (50%) patients in the A-AIH group had $S \geq 3$. Amontree et al. mentioned that the key identification between acute exacerbation of C-AIH and acute-onset AIH might be a higher globulin level [24]. Therefore, GLB and IgG might have been higher in our acute group because more acute exacerbation of C-AIH patients was included in the A-AIH group. They also found that the identification of pathological features between patients with acute exacerbation of C-AIH and acute-onset AIH could include severe liver cell necrosis and fibrosis [24]. Thus, we compared all included patients with $S < 3$ and $S \geq 3$. The results showed that patients with $S < 3$ had lower GLB [36.1 (31.7, 42.7) g/L and 40.4 (35.7, 47.3) g/L, resp., $P = 0.012$] and IgG [20.6 (16.5, 25.6) g/L and 26.8 (20.7, 32.4) g/L, resp., $P = 0.019$] levels than patients with $S \geq 3$. As a result of inflammation, AIH can cause the destruction and proliferation of bile ducts. Duct involvement was more clearly observed in A-AIH than in C-AIH [19]. In this study, 7 (23.33%) patients in the A-AIH group had multiacinar necrosis in the histological analysis, whereas only 4 (8.33%) patients in the chronic group had this condition. When comparing the two groups, we found that both ALP and GGT were higher in the acute group ($P < 0.001$ and $P = 0.003$, resp.). The severe lobulitis in A-AIH may have made the bile duct injury more apparent. This result is consistent with the above studies and indirectly confirms Czaja and Carpenter's opinion that destruction and deficiency of bile ducts cannot rule out the diagnosis of AIH [25]. Onji et al. reported that A-AIH patients had a lower positive rate of ANA than C-AIH patients [6, 10], whereas in our study the positive rate of ANA was higher in the A-AIH patients than in the C-AIH patients (87.5% and 55.3%, resp., $P = 0.042$).

This result may be due to the reason that patients with acute exacerbation of C-AIH were included in the acute group. Both the acute and chronic groups in our study included AMA (+) patients (15.6% and 2.1%, resp.). The liver functions of all of the patients were improved even when they only used the standard immunosuppressive treatment without ursodeoxycholic acid (UDCA), and their ALP and GGT levels were decreased or even returned to normal levels. Therefore, abnormal values of the above blood indicators are still likely to be due to the bile duct injury caused by inflammation in A-AIH. Leung et al. found that the AMA appearance may be caused by the oxidative stress induced by liver injury [26].

A number of studies have reported that A-AIH exhibits more severe histological characteristics than C-AIH [4, 12], and the results of our study have confirmed these reports. Many studies have speculated that centrilobular injury may be a manifestation of early AIH, and some studies have reported centrilobular necrosis in 53%–100% of A-AIH cases [4, 6, 7, 10–12, 21, 27, 28]. Hofer et al. reported that centrilobular necrosis suggested a possibility of acute-onset AIH as high as 87% [5]. We also observed that centrilobular necrosis was more obvious in the acute group than in the chronic group. Ten (33.3%) patients in our A-AIH group had centrilobular necrosis, whereas only four (8.33%) patients in the chronic group had this condition ($P = 0.005$). Eleven (78.6%) of the 14 patients had $S < 3$. Sequential liver biopsies may reveal that A-AIH with centrilobular necrosis gradually appears as a typical AIH with manifestation, thereby assisting with the diagnosis [29]. Therefore, adding centrilobular necrosis to the IAIHG diagnostic criteria should be considered to increase the diagnosis rate of A-AIH by pathologists. Our study indicated that bile duct injury was more likely to occur in A-AIH than in C-AIH. Czaja and Carpenter also reported destructive and nondestructive cholangitis and the disappearance of bile ducts in AIH [25]; thus, a liver biopsy after immunosuppressive treatment may help identify whether the disease is AIH [19, 27]. Amontree et al. reported that fibrosis and cirrhosis could be observed in A-AIH [24]. In our study, the fibrosis stage revealed no significant differences between the acute and chronic groups ($P = 0.099$), with 50% and 31.25% of patients in the acute and chronic groups, respectively, corresponding to $S \geq 3$ ($P = 0.098$). Because AIH can suddenly be exacerbated after insidious onset, determining whether acute AIH itself can appear as obvious fibrosis is difficult.

This study has several limitations. For example, the sample size of the A-AIH group was not sufficiently large. Additionally, the results of A-AIH were affected by the C-AIH. In clinical work, we have found that AIH concurrent with viral hepatitis and drug-induced AIH are not uncommon. Therefore, in this study, we also examined viral hepatitis markers in the patients and tracked their medication histories. Through long-term follow-up, we ruled out the possibility of drug-induced liver injury. Finally, patients whose IAIHG scores conformed to the possible diagnosis of AIH were included in this study, but for some patients we could not exclude an effect caused by viral hepatitis.

In conclusion, A-AIH is not uncommon and may not have features of typical AIH, and it is characterized by significantly elevated bilirubin and transaminase. Therefore, serum indicators can preliminarily distinguish A-AIH and C-AIH. Histologically, A-AIH is mainly manifested as acute lobular inflammation with clear centrilobular necrosis, and bile duct injury is not uncommon. Moreover, A-AIH may be difficult to diagnose based only on the IAIHG score. More attention should be paid to long-term follow-up, and new diagnostic criteria for A-AIH should be developed.

Ethical Approval

This study was reviewed and approved by the Ethics Committee of the West China Hospital, Sichuan University (no. 2013221).

Authors' Contributions

Yi Shen and Changli Lu contributed equally to this work.

Acknowledgments

This work was supported by grants from the National Natural Science Foundation of China [no. 81770568 to Li Yang] and the Science and Technology Department of the Sichuan Province of China [no. 2017JY0071 to Tinghong Ye].

References

[1] M. P. Manns, A. W. Lohse, and D. Vergani, "Autoimmune hepatitis," *Journal of Hepatology*, vol. 62, no. 1, supplement, pp. S100–S111, 2015.

[2] E. L. Krawitt, "Autoimmune hepatitis," *The New England Journal of Medicine*, vol. 354, no. 1, pp. 54–66, 2006.

[3] A. J. Czaja and H. A. Carpenter, "Sensitivity, specificity, and predictability of biopsy interpretations in chronic hepatitis," *Gastroenterology*, vol. 105, no. 6, pp. 1824–1832, 1993.

[4] W. R. Kessler, O. W. Cummings, G. Eckert, N. Chalasani, L. Lumeng, and P. Y. Kwo, "Fulminant hepatic failure as the initial presentation of acute autoimmune hepatitis," *Clinical Gastroenterology and Hepatology*, vol. 2, no. 7, pp. 625–631, 2004.

[5] H. Hofer, C. Oesterreicher, F. Wrba, P. Ferenci, and E. Penner, "Centrilobular necrosis in autoimmune hepatitis: A histological feature associated with acute clinical presentation," *Journal of Clinical Pathology*, vol. 59, no. 3, pp. 246–249, 2006.

[6] M. Onji, "Proposal of autoimmune hepatitis presenting with acute hepatitis, severe hepatitis and acute liver failure," *Hepatology Research*, vol. 41, no. 6, pp. 497-497, 2011.

[7] L. D. Ferrell and S. Kakar, *Liver Pathology*, vol. 517, Demos Medical Publishing, New York, NY, USA, 2011.

[8] Chinese Medical Association, "Consensus on the diagnosis and treatment of autoimmune hepatitis," *Journal of Hepatobiliary Disease*, vol. 01, pp. 9–22, 2016.

[9] M. Abe, Y. Hiasa, T. Masumoto et al., "Clinical characteristics of autoimmune hepatitis with histological features of acute hepatitis," *Hepatology Research*, vol. 21, no. 3, pp. 213–219, 2001.

[8] Chinese Medical Association, "Consensus on the diagnosis and treatment of autoimmune hepatitis," *Journal of Hepatobiliary Disease*, vol. 01, pp. 9–22, 2016.

[9] M. Abe, Y. Hiasa, T. Masumoto et al., "Clinical characteristics of autoimmune hepatitis with histological features of acute hepatitis," *Hepatology Research*, vol. 21, no. 3, pp. 213–219, 2001.

[10] Y. Miyake, Y. Iwasaki, H. Kobashi et al., "Autoimmune hepatitis with acute presentation in Japan," *Digestive and Liver Disease*, vol. 42, no. 1, pp. 51–54, 2010.

[11] H. Takahashi and M. Zeniya, "Acute presentation of autoimmune hepatitis: Does it exist? A published work review," *Hepatology Research*, vol. 41, no. 6, pp. 498–504, 2011.

[12] K. Fujiwara, M. Nakano, S. Yasui, K. Okitsu, Y. Yonemitsu, and O. Yokosuka, "Advanced histology and impaired liver regeneration are associated with disease severity in acute-onset autoimmune hepatitis," *Histopathology*, vol. 58, no. 5, pp. 693–704, 2011.

[13] J. Kogan, R. Safadi, Y. Ashur, D. Shouval, and Y. Ilan, "Prognosis of symptomatic versus asymptomatic autoimmune hepatitis: A study of 68 patients," *Journal of Clinical Gastroenterology*, vol. 35, no. 1, pp. 75–81, 2002.

[14] M. P. Manns, A. J. Czaja, J. D. Gorham et al., "Diagnosis and management of autoimmune hepatitis," *Hepatology*, vol. 51, no. 6, pp. 2193–2213, 2010.

[15] A. D. Yeoman, R. H. Westbrook, T. Al-Chalabi et al., "Diagnostic value and utility of the simplified International Autoimmune Hepatitis Group (IAIHG) criteria in acute and chronic liver disease," *Hepatology*, vol. 50, no. 2, pp. 538–545, 2009.

[16] F. Alvarez, P. A. Berg, F. B. Bianchi et al., "International autoimmune hepatitis group report: review of criteria for diagnosis of autoimmune hepatitis," *Journal of Hepatology*, vol. 31, no. 5, pp. 929–938, 1999.

[17] Y. Miyake, Y. Iwasaki, R. Terada et al., "Persistent normalization of serum alanine aminotransferase levels improves the prognosis of type 1 autoimmune hepatitis," *Journal of Hepatology*, vol. 43, no. 6, pp. 951–957, 2005.

[18] P. J. Scheuer, R. A. Standish, and A. P. Dhillon, "Scoring of chronic hepatitis," *Clinics in Liver Disease*, vol. 6, no. 2, pp. 335–347, 2002.

[19] M. Iwai, M. Jo, M. Ishii, T. Mori, and Y. Harada, "Comparison of clinical features and liver histology in acute and chronic autoimmune hepatitis," *Hepatology Research*, vol. 38, no. 8, pp. 784–789, 2008.

[20] A. Floreani, G. Niro, E. Rosa Rizzotto et al., "Type I autoimmune hepatitis: Clinical course and outcome in an Italian multicentre study," *Alimentary Pharmacology & Therapeutics*, vol. 24, no. 7, pp. 1051–1057, 2006.

[21] C. Weiler-Normann and A. W. Lohse, "Acute autoimmune hepatitis: many open questions," *Journal of Hepatology*, vol. 61, no. 4, pp. 727–729, 2014.

[22] A. J. Czaja, "Acute and acute severe (Fulminant) autoimmune hepatitis," *Digestive Diseases and Sciences*, vol. 58, no. 4, pp. 897–914, 2013.

[23] A. D. Yeoman, R. H. Westbrook, Y. Zen et al., "Prognosis of acute severe autoimmune hepatitis (AS-AIH): The role of corticosteroids in modifying outcome," *Journal of Hepatology*, vol. 61, no. 4, pp. 876–882, 2014.

[24] J. S. Amontree, T. D. Stuart, and J. E. Bredfeldt, "Autoimmune chronic active hepatitis masquerading as acute hepatitis," *Journal of Clinical Gastroenterology*, vol. 11, no. 3, pp. 303–307, 1989.

[25] A. J. Czaja and H. A. Carpenter, "Autoimmune hepatitis with incidental histologic features of bile duct injury," *Hepatology*, vol. 34, no. 4 I, pp. 659–665, 2001.

[26] P. S. C. Leung, L. Rossaro, P. A. Davis et al., "Antimitochondrial antibodies in acute liver failure: Implications for primary biliary cirrhosis," *Hepatology*, vol. 46, no. 5, pp. 1436–1442, 2007.

[27] K. Fujiwara, Y. Fukuda, and O. Yokosuka, "Precise histological evaluation of liver biopsy specimen is indispensable for diagnosis and treatment of acute-onset autoimmune hepatitis," *Journal of Gastroenterology*, vol. 43, no. 12, pp. 951–958, 2008.

[28] H. N. Canh, K. Harada, H. Ouchi et al., "Acute presentation of autoimmune hepatitis: A multicentre study with detailed histological evaluation in a large cohort of patients," *Journal of Clinical Pathology*, 2017.

[29] N. Okano, K. Yamamoto, K. Sakaguchi et al., "Clinicopathological features of acute-onset autoimmune hepatitis," *Hepatology Research*, vol. 25, no. 3, pp. 263–270, 2003.

Serum Metabonomics Analysis of Liver Failure Treated by Nonbioartificial Liver Support Systems

Chunyan Wu, Ying Zhu, and Mengqian Yu

The First Affiliated Hospital of Dalian Medical University, Dalian 116011, China

Correspondence should be addressed to Ying Zhu; zhuyingsh52@126.com

A ademic Editor: En-Qiang Chen

Objective. To analyze the small molecular metabolic compounds of nonbioartificial liver for treatment of hepatic failure and make further efforts to study the clinical efficacy, mechanism of action, and pathogenesis of hepatic failure. *Methods.* 52 patients who met the standard of artificial liver treatment for liver failure were enrolled; these patients included 6 cases of acute liver failure (11.54%), 3 cases of subacute liver failure (5.77%), acute-on-chronic liver failure in 10 cases (19.23%), and 33 cases of chronic liver failure (63.46%). Treatment modes included plasma exchange in 34 patients (65.38%), bilirubin adsorption in 9 patients (17.31%), and hemofiltration in 9 patients (17.31%). The clinical efficacy of artificial liver was assessed by monitoring the effects in the near future. Significant changes in metabolic compounds of liver failure in the treatment before and after artificial liver were screened by using Ultra-Performance Liquid Chromatography-Mass Spectrometry (UPLC-MS). Related metabolic pathways were analyzed by MetaboAnalyst. *Results.* After artificial liver treatment, the liver function and coagulation function of liver failure patients were significantly improved ($P < 0.01$), the Meld score was lower than that before treatment, and the difference was statistically significant ($P < 0.05$). Serum metabolomics identified 29 small metabolic compounds and 12 metabolic pathways with variable projection importance (VIP) greater than 1 before and after artificial liver treatment. There were 11 metabolic compounds of VIP over 1 and 7 metabolic pathways in the different modes of artificial liver treatment for chronic liver failure. Among them, bile acid metabolism, fatty acid metabolism, and amino acid metabolism are the main sources. *Conclusion.* Artificial liver treatment can effectively improve liver function and blood coagulation function and Meld score, clinical symptoms and signs in patients with liver failure; the curative effect of artificial liver was verified, which reflected the clinical value of artificial liver in the treatment of liver failure. Artificial liver treatment of liver failure on fatty acids and primary bile acid synthesis pathway was the most significant. The difference of fatty acid, primary bile acid synthesis pathway, and phenylalanine metabolic pathway in different artificial liver patterns of chronic liver failure was the most significant. This provides a new basis for understanding the mechanism of hepatic failure and the mechanism of liver failure by artificial liver treatment.

1. Introduction

Hepatic failure is a serious hepatic damage that can be caused by many factors. In China, the main cause of liver failure is hepatitis B virus (HBV), followed by drugs and hepatotoxicity [1, 2]. Treatment of liver failure includes comprehensive internal medical treatment, artificial liver support therapy, liver transplantation, and other methods. In recent years, the nonbioartificial liver technology has become one of the most effective methods for treating liver failure. It includes a variety of managements, and plasma exchange, hemofiltration, and bilirubin adsorption are the most common ones [3].

Metabolomics is a technique for studying the metabolic network of biological systems. The object which has been researched is mainly the endogenous small molecules with relative molecular mass below one thousand [4]. The most widely used and effective metabolomics techniques are gas chromatography-mass spectrometry [5] and liquid chromatography-mass spectrometry (GC-MS) [6]; the latter is used more often. At present, the use of metabonomics to analyze the changes of serum metabolites in patients with liver failure by nonbioartificial liver treatment is relatively rare. Therefore, changes of serum metabolites before and after nonbioartificial liver treatment were detected by the platform of UPLC-MS, to further analyze the pathogenesis of liver failure and investigate the effect of nonbioartificial liver in patients with liver failure metabolites. This provides a basis for further study of artificial liver technology in the treatment of liver failure. It was expected to provide a new basis for further clinical diagnosis and treatment.

2. Materials and Methods

2.1. Inclusion and Exclusion Criteria. All the patients in the group met the criteria for the diagnosis of "guideline for diagnosis and treatment of liver failure" (2012 update) and "guideline for nonbioartificial liver support systems in treatment of liver failure" (2016 update). Liver failure is a serious liver damage caused by a variety of factors and a group of clinical symptoms; the main manifestations include coagulation dysfunction, jaundice, hepatic encephalopathy, and ascites. Acute liver failure is a clinical manifestation of acute onset within 2 weeks. The clinical manifestations of subacute hepatic failure were 2-26 weeks. Acute-on-chronic liver failure is a clinical syndrome with acute or subacute liver decompensation occurring on the basis of chronic liver disease in a short time. Chronic liver failure is a progressive decline and decompensation of liver function on the basis of liver cirrhosis. Exclusion criteria included patients with active bleeding or disseminated intravascular coagulation (DIC); hemodynamic instability in patients; allergic to blood products or medications during treatment. According to the above criteria, 68 patients were evaluated, and 6 cases of active bleeding, 4 cases of allergy to blood products, 6 patients with DIC, and 52 patients with liver failure treated with nonbioartificial liver were selected from December 2015 to November 2016 at the First Affiliated Hospital of Dalian Medical University finally (Figure 1). The aetiology of individual causes of liver failure was different; there were 6 cases of drug hepatitis, 5 cases of alcoholic hepatitis, 3 cases of chronic viral hepatitis B, 2 cases of chronic viral hepatitis E, 3 cases of autoimmune hepatitis, and 33 cases of cirrhosis. According to the diagnosis and classification of hepatic failure, 52 cases were divided into acute hepatic failure in 6 cases (11.54%), subacute hepatic failure in 3 cases (5.77%), acute-on-chronic liver failure in 10 cases (19.23%), and chronic liver failure in 33 cases (63.46%).

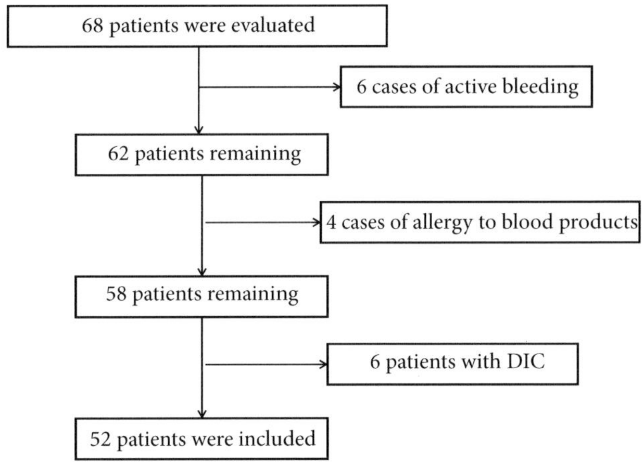

FIGURE 1: Flowchart of included patients.

2.2. Methods of Each Artificial Liver Support. Plasma exchange (PE) is to filter out the plasma containing toxins in the blood out of the membrane and back into the body with the same amount of fresh plasma or fresh frozen plasma with the blood type components that are withheld in the membrane. It can clear liver failure toxins and some pathogenic factors, supplement the essential substances such as coagulation factors that are lacking in liver failure, and correct metabolic disorders caused by liver failure. The disadvantage of PE is that it cannot effectively remove water-soluble substances from small molecules. PE has a certain risk of adverse reactions in the treatment of liver failure, mainly allergic reactions, but symptomatic treatment relieved symptoms and did not affect the treatment effect. Hemofiltration applies a membrane with larger aperture. The pressure difference between the liquid on both sides of the membrane is used as a transmembrane pressure. In the form of convection, the toxins in the blood are removed with water. Hemofiltration is more close to the function of glomerular filtration in the human kidney. If the replacement fluid is contaminated, complications such as fever and septicemia can occur, and this can be avoided by prevention and treatment. The main mechanism of bilirubin adsorption is to separate the plasma from the patient and send the plasma to the bilirubin adsorption column of BS series, so as to completely adsorb the bile acid and bilirubin in the serum and then send the purified plasma back to the human body, so as to effectively remove the blood poisoning metabolites and inflammatory cytokines. Bilirubin adsorption treatment increased the toxin clearance ability, and the safety was high. Studies have shown that PE, hemofiltration, and bilirubin adsorption are safe and effective in the treatment of liver failure and can prolong the survival time of patients.

2.3. Defining Criteria to Patients with Different Modalities of Artificial Liver Support. Plasma exchange is the most commonly used method, which can retain the relatively large molecular weight of coagulation factors, hepatocyte growth factor. Hemofiltration is suitable for all kinds of liver failure with acute kidney injury, including hepatorenal syndrome, hepatic encephalopathy, electrolyte imbalance, and acid-base imbalance. Bilirubin adsorption is applied to severe hyperbilirubinemia caused by various reasons and patients with severe cholestasis of liver disease treated by poorly internal medicine. According to the above pattern of artificial liver, 52 patients were divided into plasma exchange in 34 cases (65.38%), 9 cases were bilirubin absorption (17.31%), and 9 cases were hemofiltration (17.31%). Because chronic liver failure accounts for 63.46% of liver failure and plasma replacement is 65.38% of the artificial liver pattern, this article focuses on chronic liver failure with different artificial liver treatment and plasma exchange for liver failure.

2.4. Clinical Efficacy Observation Index. According to the guidelines, the clinical efficacy of artificial liver and the

TABLE 1: Diagnosis and classification of liver failure.

Diagnosis	acute hepatic failure	subacute hepatic failure	acute-on-chronic liver failure	chronic liver failure	Total
Cases	6	3	10	33	52
Proportion	11.54%	5.77%	19.23%	63.46%	100%

TABLE 2: Diagnosis and classification of plasma exchange for liver failure.

Diagnosis	acute hepatic failure	subacute hepatic failure	acute on chronic liver failure	Chronic liver failure	Total
Cases	6	3	10	15	34
Proportion	17.65%	8.82%	29.41%	44.12%	100%

changes of the patient's condition were evaluated by monitoring the effects in the near future, including serum bilirubin lowering, PTA or international standardization ratio improvement, MELD score decline, other laboratory indexes improvement, and digestive tract symptom improvement. The metabolic compounds of liver failure were observed before and after artificial liver by using UPLC-MS, and related metabolic pathways were analyzed by MetaboAnalyst.

2.5. Instruments and Reagents. The following reagents and instruments were used for this study: 7600 automatic biochemical analyzer from Japan's Hitachi company, blood coagulation analyzer from German BE company, Wasters UPLC-Q Exactive HF MS (Thermo Fisher Scientific, Rockford, IL, USA), centrifuge (Microfuge 22, Beckman Coulter company), vortex mixer (Vortex Genius 3, German IKA group), Acetonitrile and formic acid (from the Fisher company in the United States), ammonium acetate, and analytically pure (from the Sigma-Aldrich company in the United States), and ultrapure water was prepared by the MILLI-Q ultra purified water preparation system (US Millipore Corporation).

2.6. Samples Collection and Processing. Fasting venous blood and venous blood after treatment were taken immediately, and the serum was collected after 3500 rpm centrifugation for 8 minutes. Using a constant temperature container with dry ice for transportation, the serum finally were placed in -80 centigrade refrigerator to storage. Serum samples were thawed at room temperature, taking 50 uL serum add into 200 uL acetonitrile containing the internal standard and centrifuging at 10,000 g for 10 min. 180 μl lyophilized supernatant was taken and dissolved in 80 uL volume ratio of acetonitrile/water of 1/4, and, after whirling 30s, centrifugal supernatant was analyzed by LC-MS.

2.7. Analysis Condition. Chromatographic condition was as follows: chromatographic column: ACQUITY UPLC HSS T3 (standard: 100 mm × 2.1 mm, 1.8 μm), column temperature: 50°C, and current speed: 0.35 ml/min. Mass spectrometry condition was as follows: MS full scan range of positive ion: 80-1200 m/z; spraying voltage: 3.50 kV; anion: 70-1100; spraying voltage: 3.00 kV. Capillary temperature 300°C, auxiliary gas temperature 350°C. The velocities of sheath gas and auxiliary gas are, respectively, 45 and 10 (arbitrary units), resolution set to $12e^4$.

2.8. Data Processing and Statistical Analysis. The raw data collected by mass spectrometry was processed by SIEVE software and 80% principles were used to deal with missing values [7], and data were imported into SIMCA-P 11.5 software, pattern recognition using PLS-DA, and the VIP (Variable Importance in Projection) value of each variable in PLS-DA model was obtained, screening out potential biomarkers. Statistical software was using SPSS 17.0, and $P < 0.05$ was statistically significant.

3. Results

3.1. Classification of Liver Failure and Nonbioartificial Liver Patterns

3.1.1. Diagnosis and Classification of Liver Failure. According to the diagnosis and classification of hepatic failure, 52 cases were divided into acute hepatic failure in 6 cases (11.54%), subacute hepatic failure in 3 cases (5.77%), acute-on-chronic liver failure in 10 cases (19.23%), and chronic liver failure in 33 cases (63.46%), Table 1.

3.1.2. Diagnosis and Classification of Plasma Exchange for Liver Failure. Out of 52 patients, 34 cases (65.38%) underwent plasma exchange in the treatment of liver failure diagnosis, according to the classification, divided into 6 cases of acute liver failure (17.65%), 3 cases of subacute liver failure (8.82%), acute-on-chronic liver failure in 10 cases (29.41%), and 15 cases of chronic liver failure (44.12%), Table 2.

3.1.3. Classification of Chronic Hepatic Failure with Different Patterns of Nonbioartificial Liver Treatment. Out of 52 patients, there was chronic liver failure in 33 cases (63.46%); they are in the majority, so the following further on chronic liver failure of artificial liver pattern was analyzed, including 15 cases of plasma exchange (45.454%), 9 cases of bilirubin adsorption (27.273%), and 9 cases of hemofiltration (27.273%), Table 3.

3.1.4. Classification of Nonbioartificial Liver Treatment Patterns. According to the classification of nonbioartificial liver treatment patterns, 52 patients were divided into 34 cases of plasma exchange (65.38%), 17.31% cases were bilirubin absorption, 9 cases were hemofiltration (17.31%), Table 4.

Table 3: Classification of chronic hepatic failure with different patterns of nonbioartificial liver treatment.

therapeutic methods	plasma exchange	bilirubin adsorption	hemofiltration	Total
Cases	15	9	9	33
Proportion	45.454%	27.273%	27.273%	100%

Table 4: Classification of nonbioartificial liver models.

therapeutic method	plasma exchange	bilirubin adsorption	hemofiltration	Total
Cases	34	9	9	52
Proportion	65.38%	17.31%	17.31%	100%

Table 5: Meld score analysis of liver failure treated with nonbioartificial liver treatment.

	Before treatment	After treatment	The value of P
Meld score	23.38 ± 5.32	21.38 ± 4.81	0.001*

Note. The Meld score before and after nonbioartificial liver treatment was P ≤ 0.001, which was statistically significant.

3.2. Clinical Efficacy Analysis

3.2.1. Meld Score Analysis of Liver Failure Treated with Nonbioartificial Liver Treatment. The Meld score of all patients before and after nonbioartificial liver treatment was statistically analyzed, and the results showed that the Meld score after nonbioartificial liver treatment was lower than before; the difference was statistically significant (P = 0.001), Table 5.

3.2.2. Clinical Analysis of Liver Failure Treated by Nonbioartificial Liver Treatment. The liver function and coagulation function of the 52 patients treated with nonbioartificial liver were compared and analyzed, and the levels of AST, ALB, ALP, γ-GT, TBIL, and PT in nonbioartificial liver were significantly lower than those before nonbioartificial liver treatment (P < 0.01), with statistical significance. The level of ALT after treatment decreased but had no statistically significance (P > 0.05), Table 6.

3.2.3. Clinical Analysis of Plasma Exchange in the Treatment of Liver Failure. When the plasma exchange was used in the treatment of acute liver failure, acute-on-chronic liver failure and chronic liver failure, liver function, and blood coagulation function indicators were compared, and the levels of AST, γ-GT, TBIL, PT, and ALB after treatment were significantly lower than before (P < 0.05); the difference was statistically significant, Table 7.

3.2.4. Clinical Analysis of Different Nonbioartificial Liver Treatment Patterns in Patients with Chronic Hepatic Failure. Liver function and blood coagulation function indicators were compared in different patterns of nonbioartificial liver treatment of chronic liver failure, and the levels of AST, γ-GT, TBIL, and PT were significantly lower than that before plasma exchange treatment (P < 0.05); there was statistical significance; only TBIL was significantly decreased after bilirubin adsorption treatment (P < 0.05), and there was statistical significant differences; only PT significantly decreased after hemofiltration treatment (P < 0.05), and the difference was statistically significant, Table 8.

3.3. Serum Metabonomics Analysis

3.3.1. Serum Metabonomics Analysis of Liver Failure Treated by Nonbioartificial Liver. The LC-MS data before and after liver failure treated by nonbioartificial liver were processed, and the ion information in negative ion mode was obtained by SIEVE software. All data were processed by PLS-DA analysis and got Figures 2–4. In the scoring chart (Figure 2), the samples were distinguished before and after the nonbioartificial liver treatment, which validated the effectiveness of the nonbioartificial liver treatment; the load graph (Figure 3) showed a number of variables away from the center, indicating that these variables contributed significantly to the model, and there was a significant change before and after the nonbioartificial liver treatment; the validation model showed that R2 = (0, 0.222) and Q2 = (0, -0.228), indicating that the PLS-DA model did not have overfitting, that the prediction between groups was reliable, and that the model was successfully established. We analyzed metabolite with significant difference before and after nonbioartificial liver treatment and VIP greater than 1, which used the MetaboAnalyst analysis. Combined with Figures 2-3, we identified 29 differential metabolites and, as shown in Table 9, the fatty acids and bile acids were taken as the principal thing. Metabolic pathways were analyzed through the MetaboAnalyst analysis, and 12 metabolic pathways were identified, which relates to the proportion of fatty acid metabolites metabolism and bile acid metabolism in the highest (Figure 4, Table 10). These results indicated that nonbioartificial liver treatment had significant effects on fatty acid metabolism and bile acid metabolism.

3.3.2. Serum Metabonomics Analysis of Chronic Liver Failure Treated by Nonbioartificial Liver. The 52 patients were included, 33 cases of chronic liver failure (63.46%), among them there were 15 cases of plasma exchange (45.454%), 9 cases of bilirubin adsorption (27.273%), 9 cases of hemofiltration(27.273%). Serum LC-MS data of chronic liver failure after treatment with different nonbioartificial liver patterns were analyzed by PLS-DA, and Figures 5–7 was obtained. In the score plot (Figure 5) in different nonbioartificial liver treatment pattern distinguishing, which showed that there were obvious differences between the treatment pattern, load graphs (Figure 6) showed multiple variables

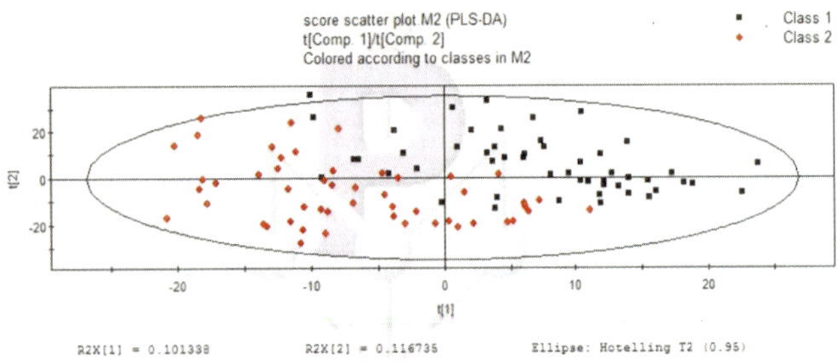

FIGURE 2: Scoring chart of PLS-DA pattern in treatment of liver failure with nonbioartificial liver. *Note.* Classl, Before nonbioartificial liver treatment; Class2, After nonbioartificial liver treatment.

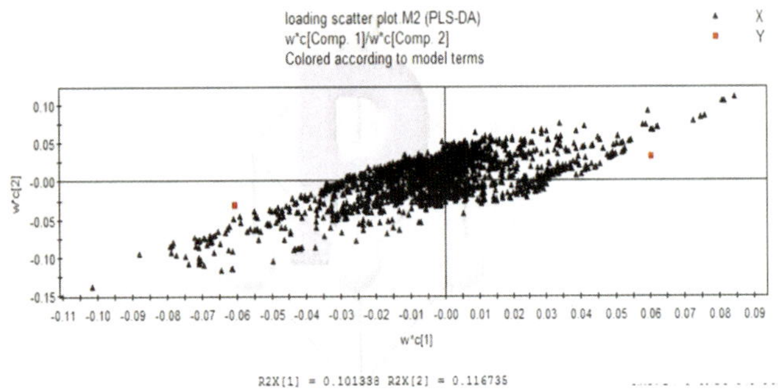

FIGURE 3: Load chart of PLS-DA pattern in treatment of liver failure with nonbioartificial liver.

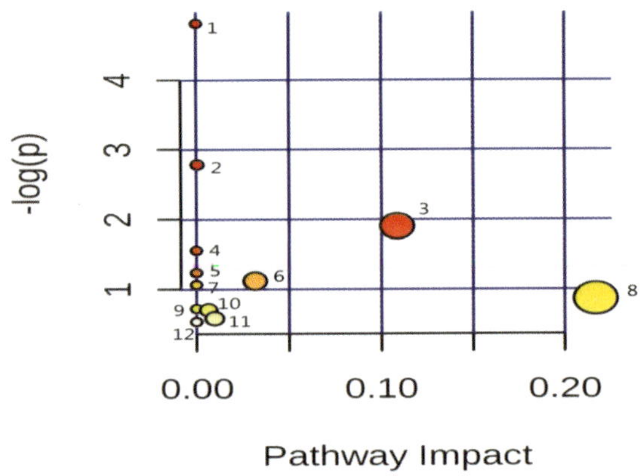

FIGURE 4: Differential metabolite related pathway. Note that numbers 1-12 represent different metabolic pathways, the name of metabolic pathways, and distribution parameters as shown in Table 10.

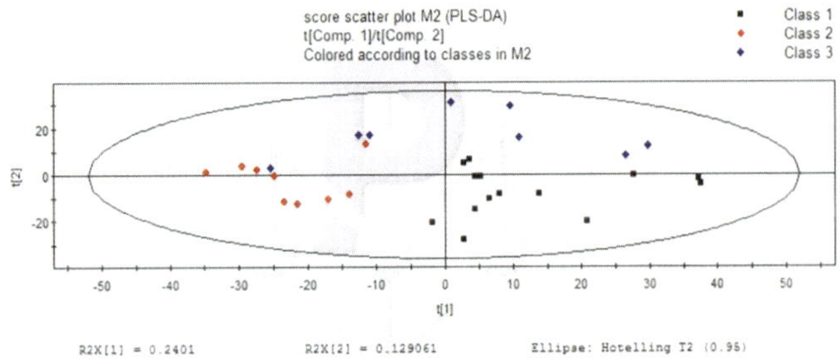

FIGURE 5: Scoring chart of PLS-DA pattern in treatment of chronic liver failure with nonbioartificial liver. Note the following: Classl: plasma exchange for chronic liver failure; Class2: treatment of chronic liver failure with bilirubin adsorption; Class3: hemofiltration in the treatment of chronic liver failure.

away from the center, indicating that these variables are important in distinguishing different treatment modalities; verification model showed that R2 = (0, 0.537) and Q2 = (0, -0.441), which indicated the PLS-DA model without overfitting; internal group prediction model was established successfully reliable. According to the variable importance projection (VIP > 1), combined with Figures 5-6, we identified 11 different metabolites, shown in Table 11, with fatty acids, bile acids, and amino acids; 7 metabolic pathways were identified through the MetaboAnalyst analysis, as shown in Figure 7 and Table 12. The proportion of metabolites involved bile acid metabolism, fatty acid metabolism, and amino acid metabolism in the metabolism was the highest. It indicated that the different treatment patterns had significant effects on bile acid metabolism, fatty acid metabolism, and amino acid metabolism.

4. Discussion

Liver failure is one of the most common serious liver disease syndromes, with high fatality rate [1]. There are three main treatment methods for liver failure: medical treatment, nonbioartificial liver support therapy, and liver transplantation treatment [7]. Because of comprehensive internal medical treatment is limited, liver transplantation improved survival rate but affected by the shortage of donor, high cost, and other factors; nonbioartificial liver support therapy can improve liver function, until you find the suitable donor liver or liver regeneration, which is particularly important in the clinical application of liver failure [8–11]. Nonbioartificial liver treatment can significantly improve liver function and coagulation indexes in the early and middle stages of liver failure. It can improve the symptoms in the late stage of liver failure and the survival time of patients waiting for liver transplantation and the survival value of patients [12–14]. In this study, we used metabonomics to analyze the changes of the organism before and after the nonbioartificial liver treatment.

Hepatic uptake of free fatty acids (FFA) plays an important role in the synthesis, storage, and transport of lipids [15]. With necrosis and apoptosis of hepatocytes, the absorbance of free fatty acids decreased and free fatty acids in serum increased liver failure patients. Studies have shown that different forms of fatty acids have different effects [16]. A protective role for endogenously generated unsaturated fatty acids was also indicated by in vivo experiments using genetically modified mice bearing an inactivating mutation in the gene encoding the enzyme stearoyl-CoA desaturase [17]. Exposure of a variety of cell types, including hepatocytes, to long-chain saturated fatty acids led to increased expression of proinflammatory cytokines, inhibition of insulin signaling, induction of endoplasmic reticulum (ER) stress, and

Table 6: Clinical analysis of hepatic failure treated by nonbioartificial liver treatment.

Index	Mean (before and after)	Standard deviation (front and back)	The value of P
ALT(U/L)	117.06, 69.60	236.50, 76.28	0.051
AST(U/L)	185.15, 141.23	250.61, 138.12	0.003*
ALB(g/L)	30.59, 28.33	4.61, 2.81	0.001**
ALP(U/L)	95.54, 86.33	33.33, 31.24	0.01*
r-GT(U/L)	60.77, 49.06	36.66, 21.87	0.003*
TBil(umol/L)	372.53, 263.53	229.01, 170.05	0.001**
PT(s)	24.66, 19.74	8.36, 5.82	0.001**

Note. *Compared with the preclinical indexes in the nonbioartificial liver treatment $P < 0.01$. **Compared with the preclinical indexes in the nonbioartificial liver treatment $P \leqslant 0.001$. There was significant statistical significance.

Table 7: Clinical analysis of plasma exchange in the treatment of liver failure.

Liver failure type	Index	Mean (before and after)	Standard deviation (front and back)	The value of P
acute hepatic failure	ALT(U/L)	130.00, 76.33	147.77, 51.69	0.08
	AST(U/L)	180.50, 100.17	117.18, 52.11	0.028*
	ALB(g/L)	31.82, 25.98	3.26, 1.06	0.042*
	ALP(U/L)	124.33, 93.00	24.19, 21.93	0.027*
	r-GT(U/L)	139.83, 79.83	30.65, 18.14	0.028*
	TBil(umol/L)	383.88, 206.82	127.49, 71.11	0.028*
	PT(s)	19.12, 16.87	2.50, 1.03	0.046*
subacute hepatic failure	ALT(U/L)	427.67, 313.67	20.79, 104.18	0.285
	AST(U/L)	343.67, 367.33	24.66, 267.99	1.00
	ALB(g/L)	34.83, 28.00	2.60, 7.43	0.109
	ALP(U/L)	117.00, 67.67	22.61, 21.50	0.109
	r-GT(U/L)	56.33, 31.67	12.50, 13.58	0.109
	TBil(umol/L)	633.90, 384.87	67.76, 80.85	0.109
	PT(s)	37.77, 20.17	4.80, 1.80	0.109
acute-on-chronic liver failure	ALT(U/L)	272.90, 88.00	469.06, 56.50	0.008**
	AST(U/L)	371.20, 187.80	506.46, 193.74	0.005**
	ALB(g/L)	33.24, 29.85	1.92, 1.74	0.007**
	ALP(U/L)	74.00, 66.00	36.24, 25.79	0.541
	r-GT(U/L)	70.50, 54.80	20.70, 13.10	0.047*
	TBil(umol/L)	559.37, 408.53	380.74, 321.44	0.005**
	PT(s)	20.24, 15.37	6.26, 1.53	0.028*
Chronic liver failure	ALT(U/L)	37.8, 37.53	27.83, 18.69	0.955
	AST(U/L)	97.20, 78.20	90.85, 76.31	0.019*
	ALB(g/L)	28.60, 27.86	6.21, 1.96	0.394
	ALP(U/L)	89.00, 80.13	28.71, 23.39	0.053
	r-GT(U/L)	41.40, 36.40	19.73, 18.53	0.033*
	TBil(umol/L)	319.73, 223.11	145.33, 79.61	0.001* * *
	PT(s)	24.06, 17.86	5.78, 2.60	0.001* * *

Note. *Compared with the preclinical indexes in the treatment of plasma exchange $P < 0.05$. **Compared with the preclinical indexes in the treatment of plasma exchange $P < 0.01$. * * *Compared with the preclinical indexes in the treatment of plasma exchange $P \leqslant 0.001$. There was significant statistical significance.

promotion of cell death, mainly by apoptosis [18]. After nonbioartificial liver treatment, the levels of various saturated fatty acids decreased and the levels of unsaturated fatty acids increased; this showed that fatty acids were involved in the process of inflammation and repair of hepatocytes. And nonbioartificial liver treatment can effectively affect the distribution of fatty acids in the environment and create conditions for the regeneration of liver cells.

Bile acid is composed of cholesterol in the cytoplasm and microsome of liver cells. Bile acids can be divided into hydrophobic and hydrophilic bile acids according to water solubility [19, 20]. Bile acid enters the cell and can inhibit the oxidative phosphorylation of mitochondria, and the ATP synthesis decreased calcium pump inactivation, extracellular Ca^{2+} influx, and activation of various proteolytic enzymes, which caused the decomposition of DNA, RNA and protein,

Table 8: Clinical analysis of different nonbioartificial liver treatment patterns in patients with chronic liver failure.

Non-bioartificial liver treatment method	Index	Mean (before and after)	Standard deviation (front and back)	The value of P
Plasma exchange	ALT(U/L)	37.80, 37.53	27.83, 18.69	0.955
	AST(U/L)	97.20, 78.20	90.85, 76.31	0.019*
	ALB(g/L)	28.60, 27.86	6.21, 1.96	0.394
	ALP(U/L)	89.00, 80.13	28.71, 23.39	0.053
	r-GT(U/L)	41.40, 36.40	19.73, 18.53	0.033*
	TBil(umol/L)	319.73, 223.11	145.33, 79.61	0.001**
	PT(s)	24.06, 17.86	5.78, 2.60	0.001**
Bilirubin adsorption	ALT(U/L)	55.33, 60.22	40.57, 38.87	0.05
	AST(U/L)	162.56, 178.33	70.30, 79.48	0.123
	ALB(g/L)	29.14, 28.82	4.32, 3.76	0.859
	ALP(U/L)	106.00, 104.78	20.71, 23.65	0.398
	r-GT(U/L)	54.00, 58.67	12.51, 13.56	0.095
	TBil(umol/L)	301.80, 210.37	90.99, 33.98	0.011*
	PT(s)	20.89, 21.38	5.76, 2.66	0.213
Hemofiltration	ALT(U/L)	25.56, 26.11	12.33, 6.95	0.767
	AST(U/L)	97.89, 109.44	85.78, 99.71	0.260
	ALB(g/L)	30.21, 28.61	3.22, 1.90	0.066
	ALP(U/L)	93.56, 102.56	40.73, 45.90	0.097
	r-GT(U/L)	37.78, 39.44	21.38, 21.15	0.233
	TBil(umol/L)	229.00, 220.31	106.43, 92.20	0.441
	PT(s)	33.64, 27.87	9.01, 8.88	0.011*

Note: *Compared with the preclinical indexes in the treatment of nonbioartificial liver in Chronic liver failure $P < 0.05$, **Compared with the preclinical indexes in the treatment of nonbioartificial liver in Chronic liver failure $P < 0.001$. There was significant statistical significance.

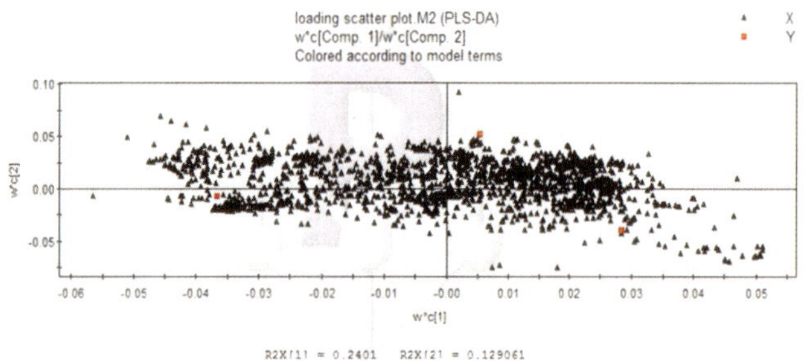

Figure 6: Load chart of PLS-DA pattern in treatment of chronic liver failure with nonbioartificial liver.

cell dysfunction, and ultimately apoptosis [21, 22]. During liver failure, a large number of liver cells were mortified and bile acid was released into the blood, resulting in elevated levels of serum bile acids, and elevated bile acids reaction on liver cells can further lead to necrosis and apoptosis of liver cells. In this study, the hydrophobic bile acid decreased and the hydrophilic bile acid increased after nonbioartificial liver treatment. The positive correlation between hydrophobic bile acids and liver injury was confirmed, and the antagonism between hydrophilic bile acids and hydrophobic bile acids was also confirmed.

The liver plays a key role in amino acid metabolism [23], liver injury can cause imbalance of amino acid metabolism

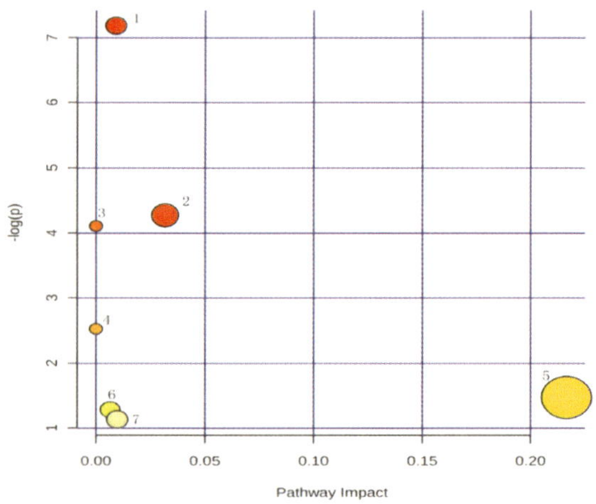

Figure 7: Differential metabolite related pathway in treatment of chronic liver failure with nonbioartificial liver. Note that numbers 1-7 represent different metabolic pathways, the name of metabolic pathways, and distribution parameters as shown in Table 12.

and change of amino acid levels in human body [24, 25]. Phenylalanine is an essential amino acid, it can synthesize proteins and be converted into nonessential amino acid tyrosine. Under the influence of hepatitis virus invasion or other physical and chemical factors, the parenchymal cells

Table 9: Identification of characteristic metabolites.

Number	Detection of mass/charge ratio	The theory of mass/charge ratio	metabolite	VIP value
1	112.1	113.1	creatinine	2.96
2	391.3	392.6	Ursodeoxycholic acid	2.74
3	367.2	288.4	Dehydroepiandrosterone	2.70
4	203.1	204.2	L- tryptophan	2.12
5	217.0	200.1	1,3 hydroxy uric acid	2.07
6	178.1	178.2	benzoyl-glycine	2.05
7	281.3	282.5	FFA 18_1	1.84
8	204.1	205.2	indolelactic acid	1.81
9	303.2	304.5	FFA 20_4	1.60
10	448.3	467.6	Glycerol deoxycholate	1.52
11	309.3	310.0	FFA 20_1	1.46
12	185.2	186.3	FFA 11_0	1.39
13	407.3	408.6	cholalic acid	1.37
14	167.0	168.1	uric acid	1.37
15	391.3	392.6	deoxycholic acid	1.35
16	157.1	158.3	FFA 9_0	1.33
17	339.3	338.6	FFA 22_0	1.32
18	286.3	284.5	FFA 18_0-d3	1.32
19	305.3	306.3	FFA 20_3	1.30
20	199.2	200.3	FFA 12_0	1.29
21	241.2	242.4	FFA 15_0	1.28
22	391.3	391.6	Ursodeoxycholic acid	1.28
23	171.1	172.3	FFA 10_0	1.25
24	295.3	296.3	FFA 19_1	1.24
25	337.3	338.4	FFA 22_1	1.23
26	301.2	302.5	FFA 20_5	1.20
27	369.2	269.4	DHES-3	1.20
28	528.3	449.4	glycoursodeoxycholic acid	1.19
29	498.3	499.7	Tauroursodeoxycholic Acid	1.18

Note. FFA: free fatty acid; DHES-3: 3-dehydro estrone; VIP: variable importance in projection.

Table 10: Metabolic pathway name and distribution parameter.

Number	Metabolic pathway name	Ordinate value (-log(p))	Abscissa value (pathway impact)
1	Fatty acid synthesis	4.8098	0.0
2	Primary bile acid synthesis	2.7816	5.4E-4
3	Tryptophan metabolism	1.8992	0.10853
4	Phenylalanine, tyrosine and tryptophan biosynthesis	1.5525	0.0
5	Nitrogen metabolism	1.233	0.0
6	Phenylalanine metabolism	1.1137	0.0315
7	Glycine, serine and threonine metabolism	1.061	0.0
8	arachidonic acid metabolism	0.85981	0.21669
9	Aminoacyl-tRNA biosynthesis	0.71939	0.0
10	Arginine and proline metabolism	0.70068	0.00645
11	Purine metabolism	0.57911	0.00969
12	Steroid hormone biosynthesis	0.53171	0.0

Note. The number of 1-12 corresponding to the 1-12 metabolic pathway in Figure 4.

Table 11: Identification of characteristic metabolites about chronic liver failure with nonbioartificial liver.

Comparison of treatment methods	Detection of mass/charge ratio	The theory of mass/charge ratio	metabolite	VIP value
Plasma exchange and Bilirubin adsorption	167.0	168.1	uric acid	2.03
	407.3	408.6	Cholic acid	1.61
	112.1	113.1	creatinine	1.58
	391.3	392.6	anthropodesoxycholic acid	1.16
	303.2	304.5	FFA 20_4	1.09
	167.0	515.7	cholaic acid	1.11
	286.3	284.5	FFA 18_0-d3	1.08
Plasma exchange and Hemofiltration	167.0	168.1	uric acid	2.03
	407.3	408.6	cholalic acid	1.61
	112.1	113.1	creatinine	1.58
	391.3	392.6	anthropodesoxycholic acid	1.16
	303.2	304.5	FFA 20_4	1.09
	281.3	282.5	FFA 18_1	1.40
	178.1	178.2	hippuric acid	1.33
	203.1	204.2	L- tryptophan	1.16
Hemofiltration and Bilirubin adsorption	281.3	282.5	FFA 18_1	1.40
	498.3	281.2	phenylacetylglutamine	1.28

Note. VIP: variable importance in projection.

Table 12: Metabolic pathway name and distribution parameter.

Number	Metabolic pathway name	Ordinate value (-log(p))	Abscissa value (pathway impact)
1	Primary bile acid synthesis	7.1808	0.009
2	Phenylalanine metabolism	4.2699	0.0315
3	Fatty acid synthesis	4.1066	0.0
4	Taurine and hypotaurine metabolism	2.5233	0.0
5	arachidonic acid metabolism	1.4694	0.21669
6	Arginine and proline metabolism	1.2801	0.00645
7	Purine metabolism	1.1293	0.00969

Note. The number of 1-7 corresponding to the 1-7 metabolic pathway in Figure 7.

of the liver are seriously damaged and even destroyed. Any of various enzymes responsible for biochemical metabolism in the liver cells that are reduced or released into the body fluid for inactivation. Thus, the catabolic pathway of aromatic amino acids slows down, and its content in the blood increases [26, 27]. After the nonbioartificial liver treatment of liver failure, the aromatic amino acids, especially phenylalanine, decreased significantly, indicating the gradual recovery of hepatocytes, which prove that the nonbioartificial liver treatment is helpful for the regeneration of liver cells and the recovery of liver function. In this study, phenylalanine metabolism in patients with chronic liver failure treated with different nonbioartificial liver models were significantly different. It was further proved that the levels of aromatic amino acids changed significantly in the treatment of chronic liver failure by nonbioartificial liver treatment.

In summary, nonbioartificial liver treatment of liver failure mainly through the impact of fatty acid synthesis pathway, primary bile acid synthesis pathway, and phenylalanine metabolic pathway affects the clinical efficacy of patients with liver failure. Through the study of metabolic changes and metabolic pathway of the organism, this study will establish the clinical basis for further study on the pathogenesis of liver failure and the mechanism of nonbioartificial liver treatment.

References

[1] "Chinese Medicine Association Infectious Diseases Branch Liver Failure and Artificial Liver," *Chinese Journal of Hepatology*, vol. 5, no. 6, pp. 321–327, 2012.

[2] M. J. W. McPhail, S. Kriese, and M. A. Heneghan, "Current management of acute liver failure," *Current Opinion in Gastroenterology*, vol. 31, no. 3, pp. 209–214, 2015.

[3] "Chinese Medical Association of Infectious Diseases Branch of liver failure and artificial liver group, Treatment of Hepatic Failure with Abiotic Artificial Liver," *Chinese Journal of Clinical Infectious Diseases*, vol. 9, no. 2, pp. 97–103, 2016.

[4] T. L. Hai, L. Lian et al., "The successful practice of metabolomics in medical research," *Progress in Modern Biomedicine*, vol. 10, pp. 1582–1584, 2007.

[5] N. Krone, B. A. Hughes, G. G. Lavery, P. M. Stewart, W. Arlt, and C. H. L. Shackleton, "Gas chromatography/mass spectrometry (GC/MS) remains a pre-eminent discovery tool in clinical steroid investigations even in the era of fast liquid chromatography tandem mass spectrometry (LC/MS/MS)," *The Journal of Steroid Biochemistry and Molecular Biology*, vol. 121, no. 3–5, pp. 496–504, 2010.

[6] D. M. Drexler, M. D. Reily, and P. A. Shipkova, "Advances in mass spectrometry applied to pharmaceutical metabolomics," *Analytical and Bioanalytical Chemistry*, vol. 399, no. 8, pp. 2645–2653, 2011.

[7] M. Zhen and W. Yun, "Treatment status of liver failureif possible," *Journal of Clinical Hepatology*, vol. 32, 2016.

[8] S. K. Sarin, C. K. Kedarisetty, Z. Abbas et al., "Acute-on-chronic liver failure: consensus recommendations of the Asian Pacific Association for the Study of the Liver (APASL) 2014," *Hepatology International*, vol. 8, no. 4, pp. 453–471, 2014.

[9] J. Lee, D. Lee, S. Lee et al., "Functional Evaluation of a Bioartificial Liver Support System Using Immobilized Hepatocyte Spheroids in a Porcine Model of Acute Liver Failure," *Scientific Reports*, vol. 7, no. 1, 2017.

[10] J. Chen, J. Huang, Q. Yang et al., "Plasma exchange-centered artificial liver support system in hepatitis B virus-related acute-on-chronic liver failure: a nationwide prospective multicenter study in China," *Hepatobiliary & Pancreatic Diseases International*, vol. 15, no. 3, pp. 275–281, 2016.

[11] M. L. Schilsky, "Acute liver failure and liver assist devices," *Transplantation Proceedings*, vol. 43, no. 3, pp. 879–883, 2011.

[12] M. Li, J. Sun, J. Li et al., "Clinical observation on the treatment of acute liver failure by combined non-biological artificial liver," *Experimental and Therapeutic Medicine*, vol. 12, no. 6, pp. 3873–3876, 2016.

[13] S. L. Nyberg, "Bridging the gap: Advances in artificial liver support," *Liver Transplantation*, vol. 18, no. S2, pp. S10–S14, 2012.

[14] X. Xu, X. Liu, Q. Ling et al., "Artificial Liver Support System Combined with Liver Transplantation in the Treatment of Patients with Acute-on-Chronic Liver Failure," *PLoS ONE*, vol. 8, no. 3, p. e58738, 2013.

[15] G. Musso, R. Gambino, and M. Cassader, "Recent insights into hepatic lipid metabolism in non-alcoholic fatty liver disease (NAFLD)," *Progress in Lipid Research*, vol. 48, no. 1, pp. 1–26, 2009.

[16] M. D. Mantzaris, E. V. Tsianos, and D. Galaris, "Interruption of triacylglycerol synthesis in the endoplasmic reticulum is the initiating event for saturated fatty acid-induced lipotoxicity in liver cells," *FEBS Journal*, vol. 278, no. 3, pp. 519–530, 2011.

[17] Z. Z. Li, M. Berk, T. M. McIntyre, and A. E. Feldstein, "Hepatic lipid partitioning and liver damage in nonalco-holic fatty liver disease: role of stearoyl-CoA desaturase," *Biological Chemistry*, vol. 284, pp. 5637–5644, 2009.

[18] Y. Akazawa, S. Cazanave, J. L. Mott et al., "Palmitoleate attenuates palmitate-induced Bim and PUMA up-regulation and hepatocyte lipoapoptosis," *Journal of Hepatology*, vol. 52, no. 4, pp. 586–593, 2010.

[19] R. E. Poupon, Y. Chrétien, R. Poupon, and G. Paumgartner, "Serum bile acids in primary biliary cirrhosis: Effect of ursodeoxycholic acid therapy," *Hepatology*, vol. 17, no. 4, pp. 599–604, 1993.

[20] H. Sagawa et al., "Protection against hydrophobic bile salt-induced cell membrance damage by liposomes and hydrophilic bile salts," *American Journal of Physiology*, vol. 264, pp. 835–839, 2001.

[21] A. P. Rolo, C. M. Palmeira, and K. B. Wallace, "Mitochondrially mediated synergistic cell killing by bile acids," *Biochimica et Biophysica Acta (BBA) - Molecular Basis of Disease*, vol. 1637, no. 1, pp. 127–132, 2003.

[22] T. Nakajima, Y. Okuda, K. Chisaki et al., " Bile acids increase intracellular Ca ," *British Journal of Pharmacology*, vol. 130, no. 7, pp. 1457–1467, 2000.

[23] B. Kinny-Köster, M. Bartels, S. Becker et al., "Plasma amino acid concentrations predict mortality in patients with end-stage liver disease," *PLoS ONE*, vol. 11, no. 7, Article ID e0159205, 2016.

[24] M. Holecek, "Ammonia and amino acid profiles in liver cirrhosis: Effects of variables leading to hepatic encephalopathy," *Nutrition Journal* , vol. 31, no. 1, pp. 14–20, 2015.

[25] M. Plauth and T. Schütz, "Branched-chain amino acids in liver disease: New aspects of long known phenomena," *Current Opinion in Clinical Nutrition & Metabolic Care*, vol. 14, no. 1, pp. 61–66, 2011.

[26] W. Jiangping, *Determination of Aromatic Amino Acids in Serum by High Performance Liquid Chromatography and Its Clinical Application*, Central South University, 2003.

[27] M. Kong, S. Hongbo, L. Bai, J. Yao, and Y. Chen, "Changes and Characteristics of Plasma Amino Acid Spectra in Patients with Hepatitis B Virus Related Chronic Hepatitis, Clinical meta," *Cirrhosis and Chronic Hepatic Failure*, vol. 7, pp. 732–735, 2016.

17

Patient Views on Advance Care Planning in Cirrhosis

Michelle Carbonneau,[1,2] Tracy Davyduke,[1] Jude Spiers,[3] Amanda Brisebois,[4,5] Kathleen Ismond,[4] and Puneeta Tandon[2,4]

[1] *Alberta Health Services, 8440 112 Street, Edmonton, AB, Canada T6G 2B7*
[2] *Cirrhosis Care Clinic, 8540 112 Street, Zeidler Ledcor Centre, Edmonton, AB, Canada T6G 2X8*
[3] *University of Alberta, Faculty of Nursing, 3-141 Edmonton Clinic Health Academy (ECHA) 11405 87 Avenue, Edmonton, AB, Canada T6G 1C9*
[4] *University of Alberta, Faculty of Medicine, 2J2.00 Walter C Mackenzie Health Sciences Centre, 8440 112 St., Edmonton, AB, Canada T6G 2R7*
[5] *University of Alberta, Department of Oncology, Division of Palliative Care, 2J2.00 Walter C Mackenzie Health Sciences Centre, 8440 112 St., Edmonton, AB, Canada T6G 2R7*

Correspondence should be addressed to Michelle Carbonneau; michelle.carbonneau@ahs.ca

Academic Editor: Michele Molinari

Aim. To investigate patient experiences and perceptions of advance care planning (ACP) process in cirrhosis. *Methods.* Purposive sampling was used to identify and recruit participants (N = 17) from discrete patient groups: compensated with no prior decompensation, decompensated and not yet listed for transplant, transplant wait listed, medical contraindications for transplant, and low socioeconomic status. Review and discussion of local ACP videos, documents, and experiences with ACP occurred in two individual interviews and four focus groups. Data were analyzed using inductive content analysis including iterative processes of open coding, categorization, and abstraction. *Results.* Three overarching categories emerged: (1) lack of understanding about disease trajectories and ACP processes, (2) roles of alternate decision makers, and (3) preferences for receiving ACP information. Most patients desired advanced care-planning conversations before the onset of decompensation (specifically hepatic encephalopathy) with a care provider with whom they had a trusting, preexisting relationship. Involvement of the alternate decision makers was of critical importance to participants, as was the use of direct, easy to understand patient education tools that address practical issues. *Conclusion.* Our findings support the need for early advance care planning in the outpatient setting. Outpatient clinicians may play a key role in facilitating these discussions.

1. Introduction

As cirrhosis progresses, patients experience frequent and sudden deteriorations in health that result in repeated hospitalizations and mortality [1]. Although time to death varies from 1 to 20 years, individuals usually progress from compensated to decompensated cirrhosis, with functional decline and complications [2]. These patients have a high symptom burden resulting in significantly impaired health related quality of life [3, 4]. Liver transplantation, the only definitive treatment option, is available to less than 10% of affected patients and approximately 20% of patients on the liver transplant wait list die or are removed from the list for being too sick [5, 6].

Palliative care minimizes symptom burden without modifying the disease trajectory [7–9]. An integral characteristic of palliative care is preparing the patient and their family with advance care planning (ACP) and end of life (EOL) options [10]. ACP is often not addressed in this population until late in the disease trajectory with one study reporting that of all the patients who had been denied liver transplant only 28% had a Goals of Care Designation (GCD) documented in their medical charts [11, 12].

TABLE 1: Goals of Care Designation Levels.

Goals of Care Designation		Chest Compressions	Intubation	ICU	Surgery	Site Transfer	Symptom Control
Resuscitative Care	1	√	√	√	√	√	√
	2	X	√	√	√	√	√
	3	X	X	√	√	√	√
Medical Care	1	X	X	X	√	√	√
	2	X	X	X	Can consider, if required for symptom control		√
Comfort Care	1	X	X	X			√
	2	X	X	X	X	X	√

From: AHS (2016) Goals of Care Designation (GCD) Pocket Card. Covenant Health Palliative Institute, August 24, 2016. Available at www.albertahealthservices.ca.

Clinician barriers to initiation of ACP conversations include concern about upsetting patients, patient cognitive capacity, lack of training or discussion aids, time limitations, and, in some situations, a focus of care on liver transplantation [7–9, 11–15]. Identifying the most appropriate time to initiate ACP/GCD discussions is difficult, as patient preferences may vary. Decisions made when one is feeling well may be different than those made when being acutely unwell [16]. Patient barriers to ACP include lack of understanding about disease trajectory, social factors, and discomfort with planning for EOL [14, 17].

1.1. Standardized ACP and GCD. In 2014, Alberta Health Services (AHS), the sole health authority for the province of Alberta, standardized ACP and GCD documentation and practices [18]. GCDs are formal clinician orders resulting from conversations and determination of preferences between the clinician and patient [19]. GCD details are divided into categories (Table 1) to describe the general focus of care, limits to interventions, and location of care [20]. The decisions are recorded on a standard form which is retained by the patient and brought to outpatient appointments or hospital admissions, to be reviewed or altered as required [20]. GCDs are most often completed in the hospital setting; however, it has been reported that less than 30% of hospitalized patients are aware they had a GCD [21].

The purpose of this study was to explore perspectives and experiences of patients regarding the processes of ACP/GCD in the setting of cirrhosis.

2. Materials and Methods

This study employed qualitative description as described by Sandelowski [22], with a goal to ensure findings reflected the participants' views in terms that remain close to the data. Interviews and focus groups allowed us to investigate patients' experiences and perceptions with ACP/GCD. We also aimed to understand how the AHS ACP/GCD resource materials, including videos and pamphlets, were perceived and if or how they had been used in the participants' own experiences. Activity oriented focus groups are particularly useful in gathering reflective data and to encourage participants to answer questions in more active ways [23]. Guiding questions were designed by the investigative team based on the current literature, and for the purposes of understanding and determining what values and information were important to participants. The study received ethics approval from the University of Alberta and was part of a larger quality improvement initiative aimed at understanding and improving ACP processes in cirrhosis.

2.1. Participants. Participants were recruited from the Cirrhosis Care Clinic at the University of Alberta Hospital. Purposive maximum variation sampling [22] was used to identify and invite a minimum of three study participants from each of the following discrete patient groups: compensated with no prior decompensation (N = 3), decompensated, not yet listed for transplant (N = 4), transplant wait listed (N = 3), medical contraindications for transplant (N = 3), and low socioeconomic status (SES) (N = 4). The low SES participants all had decompensated cirrhosis and were included in a discrete group for the purpose of understanding perspectives unique to this population. Potential participants were identified via chart review and were recruited via personal phone call by the primary investigator (PI) who is also a Nurse Practitioner in the Cirrhosis Care Clinic. Two people declined to participate; one person consented but was hospitalized the day of the focus group and could not participate. Two participants requested one on one interviews as opposed to participating in the focus groups, one of which requested to include a spouse.

2.2. Data Collection. The PI (MC), an experienced Nurse Practitioner, collected all data. The PI had professional contact with some participants but had not been involved in ACP/GCD discussions with any participant. Data collection occurred in April-August 2016, in two individual interviews (one including a spouse) and four focus groups containing 3–5 participants. All interviews and focus group meetings took place in a private meeting room within the clinic building. The focus groups were kept small due to the sensitive nature of the topic, to encourage comfort and interaction among the participants. Written consent was obtained before each interview or focus group. Interviews/focus groups were

(1) Do you have a GCD designation, personal directive, will, etc.? What do each of these mean to you?
(2) At what stage in your liver disease did you have these ACP/GCD discussions with your doctor? What were your experiences of these discussions?
(3) What other information with regard to your liver disease would you want to have in making ACP/GCD decisions? How were these things incorporated in the discussions/decisions you have already had?
(4) Before watching the videos, what was your understanding about ACP and GCD?
(5) What do you think could be changed to make these resources more useful to other people living with liver disease?
(6) What are your thoughts about the information in the video and pamphlet (probe for language, message, and GCP process)?
(7) What advice would you give your doctor in having these discussions with you?
(8) How do you think being on a liver transplant wait list would affect advance care planning and goals of care for you (asked of transplant wait-listed patients)?

Box 1: Participant demographic characteristics.

semistructured in format and consisted of two parts. In the first ten minutes, participants viewed the AHS ACP and GCD education videos [24, 25] that are used to help patients/alternate decision makers understand the concepts and start the process of thinking about their values, preferences, and options. Participants then viewed and discussed the AHS standardized ACP tracking record and GCD documentation form. Personal Directive (PD) forms were also presented for discussion. It was necessary to refresh participants' memories of these resources and documents as they may have been exposed to ACP/GCD discussions in multiple arenas including the community, hospital, intensive care, and emergency department visits over significant periods of time. Reviewing these resources allowed the participants to reflect on the messages, presentation, and language in the materials and acted as a prompt to recall their own experiences. A series of open-ended questions followed by probing questions were used to explore participants' experiences, beliefs, and attitudes about advance care planning (Box 1). Participants were also encouraged to raise their own questions and concerns beyond the topics raised through the interviewer's prompts. No restrictions were placed on the length of the interviews or focus groups (which lasted 60-90min) in order to allow participants time to freely express their individual perspectives.

2.3. Data Analysis. Data were transcribed and analysis was managed using NVivo 10©. Analysis was performed using inductive content analysis procedures including iterative processes of open coding, categorization, and abstraction [26]. Each transcript was repeatedly reviewed and independently coded by three researchers (MC, TD, and JS). Team discussions ensured consensus about interpretation and coding and the collapsing of codes into subcategories, generic categories, and main categories [26]. Analysis of focus group transcripts also included latent content coding of nonverbal behaviors that informed interpretation of the verbal information. The final analysis was reviewed by two additional team members (AB and PT). Any differences in interpretation were resolved by consensus in team discussions.

Table 2: Participant demographic characteristics.

Demographics	Participants (n = 17)
Gender	
Male	14
Female	3
Age	
40-49	2
50-59	6
60-69	8
70-79	1
Etiology	
Autoimmune Hepatitis	1
Non-alcoholic	4
Alcohol	8
Hepatitis C	2
Alcohol & Hepatitis C	1
Cryptogenic	1

3. Results

Demographic and clinical characteristics of participants are presented in Tables 2 and 3. Each participant was given a study identification number ACP 1-17, based chronologically on the date consent was signed.

Uncertainty about their disease trajectory was a major factor in participants' levels of readiness to engage in ACP discussions and decision-making. Many participants had completed legal documents such as wills and advanced directives. Few, however, appeared to understand the role and values underlying the GCD process or forms even if they did, in fact, possess a signed GCD form. Participants broadly realized the GCD process was intended to ensure their wishes were followed and to reduce decisional burden on families, although there was some indication that the GCD was seen more of a bureaucratic measure designed to safeguard the healthcare system against liability. Overall, participants indicated

TABLE 3: Participants' clinical status.

Clinical status	Number (n = 17)	MELD Score Mean (range)	Child- Pugh Class (Score)
Compensated	4	8.75 (8–10)	A (5): n= 4
Prior decompensation, not currently listed for transplant	3	13.6 (7-22)	A (5-6): n =2 C (11): n =1
Transplant Listed	3	15.3 (7-20)	A (6): n=1 B (9): n =1 C (10): n=1
Contraindication to Transplant	3	11 (8-17)	B (7-8): n =2 C (10): n =1
Low Socio-economic status	4	12.25 (9-18)	B (7-9): n=2 C (10-11): n=2

ACP/GCD discussions that occurred in acute care situations when they were experiencing an exacerbation of their condition were dispreferred. Three overarching categories emerged: (1) lack of understanding about disease trajectories and ACP processes, (2) role of family/caregivers in care and ACP decision-making, and (3) preferences for receiving ACP information.

3.1. Lack of Understanding about Disease Trajectories and ACP Processes. Participants expressed an overall lack of understanding regarding cirrhosis trajectories and the role of ACP processes. Participants with clinical decompensation wanted clinicians to clearly explain key stages in the progression of cirrhosis, treatment options, and outcomes to better manage their expectations:

> *I would've liked to have known right from the beginning, what levels are going to happen next ... If you predict when the end is near, I want to know.... You... know you have the disease and the hope is transplant later on, but [if] you know they're not going to do that ... what are the other options to manage symptoms? (Medical Contraindication to Transplant, ACP16)*

Most participants stated they were unsure about the differences between legal wills, PDs, and the GCD. Less than half of the participants had a PD and none of the low SES participants had a PD in place. Those waiting for transplant either had a PD prepared or had talked about it, as had most participants from the medical contraindication to transplant group. For these participants, working through formal ACP processes reflected their disease stage, in that wills were completed soon after diagnosis, and PDs were completed as they experienced exacerbations or were faced with transplant or the decision that transplant was not an option. Those with wills and PDs regarded them as necessary decisions that can then be *"put it aside, like an insurance you hope to never use" (Compensated, ACP1).*

Only one participant accurately articulated the intent and function of the GCD form. Interestingly, the 13 previously hospitalized participants had a GCD but were unaware of its purpose. A typical comment was, "I have one of those [GCD form] at home but I don't know what it's for." (Low SES, ACP5). Participants who had experienced decompensation typically felt that GCDs had been determined in emergency situations:

> *I was really close to dying but I pulled out of it. They gave the green sleeve [GCD form] to me at that time. Maybe it was because they thought I was going to die. (Low SES, ACP4)*

Few participants clearly recalled the ACP discussions that had led to their GCD, because the GCD had been completed during a period of acute illness. While looking at a GCD sample document, one participant vaguely remembered, but inaccurately identified it:

> *This looks familiar. I think I may have got one in hospital, on one of my trips to the hospital. Personal directive, right? (Decompensated, not yet listed for transplant, ACP15)*

A participant on the transplant wait list recounted that it was only after he had recovered that the GCD was explained:

> *I did actually get mine (GCD form) in the hospital and the nurse came and said 'you probably got this but they didn't explain what it is', and then she went through it with me...looks like it's written by an insurance company. (Transplant Wait Listed, ACP9)*

Participants were often unclear about whether the PD or the GCD held precedence. One participant from the Low SES group, who had been hospitalized numerous times, had three different GCDs. Although some knew they had a GCD, few recalled its intent.

3.2. Role of Alternate Decision Makers. Most participants had an alternate decision maker (N = 14/17), and most often named a spouse. They reported a significant reliance on their families during periods of symptom exacerbation:

> *I'm lucky that my husband was able to help, but there are times when he's found it frustrating. I'll be fine one day and then I'm gone- I can't even speak [referring to encephalopathy]. (Contraindication to Transplant, ACP16)*

Most described their alternate decision makers as having a significant role in their health decision-making as this participant described:

> *My wife, she looks after me and she knows a lot about all this stuff...what she says, they listen, so I don't have to say very much. I'm quiet. (Transplant Wait Listed, ACP10)*

Many described a personal preference for their families not to see them in an intensive care setting at EOL and saw the ACP as critical to reducing the decision-making burden on family. The existence of PDs created when the person was healthier was viewed as a way to ensure their wishes would prevail should family members disagree with their wishes:

> *Because when the time comes, then the fight starts. Maybe one of your children doesn't want to let go so when you have a personal directive that child stops, and you get to make those decisions when you're in a healthier place. (Contraindication to Transplant, ACP17)*

However, when participants felt well they appeared less motivated to initiate ACP discussions with family:

> *I've been meaning to do this for forever. It's one of those things you think, yeah that's a good idea... we've talked about my disease but I look healthy ... family look at you and think you look okay. You've never thought, sat down and said ... this is what should happen ... (Compensated, ACP2)*

Many participants spoke about difficulties in discussing EOL issues with their families. They expressed the desire for information and guidance on how to have these discussions:

> *I try to [have these discussions] with my children and they say 'you're not dying'. They don't want to think about it. It becomes very hard. It is emotional for my wife too, but she understands more. (Contraindication to Transplant, ACP17)*

Participants in the low SES group expressed concern over lack of family support and substitute decision makers:

> *My daughter doesn't talk to me. I have no family, no nothing. I don't really have any friends, so what am I supposed to do? (Low SES, ACP4)*

They were concerned about the possibility of family making poor decisions at EOL, as one person suggested, "*What if they (family) say leave him in pain forever, he owes us?" (Low SES, ACP5).*

3.3. Preferences for Receiving ACP Information. The uncertainty of determining a prognosis was a major issue for most participants. ACP conversations had occurred as a process that reflected acute changes in their illness trajectory. However, when asked when ACP/GCD conversations should occur, all agreed that discussions and GCD decisions should happen outside of hospital and not during periods when they were acutely ill:

> *We all are hoping we're going to be terrifically fine, but you don't know that's going to happen and that's why I think earlier the better because later you might not be 'all there' [referring to encephalopathy], and that's very important. (Low SES, ACP6)*

Some participants worried that situations when symptoms were worse would negatively affect their ability to pay attention and make decisions. None of the participants from the compensated group had been hospitalized in the past year or exposed to the GCD form. They felt that although having a GCD was important, their inclination was to focus on staying healthy:

> *It's always prudent to guard against the downside, deal with that, but then right away focus the vast majority of effort to on finding a solution so it doesn't come to that. (Compensated, ACP1)*

Participants wanted to feel confident their clinicians were doing everything possible to treat their disease. Some worried that ACP implied an expectation of deterioration and thus an orientation to management of symptoms rather than cure. When asked if it would be upsetting to have a clinician bring up GCD, one participant explained:

> *No. It would not upset me. I just want the goal to be recovery and not just management of deterioration. I don't want there to be an expectation of deterioration. (Compensated, ACP1)*

Participants acknowledged that ACP conversations are difficult but they preferred frank information. While some worried that such conversations could reduce hope for recovery, most preferred realistic and direct information so that they could start making decisions:

> *I want to know everything upfront. I don't want surprises. ... I'm okay with that [information] instead of sitting and waiting and wondering what is going to be the outcome. You need to know what could happen with CPR and how you will function after treatments. It's important to understand what to expect with liver problems like the toxins [encephalopathy]. (Contraindication to Transplant, ACP17)*

All participants expressed having a trusting relationship with clinicians who knew them and their medical condition as key factors in determining which clinician should initiate GCD conversations. For those who had experienced minimal complications, this was most often a family physician, and for participants with more advanced cirrhosis, it was their cirrhosis clinician. Many expressed feeling uncomfortable discussing GCD with a care provider they did not know in an acute care setting:

> *We're not all going to be the same. To know your patient, you know their personality. You know what they can take. Whereas talking to somebody you don't really know all that well, you don't know what to expect. (Low SES, ACP6)*

They explained that conversations with unfamiliar care providers could lead to lack of clarity:

> *I was in the hospital, in and out over two weeks at the holidays. One doctor would say this, one doctor would say that, nobody could tell me a straight answer, and I was like, to hell with that, I'm not doing this anymore. (Low SES, ACP4)*

Predominantly, participants acknowledged their providers' skills in difficult conversations about illness trajectories and prognosis:

> *They are very comfortable talking to me and I am very comfortable talking to them. Yes, it is hard sometimes for doctors to come out and say things, but I hope they won't feel that way. (Medical Contraindication to Transplant, ACP17)*

Participants on the transplant wait list described receiving information about risk of death on the wait list, yet none recalled discussions regarding EOL options. The focus on receiving a transplant meant that they received limited information with which to consider GCD decisions if they were no longer able to receive a transplant:

> *I think all of us have those ideas going through our heads, but that doesn't mean we have the right information to make that decision. (Transplant Wait Listed, ACP8)*

Most participants described wanting examples about treatment options and consequences rather than statistics. They expressed a desire for the GCD explanations to be made in a stepwise manner. Those who had experienced decompensation wanted more specific information, such as illness trajectory graphs, examples as they pertained to quality of life, and options regarding EOL care. For those who had not experienced decompensation, there was a preference for the information to be provided simultaneously with recommendations about maintaining or improving health.

3.4. Perceptions of ACP/GCD Resources. Participants were invited to provide feedback on the ACP/GCD resources available. Many found the generalized videos informative and helpful. All participants had recommendations for customizing the videos specific to those with cirrhosis. Participants suggested a need for new resources to help them talk about EOL with their families. Although a medical order, the GCD is meant to be easily understood. All participants commented that the language on the GCD form was too complex for them to understand:

> *I don't know if it's just me being a bit thick, but some of this [GCD form] seems too technical, and if you look at the back it doesn't help. [note: the back of the form has descriptions of each GCD level]. (Transplant Wait Listed, ACP9)*

4. Discussion

The aim of this study was to explore perceptions on ACP/GCD processes as they pertained to outpatients with cirrhosis. Lack of illness trajectory knowledge was a major barrier to ACP understanding. Limitations in patients' knowledge of cirrhosis progression and outcomes has been reported [16, 27], consistent with the findings in our study. GCD decisions at the time of hospitalization were common (n = 13/13); however, understanding the decisions or purpose of the GCD form upon recovery was sparse. Patient decision aids can help people prepare for ACP discussions. Despite being available online, there is no specific local process for providing patients with these resources, nor are the resources cirrhosis-specific. In patients with advanced cancers, decision aids are effective; however, authors likewise noted there was no process in place to standardize the use of these aids [28].

Nearly all participants mentioned involvement of family in the ACP process. They often expressed more concern over how family would cope versus themselves. In a recent review of the family experience in critical illness, many patients felt that they needed more information and that the information presented to them was confusing [29]. They also named family centered care as one of the most valuable aspects of ACP [30], validating the concerns of participants in our study. Conversely, participants who did not have an alternate decision maker expressed concern surrounding the impact this may have at EOL. Lack of alternate decision makers can present a challenge to clinicians caring for this population [31, 32] and early ACP discussions may be particularly important so there is clear understanding of the patient's wishes before complications develop [33].

Early anticipatory planning requires discussions be initiated in primary and outpatient care contexts [16]; however, there is currently no consensus on the most appropriate timing in cirrhosis. Hepatic encephalopathy is one of the most common reasons for cirrhosis hospitalization [34]. Thus, it is unsurprising that several participants listed encephalopathy as a barrier to being able to understand or remember their GCD.

For compensated participants, there was a general belief in the importance of ACP, but preference for care to be focused on improving function and providing self-health recommendations. Participants on the liver transplant list felt the focus of care was on receiving a transplant and not EOL options, even though they were aware of the significant risk of death while waiting for transplant. This dichotomy of planning for EOL while maintaining hope for a transplant is a barrier to ACP in several organ transplant candidate groups [9, 17, 35, 36].

Additionally, participants consistently preferred to have ACP discussions with a clinician who was known to them compared to an unknown hospital clinician. The importance of clinicians in providing direct, disease specific ACP information has been described in a lung disease population and our findings support this to be valid in cirrhosis [37].

To our knowledge, this is the first qualitative study examining ACP perceptions of participants at various stages of cirrhosis, allowing for analysis of experiences throughout disease trajectory. Therefore, our goal was information power [38] rather than analytic saturation for this specific topic. Individual interviews facilitated in depth identification of experiences and issues, whereas focus group participant interactions were rich and clearly elucidated where there was consensus and diversity on key concerns.

Strengths included the use of open-ended questions and encouragement of participants to raise their own questions, which was important to ensure the issues of importance to participants were elucidated. The dual role of the PI as both interviewer and clinical NP proved to be a strength, as those participants who knew her were comfortable and felt freer to express their opinions about their ACP experiences. Conversely, it is possible that participants who did not know the interviewer may have felt less comfortable expressing opinions. Several other potential limitations were noted. First, we recruited patients from a single locality and although our findings are similar to evaluations of ACP/GCD in Alberta patient populations [21], this remains a limitation. Second, there were limitations in sample size and diversity of the population. More than half of the participants (n = 9/17) had alcohol induced liver disease, a small portion (n = 3/17) were female, and none were less than 40 or more than 79 years of age. Although this can be considered fairly representative of a cirrhosis population, topics and issues specific to cirrhosis minorities, such as patients with less common cirrhosis etiologies, may not have be captured and limit the generalizability of our data. Finally, the use of focus groups provided the opportunity for interaction among participants; however, individual comfort with providing opposing opinions in a group setting may have limited the responses of some participants.

5. Conclusion

ACP conversations and GCD decisions in acute care situations may not be optimized for patients with cirrhosis and their families. These findings support the need for earlier ACP in the stable outpatient setting. Cirrhosis and primary care clinicians may play a key role in facilitating these discussions in their clinics, involving alternate decision makers, educating patients using high quality resources, and understanding their preferences.

Acknowledgments

This work was supported by a 2016 Quality Improvement Award by Alberta Health Services.

References

[1] G. D'Amico, G. Garcia-Tsao, and L. Pagliaro, "Natural history and prognostic indicators of survival in cirrhosis: a systematic review of 118 studies," *Journal of Hepatology*, vol. 44, no. 1, pp. 217–231, 2006.

[2] A. J. Muir, "Understanding the Complexities of Cirrhosis," *Clinical Therapeutics*, vol. 37, no. 8, pp. 1822–1836, 2015.

[3] N. P. de Souza, L. M. Villar, A. J. Í. Garbin, T. A. S. Rovida, and C. A. S. Garbin, "Assessment of health-related quality of life and related factors in patients with chronic liver disease," *The Brazilian Journal of Infectious Diseases*, vol. 19, no. 6, pp. 590–595, 2015.

[4] S. S. Rogal, D. Winger, K. Bielefeldt, B. L. Rollman, and E. Szigethy, "Healthcare utilization in chronic liver disease: The importance of pain and prescription opioid use," *Liver International*, vol. 33, no. 10, pp. 1497–1503, 2013.

[5] M. Sherman, M. Bilodeau, C. Cooper et al., *Liver Disease in Canada: A Crisis in the Making*, Canada, March 2013.

[6] W. R. Kim, J. R. Lake, J. M. Smith et al., "OPTN/SRTR 2015 Annual Data Report: Liver," *American Journal of Transplantation*, vol. 17, no. S1, pp. 174–251, 2017.

[7] A. M. Larson and J. R. Curtis, "Integrating palliative care for liver transplant candidates: "Too well for transplant, too sick for life"," *Journal of the American Medical Association*, vol. 295, no. 18, pp. 2168–2176, 2006.

[8] W. Sanchez and J. A. Talwalkar, "Palliative care for patients with end-stage liver disease ineligible for liver transplantation," *Gastroenterology Clinics of North America*, vol. 35, no. 1, pp. 201–219, 2006.

[9] J. Potosek, M. Curry, M. Buss, and E. Chittenden, "Integration of palliative care in end-stage liver disease and liver transplantation," *Journal of Palliative Medicine*, vol. 17, no. 11, pp. 1271–1277, 2014.

[10] X. Gómez-Batiste, S. A. Murray, K. Thomas et al., "Comprehensive and Integrated Palliative Care for People With Advanced Chronic Conditions: An Update From Several European Initiatives and Recommendations for Policy," *Journal of Pain and Symptom Management*, vol. 53, no. 3, pp. 509–517, 2017.

[11] M. O. Rakoski, R. J. McCammon, J. D. Piette et al., "Burden of cirrhosis on older Americans and their families: Analysis of the health and retirement study," *Hepatology*, vol. 55, no. 1, pp. 184–191, 2012.

[12] Z. Poonja, A. Brisebois, S. V. Van Zanten, P. Tandon, G. Meeberg, and C. J. Karvellas, "Patients With Cirrhosis and Denied Liver Transplants Rarely Receive Adequate Palliative Care or Appropriate Management," *Clinical Gastroenterology and Hepatology*, vol. 12, no. 4, pp. 692–698, 2014.

[13] K. Roth, J. Lynn, Z. Zhong, M. Borum, and N. V. Dawson, "Dying with end stage liver disease with cirrhosis: Insights from support," *Journal of the American Geriatrics Society*, vol. 48, no. 1, pp. S122–S130, 2000.

[14] Citizens Housing and Planning Council Association, *What Canadians Say: The Way Forward Survey Report, for The Way Forward initiative*, Harris/Decima, Canada, 2013.

[15] A. J. Baumann, D. S. Wheeler, M. James, R. Turner, A. Siegel, and V. J. Navarro, "Benefit of Early Palliative Care Intervention in End-Stage Liver Disease Patients Awaiting Liver Transplantation," *Journal of Pain and Symptom Management*, vol. 50, no. 6, pp. 882–886, 2015.

[16] B. Kimbell, K. Boyd, M. Kendall, J. Iredale, and S. A. Murray, "Managing uncertainty in advanced liver disease: a qualitative, multiperspective, serial interview study," *BMJ Open*, vol. 5, no. 11, p. e009241, 2015.

[17] S. Davis, J. Low, L. Greenslade, A. Marshall, D. Thorburn, and L. Jones, "What support do people with cirrhosis need from liver healthcare professionals in a liver transplant centre?" *BMJ Supportive & Palliative Care*, vol. 6, no. 3, pp. 389-390, 2016.

[18] Alberta Health Services, *Advance Care Planning and Goals of Care Designation Policy*, Alberta, Canada, 2014, Document # HCS-38, https://extranet.ahsnet.ca/teams/policydocuments/1/clp-advance-care-planning-hcs-38-policy.pdf.

[19] Alberta Health Services, *Goals of Care Designation (GCD) Order*, Alberta, Canada, 2014, http://www.albertahealthservices.ca/frm-103547.pdf.

[20] Alberta Health Services, *"Revised" Advance Care Planning/Goals of Care Designation Policy and Procedure*, Alberta, Canada, 2016, https://extranet.ahsnet.ca/teams/policydocuments/1/clp-advance-care-planning-acp-gcd-faq.pdf.

[21] M. Shaw, J. Hewson, D. B. Hogan, S. Raffin Bouchal, and J. Simon, "Characterizing Readiness for Advance Care Planning From the Perspective of Residents, Families, and Clinicians: An Interpretive Descriptive Study in Supportive Living," *The Gerontologist*, 2017.

[22] M. Sandelowski, "What's in a name? Qualitative description revisited," *Research in Nursing & Health*, vol. 33, no. 1, pp. 77–84, 2010.

[23] E. Colucci, ""Focus groups can be fun": The use of activity-oriented questions in focus group discussions," *Qualitative Health Research*, vol. 17, no. 10, pp. 1422–1433, 2007.

[24] Alberta Health Services, *Advance Care Planning*, 2016, https://www.youtube.com/watch?v=XK0xjEyjZ6E.

[25] Alberta Health Services, Goals of Care Designations, https://www.youtube.com/watch?v=fdfmostSgkM, 2016.

[26] S. Elo and H. Kyngäs, "The qualitative content analysis process," *Journal of Advanced Nursing*, vol. 62, no. 1, pp. 107–115, 2008.

[27] M. L. Volk, N. Fisher, and R. J. Fontana, "Patient knowledge about disease self-management in cirrhosis," *American Journal of Gastroenterology*, vol. 108, no. 3, pp. 302–305, 2013.

[28] J. Obel, B. Brockstein, M. Marschke et al., "Outpatient advance care planning for patients with metastatic cancer: A pilot quality improvement initiative," *Journal of Palliative Medicine*, vol. 17, no. 11, pp. 1231–1237, 2014.

[29] M. Krawczyk and R. Gallagher, "Communicating prognostic uncertainty in potential end-of-life contexts: Experiences of family members," *BMC Palliative Care*, vol. 15, no. 1, article no. 59, 2016.

[30] A. W. Schram, G. W. Hougham, D. O. Meltzer, and G. W. Ruhnke, "Palliative Care in Critical Care Settings: A Systematic Review of Communication-Based Competencies Essential for Patient and Family Satisfaction," *American Journal of Hospice and Palliative Medicine*, vol. 34, no. 9, pp. 887–895, 2017.

[31] B. D. Weiss, E. A. Berman, C. L. Howe, and R. B. Fleming, "Medical decision-making for older adults without family," *Journal of the American Geriatrics Society*, vol. 60, no. 11, pp. 2144–2150, 2012.

[32] A. Courtwright and E. Rubin, "Who should Decide for the Unrepresented?" *Bioethics*, vol. 30, no. 3, pp. 173–180, 2016.

[33] M. B. Kushel and C. Miaskowski, "End-of-life care for homeless patients: "She says she is there to help me in any situation"," *Journal of the American Medical Association*, vol. 296, no. 24, pp. 2959–2966, 2006.

[34] J. S. Bajaj, K. R. Reddy, P. Tandon et al., "The 3-month readmission rate remains unacceptably high in a large North American cohort of patients with cirrhosis," *Hepatology*, vol. 64, no. 1, pp. 200–208, 2016.

[35] A. M. Walling, S. M. Asch, K. A. Lorenz, and N. S. Wenger, "Impact of consideration of transplantation on end-of-life care for patients during a terminal hospitalization," *Transplantation*, vol. 95, no. 4, pp. 641–646, 2013.

[36] R. E. Colman, J. R. Curtis, J. E. Nelson et al., "Barriers to optimal palliative care of lung transplant candidates," *CHEST*, vol. 143, no. 3, pp. 736–743, 2013.

[37] A. E. Holland, J. F. Fiore, N. Goh et al., "Be honest and help me prepare for the future: What people with interstitial lung disease want from education in pulmonary rehabilitation," *Chronic Respiratory Disease*, vol. 12, no. 2, pp. 93–101, 2015.

[38] K. Malterud, V. D. Siersma, and A. D. Guassora, "Sample Size in Qualitative Interview Studies: Guided by Information Power," *Qualitative Health Research*, vol. 26, no. 13, pp. 1753–1760, 2016.

18

Helicobacter pylori Pathogenicity Factors Related to Gastric Cancer

Kianoosh Dadashzadeh,[1] Maikel P. Peppelenbosch,[2] and Akyala Ishaku Adamu[2]

[1] *Department of Medical Laboratory Sciences, Marand Branch, Islamic Azad University, Marand, Iran*
[2] *Erasmus MC Cancer Institute, Erasmus University Rotterdam, Rotterdam, Netherlands*

Correspondence should be addressed to Kianoosh Dadashzadeh; drkianoosh@gmail.com

Academic Editor: Yousuke Nakai

Background. Although the causal relationship between *Helicobacter pylori* infection and the development of gastric cancer is firmly established, the exact nature of the pathogenicity factors of *H. pylori* that predispose to gastric oncogenesis remains incompletely characterized. We investigated the association between *H. pylori* virulence genotypes and disease in a well-characterized cohort consisting of 109 *H. pylori* isolates from gastric biopsies originating from patients. *Methods.* The prevalence of genotype was assessed by PCR and related to clinical histopathological parameters. *Results.* The relation of *bab***A2** and *bab***B** negative and *ice***A1** positive genotype as a single genotype and the development of cases to GC was statistically significant ($P < 0.001$). The *cag***E**, *cag***A**, and *ice***A1** were found more commonly in patients with GC as compared with the other groups. The relation of the presence of *ice***A1** and the development of cases to GC was statistically significant ($P = 0.008$), but *bab***A2** and *bab***B** alleles were not detected in these patients. These apparent negative associations were still statically significant ($P = 0$ and 0.005). *Conclusion.* Our results show an elevated prevalence of infection with *H. pylori* strains carrying known virulence genotypes with high genetic diversity. This highlights the importance of identifying gene variants for an early detection of virulent genotypes.

1. Introduction

Gastric cancer remains a prevalent disease worldwide with a poor prognosis. *Helicobacter pylori* plays a major role in gastric carcinogenesis. *H. pylori* colonization leads to chronic gastritis, which predisposes to atrophic gastritis, intestinal metaplasia, dysplasia, and eventually gastric cancer. Screening, treatment, and prevention of *H. pylori* colonization can reduce the incidence of gastric cancer [1]. Other interventions that may yield a similar effect, although of smaller magnitude, include promotion of a healthy lifestyle including dietary measures, nonsmoking, low alcohol intake, and sufficient physical activity [2]. Furthermore, increasing evidence suggests that host factors, including genetic make-up, are also important determinants for carcinogenesis in *H. pylori* infection [3]. Colonization of *H. pylori* has been associated with chronic gastritis because it can trigger fulminant inflammatory response which can lead to pathological conditions such as gastric carcinoma and peptic ulcer disease [4]. Consequently a clinical need exists to stratify *H. pylori*-infected patients with respect to their propensity to develop *H. pylori*-related pathology; especially for GC this is felt as a pressing concern. The importance of *H. pylori* virulence factors is evident from the serious clinical outcome associated with bacteria positive for the vacillating cytotoxic (*vac***A**) and the cytotoxin-associated gene A (*cag***A**) antigen [5]. However, these two virulence factors are insufficient to explain the variety in clinical presentation of pathology associates with *H. pylori* infection [6, 7]. A potential *H. pylori* virulence factor possibly important to explain this variance in clinical outcome is the cag pathogenicity island (cag-PAI). The *cag***A** gene is a marker for the presence of the cag-PAI of approximately 40 kb, whose presence is associated with the more severe clinical outcomes [8, 9]. A type IV secretion system translocates *cag***A** protein into gastric epithelial cells, where it is phosphorylated. When this modification occurs, *cag***A** affects various cellular processes and signal transduction pathways, such as disruption of tight and adherent junctions that lead

Table 1: Primer sequences for polymerase chain reaction.

Gene	Primer	Nucleotide sequence	Size (bp)	Reference
*ure*C (*glm*M)	Hp-F	GGATAAGCTTTTAGGGGTGTTAGGGG	294	[13]
	HP-R	GCTTACTTTCTAACACTAACGCGC		
*cag*E	*cag*E-F	TTGAAAACTTCAAGGATAGGATAGAGC	508	[12]
	*cag*E-R	GCCTAGCGTAATATCACCATTACCC		
*bab*A2	*bab*A2-F	CCAAACGAAACAAAAAGCGT	271	[6]
	*bab*A2-R	GCTTGTGTAAAAGCCGTCGT		
*bab*B	*bab*B -F	ATGAAAAAAACCCTTTTAC	496	[14]
	*bab*B-R	CGAATTGCAAGTGATGGT		
*cag*A	*cag*A-F	AGGGATAACAGGCAAGCTTTTGA	352	[15]
	*cag*A-R	CTGCAAAAGATTGTTTGGCAGA		
*ice*A1	*ice*A1-F	GTGTTTTTAACCAAAGTATC	247	[13]
	*ice*A1-R	CTATAGCCASTYTCTTTGCA		
*ice*A2	*ice*A2-F	GTTGGGTATATCACAATTTAT	229	[13]
	*ice*A2-R	TTRCCCTATTTTCTAGTAGGT		

to proinflammatory and mitogenic responses: effects [8, 10]. One of the six cag-PAI genes is *cag***E**, located in the right half of the cag-PAI, that has been shown to induce secretion of interleukin- (IL-) 8, from infected host epithelial cells [11, 12].

Another putative virulence factor is *ice***A**, whose gene has two main allelic variants, *ice***A1** and *ice***A2**. The expression of iceA1 is upregulated on contact of *H. pylori* with human epithelial cells and may be linked with peptic ulcer disease [16, 17]. The blood group antigen binding adhesin (*bab***A**), a 78 KDa outer membrane protein encoded by the babA2 gene, binds to Lewis b antigens and ABO antigen [18, 19]. Although three *bab* alleles have been identified (*bab***A1**, *bab***A2**, and *bab***B**), only the *bab***A2** gene product is functionally active [20]. Studies in Western populations have associated the presence of the *bab***A2** gene with gastric cancer [19, 21]. The aim of this study is to assess the genotype of *H. pylori* strains infecting patients with chronic gastritis through the evaluation of the prevalence of several genes coding for virulence factors.

2. Materials and Methods

This research was approved by the regional Medical Research Ethics Committee of Azad University of Medical Science on 19 Jul 2016 (number 1311/28772) and all patients provided written informed consent for this research.

This study protocol conforms to the ethical guidelines of the 1975 Declaration of Helsinki as reflected in a prior approval by the institution's human research committee.

2.1. Patients, Bacterial Strains, and Cultivation. Our cohort consisted of 109 clinical isolates of *H. pylori;* 49 (45%) were from females and 60 from males (55%).

From male patients (sex ratio F/M: 0.82), the average age of the patients from which the isolates were obtained was 39±17 years. *H. pylori* was isolated employing gastric biopsies of patients presenting with gastritis, peptic ulcer, or gastric cancer. Patients were not exposed to antimicrobial agents at least one week before endoscopy was performed. Following collection, gastric biopsy samples were homogenized and cultured onto Brucella agar supplanted with 5% sheep blood and antibiotics (vancomycin, amphotericin B, and trimethoprim). Culture plates were incubated at microaerophilic condition, 37°C and high humidity for 5–7 days. Organisms were identified as *H. pylori* based on colony morphology, gram staining, and positive oxidase, catalase, and urease tests.

2.2. DNA Extraction from Culture. Genomic DNA of total *H. pylori* isolates was extracted using the QiAamp DNA mini kit (QIAGEN, Hilden, Germany) according to manufacturer's protocol and stored at −20°C until use.

2.3. Detection of Genes. In this study, PCR was used to detect the *H. pylori* specific *ureC* gene for confirming that the cultures represented a *bona-fide H. pylori* isolate, and the same technique was employed to establish presence or absence of *cag***E**, *cag***A**, *ice***A1**, *ice***A2** *bab***A2**, and *bab***B** genes.

All primer sets were selected from published literature (listed in Table 1). PCR reactions were performed in a volume of 50 μL containing 10 mmol/L Tris-HCl, 1.5 mmol/L $MgCl_2$, 0.2 mmol/L of each deoxynucleotide, 25 pmol of each primer, and 2.5 units of Taq polymerase (Geneone, Germany) [22, 23]. The thermal cycler program used consisted of the following steps: initial denaturation at 94°C for 3 min followed by 35 cycles of 30 seconds at 94°C (denaturation); 30 seconds at 58°C for *cag***A** and *glm***M** [24]; 30 seconds at 53°C for *cag***E**; 48°C for *bab***A2**; 49°C for *bab***B**; 57°C for *ice***A1**; and 48°C and for *ice***A2** all annealing steps, followed by 30 seconds at 72°C (extension step); and a final extension step was 3 min at 72°C [25].

2.4. Statistics Analysis. Data were analyzed by SPSS version 16. Fisher's exact test or the Chi-square test was used for analysis of categorical data. A P value of <0.05 was considered statistically significant.

TABLE 2: Relationship between clinical outcome and status of *cag*E, *bab*A2, *bab*B, *ice*A1, *ice*A2, and *Cag*A.

Genotypes	Number (%) of isolates NUD (n = 81)	PUD (n = 19)	GC (n = 9)	Total (n = 109)	P value
*cag*E	40 (49.4%)	13 (68.4%)	8 (88.9%)	61 (55.9%)	0.198
*bab*A2	60 (74%)	16 (84.2%)	0	76 (71.7%)	0.001
*bab*B	53 (65.4%)	12 (63.1%)	0	65 (61.3%)	0.005
*ice*A1	29 (35.8%)	8 (42.1%)	9 (100%)	46 (42.2%)	0.008
*ice*A2	11 (13.6%)	3 (15.8%)	0	14 (13.2%)	0.779
*cag*A	53 (65.4%)	15 (78.9%)	9 (100%)	77 (70.6%)	0.134

NUD: nonulcer dyspepsia; PUD: peptic ulcer disease; GC: gastric cancer; *Pv*: *P* value.

3. Results

3.1. Description of the Patient Cohort and Isolation of Study Samples. A total of 109 *H. pylori* samples were isolated from an initial number of 359 biopsies included in this study (yielding an apparent infection rate of 30.4%), of which 60 (55%) were derived from male patients and 49 (45%) isolates came from female patients (sex ratio F/M: 0.82). The average patients' age at the time of endoscopy was 39 ± 17 years. From the 109 patients with established *H. pylori* infection, 81 patients had presented with a nonulcer dyspepsia, nineteen patients with a peptic ulcer dyspepsia, and nine patients with GC (Signet Ring Cell Carcinoma (SRCC)). There was no significant difference between the mean age and sex of patients with and without ulcers and cancer. We concluded that our cohort would enable analysis of the link between *H. pylori* virulence factors and clinical presentation.

3.2. The Presence of Virulence Factors Is Common in the Clinical Cohort. The PCR-based amplification showed that the *cag*E, *bab*A2, and *bab*B positive strains had a prevalence of, respectively, 55.9%, 71.7%, and 61.3% in our cohort, whereas *cag*A, *ice*A1, and *ice*A2 were detected in, respectively, 70.6%, 42.2%, and 13.2% of the patients included in this study (Table 2). Thus, the virulence factors selected for this study are commonly detected in our patient cohort and allow statistical analysis as to their relation to disease manifestation.

3.3. Specific H. pylori Virulence Factors Show Trends of Being Positively or Negatively Associated with Patient's Clinical Presentation. In our study the frequency of *cag*E-positive isolates obtained from patients with nonulcer dyspepsia, peptic ulcer dyspepsia, or GC patients was 49.4%, 68.4%, and 88.9%, respectively, but this apparent positive association with more severe disease did not reach statistical significance (P = 0.198). The *bab*A2 genotype was detected in 74%, 84.2%, and 0% of isolates from NUD, PUD, and GC patients. The percentage of *bab*A2$^-$ genotype within GC patients was significantly higher than that of *cag*A$^+$ genotype ($P < 0.001$).

Also the percentage of *bab*B$^+$ was 65.4% and 63.1% for NUD and PUD cases, respectively, but for isolates from patients with GC (0%), this apparent negative association was statistically significant (P = 0.005). Conversely the prevalence of the *ice*A2 allele was observed in NUD patients (13.6%) and in PUD (15.8%) and in GC patients (0%), but no significant association was observed between *ice*A2 genotype and GC (P = 0.779). Similarly, in this study the distribution of *ice*A1 and clinical outcome was analyzed statistically and it was observed that the frequency of *ice*A1-positive isolates in NUD, PUD, and GC patients was 35.8%, 42.1%, and 100%, respectively. The relation of the presence of *ice*A1 and the development of cases to gastric cancer was statistically significant (P = 0.008).

Although the *cag*A allele was observed in NUD (65.4%) cases and in PUD patients (78.9%) and in GC patients (100%), there was not statistically significant association between *cag*A and the gastric outcomes (P = 0.134). A full overview of all virulence factors studied and their linkage to specific clinical manifestations is provided through Table 2.

It is apparent from our data that *cag*E, *cag*A, and *ice*A1 are more common in patients with gastric cancer than in the other patient groups, whereas *bab*A2 and *bab*B alleles were absent in patients with GC.

3.4. Combining Different Virulence Factors Allows Stratification of the Patient Cohort with respect to Patient Stratification. We examined eight different combinations based on analysis of *bab*A2, *bab*B, and *ice*A1 genotypes (positive and negative) in patients as a single genotype (Table 3). We were able to identify an association between these genotypes and clinical outcome. The frequency distributions of the combination genotypes of *H. pylori* showed the relation of *bab*A2 and *bab*B negative and *ice*A1 positive genotype and the development of cases to gastric cancer was statistically significant ($P < 0.001$) among the patient groups. But there was not statistically significant association between other genotype combinations and the gastric cancer ($P \geq 0.113$).

The apparent absence of *bab*A2 and *bab*B alleles in GC patients raises, however, hopes that larger studies may establish the usefulness of these alleles in guiding patient management.

4. Discussion

Various studies have observed substantial differences in incidence and/or severity of gastroduodenal pathologies related to *H. pylori* which may vary according to geographical regions [26]. Although many factors may contribute to these differences, an obvious contributing factor is the different distribution of pathogenic markers in circulating strains [27].

Table 3: Combination of *bab***A2**, *bab***B**, and *ice***A1** genotypes and clinical outcome.

*bab***A2**	*bab***B**	*ice***A1**	**GC** ($n = 9$)	**NUD** ($n = 81$)	**PUD** ($n = 19$)	**Total** ($n = 109$)	P value
Positive	Positive	Positive	0	19	6	25	0.113
Positive	Positive	Negative	0	15	3	18	0.121
Positive	Negative	Positive	0	12	2	14	0.136
Positive	Negative	Negative	0	9	4	13	0.196
Negative	Positive	Positive	3	7	1	11	0.216
Negative	Positive	Negative	0	11	2	13	0.157
Negative	Negative	Positive	6	3	1	10	0.001
Negative	Negative	Negative	0	5	0	5	0.253

Presence of a gene = positive; absence of a gene = negative; Pv: P value.

The clinical relevance of the putative virulence-associated genes of *H. pylori* and geographical region remains controversial. Other factors that influence the risks for atrophy and cancer in the presence of infection may be related to the time when infection occurred, to other environmental factors, and to the host genetic variation [28]. In particular single nucleotide polymorphisms in genes that influence bacterial handling via pattern recognition receptors appear to be involved, further strengthening the link between host risk factors, *H. pylori* incidence, and cancer [29]. In the present study we exploited this situation to study the relationship between selected virulence genes of *H. pylori* and the clinical status. Our results clearly support the notion that further studies aimed at establishing the negative predictive value of the presence of *bab***A2** and *bab***B** alleles for GC development are warranted.

The *cag*E is a pathogenicity biomarker of *H. pylori.* A survey of previous studies suggested that the *cag***E** prevalence is different around the world [30]. The general importance of *cag*E is best illustrated by its high frequency in GC patients as demonstrated by studies performed in patient populations derived from India (100%), Turkey (81.8%), and Thailand (93.8%) [31]. However, the prevalence of *cag***E** gene in this study was only 55.9%, markedly different from the results obtained in the aforementioned countries [32]. In the present study *cag***E**-positive isolates were slightly more detected in isolates from peptic ulcer dyspepsia (PUD) patients (68.4%), but the potential significance of this finding, if any, remains to be established. The prevalence of *cag***A** gene in our cohort is 70.6%, which resembles the situation in Western countries (Yamaoka et al., 2002), but is markedly lower than that observed in East Asian countries where *cag***A** is present in more than 90% of cases [32]. Like *cag***E**, *cag***A**-positive isolates were enriched in samples obtained from peptic ulcer dyspepsia patients, albeit not in a statistically significant manner. Nevertheless, our findings support previous studies [32] (Wu et al., 2003) and should prove interesting in including our data in a meta-analysis of virulence genes in this respect. Our results show that the prevalence of *ice***A1** and *ice***A2** genes in isolates was 42.2% and 13.2%, respectively. These results are in agreement with previous studies showing that the *ice***A1** gene is prevalent in Japanese, Korean, and Dutch patients [13] (Ito et al., 2000; Shiota et al., 2013); conversely the *ice***A2** allele was predominant in the United States and Colombia. In our cohort, the relation of the presence of *ice***A1** and the development of cases to gastric cancer was statistically significant ($P = 0.008$). But our data showed that there was no significant association between *ice***A2** and GC compared with PUD or NUD. However, several studies have reported different results, as the *ice***A2** gene was detected to be predominant genotype in these studies (Aghdam et al., 2014; Biernat et al., 2014).

The *bab***A** is one of the mediators for the attachment to gastric cells by *H. pylori* [33]. More recent analysis of *bab***A2** as a virulence marker has produced conflicting data on the usefulness of *bab***A2** expression in predicting clinical outcome, which is most likely dependent on the geographic origin of the *H. pylori* strains. Survey of previous studies on Portuguese, Thai, and India populations showed that *bab***A2** is not a marker for peptic ulcer disease or gastric cancer [12, 26, 34]. However, several studies have reported different results for strains isolated from Turkey or Germany [26, 35]. Our study suggests that *bab***A2**, "although quite prevalent," is associated with reduced propensity to develop GC and is thus associated with less oncogenic *H. pylori.* Similar results were obtained concerning *bab***B**.

Our results showed the relation of *bab***A2** and *bab***B** negative and *ice***A1** positive genotype and the development of cases to gastric cancer was statistically significant. Further studies are required to determine the functions of *bab***A2** and *bab***B** and their relationship with disease outcome and whether the presence of these alleles indicates the presence of bacteria unlikely to confer progression towards GC.

Disclosure

This research received no specific grant from any funding agency in the public, commercial, or not-for-profit sectors.

Acknowledgments

The authors would like to acknowledge Marand Branch, Islamic Azad University, and Erasmus MC Cancer Institute,

Erasmus University Rotterdam, Netherlands, for their support of this research.

References

[1] J. Ferlay, H. R. Shin, F. Bray, D. Forman, C. Mathers, and D. M. Parkin, "Estimates of worldwide burden of cancer in 2008: GLOBOCAN 2008," *International Journal of Cancer*, vol. 127, no. 12, pp. 2893–2917, 2010.

[2] C. M. den Hoed and E. J. Kuipers, "Gastric Cancer: How Can We Reduce the Incidence of this Disease?" *Current Fungal Infection Reports*, vol. 18, no. 7, p. 34, 2016.

[3] H. M. Malaty, L. Engstrand, N. L. Pedersen, and D. Y. Graham, "Helicobacter pylori infection: genetic and environmental influences. A study of twins," *Annals of Internal Medicine*, vol. 120, no. 12, pp. 982–986, 1994.

[4] M. A. Chiurillo, Y. Moran, M. Cañas et al., "Genotyping of *Helicobacter pylori* virulence-associated genes shows high diversity of strains infecting patients in western venezuela," *International Journal of Infectious Diseases*, vol. 17, no. 9, pp. e750–e756, 2013.

[5] S. Sahara, M. Sugimoto, R.-K. Vilaichone et al., "Role of Helicobacter pylori cagA EPIYA motif and vacA genotypes for the development of gastrointestinal diseases in Southeast Asian countries: A meta-analysis," *BMC Infectious Diseases*, vol. 12, article no. 223, 2012.

[6] J. L. Proença-Modena, G. O. Acrani, and M. Brocchi, "Helicobacter pylori: Phenotypes, genotypes and virulence genes," *Future Microbiology*, vol. 4, no. 2, pp. 223–240, 2009.

[7] V. P. Lima, M. A. P. D. Lima, M. V. P. Ferreira, M. A. P. Barros, and S. H. B. Rabenhorst, "The relationship between Helicobacter pylori genes cagE and virB11 and gastric cancer," *International Journal of Infectious Diseases*, vol. 14, no. 7, pp. e613–e617, 2010.

[8] M. J. Blaser, G. I. Perez-Perez, H. Kleanthous et al., "Infection with Helicobacter pylori strains possessing cagA is associated with an increased risk of developing adenocarcinoma of the stomach," *Cancer Research*, vol. 55, no. 10, pp. 2111–2115, 1995.

[9] J. C. Atherton, "CagA: A role at last," *Gut*, vol. 47, no. 3, pp. 330-331, 2000.

[10] S. Wen and S. F. Moss, "*Helicobacter pylori* virulence factors in gastric carcinogenesis," *Cancer Letters*, vol. 282, no. 1, pp. 1–8, 2009.

[11] M. Sozzi, M. L. Tomasini, C. Vindigni et al., "Heterogeneity of cag genotypes and clinical outcome of Helicobacter pylori infection," *Journal of Laboratory and Clinical Medicine*, vol. 146, no. 5, pp. 262–270, 2005.

[12] C. Chomvarin, W. Namwat, K. Chaicumpar et al., "Prevalence of Helicobacter pylori vacA, cagA, cagE, iceA and babA2 genotypes in Thai dyspeptic patients," *International Journal of Infectious Diseases*, vol. 12, no. 1, pp. 30–36, 2008.

[13] J. S. Ko, K. M. Kim, Y. L. Oh, and J. K. Seo, "cagA, vacA, and iceA genotypes of Helicobacter pylori in Korean children," *Pediatrics International*, vol. 50, no. 5, pp. 628–631, 2008.

[14] A. Bäckström, C. Lundberg, D. Kersulyte, D. E. Berg, T. Borén, and A. Arnqvist, "Metastability of Helicobacter pylori bab adhesin genes and dynamics in Lewis b antigen binding," *Proceedings of the National Academy of Sciences of the United States of America*, vol. 101, no. 48, pp. 16923–16928, 2004.

[15] L.-J. Van Doorn, C. Figueiredo, R. Sanna et al., "Clinical relevance of the cagA, vacA, and iceA status of *Helicobacter pylori*," *Gastroenterology*, vol. 115, no. 1, pp. 58–66, 1998.

[16] R. M. Peek Jr., S. A. Thompson, J. P. Donahue, K. T. Tham, J. C. Atherton, M. J. Blaser et al., "Adherence to gastric epithelial cells induces expression of a Helicobacter pylori gene, iceA that is associated with clinical outcome," *Proc Assoc Am Physicians*, vol. 110, no. 6, pp. 531–544, 1998.

[17] S. Shiota, M. Watada, O. Matsunari, S. Iwatani, R. Suzuki, and Y. Yamaoka, "Helicobacter pylori iceA, clinical outcomes, and correlation with cagA: A meta-analysis," *PLoS ONE*, vol. 7, no. 1, Article ID e30354, 2012.

[18] T. Borén, P. Falk, K. A. Roth, G. Larson, and S. Normark, "Attachment of Helicobacter pylori to human gastric epithelium mediated by blood group antigens," *Science*, vol. 262, no. 5141, pp. 1892–1895, 1993.

[19] M. Gerhard, N. Lehn, N. Neumayer et al., "Clinical relevance of the *Helicobacter pylori* gene for blood-group antigen-binding adhesin," *Proceedings of the National Acadamy of Sciences of the United States of America*, vol. 96, no. 22, pp. 12778–12783, 1999.

[20] D. T. Pride, R. J. Meinersmann, and M. J. Blaser, "Allelic variation within *Helicobacter pylori babA* and *babB*," *Infection & Immunity*, vol. 69, no. 2, pp. 1160–1171, 2001.

[21] L. E. Torres, K. Melián, A. Moreno et al., "Prevalence of vacA, cagA and babA2 genes in Cuban Helicobacter pylori isolates," *World Journal of Gastroenterology*, vol. 15, no. 2, pp. 204–210, 2009.

[22] K. Dadashzadeh, M. Milani, and M. H. Somi, "The prevalence of Helicobacter pylori cagA and iceA genotypes and possible clinical outcomes," *Acta Medica Mediterranea*, vol. 31, p. 1345, 2015.

[23] K. Dadashzadeh, "Relevance of Helicobacter pylori dupA and OipA genotypes and development of gastric disease," *Journal of Biomedical Research*, pp. 28-19, 2017.

[24] K. Dadashzadeh, M. Milani, M. Rahmati, and A. Akbarzadeh, "Real-time PCR detection of 16S rRNA novel mutations associated with Helicobacter pylori Tetracycline resistance in Iran," *Asian Pacific Journal of Cancer Prevention*, vol. 15, no. 20, pp. 8883–8886, 2014.

[25] Y. Yamaoka, T. Kodama, O. Gutierrez, J. G. Kim, K. Kashima, and D. Y. Graham, "Relationship between Helicobacter pylori iceA, cagA, and vacA status and clinical outcome: studies in four different countries," *Journal of Clinical Microbiology*, vol. 37, no. 7, pp. 2274–2279, 1999.

[26] P. Ghosh, A. Sarkar, M. Ganguly et al., "Helicobacter pylori strains harboring babA2 from Indian sub population are associated with increased virulence in ex vivo study," *Gut Pathogens*, vol. 8, no. 1, article no. 1, 2016.

[27] L. E. Torres, K. Melián, A. Moreno et al., "Prevalence of *vacA*, *cagA* and *babA2* genes in Cuban *Helicobacter pylori* isolates," *World Journal of Gastroenterology*, vol. 15, no. 2, pp. 204–210, 2009.

[28] E. J. Kuipers, "Review article: Exploring the link between Helicobacter pylori and gastric cancer," *Alimentary Pharmacology and Therapeutics, Supplement*, vol. 13, no. s1, pp. 3–11, 1999.

[29] J. Mayerle, C. M. den Hoed, C. Schurmann et al., "Identification of genetic loci associated with *Helicobacter pylori* serologic status," *Journal of the American Medical Association*, vol. 309, no. 18, pp. 1912–1920, 2013.

[30] A. S. Day, N. L. Jones, J. T. Lynett et al., "cagE is a virulence factor associated with Helicobacter pylori-induced duodenal ulceration in children," *The Journal of Infectious Diseases*, vol. 181, no. 4, pp. 1370–1375, 2000.

[31] V. P. Lima, I. J. D. L. Silva-Fernandes, M. K. S. Alves, and S. H. B. Rabenhorst, "Prevalence of Helicobacter pylori genotypes

(vacA, cagA, cagE and virB11) in gastric cancer in Brazilian's patients: An association with histopathological parameters," *Cancer Epidemiology*, vol. 35, no. 5, pp. e32–e37, 2011.

[32] T. Uchida, L. T. Nguyen, A. Takayama et al., "Analysis of virulence factors of Helicobacter pylori isolated from a Vietnamese population," *BMC Microbiology*, vol. 9, article no. 175, 2009.

[33] J. Yu, W. K. Leung, M. Y. Y. Go et al., "Relationship between Helicobacter pylori babA2 status with gastric epithelial cell turnover and premalignant gastric lesions," *Gut*, vol. 51, no. 4, pp. 480–484, 2002.

[34] L. L. Gatti, J. L. P. Modena, S. L. M. Payao et al., "Prevalence of *Helicobacter pylori cagA*, *iceA* and *babA2* alleles in Brazilian patients with upper gastrointestinal diseases," *Acta Tropica*, vol. 100, no. 3, pp. 232–240, 2006.

[35] Y. Erzin, V. Koksal, S. Altun et al., "Role of host interleukin 1β gene (IL-1B) and interleukin 1 receptor antagonist gene (IL-1RN) polymorphisms in clinical outcomes in Helicobacter pylori-positive Turkish patients with dyspepsia," *Journal of Gastroenterology*, vol. 43, no. 9, pp. 705–710, 2008.

19

Establishing a Porcine Model of Small for Size Syndrome following Liver Resection

Mohammad Golriz,[1] Maryam Ashrafi,[1] Elias Khajeh,[1] Ali Majlesara,[1] Christa Flechtenmacher,[2] and Arianeb Mehrabi[1]

[1] *Department of General, Visceral, and Transplantation Surgery, University of Heidelberg, Heidelberg, Germany*
[2] *Department of General Pathology, University of Heidelberg, Heidelberg, Germany*

Correspondence should be addressed to Arianeb Mehrabi; arianeb.mehrabi@med.uni-heidelberg.de

Academic Editor: Pierluigi Toniutto

Background. Small for size syndrome (SFSS) is responsible for a high proportion of mortalities and morbidities following extended liver resection. *Aim.* The aim of this study was to establish a porcine model of SFSS. *Methods.* Twenty-four Landrace pigs underwent liver resection with a remnant liver volume of 50% (group A, $n = 8$), 25% (group B, $n = 8$), and 15% (group C, $n = 8$). After resection, the animals were followed up for 8 days and clinical, laboratory, and histopathological outcomes were evaluated. *Results.* The survival rate was significantly lower in group C compared with the other groups ($p < 0.001$). The international normalized ratio, bilirubin, aspartate transaminase, alanine transaminase, and alkaline phosphatase levels increased shortly after surgery in groups B and C, but no change was observed in group A ($p < 0.05$ for all analyses). The histopathological findings in group A were mainly mild mitoses, in group B severe mitoses and hepatocyte ballooning, moderate congestion, and hemorrhage, along with mild necrosis, and in group C extended tissue damage with severe necrosis, hemorrhage, and congestion. *Conclusions.* Combination of clinical, laboratory, and histopathological evaluations is needed to confirm the diagnosis of SFSS. 75% liver resection in porcine model results in SFSS. 85% liver resection causes irreversible liver failure.

1. Introduction

Improved surgical techniques and perioperative care have increased the use of extended hepatectomy (EH) for the treatment of primary and metastatic liver lesions [1, 2]. The main limiting factor for EH in many patients is an insufficient remnant liver volume (RLV) [3]. Insufficient RLV causes posthepatectomy liver failure (PHLF), which increases postoperative morbidity and mortality [4]. The term small for size syndrome (SFSS) was first used to describe clinical manifestations of refractory ascites, coagulopathy, encephalopathy, and hyperbilirubinemia following partial liver transplantation [5, 6] and now includes PHLF with insufficient RLV [7, 8].

Human clinical trials to investigate SFSS are impractical because of the high morbidity and mortality rates and ethical concerns. Therefore, it is necessary to establish experimental models that are similar to the human condition. The anatomy and physiology of pigs are similar to humans [9, 10]; therefore porcine models of EH are well-suited to studying the pathophysiology and prediction of SFSS [11–16]. However, SFSS has not been prospectively evaluated following EH with regard to the clinical, laboratory, and histopathological findings. The aim of this study was to establish a porcine model of SFSS by analyzing the RLV following different degrees of liver resection, together with the clinical, laboratory, and histopathological outcomes.

2. Material and Methods

2.1. Study Design. Twenty-four female Landrace pigs with a body weight of 26 kg to 35 kg were used in this study. Animals were reared in the interdisciplinary biomedical research center (IBF) of the University of Heidelberg. The animals were weighed and blood samples were taken prior to surgery. Animals were allocated to one of three groups, with eight pigs in each group. In group A, 50% of the liver was resected

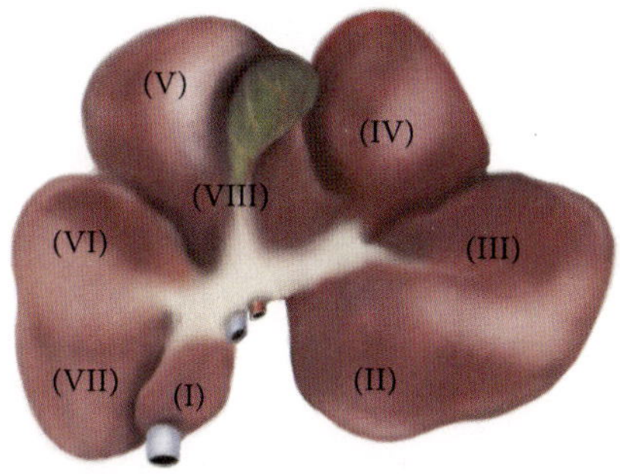

FIGURE 1: Segmental anatomy of the porcine liver. Caudate lobe: segment (I). Left lateral lobe: segments (II) and (III). Left medial lobe: segment (IV). Right medial lobe: segments (V) and (VIII). Right lateral lobe: segments (VI) and (VII).

(segments (II), (III), and (IV)). In group B, 75% of the liver was resected (segments (II), (III), (IV), (V), and (VIII)), and in group C, 85% of the liver was resected (segments (II), (III), (IV), (V), (VI), and (VIII)) (Figure 1). After resection, the pigs were observed for 8 days and clinical, laboratory, and histopathological outcomes were evaluated.

2.2. Anesthesia and Surgical Procedure. After 12 hours of fasting with free access to water, all animals underwent general anesthesia using our standard protocol [11]. Following a midline incision laparotomy, the liver was mobilized and the hepatoduodenal ligament was prepared. Liver resections were performed according to our standard method [17] using stapler (Endo GIA™ Universal Stapler, Covidien, Minneapolis, USA). After resection, electrocoagulation and hand-suturing with Polybutester 3-0 (Novafil™, Covidien, Minneapolis, USA) were performed to achieve complete hemostasis.

2.3. Postoperative Care and Assessment

2.3.1. Medications. Postoperative medication included daily intravenous (IV) administration of 3 mg buprenorphine hydrochloride (Temgesic, Reckitt Benckiser, Switzerland) and daily IV administration of 500 mg metamizole sodium (Novalgin, Sanofi-Aventis, Germany) for pain relief, prophylactic antibiotic therapy with twice daily administration of 250 mg metronidazole (Flagyl®, Sanofi-Aventis, Germany) and 375 mg sultamicillin (Unacid®, Pfizer Pharma GmbH, Berlin, Germany), and daily administration of 40 mg pantoprazole (HEXAL AG, Holzkirchen, Germany).

2.3.2. Laboratory Assessments. During the 8-day follow-up, the clinical and laboratory status of the animals were continuously assessed. Histopathological analysis was performed when the animals were sacrificed. The pigs were monitored twice daily and the general conditions, behavior, abdominal distention, food intake, and defecation were observed. Laboratory evaluation was performed before resection ($T0$), one hour after resection ($T1$), one day after resection ($T2$), and on the day of sacrifice ($T3$). Laboratory assessments included measurements of total bilirubin, aspartate transaminase (AST), alanine transaminase (ALT), alkaline phosphatase (ALP), and albumin levels and calculation of the international normalized ratio (INR).

2.3.3. Histopathological Evaluations. To evaluate histopathological changes after resection, an open wedge liver biopsy was obtained from the RLV when the animals were sacrificed. Samples were fixed in 10% formaldehyde, embedded in paraffin, and sectioned for hematoxylin and eosin (H&E) staining. The sections were reviewed by a pathologist who was blinded to the extent of liver resection. The histopathological samples were assessed for degree of mitoses, inflammation, periportal/septal edema, hepatocyte ballooning, congestion, hemorrhage, and necrosis in line with previously published studies [18–21]. Samples were graded using a severity scale ranging from 0 to +++, with 0 indicating no pathological changes, + indicating mild changes, ++ indicating moderate changes, and +++ indicating severe/significant changes. The results with significant mitosis, moderate to severe inflammation, edema, and hepatocyte ballooning were defined on behalf of SFSS. Massive necrosis and hemorrhage without mitoses and regeneration was defined as irreversible PHLF [18, 20, 21].

2.4. Statistical Analysis. Statistical analysis was performed using statistical package for social sciences (SPSS), version 23 (IBM Corp. Released 2015. IBM SPSS Statistics for Windows. Armonk, NY: IBM Corp). Continuous variables are expressed as mean ± standard deviation (SD). To analyze survival rates, the Kaplan-Meier method was applied and mean survival rates were compared using the log-rank test. Mean baseline and outcome values were compared at each time point using one-way analysis of variance (ANOVA). A repeated measures ANOVA model was used to compare the overall differences among laboratory findings between three study groups. In all tests, a p value of less than 0.05 was considered statistically significant.

2.5. Animal Rights. Animal care conformed to institutional guidelines of the Animal Care Facility at the University of Heidelberg. Animals were sacrificed under deep anesthesia at the end of the study protocol or when ethically indicated, with intravenous injection of potassium chloride (2 mmol/kg). The study protocol was approved by the German Committee for Animal Care, Karlsruhe, Germany (AZ: 35-9185.81/G-45/12).

3. Results

Twenty-four Landrace pigs with a mean body weight of 30.2±2.9 kg were divided into three groups before undergoing standard liver resection surgery: group A ($n = 8$) with 50% RLV, group B ($n = 8$) with 25% RLV, and group C ($n = 8$) with 15% RLV. There were no significant differences in body weight and baseline laboratory data between the three groups (Table 1).

TABLE 1: Body weight and laboratory results before liver resection.

	Group A (mean ± SD)	Group B (mean ± SD)	Group C (mean ± SD)	p
Body weight (kg)	30.5 ± 3.4	30.4 ± 3.3	30.0 ± 2.6	0.938
INR	1.00 ± 0.05	1.02 ± 0.04	1.06 ± 0.05	0.061
Albumin (g/l)	32.1 ± 3.3	30.4 ± 2.9	32.3 ± 3.2	0.420
Total bilirubin (μmol/l)	3.76 ± 0.86	3.42 ± 0.00	3.42 ± 0.00	0.122
AST (U/l)	46.5 ± 10.1	60.6 ± 37.6	71.6 ± 65.6	0.530
ALT (U/l)	43.6 ± 6.6	50.5 ± 10.6	53.9 ± 9.4	0.092
ALP (U/l)	170.9 ± 30.8	149.4 ± 42.0	144.4 ± 42.8	0.369

A: 50% resection; B: 75% resection; C: 85% resection; SD: standard deviation; INR: international normalized ratio; AST: aspartate transaminase; ALT: alanine transaminase; ALP: alkaline phosphatase.

TABLE 2: Laboratory findings at baseline and during the follow-up period.

	$T0$	$T1$	$T2$	$T3$	p^*
			Albumin (mean [95% CI])		
Group A	31.5 (28.8–34.1)	29.5 (26.7–32.2)	31.2 (28.3–34.1)	33.3 (31.7–34.8)	
Group B	30.7 (27.1–34.2)	23.4 (19.3–27.4)	30.2 (29.0–31.5)	27.6 (24.1–31.2)	0.016
Group C	30.1 (26.3–34.0)	28.7 (16.2–41.2)	30.7 (19.4–42.0)	26.2 (16.1–36.2)	
p^{**}	0.783	0.028	0.826	0.003	
			AST (mean [95% CI])		
Group A	46.6 (36.5–56.7)	62.9 (50.3–75.4)	59.7 (−1.9–121.4)	29.9 (25.1–34.6)	
Group B	49.0 (41.0–57.0)	249.0 (16.8–481.2)	811.2 (493.3–1129.0)	276.5 (45.4–507.6)	0.001
Group C	49.3 (37.9–60.8)	127.7 (−86.1–341.5)	502.7 (345.4–659.9)	541.3 (−610.3–1693.0)	
p^{**}	0.845	0.096	<0.001	0.017	
			ALT (mean [95% CI])		
Group A	41.2 (33.6–48.7)	39.0 (34.6–43.4)	54.0 (42.4–65.5)	37.2 (28.1–46.3)	
Group B	51.0 (39.7–62.3)	64.2 (25.7–102.6)	110.3 (79.8–140.9)	81.0 (43.7–118.3)	0.003
Group C	54.3 (35.4–73.3)	50.7 (11.8–89.5)	83.7 (51.2–116.1)	115.3 (21.2–209.5)	
p^{**}	0.116	0.307	0.004	0.010	
			ALP (mean [95% CI])		
Group A	170.7 (140.0–201.4)	168.0 (142.3–193.7)	148.1 (135.5–160.0)	101.9 (89.6–114.1)	
Group B	144.6 (85.2–204.0)	157.2 (96.5–217.9)	468.6 (341.2–596.0)	317.0 (72.5–561.5)	0.001
Group C	157.3 (121.4–193.3)	215.3 (−64.3–495.0)	435.0 (270.7–599.2)	523.0 (−405.6–1451.6)	
p^{**}	0.497	0.386	<0.001	0.020	

$^*p$ values of repeated measures ANOVA; $^{**}p$ values of one-way ANOVA; A: 50% resection; B: 75% resection; C: 85% resection; CI: confidence interval; $T0$: baseline; $T1$: one hour after resection; $T2$: one day after resection; $T3$: at sacrifice; INR: international normalized ratio; AST: aspartate transaminase; ALT: alanine transaminase; ALP: alkaline phosphatase.

3.1. Laboratory Data. Prior to and one hour after the operation, there were no significant differences in the INR between the three groups (Figure 2, $p = 0.20$ and 0.15, resp.). One day after liver resection and on the day of sacrifice, INR values were significantly lower in group A compared with groups B and C (Figure 2, $p < 0.001$). The INR reached its peak level on the first postoperative day in groups B and C. INR values decreased to near preoperative values on the day of sacrifice in group B. However, the INR did not change in group C. As depicted in Figure 2, a repeated measures ANOVA revealed that the INR was significantly lower in group A compared with groups B and C over the follow-up period ($p < 0.001$).

Mean total bilirubin levels at baseline and one hour after liver resection were not significantly different between the three groups (Figure 3, $p = 0.559$ and $p = 0.804$, resp.), but total bilirubin levels were significantly lower in group A on the first postoperative day ($p < 0.001$) and on the day of sacrifice ($p < 0.001$). The total bilirubin levels increased in groups B and C, but started to decrease slightly in group B and continued to increase in group C (Figure 3). Repeated measures ANOVA revealed that total bilirubin was significantly lower in group A during follow-up compared with the other groups ($p < 0.001$).

AST, ALT, ALP, and albumin levels for all study groups at each time point are shown in Table 2. The mean levels of AST, ALT, and ALP did not differ significantly between the three groups at baseline and one hour after liver resection but were significantly higher in groups B and C one day after resection and on the day of sacrifice. Albumin levels were significantly lower in groups B and C one hour after resection and on the day of sacrifice than group A. Repeated measures ANOVA revealed significant differences in AST, ALT, ALP,

TABLE 3: Scored pathological features.

	Mitoses	Necrosis	Congestion/hemorrhage	Inflammation	Periportal/septal edema	Hepatocyte ballooning
Group A	+	0	0	0	0	0
Group B	+++	+	++	++	++	+++
Group C	+	+++	+++	+	+	+

0: no significant changes; +: mild changes; ++: moderate changes; +++: significant (severe) changes; A: 50% resection; B: 75% resection; C: 85% resection.

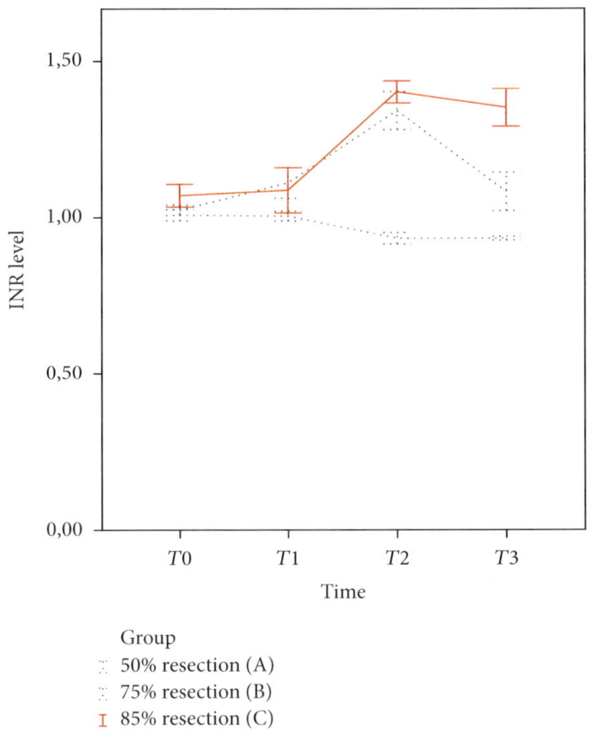

FIGURE 2: International normalized ratio (INR) levels at baseline and after liver resection. $T0$ (baseline, $p = 0.199$); $T1$ (one hour after surgery, $p = 0.148$); $T2$ (one day after surgery, $p < 0.001$); $T3$ (at sacrifice, $p < 0.001$). INR levels were significantly lower in group A compared with groups B and C ($p < 0.001$) at different time points. Error bars show standard error of the mean.

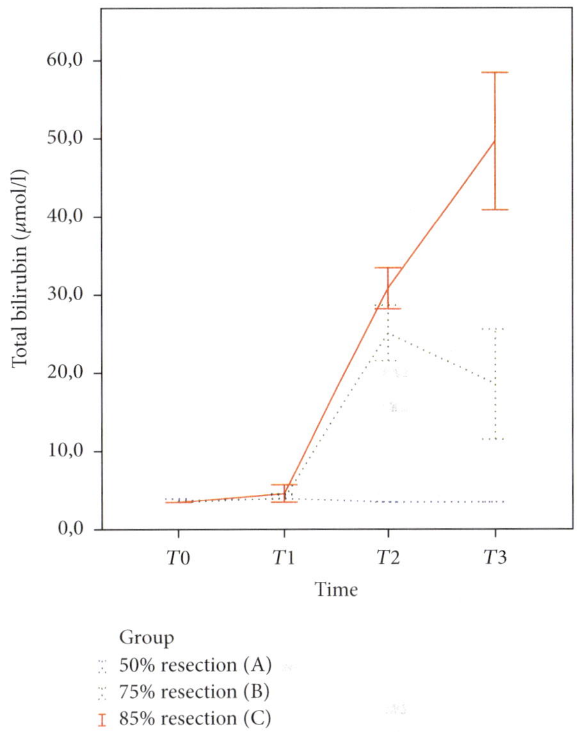

FIGURE 3: Total bilirubin levels at baseline and after liver resection. $T0$ (baseline, $p = 0.559$); $T1$ (one hour after surgery, $p = 0.804$); $T2$ (one day after surgery, $p < 0.001$); $T3$ (at sacrifice, $p < 0.001$). Total bilirubin levels were significantly lower in group A compared with groups B and C ($p < 0.001$) at different time points. Error bars show standard error of the mean.

and albumin changes between the groups during the follow-up period.

3.2. Survival. The animals were followed up for 8 days after liver resection and then sacrificed. According to the Animal Care Facility protocols, the follow-up was ended and animals were sacrificed if the clinical situation exacerbated with severe signs of acute liver failure. Seven out of eight pigs in group A survived to the end of the study period with recovered liver function; one was sacrificed on the third postoperative day due to severe ileus and abdominal distention and inability to take food. In group B, only one animal survived for 8 days; one died on the second postoperative day, and the other six survived at least 3 days (range: 3 to 6 days). In group C, seven animals died within the first 3 postoperative days, and one died on the fourth postoperative day. The log-rank test revealed that the survival rate in group C was significantly lower than the other groups ($p < 0.001$). Kaplan-Meier survival curves for each group are shown in Figure 4.

3.3. Pathologic Findings. Table 3 shows the detailed histopathological characteristics of each study group. Examination of H&E stained sections by light microscopy revealed mainly mild (+) mitoses in group A (50% RLV) (Figures 5(a), 5(b), and 5(c)). In group B (25% RLV), severe (+++) hepatocyte ballooning, moderate (++) congestion, hemorrhage, inflammation, periportal/septal edema, and mild (+) necrosis occurred (Figures 5(d), 5(e), and 5(f)). Group B livers showed significant (+++) mitoses at the time of sacrifice, but only mild (+) mitoses were seen in group C (75% RLV). Moreover, in group C, severe (+++) necrosis, hemorrhage, and congestion were observed, which reflected extensive tissue damage (Figures 5(g), 5(h), and 5(i)). Other findings in the group

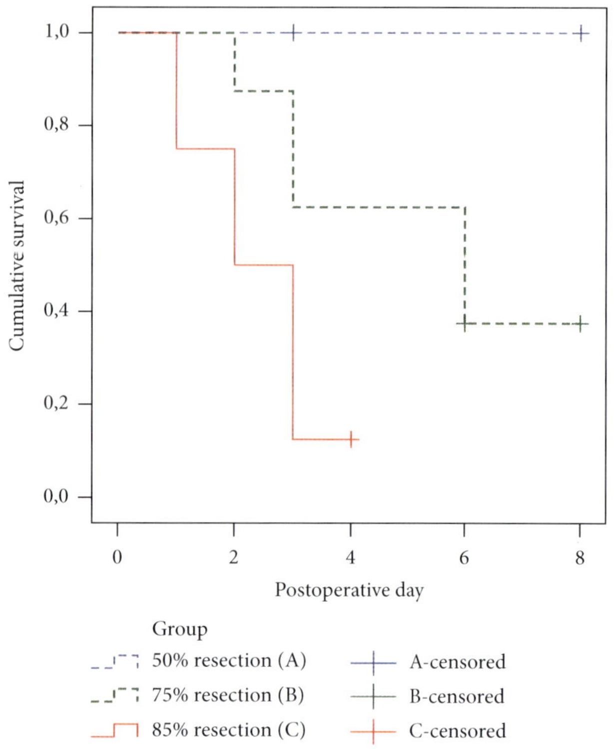

FIGURE 4: Kaplan-Meier survival graphs of the study groups. Survival rates were significantly different in three study groups (log-rank test $p < 0.001$). Censored cases died due to unknown causes or were alive at the end of the follow-up time.

C were mild (+) inflammation, periportal/septal edema, and hepatocyte ballooning.

4. Discussion

Advances in the field of hepatobiliary surgery have led to an increase in curative extended liver resection [1, 2]. However, SFSS remains a challenging issue and the size of the remnant liver is a major limiting factor of curative resection [3]. To investigate this problem, several studies have tried to develop an optimal experimental model for SFSS. [5, 12, 18, 22–25]. Even, Mohkam et al. published recently a review of literature in this regard [26]. However, the majority of published studies have focused on SFSS following partial liver transplantation and not liver resection. Also, the few studies that used a large animal model with focus of SFSS following extended liver resection [23, 25, 27, 28] did not consider the clinical evaluations, laboratory findings, and histopathological results together.

For example, in the study of Xia et al. [23] the surgical methods, survival rates, and laboratory outcomes were well described and the authors concluded that left EH plus VI segmentectomy provides a simple SFSS model. However, no differences in laboratory findings and portal pressure gradient between the left EH group and left EH plus VI segmentectomy group were found and the diagnoses of SFSS and irreversible PHLF were not confirmed by pathologic evaluation. Furthermore, the establishment of SFSS model in this previous study was based on a lower survival rate in left EH plus VI segmentectomy group compared with left EH group. In the study of Mohkam et al. [28] there is no follow-up data of the pigs after 70% and 90% resection but the authors believe that 90% hepatectomy is a reliable model for studying SFSS. An upper limit of the portal vein flow > 250 ml/min/100 g for SFSS following liver transplantation in clinical setting has been suggested by Troisi et al. [29, 30]. However, in the study of Mohkam et al. [28] the portal vein flow levels following 75% resection exceeded 250 ml/min/100 g level and it is quite likely that pigs would have developed SFSS syndrome if the follow-up continued [31]. In 2004, Court et al. [27] introduced the first porcine model of SFSS for the study of liver regeneration. They concluded that both models of 80% (trilobectomy) and 90% (subtotal) hepatectomy allow easy assessment of posthepatectomy liver function and regeneration. However, the 90% resection group with higher death rate represents a model of critical residual liver parenchyma. In a recent review of the porcine models for the study of SFSS, Mohkam et al. suggested that resection of all segments of the liver except segment 1 (subtotal hepatectomy) is the best model of SFSS after hepatectomy [26].

The most important issue in this regard that may be confusing and affect the interpretations about the volume of the resection to achieve SFSS can be explained as follows:

(1) Only based on phrasal definition, every small for size remnant liver following EH can be considered as SFSS; however, it has to be distinguished between the proper model of SFSS and the irreversible acute PHLF.

(2) It is true that a 10% RLV following EH is small for size; however, this RLV will be damaged rapidly and irreversibly following the resection.

(3) Again, only based on definition every modulation that prepares the RLV a window period for regeneration would be effective in preventing SFSS; however, in the clinical setting this window period should be tolerable and not lead to death until the liver regenerate itself. For example, following 90% liver resection the RLV will be rapidly damaged through the high portal vein flow and there is no chance for the liver to regenerate itself. Even a modulation of the transhepatic flow, which could potentially give the liver a window period for regeneration, cannot be tolerated and the animal or patient dies.

(4) Since the aim of establishment of an animal model of SFSS is a better understanding of this clinical syndrome as well as studying the possible preventive and curative methods, we strongly believe that, in a porcine model with normal parenchyma, 90% liver resection cannot be considered as SFSS model. Following 90% liver resection there is a very low chance for the liver to be rescued through any modulation.

(5) An optimal model for SFSS can be achieved following a major resection when the situation is still reversible and can be prevented or managed. In the clinical setting, it is also not logical to resect 90% of a liver

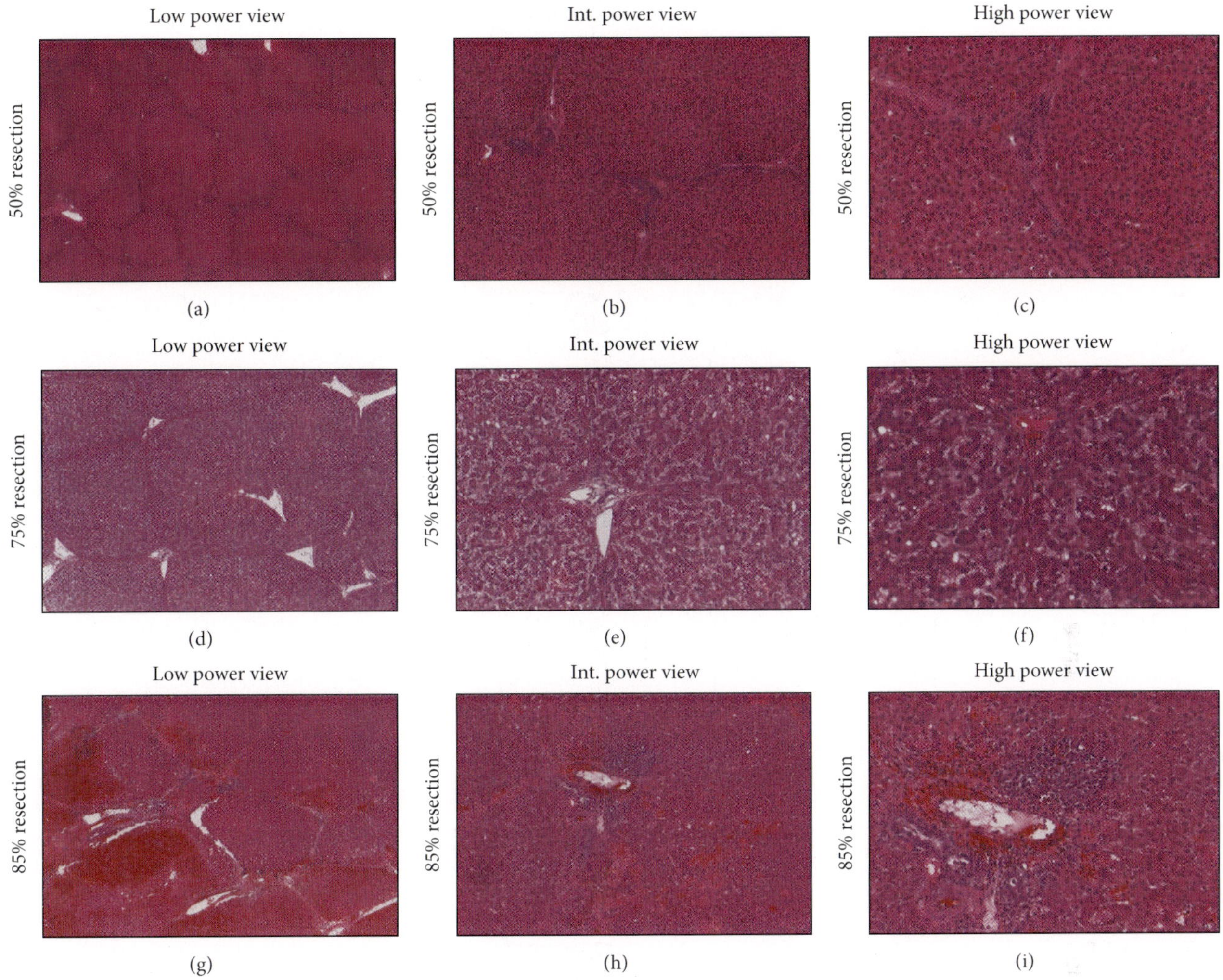

FIGURE 5: Composite of liver biopsies of 50%, 75%, and 85% liver resection at the time of sacrifice with low (a, d, and g), intermediate (b, e, and h), and high power view (c, f, and i). The low power view shows no significant change in 50% hepatectomy group. Normal hepatocytes and unchanged hepatic structures are seen (a). In the high power views only few mitoses are seen ((b) and (c)). The low power view of liver after 75% liver resection is shown in (d). Portal and periportal edema and significant elevated mitoses are prominent findings in 75% hepatectomy group ((e) and (f)). The low power view of 85% resection reveals extensive hemorrhage (g). Necrosis, bleeding, and inflammation in periportal area are shown in high power view (h and i). Int.: intermediate.

of a patient, because there is no survival chance even through hepatic inflow modulation.

In the present study, based on the experiences of Troisi et al. [29, 32] in small for size grafts in living donor liver transplantation, we established a porcine model of SFSS with consideration of the histopathologic, laboratory, and clinical findings. Histopathologic changes in 75% liver resection in our study support the establishment of SFSS in this group. We selected a porcine model because the pig liver has a similar size and anatomy to humans and therefore provides a greater scope for surgical procedures than small animal models [33, 34]. Furthermore, the segmented nature of the porcine liver makes anatomical liver resection easy to perform, similar to the human situation [9]. Since the vena cava is enclosed by the liver parenchyma in pigs, therefore it is easier and safer to perform left EH than right EH in porcine models. To compare our results with baseline data, we defined a control group and resected 50% of the liver in this group. The only histopathologic finding after 50% liver resection was mild mitoses. The laboratory findings were normal in the control group during follow-up and the survival rate was significantly higher than the other two groups. In this group only one pig was sacrificed during the follow-up due to severe ileus. However, the pathologic findings of the liver did not show any signs of liver damage. After 75% liver resection, the pigs showed histopathological signs of SFSS, including mitoses, severe hepatocyte ballooning, moderate inflammation, edema, and congestion as previously showed through Demetris et al. [20, 29]. Elevated INR, bilirubin, AST, ALT, ALP, and decreased albumin and also postoperative observation of the animals again indicated SFSS in the group with 75% resection. In this group 5 pigs survived more than 3 days and one of them survived for complete 8-day follow-up.

Among 7 pigs which died, cause of death in 5 was liver failure. These correlate with the results of Dahm et al. [5, 20, 35]. Although the mean survival rate was lower in our 75% resection group compared with previous findings of Xia et al. [23], this can be explained by our ethical policy, which did not let further follow-up of animals with severe signs and complications of SFSS.

Following 85% liver resection, the liver failed to regenerate. Histopathological evaluation revealed massive necrosis, hemorrhage, congestion, and low mitoses in all animals in group C, indicating irreversible PHLF [36]. Additional indications of irreversible PHLF were a rapid rise in INR, elevated bilirubin, impaired liver function, and a rapid deterioration of the general condition as a sign of acute irreversible PHLF [35, 36]. Only one animal survived more than 3 days in this group. The cause of death in all except one of the pigs was liver failure. Severe necrosis and microhemorrhage caused irreversible organ failure leading to early death, indicating that 15% RLV does not represent a suitable model for investigating SFSS. These findings are in agreement with previous reports that 85% liver resection causes fatal hepatic failure [14, 37, 38]. The main difference between groups B and C is the reversibility of the changes in the laboratory and pathological parameters after hepatectomy. The pathological findings revealed high rate of mitoses and regeneration in group B versus massive necrosis and only minor mitoses in group C. Thus, immediately after 85% liver resection the remnant liver starts an irreversible damage, leading to an inevitable and lethal liver failure. But after 75% liver resection some of the animals can survive only for few days (more than 3 but less than 7 days) and some others are able to overcome the acute postoperative changes while the liver regenerates itself sufficiently. Therefore, 75% liver resection is a proper model for SFSS, because the pigs have a chance to survive, and preventive and therapeutic interventions can be studied on them. We observed no differences in the laboratory results after 75% and 85% liver resection, demonstrating that laboratory findings cannot solely distinguish between SFSS and irreversible PHLF in the first postoperative days. In the case of elevated INR and bilirubin, animals should be closely observed for signs of general deterioration. In the present study, we established a porcine model of SFSS according to the RLV, clinical, laboratory, and histopathological findings. Since the transhepatic flow plays an important role in the pathophysiology of SFSS [29, 39], a limitation of our study was that we did not measure the transhepatic flow in this study. We suggest that this should be considered in all SFSS studies.

5. Conclusions

In conclusion, porcine model is a feasible and appropriate model for studying the pathophysiology, prediction, prevention, diagnosis, and management of SFSS. Resection of segments (II), (III), (IV), (V), and (VIII) of the porcine liver leaves a 25% RLV. This causes known symptoms of SFSS and can be used for experimental studies. Finally, to have an appropriate experimental model of SFSS, we suggest a comprehensive assessment of the combination of clinical, laboratory, and histopathologic findings.

Disclosure

This research did not receive any specific grant from funding agencies in the public, commercial, or not-for-profit sectors.

Acknowledgments

The authors would like to thank Dr. Omid Ghamarnejad for providing graphics (Figure 1).

References

[1] R. T. Poon, S. T. Fan, C. M. Lo et al., "Improving perioperative outcome expands the role of hepatectomy in management of benign and malignant hepatobiliary diseases: Analysis of 1222 consecutive patients from a prospective database," *Annals of Surgery*, vol. 240, no. 4, pp. 698–710, 2004.

[2] D. Dimitroulis, P. Tsaparas, S. Valsami et al., "Indications, limitations and maneuvers to enable extended hepatectomy: Current trends," *World Journal of Gastroenterology*, vol. 20, no. 24, pp. 7887–7893, 2014.

[3] J. M. Asencio, J. L. García Sabrido, and L. Olmedilla, "How to expand the safe limits in hepatic resections?" *Journal of Hepato-Biliary-Pancreatic Sciences*, vol. 21, no. 6, pp. 399–404, 2014.

[4] N. N. Rahbari, O. J. Garden, R. Padbury et al., "Posthepatectomy liver failure: a definition and grading by the International Study Group of Liver Surgery (ISGLS)," *Surgery*, vol. 149, no. 5, pp. 713–724, 2011.

[5] F. Dahm, P. Georgiev, and P.-A. Clavien, "Small-for-size syndrome after partial liver transplantation: definition, mechanisms of disease and clinical implications," *American Journal of Transplantation*, vol. 5, no. 11, pp. 2605–2610, 2005.

[6] K. Man, S.-T. Fan, C.-M. Lo et al., "Graft Injury in Relation to Graft Size in Right Lobe Live Donor Liver Transplantation: A Study of Hepatic Sinusoidal Injury in Correlation with Portal Hemodynamics and Intragraft Gene Expression," *Annals of Surgery*, vol. 237, no. 2, pp. 256–264, 2003.

[7] O. N. Tucker and N. Heaton, "The 'small for size' liver syndrome," *Current Opinion in Critical Care*, vol. 11, no. 2, pp. 150–155, 2005.

[8] N. Golse, P. O. Bucur, R. Adam, D. Castaing, A. Sa Cunha, and E. Vibert, "New Paradigms in Post-hepatectomy Liver Failure," *Journal of Gastrointestinal Surgery*, vol. 17, no. 3, pp. 593–605, 2013.

[9] F. G. Court, S. A. Wemyss-Holden, C. P. Morrison et al., "Segmental nature of the porcine liver and its potential as a model for experimental partial hepatectomy," *British Journal of Surgery*, vol. 90, no. 4, pp. 440–444, 2003.

[10] M. Golriz, H. Fonouni, A. Nickkholgh, M. Hafezi, C. Garoussi, and A. Mehrabi, "Pig kidney transplantation: An up-to-date guideline," *European Surgical Research*, vol. 49, no. 3-4, pp. 121–129, 2012.

[11] M. Golriz, S. El Sakka, A. Majlesara et al., "Hepatic Hemodynamic Changes Following Stepwise Liver Resection," *Journal of Gastrointestinal Surgery*, vol. 20, no. 3, pp. 587–594, 2016.

[12] J. Leng, H. Xing, J. Tan, K. Chen, and J. Dong, "The safe minimally ischemic liver remnant for small-for-size syndrome in porcine hepatectomy," *Transplantation Proceedings*, vol. 45, no. 6, pp. 2419–2424, 2013.

[13] J. M. Asencio, J. Vaquero, L. Olmedilla, and J. L. García Sabrido, ""Small-for-flow" syndrome: Shifting the "size" paradigm," *Medical Hypotheses*, vol. 80, no. 5, pp. 573–577, 2013.

[14] D. Pagano, F. Di Francesco, G. J. Echeverri et al., "Development of a standardized model for liver failure in pigs: Anatomopathophysiologic findings after extended liver resection," *Transplantation Proceedings*, vol. 44, no. 7, pp. 2029–2032, 2012.

[15] B. Darnis, K. Mohkam, Z. Schmitt et al., "Splenectomy and splenic artery ligation in swine: No impact on portal vein and hepatic artery flow," *HPB*, vol. 18, p. e694, 2016.

[16] M. Golriz, S. Abbasi, P. Fathi, A. Majlesara, T. Brenner, and A. Mehrabi, "Does acid-base equilibrium correlate with remnant liver volume during stepwise liver resection?" *American Journal of Physiology - Gastrointestinal and Liver Physiology*, 2017.

[17] P. Schemmer, H. Friess, U. Hinz et al., "Stapler hepatectomy is a safe dissection technique: Analysis of 300 patients," *World Journal of Surgery*, vol. 30, no. 3, pp. 419–430, 2006.

[18] D. M. Kelly, A. J. Demetris, J. J. Fung et al., "Porcine partial liver transplantaion: A novel model of the "small-for-size" liver graft," *Liver Transplantation*, vol. 10, no. 2, pp. 253–263, 2004.

[19] D. M. Kelly, X. Zhu, H. Shiba et al., "Adenosine restores the hepatic artery buffer response and improves survival in a porcine model of small-for-size syndrome," *Liver Transplantation*, vol. 15, no. 11, pp. 1448–1457, 2009.

[20] A. J. Demetris, D. M. Kelly, B. Eghtesad et al., "Pathophysiologic observations and histopathologic recognition of the portal hyperperfusion or small-for-size syndrome," *American Journal of Surgical Pathology*, vol. 30, no. 8, pp. 986–993, 2006.

[21] N. Arkadopoulos, G. Kostopanagiotou, C. Nastos et al., "Reversal of Experimental Posthepatectomy Liver Failure in Pigs: A New Application of Hepatocyte Bioreactors," *Artificial Organs*, vol. 35, no. 1, pp. 29–36, 2011.

[22] Y. Fu, H.-B. Zhang, N. Yang et al., "Porcine partial liver transplantation without veno-venous bypass: An effective model for small-for-size liver graft injury," *Transplantation Proceedings*, vol. 43, no. 5, pp. 1953–1961, 2011.

[23] Q. Xia, T. F. Lu, Z. H. Zhou et al., "Extended hepatectomy with segments I and VII as resection remnant: a simple model for small-for-size injuries in pigs," *Hepatobiliary & Pancreatic Diseases International*, vol. 7, no. 6, pp. 601–607, 2008.

[24] A. Guglielmi, A. Ruzzenente, S. Conci, A. Valdegamberi, and C. Iacono, "How much remnant is enough in liver resection?" *Digestive Surgery*, vol. 29, no. 1, pp. 6–17, 2012.

[25] A. Athanasiou, M. Kontos, E. Pikoulis et al., "Extended hepatectomy using the bipolar tissue sealer: An experimental model of small-for-size syndrome in pigs," *Journal of B.U.ON.*, vol. 21, no. 6, pp. 1403–1409, 2016.

[26] K. Mohkam, B. Darnis, and J.-Y. Mabrut, "Porcine models for the study of small-for-size syndrome and portal inflow modulation: literature review and proposal for a standardized nomenclature," *Journal of Hepato-Biliary-Pancreatic Sciences*, vol. 23, no. 11, pp. 668–680, 2016.

[27] F. G. Court, P. E. Laws, C. P. Morrison et al., "Subtotal hepatectomy: A porcine model for the study of liver regeneration," *Journal of Surgical Research*, vol. 116, no. 1, pp. 181–186, 2004.

[28] K. Mohkam, B. Darnis, Z. Schmitt, S. Duperret, C. Ducerf, and J.-Y. Mabrut, "Successful modulation of portal inflow by somatostatin in a porcine model of small-for-size syndrome," *American Journal of Surgery*, vol. 212, no. 2, pp. 321–326, 2016.

[29] R. Troisi, G. Cammu, G. Militerno et al., "Modulation of Portal Graft Inflow: A Necessity in Adult Living-Donor Liver Transplantation?," *Annals of Surgery*, vol. 237, no. 3, pp. 429–436, 2003.

[30] R. Troisi and B. de Hemptinne, "Clinical relevance of adapting portal vein flow in living donor liver transplantation in adult patients," *Liver Transplantation*, vol. 9, no. 9, pp. S36–S41, 2003.

[31] M. Golriz, A. Majlesara, E. Khajeh, and A. Mehrabi, "Reply: Hepatic Hemodynamic Changes Following Stepwise Liver Resection (Golriz et al. J Gastrointest Surg (2016) 20:587-594)," *Journal of Gastrointestinal Surgery*, vol. 20, no. 12, pp. 2109-2110, 2016.

[32] R. Troisi, M. Praet, and B. de Hemptinne, "Small-for-size syndrome: What is the problem?" *Liver Transplantation*, vol. 9, no. 9, p. S1, 2003.

[33] M. Golriz, M. Hafezi, C. Garoussi et al., "Do we need animal hands-on courses for transplantation surgery?" *Clinical Transplantation*, vol. 27, no. s25, pp. 6–15, 2013.

[34] A. C. D. A. Martins, M. A. C. Machado, and Á. A. B. Ferraz, "Porcine liver: Experimental model for the intra-hepatic glissonian approach," *Acta Cirurgica Brasileira*, vol. 23, no. 2, pp. 204–207, 2008.

[35] D. Kahn, R. Hickman, J. Terblanche, and S. von Sommoggy, "Partial hepatectomy and liver regeneration in pigs-The response to different resection sizes," *Journal of Surgical Research*, vol. 45, no. 2, pp. 176–180, 1988.

[36] Y. Panis, D. M. McMullan, and J. C. Emond, "Progressive necrosis after hepatectomy and the pathophysiology of liver failure after massive resection," *Surgery*, vol. 121, no. 2, pp. 142–149, 1997.

[37] B. Hochleitner, P. Hengster, H. Bucher et al., "Significant survival prolongation in pigs with fulminant hepatic failure treated with a novel microgravity-based bioartificial liver," *Artificial Organs*, vol. 30, no. 12, pp. 906–914, 2006.

[38] H. Wang, N. Ohkohchi, Y. Enomoto et al., "Effect of portocaval shunt on residual extreme small liver after extended hepatectomy in porcine," *World Journal of Surgery*, vol. 30, no. 11, pp. 2014–2022, 2006.

[39] M. Golriz, A. Majlesara, S. El Sakka et al., "Small for Size and Flow (SFSF) syndrome: An alternative description for posthepatectomy liver failure," *Clinics and Research in Hepatology and Gastroenterology*, vol. 40, no. 3, pp. 267–275, 2016.

Gastric Cancer Cell Lines Have Different *MYC*-Regulated Expression Patterns but Share a Common Core of Altered Genes

Jersey Heitor da S. Maués,[1] Helem Ferreira Ribeiro,[1,2] Giovanny R. Pinto,[3] Luana de Oliveira Lopes,[3] Letícia M. Lamarão,[4] Carla Mariana F. Pessoa,[5] Caroline de Fátima Aquino Moreira-Nunes,[6] Raimundo Miranda de Carvalho,[7] Paulo P. Assumpção,[5] Juan A. Rey,[8] and Rommel M. Rodríguez Burbano[7]

[1] *Human Cytogenetics Laboratory, Institute of Biological Sciences, Federal University of Pará, Belém, Brazil*
[2] *Center of Biological and Health Sciences, Department of Biomedicine, University of Amazon, Belém, Brazil*
[3] *Department of Biomedicine, Federal University of Piauí, Parnaíba, Brazil*
[4] *Laboratory of Nucleic Acids, State Center of Hematology and Hemotherapy, Belém, Brazil*
[5] *Oncology Research Nucleus, University Hospital João de Barros Barreto, Federal University of Pará, Belém, Brazil*
[6] *Laboratory of Pharmacogenetics, Drug Research and Development Center, Federal University of Ceará, Fortaleza, Brazil*
[7] *Laboratory of Molecular Biology, Ophir Loyola Hospital, Belém, Brazil*
[8] *Molecular Oncogenetics Laboratory, Research Unit, Hospital Universitario La Paz, Madrid, Spain*

Correspondence should be addressed to Jersey Heitor da S. Maués; jerseymaues@gmail.com

Guest Editor: Kiran L. Sharma

MYC is an oncogene responsible for excessive cell growth in cancer, enabling transcriptional activation of genes involved in cell cycle regulation, metabolism, and apoptosis, and is usually overexpressed in gastric cancer (GC). By using siRNA and Next-Generation Sequencing (NGS), we identified *MYC*-regulated differentially expressed Genes (DEGs) in three Brazilian gastric cancer cell lines representing the histological subtypes of GC (diffuse, intestinal, and metastasis). The DEGs were picked using *Sailfish* software, followed by Gene Set Enrichment Analysis (GSEA) and Kyoto Encyclopedia of Gene and Genome (KEGG) pathway analysis using KEGG. We found 11 significantly enriched gene sets by using enrichment score (ES), False Discovery Rate (FDR), and nominal P-values. We identified a total of 5.471 DEGs with correlation over (80%). In diffuse-type and in metastatic GC cell lines, *MYC*-silencing caused DEGs downregulation, while the intestinal-type GC cells presented overall DEGs upregulation after *MYC* siRNA depletion. We were able to detect 11 significant gene sets when comparing our samples to the hallmark collection of gene expression, enriched mostly for the following hallmarks: proliferation, pathway, signaling, metabolic, and DNA damage response. When we analyzed our DEGs considering KEGG metabolic pathways, we found 12 common branches covering a wide range of biological functions, and three of them were common to all three cell lines: ubiquitin-mediated proteolysis, ribosomes, and system and epithelial cell signaling in *Helicobacter pylori* infection. The GC cell lines used in this study share 14 *MYC*-regulated genes, but their gene expression profile is different for each histological subtype of GC. Our results present a computational analysis of *MYC*-related signatures in GC, and we present evidence that GC cell lines representing distinct histological subtypes of this disease have different *MYC*-regulated expression profiles but share a common core of altered genes. This is an important step towards the understanding of *MYC*'s role in gastric carcinogenesis and an indication of probable new drug targets in stomach cancer.

1. Introduction

Gastric cancer (GC) remains as an important cause of cancer-related morbidity and mortality worldwide, with recent estimates accounting for over 950.000 new diagnosis and 720.000 deaths each year [1]. Treatment of GC at advanced stages remains difficult, and the prognosis is still poor, partly as a result of local recurrence, tumor invasion, and/or metastasis [2]

The *MYC* oncogene, located at 8q24, is a key oncogene in gastric carcinogenesis, and an increase in both copy number

Table 1: Samples used in this study. Control siRNA samples are labeled as C and MYC-siRNA as M.

Cell line	Samples (GEO)	Sample Name	GC Histological subtype
AGP01	GSM2147866	1C	Ascitic fluid of intestinal GC
	GSM2147867	1M	Ascitic fluid of intestinal GC
ACP02	GSM2147868	2C	Diffuse
	GSM2147869	2M	Diffuse
ACP03	GSM2147870	3C	Intestinal
	GSM2147871	3M	Intestinal

and mRNA expression was classified as one of the driver mutations in gastric tumors [3]. *MYC* amplification and overexpression are present in 6-58% of all sporadic gastric tumors [4–6], being more frequent in Brazilian samples [7–9], usually as a result from gene amplification and chromosomal translocations [2, 10].

Our research group previously reported that MYC mRNA and protein overexpression is a common finding in GC samples and in some preneoplastic gastric lesions [7, 11–14] from a Brazilian population, as well as in nonhuman primate models of gastric carcinogenesis [15]. We also established and characterized three GC cell lines, AGP01, ACP02, and ACP03, obtained from intestinal-type GC metastasis, diffuse-type GC, and intestinal-type GC, respectively (Leal et al. 2009). Those cell lines also carry genetic alterations commonly found in Brazilian GC patients, such as *MYC* amplification and overexpression and *TP53* deletion [7, 13, 16].

Some consequences of excessive intracellular *MYC* levels are genomic instability [17] and error-prone DNA replication caused by oncogene-induced replicative stress [18]. Even though there is an association between an increase in *MYC* expression and gastric cancer, its exact role in gastric tumorigenesis is not yet fully understood [19, 20] and most of the high-throughput studies carried so far concerning gastric cancer genetics overlook *MYC*'s importance in this process [2, 3, 21–24]

Bioinformatics has mostly been applied in basic science research. Following the completion of human genome sequencing, it has also facilitated numerous discoveries in basic medicine, and several clinical applications of bioinformatics have been reported, including clinical sequencing, an emerging field of precision medicine [25]. In cancer research, bioinformatics has been used to study cancer transcriptome, early diagnosis, cancer grading, and prognosis prediction [26].

In this study, we used RNA interference (RNAi) to block *MYC*'s mRNA translation, followed by Ion Proton™ semiconductor sequencing, in order to identify *MYC*'s regulation signature in AGP01, ACP02, and ACP03 cell lines. We found 11 common pathways for the GC cell lines, which we believe can help in the understanding of expression signatures in different GC histological subtypes.

2. Materials and Methods

2.1. Cell Lines and siRNA Transfection. Three GC cell lines previously established and characterized by our group were used: AGP01, ACP02, and ACP03 [27]. The three cell lines present chromosome 8 trisomy, *MYC* amplification [13, 27], and *TP53* deletion, which are common genetic alterations in Brazilian gastric cancer patients [28] and in another GC cell line developed in Brazil [29]. A cell culture of nonneoplastic gastric mucosa cells (MNP01, Normal Gastric Mucosa Cell Line 01) pooled from 10 patients without gastric cancer or any other gastric disease, was also used to evaluate the gene and protein expression after *MYC*-silencing and to validate the knockdown results, as well as the *MYC*-regulated genes identified after NGS.

A total of $3x10^5$ cells were seeded into $6\,cm^2$ plates for each cell line for 24 h before transfection. Small interfering RNAs (siRNA) targeting *MYC* (ON-TARGETplus Human MYC (4609) siRNA Dharmacon, EUA) or scrambled control siRNAs (ON-TARGETplus Non-Targeting Pool, Dharmacon, EUA) were transfected into AGP01, ACP02, and ACP03 cell lines using Lipofectamine RNAiMAX Transfection Reagent (Thermo Fisher Scientific, EUA). Optimal transfection was reached after 48 h, and total RNA and proteins were extracted with TRIzol reagent (Thermo Fisher Scientific, EUA). All siRNA experiments were performed three times. The sample names and GEO access codes are shown in Table 1. All siRNA experiments were carried out in biological triplicates.

2.2. Semiconductor Sequencing and Data Pretreatment. Total RNA samples were first treated with DNAse-I to remove any possible DNA contamination, and then the mRNA was enriched using Dynabeads Oligo$(dt)_{25}$ (Thermo Fisher Scientific, USA). The enriched mRNA was fragmented in smaller fragments of 200 bps approximately, which were attached to adapters with known sequences that were unique for each sample. Samples were connected to magnetic beads containing complementary sequences for the adapters and then inserted in microwells where an emulsion-PCR for cDNA synthesis was carried (illustra Ready-To-Go RT-PCR Beads, GE Lifesciences). Our six cDNA libraries were submitted to quantification and quality control using Agilent 2100 Bioanalyzer and were then loaded in Ion Proton V2 PI chip using the Ion PI™ 200 Sequencing Kit v3 and sequenced using Ion Proton™ (Thermo Fisher Scientific, EUA) platform in a single multiplex run.

Raw data reads obtained by primary sequencing using Ion Proton™ were submitted to quality control to calculate alignment and to assess how the reads behave when compared to the reference human genome (Hg19/GRCh37). The aligned reads were mapped and quantified using TMAP (*Torrent Mapping Alignment Program*), which supports different alignment algorithms [30–32]. Processed datasets were

TABLE 2: Reads quantification after *MYC*-siRNA.

Sample name	Total Reads	Total Mapped Reads	Gene mapping rate	Expressed genes
1C	13.319.736	12.944.452	97.18%	14.594
1M	11.043.607	10.771.298	97.53%	10.709
2C	12.021.142	11.751.830	97.76%	9.859
2M	11.701.695	11.481.863	98.12%	8.793
3C	12.772.535	12.546.479	98.23%	7.988
3M	12.430.807	12.112.157	97.44%	10.685

uploaded to GEO (Gene Expression Omnibus) under the access number GSE81265.

2.3. Identification and Statistical Analysis of DEGs. Sailfish software pack [33] and the RPKM (Reads Per Kilobase per million mapped reads) [34, 35] were used to significance analysis of DEGs between control and *MYC*-silenced samples. To identify the DEGs between two paired samples, we used the Audic-Claverie test [36]. Fold-change (FC) was calculated as the $\log_2$ ratio between the silenced (M) and the control (C) sample. We used a p-value correction corresponding to differential expression tests using Bonferroni correction [37]. Our cut-off for DEGs definition was established as a False Discovery Rate (FDR) < 0.05 [38] and |log2 (FC)| > 1. DEGs were plotted using Multiplot v2, which exhibits personalized gene expression profiles (http://software.broadinstitute.org/cancer/software/genepattern/modules/docs/multiplot/2).

2.4. Functional Enrichment Analysis. We used Gene Set Enrichment Analysis (GSEA) [39] to identify significantly enriched gene sets between siRNA control versus MYC-silenced and vice versa. The gene expression changes perceived by DEGs were related to biologically enriched pathways found in GSEA. The gene expression datasets used were collections H (Hallmark gene set) [40] and C2 (curated gene set: KEGG), publicly available at MsigDB [41]. The standard parameters defined by Subramanian et al. were used in our analysis. The statistical significance of GSEA analysis was determined by 100 permutations, the enrichment maps were created to significant ($P < 0.05$ and False Discovery Rate (FDR) < 0.25) gene sets, and GraphPad Prism™ Software was used to graphically represent our data.

2.5. Real-Time Quantitative PCR (RT-qPCR). To confirm the silencing effect of siRNA on *MYC* expression, we used real-time quantitative PCR to evaluate its expression in relation to the expression found for the normal gastric mucosa cell line MN01. All tests were made in triplicate and using TaqMan® probes as assays-on-demand products for gene expression (Life Technologies, EUA) (*MYC:* Hs00153408_m1). The fourteen DEGs identified by our analysis (*SKIV2L2:* Hs00299011_m1, *SRPRB:* Hs00253639_m1, *JUNB:* Hs00357891_s1, *BNIP3:* Hs00969291_m1, *RAB22A:* Hs00221082_m1, *TMED2:* Hs00607277_m1, *ACAT1:* Hs00608002_m1, *NDUFV2:* Hs00221478_m1, *LBR:* Hs01032700_m1, *NCL:* Hs01066668_m1, *AAAS:* Hs00210351_m1, *ATXN2:* Hs00268077_m1, *LGMN:* Hs00271599_m1, and *CDKN1B:* Hs00153277_m1) were also analyzed and validated by real-time quantitative PCR. The expression of those genes was calculated relative to their expression in the normal gastric mucosa cell line MN01.

3. Results

3.1. Quantification of GCs Transcripts and Identification of DEGs Using NGS. In this study, we used next-generation sequencing based in semiconductors, as well as RNA-Seq, to quantify the transcripts and its isoforms in three gastric cancer cell lines, ACP02, ACP03, and AGP01, before and after *MYC*-silencing using siRNA. The use of siRNA to reduce *MYC* expression in the three gastric cancer cell line used in this study was very effective, reducing *MYC* mRNA expression in 73% for AGP01, in 84% for ACP02, and in 77% for ACP03.

Our NGS sequencing of six libraries generated over 75 million reads, which, after enrichment, were mapped within the reference genome in over 99% of the samples and in over 98% of the reference transcriptome (Table 2), and the distribution of the amplified segments was consistent in all samples. Table 2 also shows in average how many genes were identified for each sample. The average reads produced by Ion Proton™ ranged between 125 and 130 bps.

According to our cut-off (FDR < 0.05 and $|\log_2 (FC)| > 1$), we obtained a distinct amount of DEGs between siRNA control versus *MYC* -silenced samples. Using Multiplot (v2), we identified 1.556 downregulated and 917 upregulated DEGs for AGP01; for the diffuse-type cell line (ACP02), we found 4.098 downregulated versus 1.229 upregulated DEGs; finally, for ACP03, an intestinal-type cell line, we identified 3.272 upregulated versus 842 downregulated DEGs (Figure 1). Our results indicate that it is possible to discern histological subtypes of GC by analyzing its *MYC*-related gene expression pattern.

A total of 16.777 genes from our six datasets obtained by RNA-Seq (GSE81265) were inserted in an expression matrix normalized by RPKM and, after that, used for enrichment comparing with expression datasets from collections H and C2. By applying GSEA, we looked for gene sets which presented enrichment only in siRNA control samples, but not in *MYC* -silenced samples, likely *MYC* targets, and found 11 significant gene sets ($P < 0.05$ and FDR < 0.25), as shown in Table 3. We found a total of 7903 genes, and 5471 (69.2%) are enriched in siRNA control samples, presenting a very high correlation between biological replicates and libraries (80%).

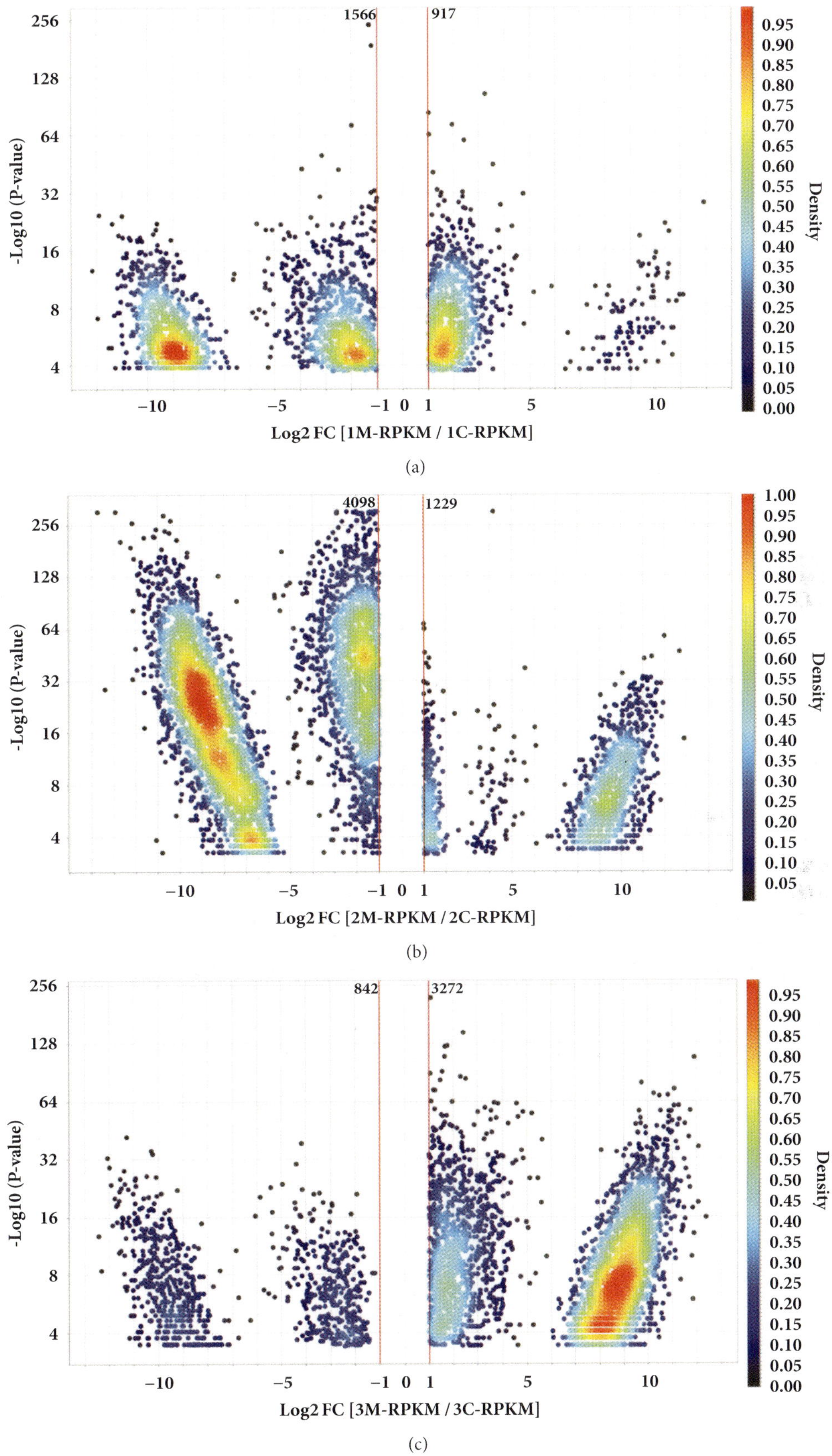

FIGURE 1: Volcano plots of DEGs for three GC cell lines after *MYC*-silencing. $\log_2$ Fold-change and P-values ($-\log_{10}$) are shown for DEGs with ($|\log_2 (FC)| > 1$ and $p \leq 0.05$). (a) DEGs for AGP01. (b) DEGs for ACP02. (c) DEGs for ACP03. Density is a special-case calculation which is only used in advanced shading. It considers only the operands for this calculation are the X and Y values of the graph axes.

TABLE 3: Enriched hallmark gene sets for DEGs after *MYC*-siRNa in three GC cell lines.

Hallmark Name:	Process category	Description	Size*	ES	NES	Nom. P-value	FDR	Max. Rank
MYC_TARGETS_V1	Proliferation	MYC targets, variant 1	100/44	0.59	1.89	0.00	0.000	1368
REACTIVE_OXIGEN_SPECIES_PATHWAY	Pathway	Reactive oxygen species pathway	25/13	0.55	1.42	0.00	0.000	2316
UNFOLDED_PROTEIN_RESPONSE	Pathway	Unfolded protein response; ER stress	50/22	0.55	1.56	0.00	0.000	1891
PROTEIN_SECRETION	Pathway	Protein secretion	44/26	0.55	1.70	0.00	0.000	2376
G2M_CHECKPOINT	Proliferation	Cell cycle progression: G2/M checkpoint	97/40	0.52	1.67	0.00	0.000	1813
MTORC1_SIGNALING	Signaling	mTORC1 signaling	102/43	0.50	1.46	0.00	0.044	2021
E2F_TARGETS	Proliferation	Cell cycle progression: E2F targets	89/35	0.48	1.42	0.00	0.052	1607
OXIDATIVE_PHOSPHORYLATION	Metabolic	Oxidative phosphorylation and citric acid cycle	118/57	0.48	1.46	0.00	0.062	2284
CHOLESTEROL_HOMEOSTASIS	Metabolic	Cholesterol homeostasis	39/14	0.48	1.48	0.00	0.069	1671
DNA_REPAIR	DNA damage	DNA repair	80/38	0.46	1.42	0.00	0.077	2337
APOPTOSIS	Pathway	Programmed cell death; caspase pathway	66/29	0.42	1.31	0.20	0.190	2405

*Number of genes found for each gene set after curating data. ES: enrichment score. NES: normalized enrichment score. Nom. P-value: nominal P-values for each gene set. FDR: false discovery rate. Max. rank: maximum rank numbers for each gene sets.

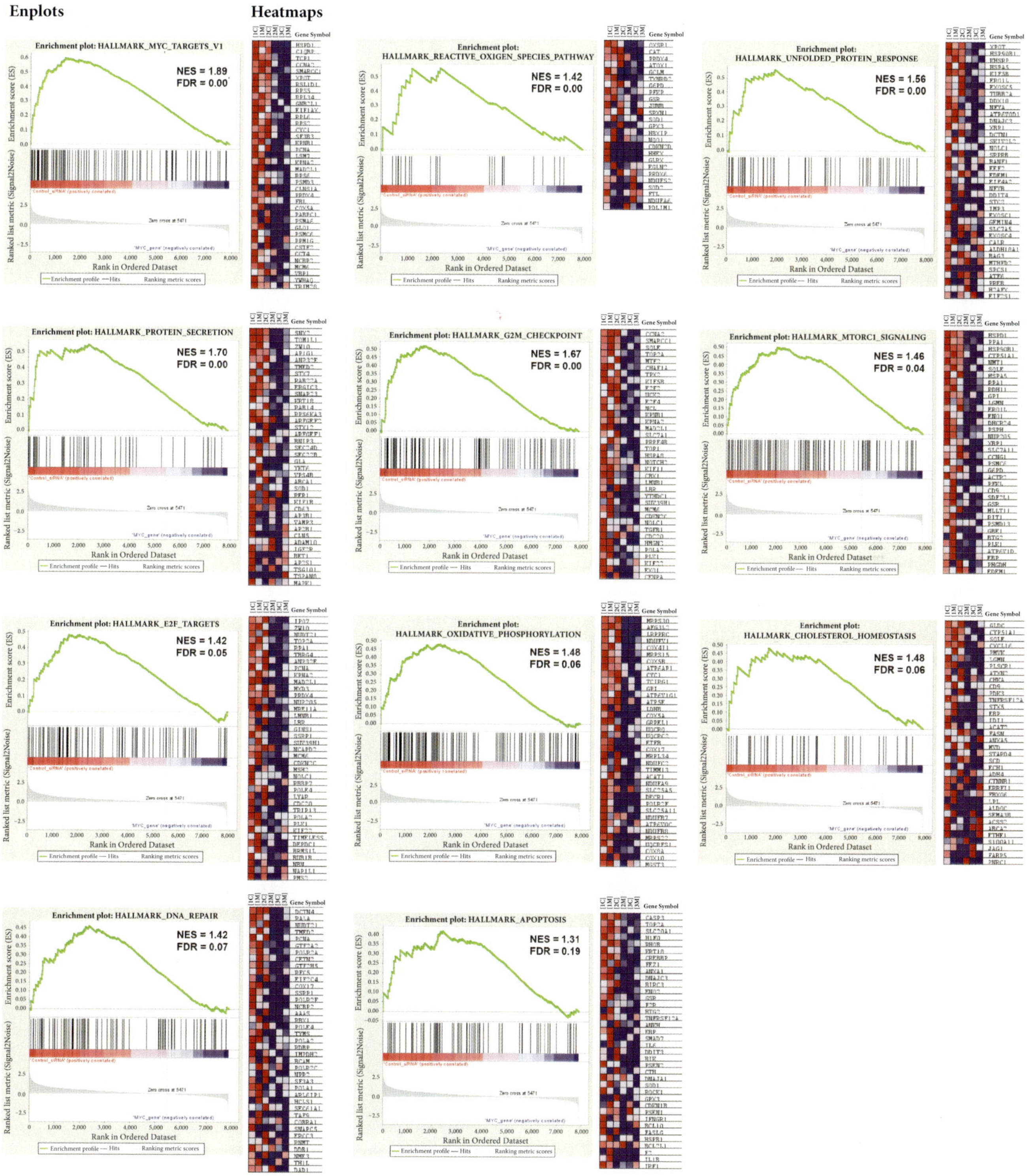

FIGURE 2: Panel with 11 gene sets enriched for three GC cell lines after *MYC*-silencing. Each gene set was represented on the Enplot by its normalized enrichment score (NES) and False Discovery Rate (FDR), along with its heatmap showing the gene expression for each gene.

The enrichment maps obtained are shown in Figure 2, where we created a panel of 11 gene sets significantly enriched.

3.2. MYC-Silenced GC Cells Lines from Different Histological Subtypes Show Distinct MYC-Dependent Expression Profiles. We then evaluated the metabolic pathways more likely to be *MYC*-regulated as shown by GSEA, listing those genes in the categories described as hallmarks of gene expression [40] and found that they are related to cellular proliferation, pathway, cellular signaling, metabolic processes, and response to DNA

Table 4: The 14 common DEGs for three GC cell lines after *MYC*-siRNA and the gene set hallmarks they were enriched in.

Hallmark Name:	Gene Symbol	Rank in Gene List	Rank Metric Score	Running (ES)
PROTEIN_SECRETION	*BNIP3*	1438	6.0E-01	0.522
UNFOLDED_PROTEIN_RESPONSE	*SKIV2L2*	1051	7.2E-01	0.508
UNFOLDED_PROTEIN_RESPONSE	*SRPRB*	1442	6.0E-01	0.506
REACTIVE_OXIGEN_SPECIES_PATHWAY	*JUNB*	1969	4.8E-01	0.491
G2M_CHECKPOINT	*LBR*	817	8.2E-01	0.451
OXIDATIVE_PHOSPHORYLATION	*NDUFV2*	1542	5.7E-01	0.444
APOPTOSIS	*CDKN1B*	2405	4.0E-01	0.420
PROTEIN_SECRETION	*RAB22A*	289	1.2E+15	0.408
CHOLESTEROL_HOMEOSTASIS	*ATXN2*	945	7.6E-01	0.382
CHOLESTEROL_HOMEOSTASIS	*LGMN*	445	1.1E+16	0.367
OXIDATIVE_PHOSPHORYLATION	*ACAT1*	840	8.1E-01	0.367
PROTEIN_SECRETION	*TMED2*	254	1.3E+16	0.326
DNA_REPAIR	*AAAS*	1109	7.0E-01	0.313
G2M_CHECKPOINT	*NCL*	328	1.2E+13	0.289

ES: enrichment score.

damage (Table 3). We refined the raw data sets obtained from our GC cell lines, identifying the DEGs for each of the 11 gene sets for collection H that were enriched for the Control_siRNA phenotype. Figure 3 shows the ranks for enriched DEGs when compared to collection H with their average enrichment score (ES) for each analysis. Part of these results generated in this analysis is in Table 1 (see Supplementary Materials), which show the most enriched DEGs in the set gene MYC TARGETS V1.

The diffuse-type cell line (ACP02) presented 149 enriched DEGs by GSEA, 3 up- and 146 downregulated. Genes enriched with ranks above 15.000 fit the downregulated profile and were emphasized for gene sets such as *MYC* target V1, protein secretion, and reactive oxygen species pathway (Figure 3(a)). On the other hand, ranks above 30.000 were enriched for downregulated DEGs, presenting gene sets described as protein secretion, *MYC* target V1, unfolded protein response, and reactive oxygen species pathway (Figure 3(b)). Meanwhile, the intestinal-type cells (ACP03) showed 85 DEGs, 76 up- and 9 downregulated; genes with ranks above 20.000 were upregulated for pathways such as protein secretion, *MYC* target V1, and reactive oxygen species pathway (Figure 3(c)); downregulated genes with ranks above 15.000 presented enrichment emphasis for GM2-checkpoint, protein secretion, *MYC* target V1, reactive oxygen species pathway, and unfolded protein response (Figure 3(d)). For the metastatic samples (AGP01), 65 enriched DEGs were identified by GSEA, 25 up- and 40 downregulated, and the gene sets were enriched with ranks above 20.000 for both DEGs profiles. Upregulated sets (Figure 3(e)) were enriched for GM2-checkpoint, protein secretion, *MYC* target V1, and reactive oxygen species pathway, while the downregulated profile had emphasis for Oxidative_Phosphorylation, *MYC* target V1, protein secretion, and reactive oxygen species pathway (Figure 3(f)).

In the 11 gene sets from collection H that were used for DEGs enrichment, we identified the genes with higher ES. We used this strategy to identify similar genes that overlap as a consensus grouping as described elsewhere [40], so it would be easier to identify *MYC*-regulated genes. We identified DEGs for the three GC cell lines that were enriched when compared to collection H, with ranks above 2.000. The MYC target V1 gene set was identified as the most enriched for our studied cell lines, with higher ES scores for the genes *SNRPD2* and *TYMS*. When we compared the enriched genes found for collection H for ACP02 and ACP03, we noticed that some genes presented enrichment ranks that were also common for the metastatic cells (AGP01) (Figures 4(a)–4(c)).

The same analysis was applied to identify enriched DEGs found for KEGG pathways, to deepen our understanding about the genes involved in the *MYC*-related carcinogenesis for the stomach. The enrichment maps for KEGG [42] are shown in Figures 4(d)–4(f), presenting 12 significantly enriched pathways found using GSEA, suggesting that GC has multiple altered pathways that lead normal gastric mucosa into the carcinogenic process. These pathways were defined by a normalized enrichment score (NES) > 1.47. The average t-statistic for the genes was calculated for each KEGG pathway using permutation tests with 100 repetitions. The enrichment plot for three common pathways altered in all our cell lines is presented in Figure 4(g) (ribosome-hsa03010), which presented the highest ES among the cells, Figure 4(h) (ubiquitin-mediated proteolysis-hsa04120), with the highest ranks in our gene list, and Figure 4(i) (epithelial cell signaling in *Helicobacter pylori* infection-hsa05120). For more details on the DEGs enriched with KEGG, see Table 2 in Supplementary Materials.

We identified enriched DEGs common to all three GC cell lines used in this study and represent them as Venn diagrams constructed by the InteractiVenn platform [43]. We found 14 DEGs that are shared enriched in both AGP01, ACP02, and ACP03 cell lines (Figure 5(a)), which are likely to be *MYC* targets according to our analysis. When we search for gene function in different databases (Figure 5(b)), most of them (14.78%) are involved in protein secretion, followed by unfolded protein response (14.39%) and reactive oxygen species pathway (13.91%). Table 4 shows the 14 individual

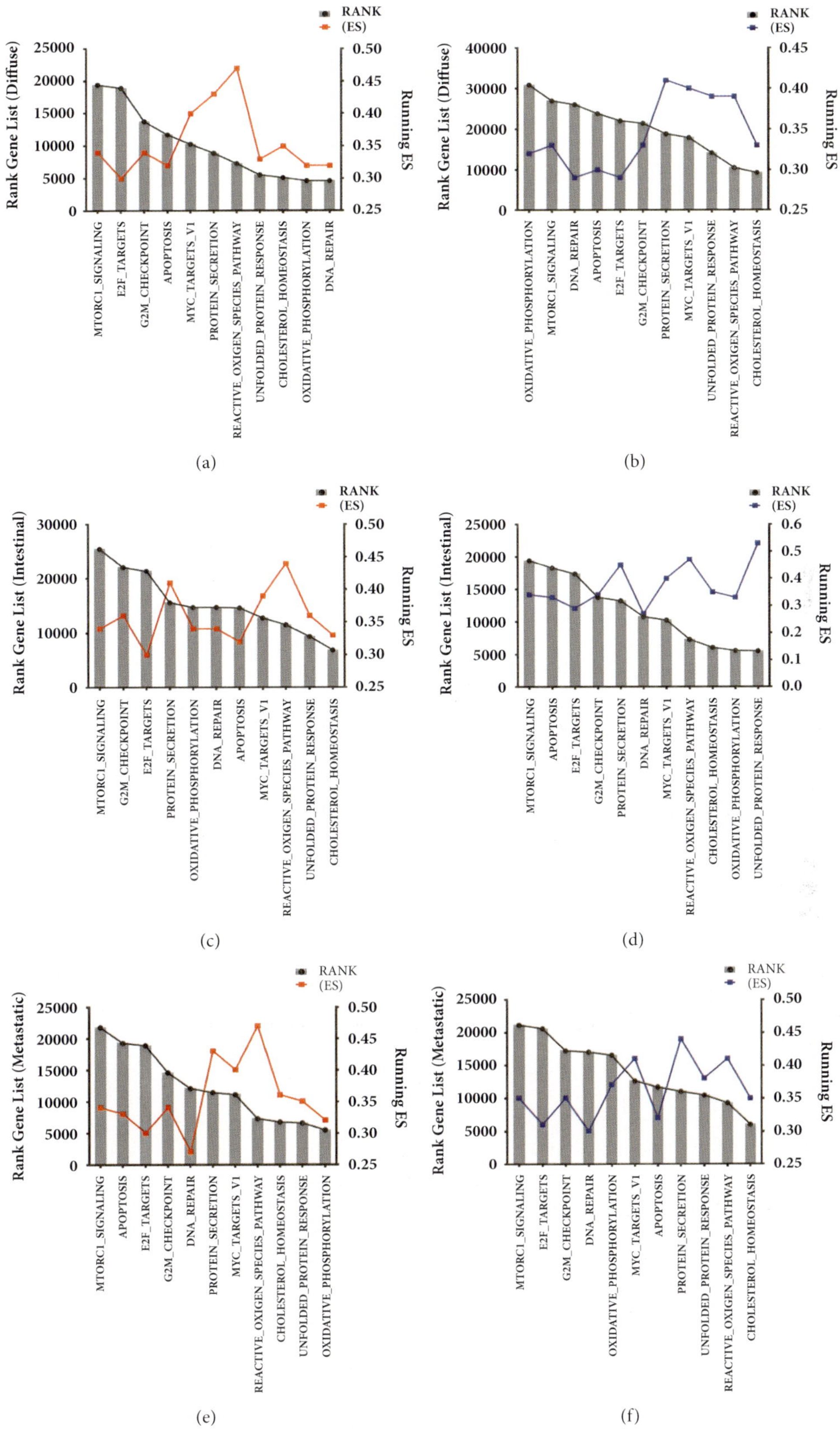

FIGURE 3: Ranks for enriched DEGs when compared to collection H with their average enrichment score (ES) for each analysis. (a) ACP02 upregulated DEGs, ranks (4.640 to 19.433), and ES (0.30 to 0.47). (b) ACP02 downregulated DEGs, ranks (9.245 to 30.875), and ES (0.29 to 0.41). (c) ACP03 upregulated DEGs, ranks (6.853 to 25.475), and ES (0.30 to 0.47). (d) ACP03 downregulated DEGs, ranks (5.530 to 19.433), and ES (0.27 to 0.53). (e) AGP01 upregulated DEGs, ranks (5.480 to 21.804), and ES (0.27 a 0.47). (f) AGP01 downregulated DEGs, ranks (6.060 to 21.134), and ES (0.30 a 0.44).

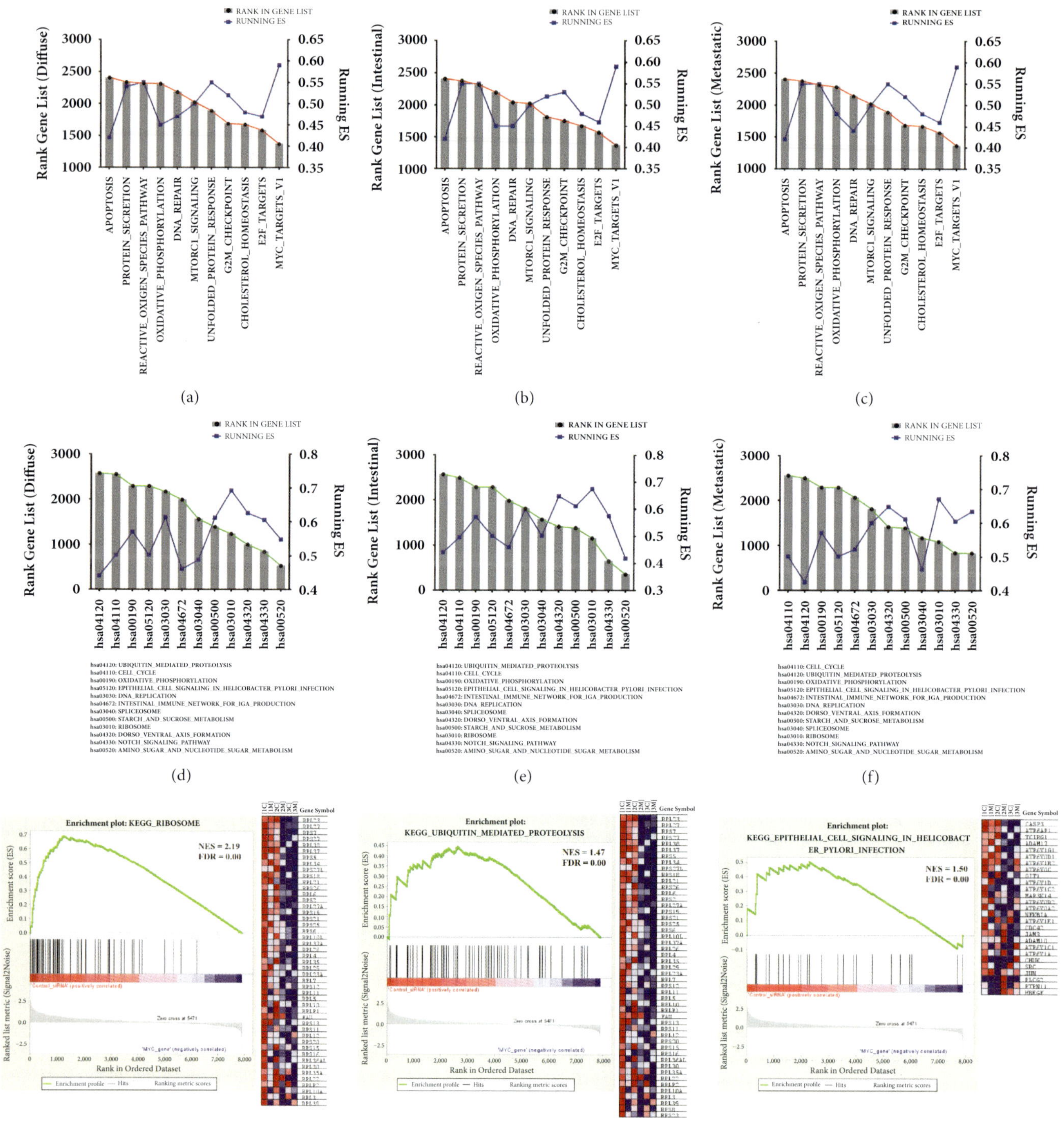

FIGURE 4: Identification of individual genes in the enriched DEG datasets with the higher ES. (a) DEGs enrichment for ACP02. (b) DEGs enrichment for ACP03. (c) DEGs enrichment for AGP01. The most enriched hallmark for the three cell lines as MYC_Target_V1 with an ES = 0.59. (d) KEGG pathway identification for ACP02. (e) KEGG pathway identification for ACP03. (f) KEGG pathway identification for AGP01. Enplot and heatmap for the pathways with the highest ES scores among the three GC cell lines can be seen in (g) for ACP02, in (h) for ACP03, and in (i) for AGP01.

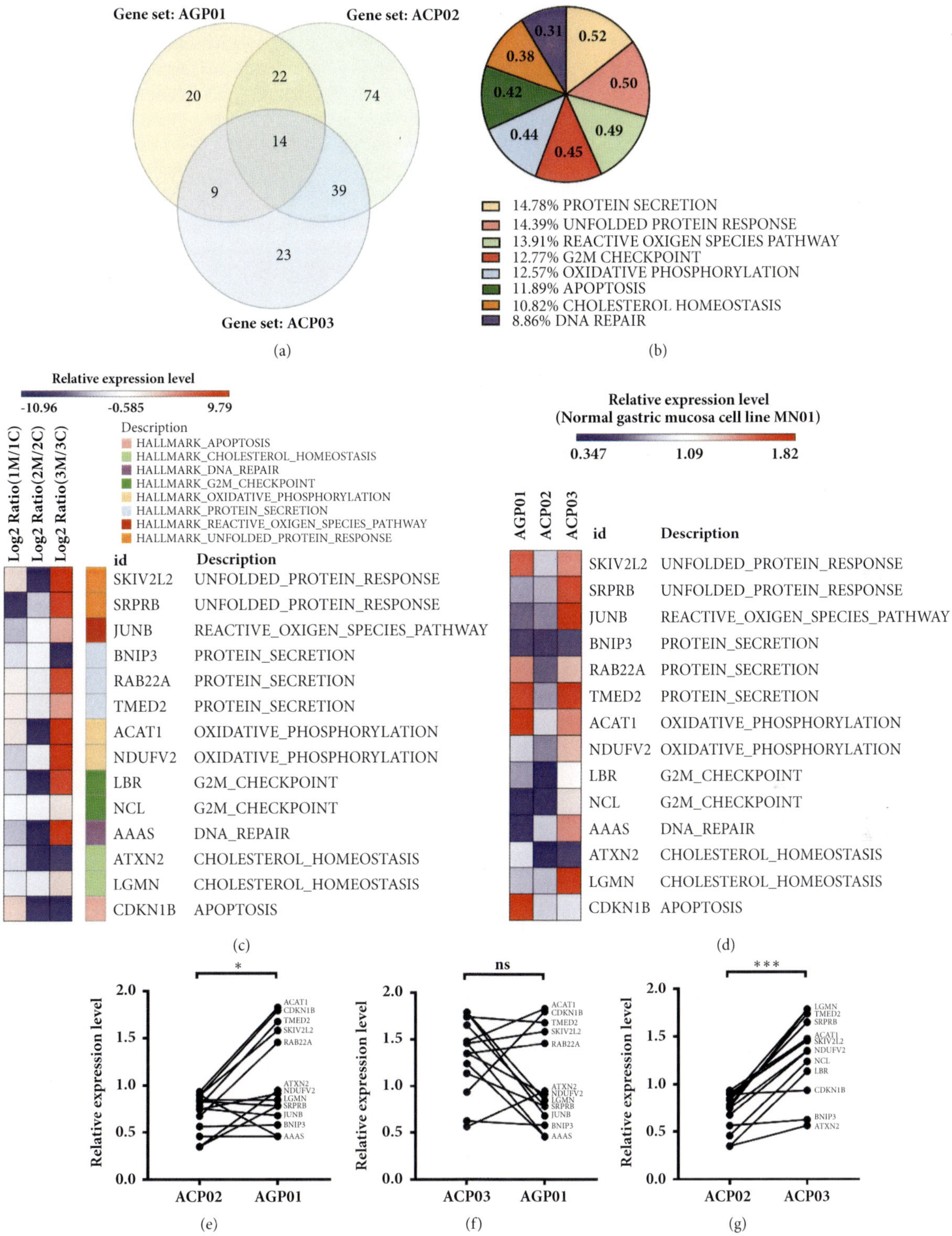

FIGURE 5: Common DEGs enriched in three GC cell lines after *MYC*-silencing. (a) Using Venn diagram, we were able to identify 14 common DEGs among AGP01, ACP02, and ACP03, but each one of them also has a unique set of DEGs. (b) Identification of the 14 common DEGs in 8 enriched hallmarks of collection H, represented by the % of its correspondent ES, ES scores are shown inside the pie chart for each hallmark. (c). Heatmap for the expression of the 14 common DEGs shared for three GC cell lines after *MYC*-silencing. Blue represents downregulation while red means upregulation. Notice that, even for the 14 common genes, each cell line has a different expression pattern. Relative read expression was normalized using $\log_2$ Fold-change between *MYC*-silenced/control siRNA. (d) Heatmap for the relative gene expression obtained by RT-qPCR for the 14 identified DEGS for the AGP01, ACP02, and ACP03 cell lines. (e) The overall expression for the 14 DEGs is downregulated in the ACP02 cell line when compared to AGP01 cells. (f) The gene expression levels were increased in ACP03 cell line, but no statistical difference was found. (g) Relative gene expression was increased for ACP03 when compared to ACP02. Wilcoxon matched-pairs signed rank test was used to compare the relative gene expression levels ($^{*}P < 0.05$, ns: not significant, and $^{***}P < 0.0001$).

DEGs as well as the gene expression hallmarks they are involved, ranks and ES. We show a heatmap (Figure 5(c)) of the 14 shared DEGs in clusters grouped using the GENE E tool (https://software.broadinstitute.org/GENE-E/), where downregulation is expressed in blue and upregulation in red. Most genes for ACP02 (diffuse-type GC) presented downregulation, while for ACP03 (intestinal-type GC) the same genes presented themselves as upregulated. The metastatic cell line AGP01, even though its original tumor was intestinal-type, presented mixed expression patterns with predominant downregulation.

3.3. The 14 MYC-Regulated DEGs Show Distinct Expression Profiles for Each GC Histological Subtype. Our *in silico* analysis identified a core set of 14 DEGs (Figure 5(a)) who are *MYC*-regulated, but whose expression profile is distinct for each GC cell line since they represent different histological subtypes. We validated the gene expression profiles presented by the AGP01, ACP02, and ACP03 after *MYC*-silencing by RT-qPCR in the cDNA obtained originally for each cell line and compared them with their expression in the MN01 cell line. Our results point out that the 14 identified DEGs are under *MYC* transcriptional regulation (Figure 5(d)). The ACP02 cell line presented mostly downregulation for the expression of the 14 DEGs (Figure 5(c)); on the other hand, ACP03, the same 14 genes, were upregulated; AGP01 results were mixed, with some genes showing downregulation and others showing downregulation. Our gene expression results (Figure 5(d)) confirm our *in silico* analysis (Figure 5(c)).

Each cell line used in this study represents a GC histological subtype: AGP01 was obtained from the ascitic fluid of intestinal-type GC, representing a metastatic disease, while ACP02 was developed from a diffuse-type stomach cancer patient and ACP03 origin was an intestinal-type gastric tumor.

We compared the mRNA expression measured by RT-qPCR for our identified DEGs to assess whether the gene expression of those 14 genes was enough to statistically distinguish each cell line. When comparing ACP02 versus AGP01 (Figure 5(e)), we noticed a significant gene expression downregulation for ACP02; confronting ACP03 versus AGP01 indicated an increase in mRNA relative quantification (Figure 5(f)) for ACP03; however, those results were not significant; the comparison between ACP02 versus ACP03 confirmed that the 14 *MYC*-regulated DEGs are significantly more expressed in the ACP03, the intestinal-type cell line, than in ACP02 (Figure 5(g)).

Taken together, our results indicate that, even though *MYC*-related carcinogenesis alters the same 14 genes in GC cell lines representing the most common histological subtypes, how *MYC* causes GC carcinogenesis is different for each disease presentation and it is possible to distinct them by using expression signatures.

4. Discussion

A key goal of cancer studies is to systematically characterize the cellular and molecular mechanisms involved in the disease and its distinct stages, to identify both potential biomarkers and new probable drug targets [44]. The molecular profile of gastric cancer is heterogeneous, partly due to different classification systems [45] and, in order to clarify the true molecular origins of GC, both the Cancer Genome Atlas [22] and the Asian Cancer Research Group [46] published the molecular subtypes of gastric cancer, with remarkable overlap between the two models. Therefore, several genes have been implied as biomarkers for GC subtypes, such as *RHOA, EGFR, PDL, CDH1, TP53,* and *JAK2*. However, those studies use samples from populations in which the disease incidence is highest, and few studies have examined populations in which the incidence of this disease is lower, such as Brazil [47]. There is evidence that GC incidence varies between countries greatly because the genetic heterogeneity exhibited by human populations [48], and it has already been showed that there is a unique gene expression signature for Brazilian cases of intestinal-type GC [47]. Our study helps to highlight the molecular profiles of Brazilian GC cell lines, which can help greatly our understanding about the molecular basis of GC in South America.

Most NGS studies investigate GC by comparing tumor versus nontumoral tissue, analyzing global gene expression patterns, copy number variation, and other molecular characteristics, and most of the high-throughput studies carried so far concerning gastric cancer genetics overlook *MYC*'s importance in this process [2, 3, 21–24]. Our results are relevant because *MYC* overexpression is a key finding in Brazilian GC samples [8]. Therefore, we reduced the expression of this gene using siRNA to identify the *MYC*-related signature in GC cell lines, comparing nonsilenced with silenced samples. We identified a total of 5.471 DEGs, and 11 significant gene sets, including classic *MYC* targets represented by *MYC* target V1.

We hereby present the computational analysis of gene sets identified after *MYC*-silencing in Brazilian GC cell lines [13, 27], who carry genetic alterations commonly found in Brazilian GC patients [7, 13, 16]. This oncogene promotes cell growth acting as a transcription factor regulating cell cycle, metabolism, and cell survival [49]. We found DEGs upregulation only for the intestinal-type cell line (ACP03), while the diffuse-type (ACP02) and the metastatic GC cells (AGP01) presented overall gene expression downregulation; when looking at individual genes between ACP02 and AGP01, it is still possible to distinguish between them by *MYC*-related gene expression. It is important to notice that *MYC* has a dual-role in the carcinogenic process, selectively activating and inactivating different gene sets [50–52]. Taken together, we present evidences supporting the fact that *MYC* deregulation has an important role in gastric carcinogenesis [14] and that *MYC*-related signatures in gastric cancer are different for each histological subtype of this disease, which is clinically relevant [47, 53].

One of the main forms of MYC protein regulation in normal cells is through its targeted degradation by the ubiquitin-proteasome system [54], which was one of the KEGG enriched pathways found in our analysis (Figure 4). This means that, in a *MYC*-overexpression condition, like GC [7], not only this gene and its protein are more produced, but they are also less destroyed because it diminishes the expression of E3 ubiquitin-ligases, such as Fbw7 and HectH9, contributing to prolonged MYC protein half-life and amplification of its effects [55]. Ubiquitin-ligases, including the MYC-regulated Fbw7, have recently evolved as promising therapeutic targets for the development of novel anticancer drugs [56].

Other pathways involved in MYC-related gastric carcinogenesis found by our study are known targets, such as ribosome and cell cycle control genes, which are hardly druggable. When taken together, the 12 different pathways we found under *MYC* control for gastric carcinogenesis represent many biological functions, meaning that *MYC* overexpression in GC disturbs almost all the regular cellular processes in favor of tumor development [52]. Another interesting gene set includes glucose metabolism, which is an area of growing interest in cancer research [57], and it has been shown that *MYC* directs the activation of aerobic glycolysis, a hallmark of cancer metabolism known as Warburg effect, and pretty much all genes involved in glycolysis and most of the ones responsible for glutaminolysis [57, 58].

We were also able to pinpoint 14 enriched DEGs in all the three GC cell lines used in this study that might represent the common set of *MYC*-regulated genes in gastric carcinogenesis (Table 4). This is important because it shows that, even though we have represented distinct GC histological subtypes and disease stages, there is still a core set of genes regulated by MYC involved in the carcinogenic process. We also did not find other reports in the literature concerning those 14 genes and high-throughput analysis of gastric cancer [1, 22, 26, 44–46, 53, 59–64]. Even when we consider the molecular signatures presented by Brazilian intestinal-type GC [47], we could not find any concordance for the 14 genes found by our study, but it is important to consider that Binato et al. [47] did not take into account *MYC* overexpression in their samples. Therefore, the unique DEGs found in this paper represent new and important findings concerning the process of gastric carcinogenesis regulated by MYC in the Brazilian population.

Even though additional studies are needed to validate our results, we present strong evidence that MYC-regulated genes in GC have different expression patterns when we consider histological and disease stage differences; however, they still share pathways and core genes involved in the carcinogenic process.

Authors' Contributions

Jersey Heitor da S. Maués, Helem Ferreira Ribeiro, Caroline de Fátima Aquino Moreira-Nunes, and Giovanny R. Pinto conceived and designed the study. Helem Ferreira Ribeiro, Luana de Oliveira Lopes, Giovanny R. Pinto, Letícia M. Lamarão, and Carla Mariana F. Pessoa conducted the study and participated in laboratory analysis. Raimundo Miranda de Carvalho, Jersey Heitor da S. Maués, Helem Ferreira Ribeiro, Juan A. Rey, and Paulo P. Assumpção conducted the RT-qPCR analysis. Jersey Heitor da S. Maués, Caroline de Fátima Aquino Moreira-Nunes, and Rommel M. Rodríguez Burbano conducted bioinformatic analysis and analyzed the data. Jersey Heitor da S. Maués, Helem Ferreira Ribeiro, and Rommel M. Rodríguez Burbano wrote the paper. All authors read and approved the final manuscript.

Acknowledgments

This work was supported by CNPq, Process no. 402283/2013 and Process no. 471072/2012-5; by FAPESPA, Process no. ICAAF 123/2014; by CAPES, Process no. 17704/12-0.

References

[1] B. W. Katona and A. K. Rustgi, "Gastric cancer genomics: advances and future directions," *Cellular and Molecular Gastroenterology and Hepatology*, vol. 3, no. 2, pp. 211–217, 2017.

[2] M. H. McLean and E. M. El-Omar, "Genetics of gastric cancer," *Nature Reviews Gastroenterology & Hepatology*, vol. 11, no. 11, pp. 664–674, 2014.

[3] K. Wang, S. T. Yuen, J. Xu et al., "Whole-genome sequencing and comprehensive molecular profiling identify new driver mutations in gastric cancer," *Nature Genetics*, vol. 46, no. 6, pp. 573–582, 2014.

[4] A. D. Panani, "Cytogenetic and molecular aspects of gastric cancer: Clinical implications," *Cancer Letters*, vol. 266, no. 2, pp. 99–115, 2008.

[5] X. Liu, H. Cai, H. Huang et al., "The prognostic significance of apoptosis-related biological markers in chinese gastric cancer patients," *PLoS ONE*, vol. 6, no. 12, 2011.

[6] J.-S. Choi, J. Seo, E. J. Jung, E. J. Kim, G. K. Lee, and W. H. Kim, "c-MYC amplification in mucinous gastric carcinoma: A possible genetic alteration leading to deeply invasive tumors," *Anticancer Reseach*, vol. 32, no. 11, pp. 5031–5038, 2012.

[7] D. Q. Calcagno, V. M. Freitas, M. F. Leal et al., "MYC, FBXW7 and TP53 copy number variation and expression in Gastric Cancer," *BMC Gastroenterology*, vol. 13, no. 1, 2013.

[8] M. F. Leal, H. F. Ribeiro, J. A. Rey et al., "YWHAE silencing induces cell proliferation, invasion and migration through the up-regulation of CDC25B and MYC in gastric cancer cells: New insights about YWHAE role in the tumor development and metastasis process," *Oncotarget* , vol. 7, no. 51, pp. 85393–85410, 2016.

[9] A. A. Mello, M. F. Leal, J. A. Rey et al., "Deregulated expression of SRC, LYN and CKB kinases by DNA methylation and its potential role in gastric cancer invasiveness and metastasis," *PLoS ONE*, vol. 10, no. 10, 2015.

[10] W. P. Tansey, "Mammalian MYC Proteins and Cancer," *New Journal of Science*, vol. 2014, Article ID 757534, 27 pages, 2014.

[11] L. C. Costa Raiol, E. C. Figueira Silva, D. Mendes da Fonseca et al., "Interrelationship between MYC gene numerical aberrations and protein expression in individuals from northern Brazil with early gastric adenocarcinoma," *Cancer Genetics and Cytogenetics*, vol. 181, no. 1, pp. 31–35, 2008.

[12] D. Q. Calcagno, M. F. Leal, S. Demachki et al., "MYC in gastric carcinoma and intestinal metaplasia of young adults," *Cancer Genetics and Cytogenetics*, vol. 202, no. 1, pp. 63–66, 2010.

[13] M. F. Leal, D. Q. Calcagno et al., "*MYC, TP53,* and chromosome 17 copy-number alterations in multiple gastric cancer cell lines and in their parental primary tumors," *Journal of Biomedicine and Biotechnology*, vol. 2011, Article ID 631268, 8 pages, 2011.

[14] C. R. T. De Souza et al., "MYC deregulation in gastric cancer and its clinicopathological implications," *PLoS One*, vol. 8, no. 5, 2013.

[15] J. D. F. F. Borges Da Costa et al., "Experimental gastric carcinogenesis in cebus apella nonhuman primates," *PLoS One*, vol. 6, no. 7, p. 13, 2011.

[16] F. Wisnieski, D. Q. Calcagno, M. F. Leal et al., "Reference genes for quantitative RT-PCR data in gastric tissues and cell lines," *World Journal of Gastroenterology*, vol. 19, no. 41, pp. 7121–7128, 2013.

[17] J. R. Whitfield and L. Soucek, "Tumor microenvironment: Becoming sick of Myc," *Cellular and Molecular Life Sciences*, vol. 69, no. 6, pp. 931–934, 2012.

[18] S. A. Hills and J. F. X. Diffley, "DNA replication and oncogene-induced replicative stress," *Current Biology*, vol. 24, no. 10, pp. R435–R444, 2014.

[19] L. Zhang, Y. Hou, H. Ashktorab et al., "The impact of C-MYC gene expression on gastric cancer cell," *Molecular and Cellular Biochemistry*, vol. 344, no. 1-2, pp. 125–135, 2010.

[20] S. Walz and M. Eilers, "Unlocking the mysterious mechanisms of Myc," *Nature Medicine*, vol. 19, no. 1, pp. 26-27, 2013.

[21] P. Karimi, F. Islami, S. Anandasabapathy, N. D. Freedman, and F. Kamangar, "Gastric cancer: descriptive epidemiology, risk factors, screening, and prevention," *Cancer Epidemiology Biomarkers & Prevention*, vol. 23, no. 5, pp. 700–713, 2014.

[22] A. J. Bass et al., "Comprehensive molecular characterization of gastric adenocarcinoma," *Nature*, vol. 513, no. 7517, pp. 202–209, 2014.

[23] C. Figueiredo, M. C. Camargo, M. Leite, E. M. Fuentes-Pananá, C. S. Rabkin, and J. C. Machado, *Pathogenesis of Gastric Cancer: Genetics and Molecular Classification BT - Molecular Pathogenesis and Signal Transduction by Helicobacter pylori*, N. Tegtmeyer and S. Backert, Eds., vol. 400 of *Current Topics in Microbiology and Immunology*, Springer International Publishing, 2017.

[24] J. Cools-Lartigue, L. Baker, and L. E. Ferri, *Molecular Mechanisms in Gastric Carcinogenesis BT - Gastric Cancer: Principles and Practice*, V. E. Strong, Ed., Springer International Publishing, 2015.

[25] M. Kato, "Bioinformatics in cancer clinical sequencing–an emerging field of cancer personalized medicine," *Gan To Kagaku Ryoho*, vol. 43, no. 4, pp. 391–397, 2016.

[26] C. Sun, Q. Yuan, D. Wu, X. Meng, and B. Wang, "Identification of core genes and outcome in gastric cancer using bioinformatics analysis," *Oncotarget* , vol. 8, no. 41, pp. 70271–70280, 2017.

[27] M. F. Leal, J. L. Martins do Nascimento, C. E. A. da Silva et al., "Establishment and conventional cytogenetic characterization of three gastric cancer cell lines," *Cancer Genetics and Cytogenetics*, vol. 195, no. 1, pp. 85–91, 2009.

[28] A. S. Khayat, A. C. Guimarães, D. Q. Calcagno et al., "Interrelationship between TP53 gene deletion, protein expression and chromosome 17 aneusomy in gastric adenocarcinoma," *BMC Gastroenterology*, vol. 9, no. 1, 2009.

[29] H. F. Ribeiro, D. F. A. Alcântara, L. A. Matos et al., "Cytogenetic characterization and evaluation of c-MYC gene amplification in PG100, a new Brazilian gastric cancer cell line," *Brazilian Journal of Medical and Biological Research*, vol. 43, no. 8, pp. 717–721, 2010.

[30] H. Li and R. Durbin, "Fast and accurate long-read alignment with Burrows-Wheeler transform," *Bioinformatics*, vol. 26, no. 5, pp. 589–595, 2010.

[31] N. Leng, J. A. Dawson, J. A. Thomson et al., "EBSeq: an empirical Bayes hierarchical model for inference in RNA-seq experiments," *Bioinformatics*, vol. 29, no. 8, pp. 1035–1043, 2013.

[32] H. Li, "Exploring single-sample snp and indel calling with whole-genome de novo assembly," *Bioinformatics*, vol. 28, no. 14, Article ID bts280, pp. 1838–1844, 2012.

[33] R. Patro, S. M. Mount, and C. Kingsford, "Sailfish enables alignment-free isoform quantification from RNA-seq reads using lightweight algorithms," *Nature Biotechnology*, vol. 32, no. 5, pp. 462–464, 2014.

[34] C. Trapnell, B. A. Williams, G. Pertea et al., "Transcript assembly and quantification by RNA-Seq reveals unannotated transcripts and isoform switching during cell differentiation," *Nature Biotechnology*, vol. 28, no. 5, pp. 511–515, 2010.

[35] M. Garber, M. G. Grabherr, M. Guttman, and C. Trapnell, "Computational methods for transcriptome annotation and quantification using RNA-seq," *Nature Methods*, vol. 8, no. 6, pp. 469–477, 2011.

[36] S. Audic and J.-M. Claverie, "The significance of digital gene expression profiles," *Genome Research*, vol. 7, no. 10, pp. 986–995, 1997.

[37] H. Abdi, "The Bonferonni and Šidák Corrections for Multiple Comparisons," pp. 1–9, 2007.

[38] Y. Benjamini and D. Yekutieli, "The control of the false discovery rate in multiple testing under dependency," *The Annals of Statistics*, vol. 29, no. 4, pp. 1165–1188, 2001.

[39] A. Subramanian, P. Tamayo, V. K. Mootha, S. Mukherjee, and B. L. Ebert, "Gene set enrichment analysis: a knowledge-based approach for interpreting genome-wide," 2005.

[40] A. Liberzon, C. Birger, H. Thorvaldsdóttir, M. Ghandi, J. P. Mesirov, and P. Tamayo, "The molecular signatures database hallmark gene set collection," *Cell Systems*, vol. 1, no. 6, pp. 417–425, 2015.

[41] A. Liberzon, A. Subramanian, R. Pinchback, H. Thorvaldsdóttir, P. Tamayo, and J. P. Mesirov, "Molecular signatures database (MSigDB) 3.0," *Bioinformatics*, vol. 27, no. 12, pp. 1739-1740, 2011.

[42] M. Kanehisa, S. Goto, Y. Sato, M. Furumichi, and M. Tanabe, "KEGG for integration and interpretation of large-scale molecular data sets," *Nucleic Acids Research*, vol. 40, no. 1, pp. D109–D114, 2012.

[43] H. Heberle, V. G. Meirelles, F. R. da Silva, G. P. Telles, and R. Minghim, "InteractiVenn: a web-based tool for the analysis of sets through Venn diagrams," *BMC Bioinformatics*, vol. 16, no. 1, article 169, 2015.

[44] J. Y. Cho, "Molecular diagnosis for personalized target therapy in gastric cancer," *Gastric Cancer*, vol. 13, no. 3, pp. 129–135, 2013.

[45] M. Rugge, M. Fassan, and D. Y. Graham, "Epidemiology of gastric cancer," *Gastric Cancer: Principles and Practice*, pp. 23–34, 2015.

[46] R. Cristescu, J. Lee, M. Nebozhyn et al., "Molecular analysis of gastric cancer identifies subtypes associated with distinct clinical outcomes," *Nature Medicine*, vol. 21, no. 5, pp. 449–456, 2015.

[47] R. Binato, E. C. Santos, M. Boroni, S. Demachki, P. Assumpção, and E. Abdelhay, "A common molecular signature of intestinal-type gastric carcinoma indicates processes related to gastric carcinogenesis," *Oncotarget* , vol. 9, no. 7, pp. 7359–7371, 2018.

[48] T. E. Buffart, M. Louw, N. C. van Grieken et al., "Gastric cancers of Western European and African patients show different patterns of genomic instability," *BMC Medical Genomics*, vol. 4, no. 1, 2011.

[49] V. Posternak and M. D. Cole, "Strategically targeting MYC in cancer," *F1000Research*, vol. 5, 2016.

[50] S. Walz, F. Lorenzin, J. Morton et al., "Activation and repression by oncogenic MYC shape tumour-specific gene expression profiles," *Nature*, vol. 511, no. 7510, pp. 483–487, 2014.

[51] T. R. Kress, A. Sabò, and B. Amati, "MYC: Connecting selective transcriptional control to global RNA production," *Nature Reviews Cancer*, vol. 15, no. 10, pp. 593–607, 2015.

[52] T. R. Kress, P. Pellanda, L. Pellegrinet et al., "Identification of MYC-dependent transcriptional programs in oncogene-addicted liver tumors," *Cancer Research*, vol. 76, no. 12, pp. 3463–3472, 2016.

[53] S. Zang, R. Guo, R. Xing et al., "Identification of differentially-expressed genes in intestinal gastric cancer by microarray analysis," *Genomics, Proteomics & Bioinformatics*, vol. 12, no. 6, pp. 276–283, 2014.

[54] A. S. Farrell and R. C. Sears, "MYC degradation," *Cold Spring Harbor Perspectives in Medicine*, vol. 4, no. 3, Article ID a014365, 2014.

[55] B. King, T. Trimarchi, L. Reavie et al., "The ubiquitin ligase FBXW7 modulates leukemia-initiating cell activity by regulating MYC stability," *Cell*, vol. 153, no. 7, pp. 1552–1566, 2013.

[56] J. Liu, S. Shaik, X. Dai et al., "Targeting the ubiquitin pathway for cancer treatment," *Biochimica et Biophysica Acta (BBA) - Reviews on Cancer*, vol. 1855, no. 1, pp. 50–60, 2015.

[57] C. V. Dang, "MYC, metabolism, cell growth, and tumorigenesis," *Cold Spring Harbor Perspectives in Medicine*, vol. 3, no. 8, 2013.

[58] Z. E. Stine, Z. E. Walton, B. J. Altman, A. L. Hsieh, and C. V. Dang, "MYC, metabolism, and cancer," *Cancer Discovery*, vol. 5, no. 10, pp. 1024–1039, 2015.

[59] S. S. Wong, K. Kim, J. C. Ting et al., "Genomic landscape and genetic heterogeneity in gastric adenocarcinoma revealed by whole-genome sequencing," *Nature Communications*, vol. 5, no. 1, 2014.

[60] S. K. Garattini, D. Basile, M. Cattaneo et al., "Molecular classifications of gastric cancers: Novel insights and possible future applications," *World Journal of Gastrointestinal Oncology*, vol. 9, no. 5, pp. 194–208, 2017.

[61] E. Bria, S. Pilotto, M. Simbolo et al., "Comprehensive molecular portrait using next generation sequencing of resected intestinal-type gastric cancer patients dichotomized according to prognosis," *Scientific Reports*, vol. 6, no. 1, 2016.

[62] Y. Lin, Z. Wu, W. Guo, and J. Li, "Gene mutations in gastric cancer: a review of recent next-generation sequencing studies," *Tumor Biology*, vol. 36, no. 10, pp. 7385–7394, 2015.

[63] J. Cools-Lartigue, L. Baker, and L. E. Ferri, "Molecular mechanisms in gastric carcinogenesis," *Gastric Cancer: Principles and Practice*, pp. 35–56, 2015.

[64] M. Kanda and Y. Kodera, "Recent advances in the molecular diagnostics of gastric cancer," *World Journal of Gastroenterology*, vol. 21, no. 34, pp. 9838–9852, 2015.

21

Diagnostic Accuracy of Platelet Count and Platelet Indices in Noninvasive Assessment of Fibrosis in Nonalcoholic Fatty Liver Disease Patients

Tamara Milovanovic Alempijevic,[1,2] Milica Stojkovic Lalosevic,[1] Igor Dumic,[3,4] Nevena Jocic,[1] Aleksandra Pavlovic Markovic,[1,2] Sanja Dragasevic,[1] Ivana Jovicic,[1] Snezana Lukic,[1,2] Dragan Popovic,[1,2] and Tomica Milosavljevic[1,2]

[1]*Clinic of Gastroenterology and Hepatology, Clinical Center of Serbia, 11000 Belgrade, Serbia*
[2]*Faculty of Medicine, University of Belgrade, 11000 Belgrade, Serbia*
[3]*Mayo Clinic College of Medicine and Sciences, Rochester, MN, USA*
[4]*Mayo Clinic Health System, Eau Claire, WI, USA*

Correspondence should be addressed to Tamara Milovanovic Alempijevic; tamara.alempijevic@med.bg.ac.rs

Academic Editor: Dan Dumitrascu

Objective. Keeping in mind the rising prevalence of nonalcoholic fatty liver disease (NAFLD) and the need to establish noninvasive tests for its detection, the aim of our study was to investigate whether platelet count (PC), mean platelet volume (MPV), and platelet distribution width (PDW) can predict the presence of liver fibrosis in this group of patients. *Methods.* In 98 patients with NAFLD and 60 healthy volunteers, complete blood counts with automated differential counts were performed and values of PC, PDW, MPV, and PCT were analyzed. *Results.* Patients with NAFLD had lower PC and higher MPV, PCT, and PDW compared to the controls ($P < 0.05$). When NAFLD group was stratified according to severity of liver fibrosis, there was a statistically significant difference in the average values of PDW and PC between the groups ($P < 0.05$). *Conclusion.* Patients with NAFLD have significantly higher values of PCT, PDW, and MPV when compared to the healthy controls. Further studies are needed to establish their potential use for prediction of the degree of liver steatosis and fibrosis in NAFLD patients.

1. Introduction

Nonalcoholic fatty liver disease (NAFLD) is the leading cause of chronic liver disease worldwide, affecting 20–30% of population in Western countries [1]. NAFLD is a spectrum from simple steatosis with favorable prognosis to nonalcoholic steatohepatitis (NASH), which may progress to cirrhosis and its complications [2]. The hallmark of NAFLD is intrahepatic deposition of triglycerides and the leading factors in this process are insulin resistance and energy misbalance. NAFLD is considered as hepatic manifestation of the metabolic syndrome [3]. Although a liver biopsy is the gold standard for establishing the diagnosis of NAFLD, we must be aware of its invasiveness, patients' discomfort, risk of severe complications, and its high cost. Bearing in mind the rising prevalence of NAFLD and the fact that it has become one of the most common indications for liver transplantation, there is a need to establish noninvasive diagnostic markers for early detection and monitoring of the disease progression [4–6]. Several noninvasive scores for predicting liver fibrosis have already been described: the aspartate aminotransferase to alanine aminotransferase ratio (AAR), the aspartate aminotransferase to platelet ratio index (APRI), fibrosis index (FI), fibrosis-cirrhosis index (FCI), and FIB-4 index (based on age, aspartate and alanine aminotransferase, and platelet counts). Despite the suggestion that these scores correlate with degree of liver fibrosis, there is no sufficient data supporting their everyday use, yet.

Platelets, along their well-known role in hemostasis, are active participants in the process of liver inflammation. They promote leukocyte recruitment through hepatic sinusoids and activate effector cells [7]. Additionally, there are studies suggesting that function and morphology of platelets are altered in patients with diabetes mellitus and metabolic syndrome [8]. MPV, PDW, and PCT (platelet indices) are the indicators of platelet function and activation. It has been suggested that values of platelet indices closely correlate with the presence of insulin resistance and its severity and complications [9, 10].

The aim of our cross-sectional case control study was to evaluate whether platelet count and platelet indices can accurately predict severe steatosis and liver fibrosis in patients with NAFLD patients and to compare their diagnostic accuracy with the other noninvasive scores that have been already published and validated.

2. Patients and Methods

A total of 98 patients diagnosed with NAFLD and 60 sex- and age-matched healthy volunteers without NAFLD were included in this prospective study from March to September 2016. All patients were diagnosed with NAFLD based on history, physical examination, laboratory testing, and ultrasound imaging. The diagnosis of NAFLD required the exclusion of secondary causes of liver disease and daily alcohol consumption (≥20 g for men and >10 g for women) [2]. The exclusion criteria were the following: age < 18 years, presence of any other chronic liver disease (CLD), hepatocellular carcinoma, severe chronic extrahepatic disease, hospital admission due to other chronic illnesses, or presence of human immunodeficiency virus infection. All patients provided a written informed consent prior to inclusion in the study.

Data necessary for the diagnosis of the metabolic syndrome [2] were collected from the patients' records. Physical examination of each patient included body weight, height, waist circumference, calculation of body mass index (BMI), and measurement of blood pressure (BP).

Blood samples were collected after 12 hours of fasting. Analyses included PC, platelet indices, liver function tests (AST, ALT, gamma-glutamyl transferase (GGT), and alkaline phosphatase (ALP)), lipid profile, and fasting blood sugar and insulin levels. Analysis of hematological parameters along with platelets and their indices was performed in whole blood anticoagulated with EDTA within 4 hours after collection, using Coulter® LH 750 Hematology Analyzer (Beckman Coulter, USA). Analysis of biochemical parameters was performed using Olympus AU2700 (Olympus Co. Ltd., Tokyo, Japan). For each patient, we calculated homeostasis model assessment-estimated insulin resistance (HOMA-IR) [11].

Sonographic evaluation (US) of hepatic steatosis was performed using five criteria: parenchymal brightness, liver to kidney contrast, deep beam attenuation, bright vessel walls, and gallbladder wall definition [12]. Grading of diffuse hepatic steatosis was used to evaluate the extent of fatty changes in the liver. Grades I to III were defined as follows:

Grade I: increased hepatic echogenicity with visible periportal and diaphragmatic echogenicity

Grade II: increased hepatic echogenicity with imperceptible periportal echogenicity, without obscuration of diaphragm

Grade III: increased hepatic echogenicity with imperceptible periportal echogenicity and obscuration of the diaphragm [13]

For the assessment of steatosis, we used hepatic steatosis index (HSI) and NAFLD liver fat score (NAFLD-LFS) and we used NAFLD fibrosis score (NFS), APRI, FIB-4 index, and BARD score (which takes into account BMI, AAR, and presence of type II diabetes mellitus) for the assessment of fibrosis. All the above scores were calculated using standard formulas on admission (Tables 1 and 2) [11, 12].

We stratified patients with NAFLD into the two groups based on the US findings. Group 1 included patients with mild and moderate steatosis, while group 2 included patients with severe steatosis and possible fibrosis. In the absence of results from a liver biopsy, we used APRI score as validated "gold noninvasive score" to stratify our patients according to the severity of steatosis and fibrosis [11, 12, 14].

A statistical analysis was performed using SPSS 22.0 (SPSS Inc., Chicago, IL, USA). Basic descriptive statistics included the means, standard deviations, ranges, and percentages. Normality of the distribution was examined by the Kolmogorov-Smirnov test. The differences were considered as statistically significant if the two-tailed P value was less than 0.05. The sensitivity and specificity as well as the best cut-off value for the platelet indexes were calculated using ROC curves (AUROC).

This study was approved by the Ethics Committee of our institution in keeping with the principles of the Declaration of Helsinki (2000 revision of Edinburgh).

3. Results

Clinical, laboratory, and demographic data of patients were summarized in Table 3.

Gender, age, and mean diastolic blood pressure were similar among the NAFLD patients and the control group ($P > 0.05$). NAFLD patients had significantly higher systolic blood pressure, waist circumference, and BMI compared to the controls ($P < 0.01$). Among the biochemical variables, fasting plasma glucose, insulin levels, and triglycerides were significantly higher and high-density lipoprotein was significantly lower in NAFLD group ($P < 0.01$). NAFLD group also had lower PC and higher MPV, PCT, and PDW ($P < 0.05$).

When we stratified NAFLD patients into the two groups, we found a statistically significant difference in the average values of PDW and PC between the groups ($P = 0.04$, $P = 0.03$, and $P < 0.05$) with PDW cut-off value of 16.18 for the presence of severe steatosis and possible fibrosis with sensitivity of 88.1% and specificity of 32.6% and AUROC of 0.688 (Figure 1). There were no differences between these groups with regard to MPV and PCT ($P > 0.05$).

When these groups were further stratified according to APRI score (more than or equal to 0.7), we found a statistically significant difference in values of PC, PDW, and

TABLE 1: Formulas for calculating noninvasive scores for steatosis.

Noninvasive index of steatosis	Formula
HSI	8 ∗ ALT/AST + BMI + 2 if DM + 2 if female
NAFLD-LFS	−2.89 + 1.18 ∗ metabolic syndrome (yes = 1, no = 0) + 0.45 ∗ type 2 DM (yes = 1, no = 0) + 0.15Io + 0.04 ∗ AST − 0.94 ∗ AST/ALT

HSI: hepatic steatosis index; NAFLD-LFS: NAFLD liver fat score.

TABLE 2: Formulas for calculating noninvasive scores for fibrosis [12, 13].

Noninvasive index of fibrosis	Formula
NFS	1.675 + 0.037 × age (years) + 0.094 × BMI (kg/m^2) + 1.13 × IFG/diabetes (yes = 1, no = 0) + 0.99 × AST/ALT ratio − 0.013 × platelet (×10^9/l) − 0.66 × albumin (g/dl)
APRI	[(AST/upper normal limit AST) × 100]/platelets (10^9/L)
FIB-4	(Age × AST)/(platelets × sqr (ALT))
BARD	BMI ≥ 28 = 1p, AST/ALT ratio (AAR) ≥ 0.8 = 2p, DM = 1p

NFS: NAFLD fibrosis score; APRI: AST platelet ratio index; FIB-4: fibrosis-4; BARD: BMI, AST/ALT ratio, and diabetes [12, 13].

TABLE 3: Clinical, laboratory, and demographic data of NAFLD patients compared to controls.

	NAFLD	Control cases	*P* value
Age	51.8 ± 14.6	50.4 ± 14.1	>0.05
Gender: *male/female*	56/42	32/28	>0.05
BMI	29.3 ± 4.7	26.2 ± 3.6	<0.01
Waist circumference	109.4 ± 8.9	108.2 ± 6.6	<0.05
Systolic BP	130.3 ± 8.9	124 ± 6.6	<0.01
Diastolic BP	82.6 ± 6.4	81.5 ± 4.4	>0.05
Glucose	6.6 ± 2.04	5.8 ± 1.5	<0.01
Urea	6.5 ± 5.9	6.6 ± 7.5	>0.05
Creatinine	77.5 ± 15.2	73.3 ± 21.1	>0.05
Total cholesterol	5.78 ± 1.1	5.72 ± 1.4	>0.05
LDL cholesterol	3.6 ± 0.9	2.6 ± 1.1	<0.01
HDL cholesterol	1.2 ± 0.6	1.7 ± 0.4	<0.01
Triglyceride	2.4 ± 1.7	1.7 ± 0.9	<0.01
AST	33.1 ± 19.3	22.3 ± 11.2	<0.01
ALT	46.1 ± 25.8	22.1 ± 7.8	<0.01
ALP	72.3 ± 23.0	73 ± 19.2	>0.05
GGT	73.6 ± 82.9	44 ± 12.1	<0.01
WBC	7.02 ± 1.7	7.2 ± 2.6	>0.05
PC	218.4 ± 56.8	255.3 ± 77.9	<0.01
MPV	9.1 ± 1.3	7.6 ± 1.1	<0.01
PDW	16.7 ± 0.7	15.9 ± 0.7	<0.01
PCT	0.2 ± 0.1	0.1 ± 0.0	<0.01

PCT between the two groups ($P = 0.00$, $P = 0.00$, $P = 0.006$, and $P < 0.05$) (Table 4).

We found a statistically significant negative correlation between PC and APRI ($P = 0.00$; $r = -0.530$), FIB-4 ($P = 0.00$; $r = -0.480$), and NFS ($P = 0.00$; $r = -0.320$) scores, respectively. Additionally, we found statistically significant negative correlations between PDW and APRI ($P = 0.00$; $r = -0.5629$), FIB-4 ($P = 0.00$; $r = -0.553$), and NFS ($P = 0.00$; $r = -0.346$) scores, respectively.

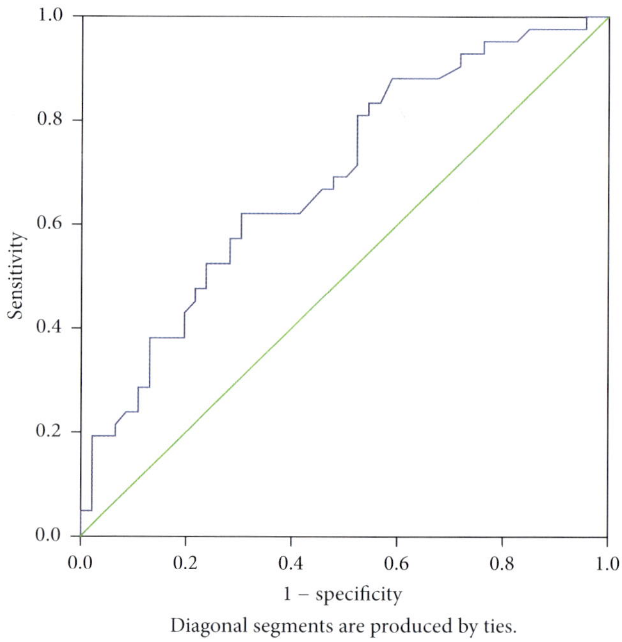

FIGURE 1: ROC curve 1. Receiver Operating Characteristic (ROC) Curve illustrates sensitivity and specificity of mean PDW values for detection of mild, moderate, and severe steatosis.

The results of our study suggest that there is a statistically significant negative correlation between PCT and PDW ($P = 0.06$; $r = -0.252$), as well as a significant positive correlation between PDW and MPV ($P = 0.04$; $r = 0.261$).

4. Discussion

The ability to determine the degree of the liver steatosis and fibrosis as well as to predict the progression of disease is

TABLE 4: APRI score according to platelet count and indices.

	APRI ≥ 0.7	APRI < 0.7	*P*
PC (mean ± SD)	154.71 ± 44.92	226.91 ± 52.90	<0.01
MVP (mean ± SD)	9.21 ± 1.05	9.04 ± 1.46	0.581
PCT (mean ± SD)	0.14 ± 0.03	0.22 ± 0.16	<0.01
PDW (mean ± SD)	16.91 ± 0.35	16.55 ± 0.77	<0.01

essential in the management of patients with NAFLD. A liver biopsy has been used as a gold standard for this purpose over many years. However, its invasive nature, high cost, and risk for development of severe complications (bleeding in particular) resulted in the development of noninvasive tests. These tests consist of different scores derived from various combinations of serologic markers as well as noninvasive imaging modalities [15]. Over the last decade, particularly promising imaging modality has emerged, ultrasound-based transient elastography (TE) with controlled attenuation parameter (CAP). This technique is based on mechanical excitation of the hepatic tissue with monitoring of the resulting tissue response. The fact that fibrotic tissue differs from healthy tissue in the way that it responds to excitation is used to determine level of steatosis and fibrosis. This technique is particularly useful, since it eliminates sampling errors, which was common with liver biopsy, in addition to its noninvasiveness [16, 17]. However, while it is being used more commonly, high cost of the machine is still an obstacle for use in many developing countries. Hence, there is an ongoing interest for discovery of the cheaper and easily available serologic tests for detection of liver steatosis and fibrosis and estimation of the severity grades. Multiple serologic markers reflective of liver function (AST, ALT, bilirubin, PC, GGT, ALP, and haptoglobin) have been used in combination to formulate diagnostic and prognostic scores that would be an alternative to liver biopsy. While some of them are more simple (AAR), some of them include complicated algorithms and multiple variables (FibroTest).

The current research studies suggest that platelets have a role in the process of liver fibrosis by decreasing expression of the principal fibrogenic cytokine TGF-β and by increasing expression of matrix metalloproteinases [18, 19]. Subsequently, an inverse correlation occurs between progression of liver fibrosis and platelets. Taking this into account, PC is presently included in many prognostic scores for fibrosis and cirrhosis of the liver. Some previous studies have described that lower PC is related to the more advanced fibrosis; however, only few of these studies assessed PC in NAFLD patients [20]. Unlike platelets, the platelet indices are not widely investigated as the markers of liver steatosis and fibrosis. They might prove to be very useful in the future as a part of diagnostic scores for detection of liver steatosis and fibrosis in patients with NAFLD.

Our study aimed to determine the association between PC and platelet indices with the presence of fibrosis in NAFLD patients and we found an inverse correlation between PC and liver fibrosis, similar to previously published data [18, 19].

Platelet functions can be affected by platelet size, density, other comorbidities, and age. Larger platelets have higher quantity of granules and adhesion receptors, which results in an increase in platelet activation [21]. PDW directly refers to platelet size, changes with platelet activation, and reflects the heterogeneity in platelet morphology [7]. Our study suggests that NAFLD patients have higher values of PDW compared to controls. Study of Cao et al. showed that PC and PDW negatively correlate with the stage of fibrosis, which is in accordance with results that we found in the present study [22].

The results of Ozhan et al. suggest that lower PC and higher MPV are independent predictors of NAFLD [23]. Several independent studies have reported that steatosis was associated with an elevation in MPV [23–27]. A large Korean study has demonstrated a significant association between the presence of NAFLD and higher MPV values in 628 obese volunteers [24]. In our study, the NAFLD group had significantly higher values of MPV compared to the controls, which is similar to the published data.

To the best of our knowledge, there are no studies that investigated potential use of PCT for estimation of the degree of liver steatosis/fibrosis in patients with NAFLD. In the current study, we have not found any significant difference in the values of PCT between NAFLD groups 1 and 2; however, we have found significant difference in the values of PCT between NAFLD patients and the controls. This can be potentially useful as quick and simple parameter for orientation towards patients with suspected NAFLD.

5. Conclusion

In conclusion, our study demonstrates that patients with NAFLD have significant increase in the values of PCT, PDW, and MPV. We will need larger studies to investigate potential use of PC and platelet indices and their inclusion in the diagnostic algorithms for noninvasive assessment of degree of steatosis and fibrosis in NAFLD patients. Their use may be beneficial considering that they are simple, easy to measure, and cost-effective and are routinely checked in everyday practice.

Additional Points

Limitations of the Study. NAFLD diagnosis was not confirmed by liver biopsy and baseline analyses may not reflect patient's condition over prolonged period of time. Additionally, low AUROC suggest that there is a need for a larger cohort.

References

[1] S. A. Madan, F. John, and C. S. Pitchumoni, "Nonalcoholic Fatty Liver Disease and Mean Platelet Volume: A Systemic Review and Meta-analysis," *Journal of Clinical Gastroenterology*, vol. 50, no. 1, pp. 69–74, 2016.

[2] M. Cengiz, B. A. Candir, G. Yilmaz, G. Akyol, and S. Ozenirler, "Is increased red cell distribution width an indicating marker of nonalcoholic steatohepatitis and fibrotic stage?" *World Journal of Gastroenterology*, vol. 19, no. 42, pp. 7412–7418, 2013.

[3] European Association for the Study of the Liver (EASL), "EASL–EASD–EASO Clinical Practice Guidelines for the management of non-alcoholic fatty liver disease," *Diabetologia*, vol. 59, no. 6, pp. 1121–1140, 2016.

[4] D. R. LaBrecque, Z. Abbas, F. Anania et al., "World gastroenterology organisation global guidelines: nonalcoholic fatty liver disease and nonalcoholic steatohepatitis," *Journal of Clinical Gastroenterology*, vol. 48, no. 6, pp. 467–473, 2014.

[5] S. Bellentani, F. Scaglioni, M. Marino, and G. Bedogni, "Epidemiology of non-alcoholic fatty liver disease," *Digestive Diseases*, vol. 28, no. 1, pp. 155–161, 2010.

[6] S. Milić, I. Mikolasevic, and I. Krznaric-Zrnic, "Nonalcoholic steatohepatitis: emerging targeted therapies to optimize treatment options," *Drug Design, Development and Therapy*, vol. 9, pp. 4835–4845, 2015.

[7] A. Chauhan, D. H. Adams, S. P. Watson, and P. F. Lalor, "Platelets: No longer bystanders in liver disease," *Hepatology*, vol. 64, no. 5, pp. 1774–1784, 2016.

[8] A. Koneti Rao, R. E. Goldberg, and P. N. Walsh, "Platelet coagulant activities in diabetes mellitus. Evidence for relationship between platelet coagulant hyperactivity and platelet volume," *Journal of Laboratory and Clinical Medicine*, vol. 103, no. 1, pp. 82–92, 1984.

[9] Y. U. Budak, M. Polat, and K. Huysal, "The use of platelet indices, plateletcrit, mean platelet volume and platelet distribution width in emergency non-traumatic abdominal surgery: a systematic review," *Biochemia Medica*, vol. 26, no. 2, pp. 178–193, 2016.

[10] A. T. Eminler, M. I. Uslan, T. Ayyildiz et al., "Mean platelet volume is an important predictor of hepatitis C but not hepatitis B liver damage," *Journal of Research in Medical Sciences*, vol. 20, no. 9, pp. 865–870, 2015.

[11] T. Alempijevic, A. Sokic-Milutinovic, A. P. Markovic et al., "Assessment of metabolic syndrome in patients with primary biliary cirrhosis," *Wiener Klinische Wochenschrift*, vol. 124, no. 7-8, pp. 251–255, 2012.

[12] S. Kahl, K. Straßburger, B. Nowotny et al., "Comparison of liver fat indices for the diagnosis of hepatic steatosis and insulin resistance," *PLoS ONE*, vol. 9, no. 4, Article ID A1453, 2014.

[13] C. Das, M. Baruah, and D. Singh, "Imaging of non alcoholic fatty liver disease: A road less travelled," *Indian Journal of Endocrinology and Metabolism*, vol. 17, no. 6, p. 990, 2013.

[14] A. Unalp-Arida and C. E. Ruhl, "Noninvasive fatty liver markers predict liver disease mortality in the U.S. population," *Hepatology*, vol. 63, no. 4, pp. 1170–1183, 2016.

[15] A. Wieckowska and A. E. Feldstein, "Diagnosis of nonalcoholic fatty liver disease: Invasive versus noninvasive," *Seminars in Liver Disease*, vol. 28, no. 4, pp. 386–395, 2008.

[16] J. Foucher, E. Chanteloup, J. Vergniol et al., "Diagnosis of cirrhosis by transient elastography (FibroScan): a prospective study," *Gut*, vol. 55, no. 3, pp. 403–408, 2006.

[17] J. Ophir, I. Céspedes, H. Ponnekanti, Y. Yazdi, and X. Li, "Elastography: a quantitative method for imaging the elasticity of biological tissues," *Ultrasonic Imaging*, vol. 13, no. 2, pp. 111–134, 1991.

[18] C. Fierbinteanu-Braticevici, I. Dina, A. Petrisor, L. Tribus, L. Negreanu, and C. Carstoiu, "Noninvasive investigations for non alcoholic fatty liver disease and liver fibrosis," *World Journal of Gastroenterology*, vol. 16, no. 38, pp. 4784–4791, 2010.

[19] A. Gülali, A. Aytekin, K. Buket et al., "Mean Platelet Volume and Red Cell distribution width in Hepatosteatosis," *National Journal of Medical Research*, vol. 3, no. 3, pp. 264–266, 2013.

[20] Z. Saremi, M. Rastgoo, M. Mohammadifard, B. Bijari, and E. Akbari, "Comparison of platelet number and function between nonalcoholic fatty liver disease and normal individuals," *Journal of Research in Medical Sciences*, vol. 22, no. 1, p. 75, 2017.

[21] C. H. Kim, S. J. Kim, M. J. Lee et al., "An increase in mean platelet volume from baseline is associated with mortality in patients with severe sepsis or septic shock," *PLoS ONE*, vol. 10, no. 3, Article ID e0119437, 2015.

[22] W. Cao, C. Zhao, C. Shen, and Y. Wang, "Cytokeratin 18, alanine aminotransferase, platelets and triglycerides predict the presence of nonalcoholic steatohepatitis," *PLoS ONE*, vol. 8, no. 12, Article ID e82092, 2013.

[23] H. Ozhan, M. Aydin, M. Yazici et al., "Mean platelet volume in patients with non-alcoholic fatty liver disease," *Platelets*, vol. 21, no. 1, pp. 29–32, 2010.

[24] W.-Y. Shin, D.-H. Jung, J.-Y. Shim, and H.-R. Lee, "The association between non-alcoholic hepatic steatosis and mean platelet volume in an obese Korean population," *Platelets*, vol. 22, no. 6, pp. 442–446, 2011.

[25] K. Fang, Y. Cheng, C. Su et al., "Higher platelet counts are associated with metabolic syndrome independent of fatty liver diagnosis," *Journal of the Chinese Medical Association*, vol. 80, no. 3, pp. 125–132, 2017.

[26] S. Arundhathi, S. Sunitha, and R. Gandham, "Mean Platelet Volume in Non-Alcoholic Fatty Liver Disease in Type 2 Diabetes Mellitus - A Marker of Cardiovascular Risk," *International Journal of Biomedical and Advance Research*, vol. 7, no. 2, pp. 76–78, 2016.

[27] M. Aydin, M. Yazici, O. Yazgan et al., "Mean platelet volume in patients with non-alcoholic fatty liver disease," *Platelets*, vol. 21, pp. 29–32, 2010.

22

Outcomes following Serial Intragastric Balloon Therapy for Obesity and Nonalcoholic Fatty Liver Disease in a Single Centre

Vi Nguyen,[1,2] Jiawei Li,[1] Jaslyn Gan,[1] Paul Cordero,[1] Shuvra Ray,[1,2] Alessandro Solis-Cuevas,[3] Mai Khatib,[3] and Jude A. Oben[1,2]

[1] *Institute for Liver and Digestive Health, University College London, Royal Free Hospital, Rowland Hill Street, London NW3 2PF, UK*
[2] *Department of Gastroenterology and Hepatology, Guy's and St Thomas' Hospital, NHS Foundation Trust, Westminster Bridge Rd., London SE1 7EH, UK*
[3] *Department of Biological Sciences, University College London, Gower St., Bloomsbury, London WC1E 6BT, UK*

Correspondence should be addressed to Paul Cordero; paul.sanchez@ucl.ac.uk and Jude A. Oben; j.oben@ucl.ac.uk

Academic Editor: Branka Filipović

Background. The incidence of nonalcoholic fatty liver disease (NAFLD) continues to parallel the rise in obesity rates. Endobariatric devices such as the intragastric balloon (IGB) may provide an alternative treatment option. *Methods.* Outcomes following IGB treatment in 135 patients with obesity and NAFLD (mean baseline weight 117.9 kg; BMI 41.7 kg/m^2; HOMA-IR 3.6) were retrospectively examined. Clinical, anthropometric, and biochemical changes were analysed at six months and after consecutive treatment with two and three serial IGBs. *Results.* After six months, significant changes were seen with weight and BMI (mean reductions of 11.3 kg and 4.1 kg/m^2, resp., $p < 0.01$ for both). Significant improvements were also seen with ALT, GGT, and HOMA-IR, with all changes corresponding with weight loss. Forty-eight patients received two IGBs, and 20 were treated with three serial IGBs. The greatest amount of total weight loss was observed after the first 6 months (mean weight lost 7.4 kg, versus 3.6 kg and 1.9 kg with two and three IGBs, resp.). *Conclusions.* IGB therapy is an effective, alternative nonsurgical means for weight loss in the management of obesity and NAFLD over the short term, with greatest outcomes observed after six months. Improvements in insulin resistance and hepatic transaminases correlated with weight change.

1. Introduction

Nonalcoholic fatty liver disease (NAFLD) is now the leading cause of chronic liver disease in most affluent and several emerging economies [1]. It is expected that NAFLD will become the main indication for liver transplantation by 2020 [2].

NAFLD is invariably linked with obesity and closely associated with other complications of the metabolic syndrome (impaired glucose tolerance, hypertension, and dyslipidaemia) [3, 4]. The estimated prevalence of NAFLD largely parallels the obesity epidemic, and although it varies across different regions of the world, the unifying trend is a rapidly increasing rate being observed worldwide [2].

Obesity is primarily caused by an imbalance in energy homeostasis, with nutrient intake exceeding energy expenditure. However, this disequilibrium likely encompasses complex interactions with several other factors, including physical activity levels, genetics, hormonal changes, maternal and perinatal nutrition, and the gut microbiota [5–7]. The prevalence of obesity, together with its associated metabolic comorbidities, is now recognised as perhaps the most important health pandemic of the 21st century [8, 9].

Although the individual natural history of NAFLD is largely uncertain, up to 30% of patients can progress to develop nonalcoholic steatohepatitis (NASH) [10], with approximately 5% of these patients at further risk of long-term progression to cirrhosis and end-stage liver disease, including hepatocellular cancer [11, 12]. Moreover, the presence of NAFLD is itself associated with a broader range of complications, including a higher risk of cardiovascular disease (CVD) and early mortality, as well as a greater risk of extrahepatic malignancies [13, 14]. The leading cause of morbidity and death among patients with NAFLD/NASH remains adverse cardiovascular events [15].

There is currently no single, reliable treatment for NAFLD/NASH. While several potential therapeutic options are under development, lifestyle interventions remain the most effective treatment modality. Unfortunately, effective weight loss maintenance following lifestyle interventions remains elusive for most, with the majority returning to their baseline weight by 18–24-month follow-up [16, 17].

Weight loss surgeries (such as gastric bypass, sleeve gastrectomy, and gastric banding) have been shown to improve hepatosteatosis, inflammatory changes, and fibrosis in NASH patients and are currently the only treatments that have demonstrated significant, durable weight loss over the longer term [18]. Not all patients, however, are suitable or eligible for bariatric surgery, especially given the higher risk of complications with formal surgery and general anaesthesia, as well as the greater risk of impaired wound healing in obese patients. Interim or definitive endoscopic procedures such as the intragastric balloon (IGB) may therefore offer less-invasive, reversible alternatives to effect weight loss in instances where lifestyle interventions have failed and/or the patient is not a candidate for bariatric surgery.

Several prospective studies have demonstrated the efficacy of IGBs in achieving significant weight loss. Results from a meta-analysis of 15 trials (13 cohort, 2 controlled trials) studying the efficacy of IGBs in 3608 patients reported an average 34% excess weight loss (EWL) in those receiving IGB insertion for 3–6 months, associated with mean body mass index (BMI) reduction of approximately 3.2 kg/m^2 [19]. A few more, albeit relatively small, studies have also reported associated improvements with features of the metabolic syndrome [20], as well as liver transaminases and indexes of insulin resistance in obese patients with NAFLD over the short-medium term [21–23].

The aim of this current analysis was to report on the experience of IGB therapy as it is offered for the treatment of obesity and NAFLD. Our primary aim was to examine the efficacy of IGBs, and serial IGB therapy in particular, as an alternative or adjunctive treatment for patients with obesity and insulin resistance, focusing on weight reduction, and associated changes in metabolic and hepatic indices, as well as safety outcomes.

2. Materials and Methods

2.1. Participants. From 2005 to 2015, 135 obese patients with NAFLD received treatment with the BioEnterics Intragastric Balloon (BIB; Allergan, Goleta, CA, USA) at a single tertiary hospital (Guy's and St Thomas' Hospital, London, UK). Patients were eligible for IGB insertion if they were ≥18 years of age, with a BMI ≥ 27 kg/m^2. The majority of patients were also insulin resistant at baseline (HOMA-IR score > 2.50), and most had failed previous attempts at weight loss through lifestyle interventions or medical therapy alone. IGB therapy was contraindicated in those with a hiatus hernia > 5 cm, previous gastric surgery, significant gastric erosions or ulceration, >Grade 1 oesophagitis, active coagulopathies (including anticoagulants that could not be withheld), pregnancy, decompensated cirrhosis, contraindications to sedation for endoscopy, and an inability to provide informed consent.

The efficacy of IGB therapy in subjects with a BMI >27–35 kg/m^2, who may not qualify for formal bariatric surgery, has been demonstrated [24]. A BMI cut-off of >27 kg/m^2 was therefore chosen for patient selection in this unit.

The presence of NAFLD was determined on the basis of retrospective liver biopsies confirming >5% hepatic steatosis, formal reports of hepatic steatosis on liver ultrasound (performed within six months from the time of IGB insertion), or a raised controlled attenuation parameter (CAP) reading of >268 dB/m on FibroScan-CAP [25].

All experiments were conducted in accordance with the Declaration of Helsinki, and all procedures were carried out with well-informed and written consent.

2.2. IGB Insertion. Patients initially underwent gastroscopy under conscious sedation with midazolam and fentanyl. The IGB was inserted orally in deflated form into the stomach and filled under direct endoscopic vision with 500–600 mL of normal saline and 10 mL of methylene blue fluid. At approximately 6 months following insertion, each IGB was removed during another endoscopic procedure during which balloon puncture, fluid removal, and transoral retrieval of the deflated device were undertaken using specifically designed instruments. Both IGB insertion and removal were carried out as day-only procedures, with patients discharged on the same day, provided no complications were encountered. The serial (second and/or third) IGBs were placed approximately 1-2 weeks following removal of the previous balloon, using insertion and removal procedures identical to those described above. Approval for a subsequent IGB was dependent on weight loss achieved with the first balloon, patient tolerance, and preference.

2.3. Clinical, Anthropometric, and Biochemical Measurements. Clinical, anthropometric, and biochemical data were examined retrospectively for each patient where available, and differences in outcomes were compared between baseline (prior to the first IGB insertion) and at three separate time points where appropriate: T1; after the removal of the first 1st IGB, T2; after the removal of the 2nd IGB, and T3; after removal of the 3rd IGB. The primary outcome measure was weight loss, with secondary outcome measures including any significant changes in liver function, insulin resistance, and lipid profiles. Safety outcomes were also analysed.

Weight and height measurements were undertaken using standard protocols in the endoscopy suite at baseline (just prior to the IGB insertion procedure) and following IGB removal [26]. Waist circumference was also measured using standard techniques in the outpatient clinics, usually at the time of a follow-up consultation before/after IGB insertion.

Fasting blood samples were collected at baseline and at the time of IGB removal, usually following an outpatient clinic review performed within two weeks before/after the IGB insertion. The following biochemical assays were performed: full blood count, liver function tests, renal function, total cholesterol, high-density lipoprotein (HDL), low-density lipoprotein (LDL), triglycerides, glucose, insulin,

HbA1c, vitamin D, and CRP. Serum biochemistry was performed by the diagnostic testing laboratory at St Thomas' Hospital, London, United Kingdom.

Insulin resistance was calculated using the Homeostasis Model Assessment- (HOMA-) IR score, equation: HOMA-IR = [mean fasting insulin (mIU/L) × mean fasting glucose (mmol/L)] ÷ 22.5. A HOMA-IR score of >2.0 has been demonstrated to accurately correlate with more invasive measures of insulin resistance, as determined through euglycemic clamps and intravenous glucose tolerance tests [27].

Controlled attenuation parameter (CAP) refers to an ultrasonographic coefficient that is affected by and directly proportional to the amount of liver fat. Consequently, CAP readings are commonly measured in conjunction with transient elastography, to quantitate hepatic steatosis. CAP values range from 100 to 400 dB/m, with higher values indicating a greater degree of liver fat. CAP measurement has now also been demonstrated to provide a further useful tool in the diagnosis and staging of NAFLD, with cut-off values > 268 dB/m accurately correlating with steatosis grades > 5–33% [25]. FibroScan-CAP measurements (performed at the discretion of the clinician) where available in the clinical notes were collated for review as part of outcomes before/after IGB insertion and part of the process for identifying obese patients with NAFLD who could be included into this analysis.

2.4. Statistical Analysis. Statistical analysis was performed using SPSS software (SPSS version 20.0, Chicago, IL, USA). Continuous variables were analysed using one-way ANOVA and nonparametric testing, while categorical variables were assessed via Chi-square and Fisher's exact analyses. Two-tailed p values of <0.05 were regarded as significant throughout.

3. Results

3.1. Baseline Characteristics. Follow-up data from a total number of 135 patients were available for analysis (Table 1). The majority were women (71%), of Caucasian background (66%), with a mean age of 47 ± 12 years. The mean baseline weight was 117.9 ± 22.0 kg (M: 122.7 kg; F: 115.7 kg), with baseline BMI of 41.7 ± 6.6 kg/m^2 (M: 39.7 kg/m^2; F: 42.8 kg/m^2). Waist circumference measurements were also available in a subset of patients (n = 33), with an average recording of 124.2 ± 13.6 cm (accepted normal values being ≤94 cm for men and ≤80 cm for women). The majority of patients were insulin resistant, with a median HOMA-IR score of 3.6 and moderately abnormal liver function tests and adverse lipid profiles also apparent at baseline (Table 1). The majority of patients also had concurrent features of the metabolic syndrome (60/134, 45%), and 29% already required medical treatments for Type 2 diabetes (Table 1).

3.2. Clinical Outcomes at 6 Months (T1). The mean time at IGB removal was 5.8 ± 1.7 months following insertion (Table 1). At the end of follow-up, significant reductions were seen in both weight and BMI for the majority of the cohort, with mean weight loss of 11.3 kg (117.9 kg to 106.6 kg, $p < 0.01$) and mean BMI reduction of 4.1 kg/m^2 (41.7 to 37.6 kg/m^2, $p < 0.01$), respectively (Table 2). In those with paired waist circumference measurements (n = 33), recordings also improved significantly following IGB therapy, 124.2 cm to 101.1 cm (mean reduction of 23.1 cm, $p < 0.05$).

Although there was a trend in the reduction of fasting serum lipids following IGB therapy, the results did not reach statistical significance (Table 2).

3.3. Clinical Outcomes following Serial IGB Therapy (T2 and T3). In this cohort of 135 patients, 67 had received only one IGB during the study period, while 48 patients received two serial IGBs, and 20 patients received three IGBs. The greatest amount of total weight loss was observed in the

TABLE 1: Baseline characteristics.

Clinical parameter	Patient numbers (n = 135)
Age (years), mean ± SD	47.1 (12.2)
Sex	M 39 (29%), F 96 (71%)
Ethnicity	
(i) Caucasian	89 (66%)
(ii) Black	27 (20%)
(iii) Asian (Indian)	2 (2%)
(iv) Asian (oriental)	2 (2%)
(v) Latino	6 (4%)
(vi) Mixed	3 (2%)
Diabetes	39/134 (29%)
Other MetSy features	60/134 (45%)
Taking ACE-inhibitor medication	94/133 (71%)
Fasting BSL [n = 96] (mmol/L), mean ± SD	6.0 ± 2.7
Weight [n = 134] (kg), mean ± SD	117.9 ± 22.0
BMI [n = 96] (kg/m^2), mean ± SD	41.7 ± 6.6
Waist circumference [n = 33] (cm), mean ± SD	124.2 ± 13.6
Fasting cholesterol [n = 50] (mmol/L), mean ± SD	4.8 ± 1.4
Fasting LDL [n = 41] (mmol/L), mean ± SD	2.7 ± 1.1
Fasting HDL [n = 41] (mmol/L), mean ± SD	1.2 ± 0.3
Fasting triglycerides [n = 41] (mmol/L), mean ± SD	1.8 ± 1.0
Fasting insulin [n = 83] (mIU/L), mean ± SD	136.0 ± 169.0
HOMA-IR [n = 78], median (range)*	3.6 (2.1–5.9)
ALT [n = 108] (IU/L), mean ± SD	38.9 ± 30.6
AST [n = 16] (IU/L), mean ± SD	35.1 ± 25.2
GGT [n = 82] (IU/L), mean ± SD	62.6 ± 74.9
Fib-4 score [n = 12], mean ± SD	1.5 ± 0.7
Period of 1st IGB placement (months), mean ± SD	5.8 ± 1.7
Total number of balloons	One = 135, two = 48, three =20

*25–75% interquartile ranges expressed.

Table 2: Clinical outcomes at 6 months.

Clinical parameter	Baseline	6 months (after IGB removal)	Mean difference	p value
Weight (kg)	*117.9*	*106.6*	*11.3*	*<0.01*
BMI (kg/m²)	*41.7*	*37.6*	*4.1*	*<0.01*
Waist circumference (cm)	*124.2*	*101.1*	*23.1*	*0.04*
Fasting BSL (mmol/L)	6.0	5.4	0.6	0.12
Fasting insulin (mIU/L)	136.0	96.5	39.5	0.12
*HOMA-IR**	*3.6*	*2.6*	*1.0*	*0.03*
*ALT (IU/L)**	*38.9*	*31.0*	*7.9*	*<0.01*
AST (IU/L)	35.1	32.8	2.3	0.11
*GGT (IU/L)**	*62.6*	*39.1*	*23.5*	*<0.01*
Fasting cholesterol (mmol/L)	4.8	5.1	−0.3	0.08
Fasting LDL (mmol/L)	2.7	2.8	−0.1	0.09
Fasting HDL (mmol/L)	1.2	1.5	−0.3	0.39
Fasting triglycerides (mmol/L)	1.8	1.4	0.4	0.22

*A significant difference in ALT and GGT was noted at follow-up in those with an elevated HOMA-IR score (i.e., insulin resistance) at baseline.

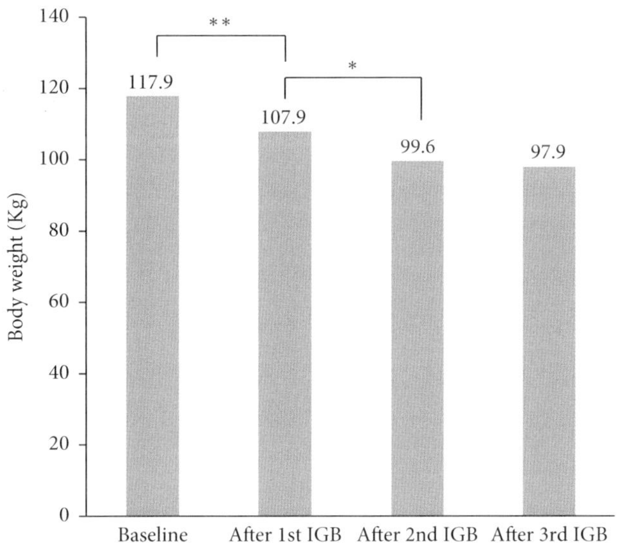

Figure 1: Incremental weight loss following serial IGB therapy ($^{*}p < 0.05$; $^{**}p < 0.01$).

first 6 months after treatment with one IGB (T1), whereas the additional amount of weight loss achieved in those who received a 2nd (T2) and 3rd (T3) IGB were not as significant (mean weight loss of 7.4 kg versus 3.6 kg and 1.9 kg, resp.; $p = 0.05$) (Table 3). Furthermore, while the incremental weight decline following a second IGB was statistically significant, no further significant weight losses were observed in those who underwent treatment with a third IGB (Figure 1).

3.4. Changes in NAFLD Indices after IGB Treatment. After six months of IGB therapy, HOMA-IR scores were observed to significantly improve in a total of 78 patients with paired readings at baseline and final follow-up, 3.6 compared with 2.6 ($p < 0.05$). Significant improvements in serum ALT and GGT were also noted, but only when analysed in those with an elevated HOMA-IR score at baseline. The prevalence of elevated plasma ALT and GGT concentrations decreased from 42% to 22% and from 57% to 34%, respectively, after IGB therapy at six months (Table 2). Similar findings were noted with observed changes in BMI and ALT across the groups who received serial treatment with two or three IGBs, but no further significant reductions in HOMA-IR scores were observed (Table 3).

3.5. Long-Term Follow-Up after IGB Treatment. The average period of follow-up for the total cohort was approximately 20 months. During this time, 58% ($n = 78$) of patients were lost to follow-up, and 20% ($n = 27$) were eventually referred for bariatric surgery. Of those who continued in clinical follow-up for whom data were available ($n = 37$), the mean final weight and total % of baseline weight lost at final follow-up were 108.8 kg and 6.3% for T1, 107.5 kg and 9.0% for T2, and 115.3 kg and 7.5% for T3, respectively ($p = 0.05$).

3.6. Safety Outcomes. The majority of patients tolerated IGB therapy. The most common adverse symptoms reported were nausea and vomiting (20.7%) and abdominal cramps, experienced primarily in the first few weeks after IGB insertion. During this time period, only one patient required emergency balloon removal for an unexpected gastrointestinal obstruction [28], and 14 patients (10.4%) had their IGB removed prematurely for intolerance (Table 4). There were no predominant clinical factors that predicted IGB intolerance, including gender or age.

In the patient who experienced an unexpected obstruction, the IGB was found to be significantly distended with air and fluid while still within the stomach. Balloon puncture and retrieval were performed in the standard manner, with the patient making a swift recovery after balloon extraction. Prolonged cultures of the IGB fluid did not reveal any infective (gas-forming) organisms, which raised the possibility of a defective valve potentially allowing entry of air into the device, with consequent distension.

TABLE 3: Anthropometric and ALT changes following serial IGB therapy.

Clinical parameter	After 1st IGB (T1) [$n = 67$]	After 2nd IGB (T2) [$n = 48$]	After 3rd IGB (T3) [$n = 20$]	p value
Final weight (kg)	107.9 ± 23.5	99.6 ± 17.1	97.9 ± 43.4	0.18
Incremental weight change*	−7.4	−3.6	−1.9	0.05$
Total weight change**	−6.9	−10.6	−9.4	<0.01$
Final BMI (kg/m^2)	39.0	35.5	38.2	0.15
Total change in BMI**	−2.0	−5.7	−5.5	<0.01$
Final HOMA-IR	4.27	1.89	2.71	0.21
Total change in HOMA-IR**	−1.17	−1.37	−3.00	0.71
Final ALT (IU/L)	31.7	27.9	26.3	0.57
Total change in ALT**	−5.8	−4.2	21.8¶	<0.01$
Total follow-up (months)	17.1	18.8	26.6	
Final outcomes:				
(i) Loss to follow-up	44	25	9	
(ii) Referred for surgery	12	10	5	0.65
(iii) Still in active follow-up	11	13	6	

*Changes compared with the start weight prior to IGB insertion, and the end of the treatment period (T1/T2/T3). **Changes compared with baseline (prior to placement of the 1st IGB), and final follow-up. ¶Data only available in 5 cases. $Significant changes were observed in outcomes between T1 and T2, but not between T2 and T3.

TABLE 4: Adverse outcomes.

Side effect	Number of patients
Nausea and vomiting	28 (20.7%)
Abdominal pain	8 (5.9%)
Abdominal bloating/flatulence	16 (11.9%)
Constipation or diarrhoea	6 (4.4%)
Gastroesophageal reflux	9 (6.7%)
Erosive gastritis or oesophagitis	2 (1.5%)
Deflation or displacement of IGB	1 (0.7%)
Gastrointestinal obstruction	1 (0.7%)
Premature removal	15 (10.4%)

4. Discussion

Over the next decade, obesity and its related complications will continue to instigate overwhelming health-related population and cost burdens for most economies of the world [29]. Although there is increasing recognition of this burgeoning problem, more effective treatment modalities are still desperately needed. While lifestyle interventions, focusing on dietary changes and increased exercise, remain the primary treatment recommendation, endoscopic bariatric devices such as the IGB are fast becoming a viable option for improved management through assisted weight loss [30].

To date, several studies have reported on the efficacy of IGBs in inducing significant weight loss over the short to medium term [31, 32]. Similarly, we found that IGB therapy resulted in an average weight loss of 11.3 kg and BMI reduction of 4.1 kg/m^2 over the initial 6 months, approximating to an average EWL (excess weight loss) of 22.5%. These findings are in keeping with figures reported by Imaz et al. [19] in their meta-analysis of several earlier studies examining the efficacy of IGB therapy, with pooled weight and BMI losses of 14.7 kg and 5.7 kg/m^2, respectively.

In addition to the management of obesity and excess weight, IGB therapy appears to offer a promising adjunctive treatment modality for NAFLD/NASH, even independent of weight changes [21]. To date, only a few, relatively small studies have focused on the efficacy of IGB therapy in reducing hepatic steatosis. Forlano et al. [22] demonstrated a significant reduction in liver steatosis on serial abdominal ultrasonography in 91 "responder" patients who achieved significant weight loss after IGB treatment over 6 months. This correlated with a significant reduction in HOMA-IR scores (3.8 to 1.6, $p < 0.001$) and presumably improved insulin resistance. Similarly, Folini and colleagues [21] quantified improved hepatic steatosis on serial hepatic magnetic resonance imaging (MRI) in 18 patients who underwent IGB placement (or laparoscopic gastric banding) for 6 months, compared with no significant changes seen in 13 controls. Again, these changes correlated with improved BMI and significant reductions in weight and waist circumference.

Furthermore, in a prospective sham-controlled trial including 18 patients with obesity and NAFLD who underwent serial liver biopsies before and after 6 months of IGB placement, or sham therapy, liver histology demonstrated improved NAFLD Activity Scores (NAS) [33] in those who received IGB therapy versus no improvement in those who received sham treatment (intragastric normal saline solution infusion) [34]. However, no improvements in median lobular inflammation, ballooning, or fibrosis scores were seen in either group, although this may have been due to the short duration of treatment.

In our cohort, we also found improved insulin resistance through reduced HOMA-IR scores in those who achieved significant weight losses, which correlated with significant improvements in liver function tests (i.e., serum ALT and GGT) [4]. We also observed several cases of improved hepatic NASH fibrosis with IGB therapy, as measured though serial FibroScan recordings (results not shown) in a few patients and verified with serial liver biopsy results in one case. In this particular case, originally diagnosed with decompensated cirrhosis with portal hypertension from NASH, serial IGB treatment resulted in a total weight loss of 54 kg over 19 months, with improved portal inflammation and steatosis, and fibrosis remodelling thought to indicate early cirrhosis reversal on follow-up histology. To our knowledge, this case is the first to report on regression of cirrhosis following weight loss through nonsurgical means. This case is also more significant as it demonstrates how IGB therapy can provide an alternative weight loss tool for those with advanced liver disease, and often poor levels of medical and physical fitness, for whom treatment options are often severely limited.

This study is the first to document outcomes with serial (more than two) periods of IGB therapy. In their publication examining weight loss following two IGB treatments, Genco and colleagues [35] found improved and prolonged weight loss in 50 patients who underwent a second IGB following weight loss achieved with a primary balloon, as compared with control patients who were randomised to receive only dietary therapy following their initial IGB. In the group who received two serial IGBs, the mean BMI was 30.9 versus 35.9 kg/m^2 ($p < 0.05$) in the control cohort at the end of approximately 13 months. In our analysis, we observed the greatest degree of weight loss following treatment with the 1st IGB (average weight loss of 7 kg posttherapy), while the amount of weight lost following the second and third IGBs was not as significant (mean weight loss of 3.6 kg and 1.9 kg, resp.), as compared with the start weights prior to each insertion period. Indeed, weight regain was actually observed in a few patients after their third IGB, which would suggest that optimal weight loss is likely achieved following two IGBs, over 12 months, while the third IGB may help to promote weight loss "maintenance" rather than further weight decline. Again, a greater magnitude of weight loss again correlated with the most significant changes in ALT, although we did not observe any concurrent improvements in HOMA-IR scores over the extended treatment period beyond the initial 6 months, likely due to the smaller degrees of weight change achieved during these later time points.

Although these results provide a promising outlook for short-medium term outcomes, the longer-term utility of IGB therapy still requires elucidation. Currently, there are few studies that report on the outcomes with IGBs beyond 12 months and none reporting on long-term outcomes with serial IGB treatments. In their report comparing weight loss outcomes on 130 patients who had retrospectively received IGB versus a matched cohort of controls who received only prospective, specialised dietary interventions, Genco et al. [36] found more significant maintenance of weight loss endpoints in the IGB group as compared with controls at both 6 months and 24 months. Similarly, a prospective analysis by Mitura and Garnysz [37] found that of 70 patients who received one IGB, at two-year follow-up, 45 patients still maintained their reduced weight, while 7 had returned to their baseline weight, and 18 patients had experienced a "yo-yo" effect with an average weight gain of 2.7 kg.

In our cohort, over an average longer-term follow-up period of 20 months, we found that 20% of patients were unable to maintain their initial weight loss, which necessitated a referral for bariatric surgery for most. The number of IGB treatments did not appear to significantly affect the long-term outcomes in this regard, although it should be noted that almost 50% of each group had chosen to discontinue their clinical follow-up during the study period. For those in follow-up who maintained their weight loss, this seemed to plateau at 12 months (with approx. 9% of baseline weight loss) and then decline following this period. While these results might suggest that the durability of weight loss outcomes with IGB treatment can be limited in the longer term, findings to date certainly demonstrate improved weight loss maintenance as compared with current standard of care (i.e., lifestyle interventions alone) and highlight the need for more prospective, controlled trials examining the efficacy of serial IGB therapy in the long-term treatment of obesity and NAFLD. Furthermore, it reinforces the important need for supplementary, holistic measures (psychological support) to optimise the management of obesity and other metabolic diseases.

The safety of IGB therapy has been verified in several earlier studies. Although our analysis revealed a 10% premature removal rate (due primarily to intolerance), which is higher than that reported in previous publications [19], the majority of patients underwent successful, uncomplicated insertions. The main side effects of nausea, vomiting, bloating, and abdominal cramping were reported to relent by 1–3 weeks following the point of insertion.

There are several limitations to our study. Firstly, this was an uncontrolled, retrospective review; therefore, we could not directly compare our outcomes with an untreated group, and some biochemical and anthropometric indices were not available in a substantive number of patients to enable a robust analysis on such changes beyond six months of follow-up. Furthermore, the number of patients who had received two and three serial IGBs was not comparable with those who had received only one IGB, which may have diminished the statistical significance of some outcome measures. Nonetheless, our results at six and twelve months are consistent with findings described in previous reports [19, 32]. Prospective studies examining longer-term outcomes, involving two or more serial IGBs, are indeed required to further validate these important endpoints and the potential utility of IGB therapy in the management of obesity and NAFLD.

In conclusion, obesity and its related complications, including NAFLD/NASH, will continue to present a major health burden if rates continue to rise over the next decade. Weight loss remains the primary treatment recommendation for most, but modalities to affect successful and durable weight loss are limited. While medical therapies are awaited, and bariatric surgery is not a viable option for all, endoscopic bariatric devices, such as the IGB, provide an alternative or adjunctive treatment with proven efficacy in the short-medium term, with an acceptable safety profile. More studies will be required to determine their potential role as a therapeutic weight loss option in the longer term and whether advanced metabolic liver diseases can definitely regress following effective treatment.

Acknowledgments

The authors acknowledge the support of the Obesity Action Campaign, as well as all the patients for their participation in the study.

References

[1] S. Bellentani, F. Scaglioni, M. Marino, and G. Bedogni, "Epidemiology of non-alcoholic fatty liver disease," *Digestive Diseases*, vol. 28, no. 1, pp. 155–161, 2010.

[2] M. R. Charlton, J. M. Burns, R. A. Pedersen, K. D. Watt, J. K. Heimbach, and R. A. Dierkhising, "Frequency and outcomes of liver transplantation for nonalcoholic steatohepatitis in the United States," *Gastroenterology*, vol. 141, no. 4, pp. 1249–1253, 2011.

[3] P. Dietrich and C. Hellerbrand, "Non-alcoholic fatty liver disease, obesity and the metabolic syndrome," *Best Practice & Research Clinical Gastroenterology*, vol. 28, no. 4, pp. 637–653, 2014.

[4] J. L. Temple, P. Cordero, J. Li, V. Nguyen, and J. A. Oben, "A guide to non-alcoholic fatty liver disease in childhood and adolescence," *International Journal of Molecular Sciences*, vol. 17, no. 6, article no. 947, 2016.

[5] P. Cordero, P. Gonzalez-Muniesa, F. I. Milagro, J. Campion, and J. A. Martinez, "Perinatal maternal feeding with an energy dense diet and/or micronutrient mixture drives offspring fat distribution depending on the sex and growth stage," *Journal of Animal Physiology and Animal Nutrition*, vol. 99, no. 5, pp. 834–840, 2015.

[6] P. Cordero, J. Li, and J. A. Oben, "Epigenetics of obesity: beyond the genome sequence," *Current Opinion in Clinical Nutrition & Metabolic Care*, vol. 18, no. 4, pp. 361–366, 2015.

[7] P. Manna and S. K. Jain, "Obesity, oxidative stress, adipose tissue dysfunction, and the associated health risks: causes and therapeutic strategies," *Metabolic Syndrome and Related Disorders*, vol. 13, no. 10, pp. 423–444, 2015.

[8] M. Ng, T. Fleming, M. Robinson, and et al, "Global, regional, and national prevalence of overweight and obesity in children and adults during 1980–2013: a systematic analysis for the Global Burden of Disease Study 2013," *The Lancet*, vol. 384, no. 9945, pp. 766–781, 2014.

[9] P. Gonzalez-Muniesa, M. Mártinez-González, F. B. Hu et al., "Obesity," *Nature Reviews Disease Primers*, vol. 3, p. 17034, 2017.

[10] C. D. Williams, J. Stengel, M. I. Asike et al., "Prevalence of nonalcoholic fatty liver disease and nonalcoholic steatohepatitis among a largely middle-aged population utilizing ultrasound and liver biopsy: a prospective study," *Gastroenterology*, vol. 140, no. 1, pp. 124–131, 2011.

[11] M. Ekstedt, L. E. Franzén, U. L. Mathiesen et al., "Long-term follow-up of patients with NAFLD and elevated liver enzymes," *Hepatology*, vol. 44, no. 4, pp. 865–873, 2006.

[12] D. L. White, F. Kanwal, and H. B. El-Serag, "Association between nonalcoholic fatty liver disease and risk for hepatocellular cancer, based on systematic review," *Clinical Gastroenterology and Hepatology*, vol. 10, no. 12, pp. 1342.e2–1359.e2, 2012.

[13] L. A. Adams, J. F. Lymp, J. St. Sauver et al., "The natural history of nonalcoholic fatty liver disease: a population-based cohort study," *Gastroenterology*, vol. 129, no. 1, pp. 113–121, 2005.

[14] E. E. Calle, C. Rodriguez, K. Walker-Thurmond, and M. J. Thun, "Overweight, obesity, and mortality from cancer in a prospectively studied cohort of U.S. adults," *The New England Journal of Medicine*, vol. 348, no. 17, pp. 1625–1638, 2003.

[15] M. Lazo, R. Hernaez, S. Bonekamp et al., "Non-alcoholic fatty liver disease and mortality among US adults: prospective cohort study," *BMJ*, vol. 343, no. 7836, Article ID d6891, p. 1245, 2011.

[16] S. Byrne, Z. Cooper, and C. Fairburn, "Weight maintenance and relapse in obesity: A qualitative study," *International Journal of Obesity*, vol. 27, no. 8, pp. 955–962, 2003.

[17] S. Phelan, J. O. Hill, W. Lang et al., "Recovery from relapse among successful weight maintainers," *American Journal of Clinical Nutrition*, vol. 78, pp. 1079–1084, 2003.

[18] L. Sjoström, M. Peltonen, P. Jacobson et al., "Association of bariatric surgery with long-term remission of type 2 diabetes and with microvascular and macrovascular complications," *Journal of the American Medical Association*, vol. 311, no. 22, pp. 2297–2304, 2014.

[19] I. Imaz, C. Martinez-Cervell, E. E. García-Álvarez, J. M. Sendra-Gutiérrez, and J. González-Enríquez, "Safety and effectiveness of the intragastric balloon for obesity. A meta-analysis," *Obesity Surgery*, vol. 18, no. 7, pp. 841–846, 2008.

[20] A. Genco, T. Bruni, S. B. Doldi et al., "BioEnterics intragastric balloon: the Italian experience with 2,515 patients," *Obesity Surgery*, vol. 15, no. 8, pp. 1161–1164, 2005.

[21] L. Folini, A. Veronelli, A. Benetti et al., "Liver steatosis (LS) evaluated through chemical-shift magnetic resonance imaging liver enzymes in morbid obesity; effect of weight loss obtained with intragastric balloon gastric banding," *Acta Diabetologica*, vol. 51, no. 3, pp. 361–368, 2014.

[22] R. Forlano, A. M. Ippolito, A. Iacobellis et al., "Effect of the BioEnterics intragastric balloon on weight, insulin resistance, and liver steatosis in obese patients," *Gastrointestinal Endoscopy*, vol. 71, no. 6, pp. 927–933, 2010.

[23] J. Li, P. Cordero, V. Nguyen, and J. A. Oben, "The role of vitamins in the pathogenesis of non-alcoholic fatty liver disease," *Integrative Medicine Insights*, vol. 11, pp. 19–25, 2016.

[24] G. C. Nunes, D. Pajecki, M. E. de Melo, M. C. Mancini, R. de Cleva, and M. A. Santo, "Assessment of Weight Loss With the Intragastric Balloon in Patients With Different Degrees of Obesity," *Surgical Laparoscopy, Endoscopy & Percutaneous Techniques*, vol. 27, no. 4, pp. e83–e86, 2017.

[25] T. Karlas, D. Petroff, M. Sasso et al., "Individual patient data meta-analysis of controlled attenuation parameter (CAP) technology for assessing steatosis," *Journal of Hepatology*, vol. 66, no. 5, pp. 1022–1030, 2017.

[26] M. Marfell-Jones, "Preface," *Kinanthropometry VIII: Proceedings of the 8th International Conference of the International Society for the Advancement of Kinanthropometry (ISAK)*, p. viii, 2003.

[27] D. R. Matthews, J. P. Hosker, A. S. Rudenski, B. A. Naylor, D. F. Treacher, and R. C. Turner, "Homeostasis model assessment: insulin resistance and β-cell function from fasting plasma glucose and insulin concentrations in man," *Diabetologia*, vol. 28, no. 7, pp. 412–419, 1985.

[28] K. V. Patel, J. Ooi, S. Ray, N. Griffin, and J. A. Oben, "Abdominal pain following obesity treatment," *Gut*, vol. 63, no. 2, pp. 364-365, 2014.

[29] A. Dee, K. Kearns, C. O'Neill et al., "The direct and indirect costs of both overweight and obesity: A systematic review," *BMC Research Notes*, vol. 7, no. 1, article no. 242, 2014.

[30] A. Genco, G. López-Nava, C. Wahlen et al., "Multi-Centre european experience with intragastric balloon in overweight populations: 13 years of experience," *Obesity Surgery*, vol. 23, no. 4, pp. 515–521, 2013.

[31] A. Genco, M. Cipriano, V. Bacci et al., "BioEnterics® Intragastric Balloon (BIB®): A short-term, double-blind, randomised, controlled, crossover study on weight reduction in morbidly obese patients," *International Journal of Obesity*, vol. 30, no. 1, pp. 129–133, 2006.

[32] E. M. H. Mathus-Vliegen and G. N. J. Tytgat, "Intragastric balloon for treatment-resistant obesity: Safety, tolerance, and efficacy of 1-year balloon treatment followed by a 1-year balloon-free follow-up," *Gastrointestinal Endoscopy*, vol. 61, no. 1, pp. 19–27, 2005.

[33] E. M. Brunt, D. E. Kleiner, L. A. Wilson, P. Belt, and B. A. Neuschwander-Tetri, "Nonalcoholic fatty liver disease (NAFLD) activity score and the histopathologic diagnosis in NAFLD: distinct clinicopathologic meanings," *Hepatology*, vol. 53, no. 3, pp. 810–820, 2011.

[34] Y.-M. Lee, H. C. Low, L. G. Lim et al., "Intragastric balloon significantly improves nonalcoholic fatty liver disease activity score in obese patients with nonalcoholic steatohepatitis: A pilot study," *Gastrointestinal Endoscopy*, vol. 76, no. 4, pp. 756–760, 2012.

[35] A. Genco, M. Cipriano, V. Bacci et al., "Intragastric balloon followed by diet vs intragastric balloon followed by another balloon: A prospective study on 100 patients," *Obesity Surgery*, vol. 20, no. 11, pp. 1496–1500, 2010.

[36] A. Genco, S. Balducci, V. Bacci et al., "Intragastric balloon or diet alone? A retrospective evaluation," *Obesity Surgery*, vol. 18, no. 8, pp. 989–992, 2008.

[37] K. Mitura and K. Garnysz, "In search of the ideal patient for the intragastric balloon - Short- and long-term results in 70 obese patients," *Wideochirurgia i Inne Techniki Maloinwazyjne*, vol. 10, no. 4, pp. 541–547, 2015.

23

Indications for Endoscopic Ultrasound-Guided Pancreatic Drainage: For Benign or Malignant Cases?

Daisuke Uchida, Hironari Kato, Yosuke Saragai, Saimon Takada, Sho Mizukawa, Shinichiro Muro, Yutaka Akimoto, Takeshi Tomoda, Kazuyuki Matsumoto, Shigeru Horiguchi, and Hiroyuki Okada

Department of Gastroenterology, Okayama University Hospital, 2-5-1 Shikata-cho, Kita-ku, Okayama 700-8558, Japan

Correspondence should be addressed to Daisuke Uchida; d.uchida0309@gmail.com

Academic Editor: Yousuke Nakai

Background and Aims. Recurrent pancreatitis associated with pancreatic strictures requires treatment with endoscopic retrograde pancreatography (ERP), but it is sometimes technically unsuccessful. Endoscopic ultrasound-guided pancreatic drainage (EUS-PD) was developed as an alternative to a surgical approach after failed ERP; however, the indications for EUS-PD are unclear. In this study, we evaluated the outcomes of EUS-PD and established the indications for EUS-PD. *Methods.* A total of 15 patients had indications for EUS-PD for recurrent pancreatitis due to pancreatic strictures. There were eight patients with benign pancreatic strictures and seven with malignant pancreatic strictures. The success rate, adverse events, and long-term outcomes were evaluated. *Results.* The technical success rates of benign and malignant strictures were 75% (6/8) and 100% (7/7), respectively, and clinical success was achieved in 100% (6/6) and 87.5% of cases (6/7), respectively. Rendezvous procedures were performed in two patients with benign strictures. The adverse event (AE) rate was 26.7% (4/15) and included cases of peritonitis, bleeding, and stent migration. Reinterventions were performed in three patients with benign strictures and two with malignant strictures. *Conclusions.* EUS-PD was an appropriate treatment for not only benign strictures but also malignant strictures with recurrent pancreatitis after failed ERP. However, the AE rate was high, and reinterventions were required in some cases during long-term follow-up. The indications for EUS-PD should be considered carefully, and careful follow-up is needed.

1. Introduction

Symptomatic pancreatic strictures are troubling problems associated with pancreatic diseases. Benign pancreatic strictures have various causes, such as chronic pancreatitis, anastomotic strictures after pancreaticoduodenectomy, and traumatic pancreatic injuries. Endoscopic retrograde pancreatography (ERP) and drainage are feasible treatments for benign strictures [1–3]. Recently, ERP in altered anatomy using a balloon-assisted enteroscope was developed, and anastomotic strictures after surgery can now be treated without surgical treatment [4]. Malignant pancreatic strictures with recurrent pancreatitis are rare but sometimes occur in cases with pancreatic head tumors. ERP is the standard approach for symptomatic malignant strictures, as with benign ones; however, some patients require a surgical approach [5–7]. Surgical treatment is a gold standard therapy for uncontrollable recurrent pancreatitis but is an invasive treatment with a high adverse event (AE) rate [8, 9].

Endoscopic ultrasound- (EUS-) guided pancreatic drainage (EUS-PD) was developed as an alternative to a surgical approach after failed ERP; however, the indications for EUS-PD remain controversial [10, 11]. It is a feasible treatment but is technically challenging, and the AE rate is relatively high [10, 12, 13]. In this study, we evaluated the outcomes of EUS-PD and considered the indications.

2. Materials and Methods

2.1. Patients. Fifteen patients with recurrent pancreatitis who were admitted to Okayama University Hospital from September 2012 to December 2017 were enrolled. Conventional ERP had been attempted in all patients, but drainage could not be achieved. EUS-PD was carried out

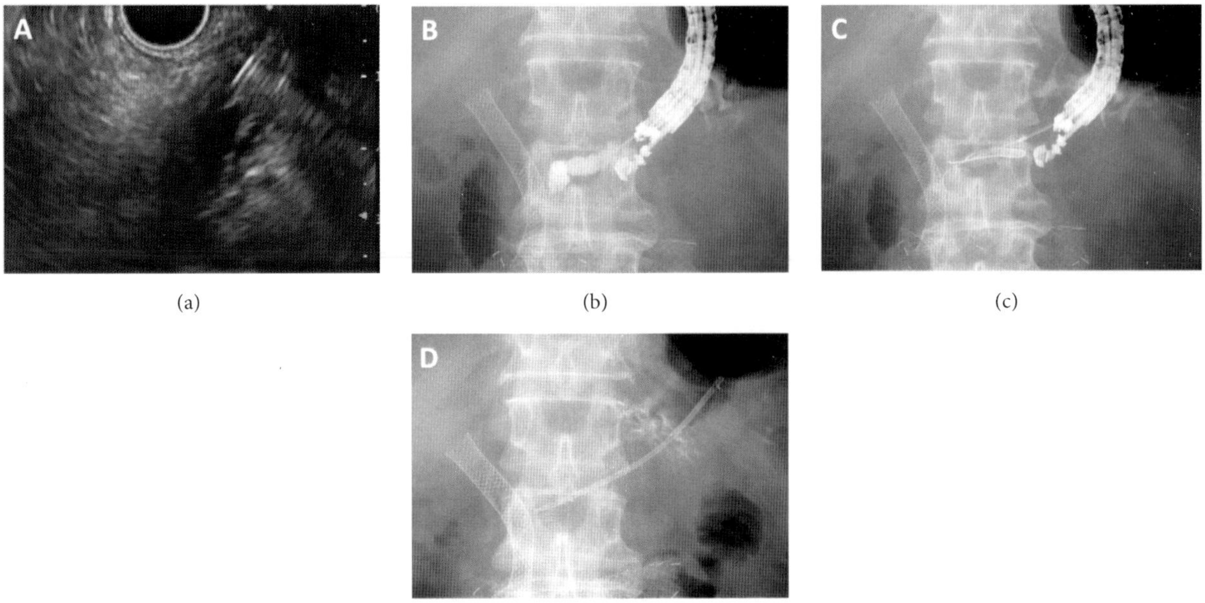

(a) (b) (c) (d)

Figure 1: The EUS-PD procedure for a patient with obstructive pancreatitis due to pancreatic head cancer. (a) The pancreatic duct was punctured via the stomach with a 19-gauge needle under EUS guidance. (b) The pancreatogram was obtained by the injection of contrast agent. (c) A 0.025-inch guidewire was advanced into the pancreatic duct, and the tract was dilated using a long-tapered catheter or a diathermy catheter. (d) A 7-Fr plastic stent was inserted over the guidewire.

after failed ERP and after obtaining written informed consent. There were nine patients with benign pancreatic strictures. Pancreatic drainage was required for strictures of pancreatodigestive anastomosis after pancreatoduodenectomy in six patients and chronic pancreatitis in two patients. In contrast, there were seven patients with malignant pancreatic strictures associated with pancreatic head tumors, six patients with pancreatic cancer, and one patient with cholangiocarcinoma (Table 1). All of them had distant metastasis and were not indicated for surgical treatments.

2.2. EUS-PD Procedure. The EUS-PD procedure is shown in Figure 1. The dilated pancreatic duct was punctured anterogradely via the stomach by a 19-gauge needle under EUS guidance. The 0.025-inch guidewire (Visiglide2; Olympus, Tokyo, Japan) was advanced as far as possible. The puncture tract was then dilated by a long-tapered catheter (3.5Fr; PR-V220Q, Olympus, Tokyo, Japan). If this dilation failed, a diathermy catheter was used to dilate the tract. Finally, a 7-Fr plastic stent (Flexima; Boston Scientific Japan, Tokyo, or Advanix; Boston Scientific Japan, Tokyo, or Cotton-Leung; COOK Japan, Tokyo) was placed into the pancreatic duct. In patients with benign strictures, stents were placed across the papilla or at the anastomotic sites if feasible.

2.3. Definition of Success. Technical success was defined as the placement of a plastic stent into the pancreatic duct. Clinical success was defined as the improvement of symptoms and pancreatitis within a week.

3. Results

The patients' characteristics and outcomes are shown in Table 1. The technical success rate was 86.7% (13/15), and clinical success was achieved in 92.3% (12/13) of cases. The technical and clinical success rates of benign strictures were 75% (6/8) and 100% (6/6), respectively, and those of malignant strictures were 100% (7/7) and 85.7% (6/7), respectively. There were two technical failures in benign cases. In both patients, EUS-PD was attempted because anastomotic strictures developed after pancreaticoduodenectomy, but plastic stents could not be placed because of unsuccessful advancement of the guidewire after puncture (cases 1 and 2). They were treated with a percutaneous approach and ultimately improved. Clinical success was not achieved in one patient with malignant stricture (case 13). He underwent EUS-PD for obstructive pancreatitis with pancreatic head cancer and failed to regain the ability for oral intake until his death due to his poor general condition.

The median follow-up period was 223 days (benign: 503 days, malignant: 116 days). AEs occurred in 4 cases (26.7%) during the follow-up period, including 3 benign cases and 1 malignant case. In the benign cases, bleeding, stent migration, and peritonitis occurred. Peritonitis occurred in case 8 the day after the procedure. He was suspected of having pancreatic juice leakage from the side holes of the plastic stent, and he required replacement of a plastic stent. Stent migration into the stomach was detected incidentally at the 97th day after the procedure in case 4. He was followed up with conservative treatment because he had no symptoms. Bleeding from the puncture tract occurred at the 371st day

TABLE 1: Patients' characteristics and outcomes of EUS-PD.

Case no.	Sex	Age (years)	Indication	Benign or malignant	Diameter of PD (mm)	Technical success	Clinical success	Rendezvous procedure	Adverse events	Reintervention
1	M	75	Anastomotic stricture after pancreaticojejunostomy	Benign	4	No	NA	NA	None	NA
2	M	67	Anastomotic stricture after pancreaticojejunostomy	Benign	4	No	NA	NA	None	NA
3	M	64	Pancreatic stricture with chronic pancreatitis	Benign	21	Yes	Yes	No	Bleeding	Yes
4	M	70	Anastomotic stricture after pancreaticogastrostomy	Benign	8	Yes	Yes	Yes	Stent migration	No
5	M	47	Pancreatic stricture with chronic pancreatitis	Benign	10	Yes	Yes	Yes	None	Yes
6	M	78	Anastomotic stricture after pancreaticogastrostomy	Benign	18	Yes	Yes	No	None	No
7	F	66	Anastomotic stricture after pancreaticojejunostomy	Benign	6	Yes	Yes	No	None	Yes
8	M	43	Anastomotic stricture after pancreaticojejunostomy	Benign	4	Yes	Yes	No	Peritonitis	Yes
9	M	70	Obstructive pancreatitis with pancreatic cancer	Malignant	7	Yes	Yes	No	None	No
10	F	83	Obstructive pancreatitis with pancreatic cancer	Malignant	9	Yes	Yes	No	None	Yes
11	M	64	Obstructive pancreatitis with pancreatic cancer	Malignant	7	Yes	Yes	No	None	No
12	F	82	Obstructive pancreatitis with pancreatic cancer	Malignant	12	Yes	Yes	No	None	No
13	M	88	Obstructive pancreatitis with pancreatic cancer	Malignant	7	Yes	No	No	None	No
14	M	77	Obstructive pancreatitis with cholangiocarcinoma	Malignant	5	Yes	Yes	No	None	No
15	F	66	Obstructive pancreatitis with pancreatic cancer	Malignant	4	Yes	Yes	No	Peritonitis	No

EUS-PD, endoscopic ultrasound-guided pancreatic duct drainage; PD, pancreatic duct; NA, not available.

Table 2: Results of previous studies performed on EUS-PD.

Reference	Study design	Number of patients	Technical success (%)	Clinical success (%)	Adverse events (%)
Tvberg et al. [13]	Prospective observational	80	89	81	20
Fujii et al. [12]	Retrospective	45	74	83	6
Tessier et al. [10]	Retrospective	36	92	70	14
Oh et al. [14]	Prospective observational	25	100	100	20
Ergun et al. [15]	Retrospective	20	90	72	10
Kurihara et al. [16]	Retrospective	17	88	100	6

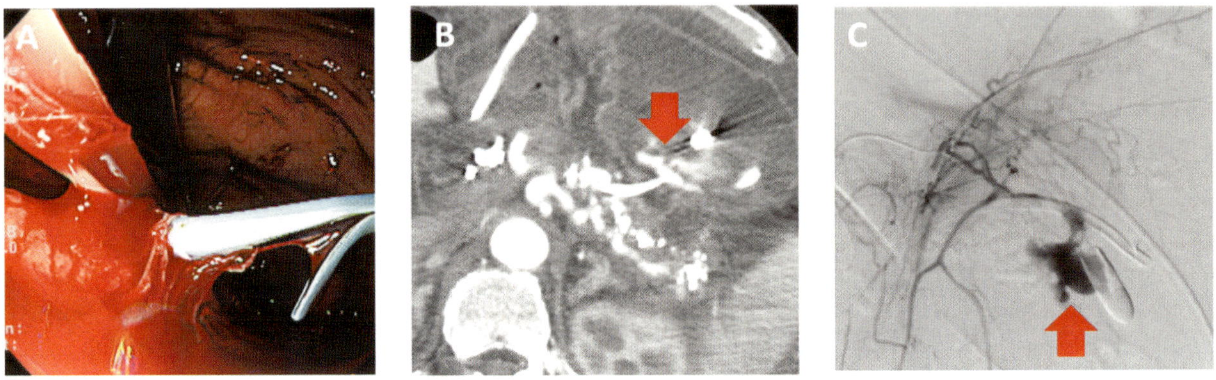

(a) (b) (c)

Figure 2: Bleeding occurred at the 371st day after EUS-PD in case 3. (a) Arterial bleeding from the transgastric puncture tract. (b) Contrast-enhanced computed tomography revealed extravasation into the stomach (arrow). (c) Interventional radiology revealed a pseudoaneurysm from the left gastric artery (arrow), and arterial embolization was performed.

after EUS-PD in case 3 (Figure 2). In this case, a rendezvous procedure failed, and periodic stent replacement via the puncture tract was performed because of recurrent pancreatitis due to stent occlusion. He had a bleeding from puncture tract and required arterial embolization with interventional radiology. In the malignant cases, only one AE (peritonitis) occurred the day after the procedure; however, the patient's condition improved with conservative treatment (case 15).

Reinterventions were performed in four patients (cases 3, 5, 8, and 10). Cases 3 and 10 underwent stent replacement because of recurrent pancreatitis associated with stent occlusion (patency times: 54 and 224 days, respectively). All of them achieved technical and clinical success, but they still require periodic stent replacement. Case 5 underwent rendezvous procedure for benign stricture with chronic pancreatitis. He was also treated with transpapillary stent replacements at regular intervals. Case 8 developed peritonitis the day after EUS-PD, which might have been caused by pancreatic juice leakage via the puncture tract. The stent was then exchanged to a different type of plastic stent without side holes (Through Pass TYPE-IT; Gadelius Medical, Tokyo, Japan). After reintervention, the patient's peritonitis improved.

4. Discussion

Recurrent pancreatitis is a troubling problem associated with pancreatic disease and is caused by pancreatic stricture in most cases. There are various causes of stricture, such as chronic pancreatitis, anastomotic stenosis after surgery, and malignant tumor. A retrograde approach with ERP is most common treatment for these strictures [1–6]. However, ERP sometimes fails because of technical difficulties, and a percutaneous or surgical approach is required. EUS-PD was developed as an alternative treatment to these invasive approaches after failed ERP [10, 11, 15, 17, 18]. While this is an innovative and useful procedure, it remains technically challenging and is associated with a high AE rate. Tyberg et al. reported the findings of a multicenter retrospective study of EUS-PD [13]. They found a high success rate, although the AE rate was as high as 20%. Various AEs were noted, including severe ones that required surgical treatment. The study was a relatively large-scale study of 80 patients; however, no predictors of AE were identified. Oh et al. reported a high success rate of EUS-PD with a fully covered self-expandable metal stent, but the AE rate was also high in that study (Table 2) [14]. There are some other reports, but the indication for EUS-PD is still unclear [10, 12, 15, 19]. We evaluated our case series and considered the indications for EUS-PD.

Anastomotic structure after failed balloon-assisted ERP is a candidate for EUS-PD. The recently developed balloon-assisted ERCP technique has allowed anastomotic pancreatic and biliary strictures after surgery to be treated without a percutaneous or surgical approach [4, 16, 20]. However, pancreatic anastomosis is often more difficult than biliary anastomosis. In our study, 6 of 15 patients underwent EUS-PD after failed balloon-assisted ERP. Two of these patients failed their procedure due to the operator's inexperience and required percutaneous treatments, while the other four achieved clinical success and benefitted significantly from EUS-PD.

We consider that obstructive pancreatitis associated with pancreatic tumor is also a candidate indication for EUS-PD. In our series, there were seven patients with malignant pancreatic strictures. All of them achieved technical success, and six of them achieved clinical success. Peritonitis occurred in case 15, but her condition improved with conservative treatment. Stent occlusion occurred in case 10 at the 224th day after EUS-PD, and reintervention was performed. Recurrent pancreatitis did not occur due to periodic stent replacement after stent occlusion. AEs, including stent occlusion, were rarer in cases with malignant strictures (12.5%) than in those with benign strictures (37.5%), though not to a significant degree (P=0.12). This discrepancy might have been caused by the difference in the follow-up period (116 days and 503 days). EUS-PD may be feasible as a palliative treatment for patients with malignant strictures.

Chronic pancreatitis is the most common disease causing troubling pancreatic strictures. In this study, two patients with chronic pancreatitis underwent EUS-PD after failed ERP. Both achieved technical and clinical success, but bleeding from a fistula associated with pseudoaneurysm occurred at the 371st day after EUS-PD in case 3. He underwent periodic stent replacement because a rendezvous procedure failed due to pancreatic stones. Therefore, case 3 required long-term stent placement via the puncture tract. Pseudoaneurysm from the gastric artery might be induced by mechanical stimulation with long-term stent placement and inflammation of chronic pancreatitis. Kurihara et al. also reported the occurrence of aneurysms associated with the EUS-PD procedure in patients with recurrent pancreatitis [19]. Stent removal should be considered in cases with chronic pancreatitis. If stent removal is impossible, a surgical approach should be considered.

In our cases series, benign strictures requiring long-term stent placement might be predictors of AEs, such as bleeding or stent migration. However, this study is limited by the small number of patients and its retrospective design, and further prospective evaluations should be performed.

In conclusion, EUS-PD conferred benefits on patients with uncontrollable recurrent pancreatitis. In cases of benign strictures, especially with chronic pancreatitis, rendezvous procedures and eventual stent removal should be considered to avoid late adverse events. In cases with malignant strictures, a high success rate was achieved, and severe AEs did not occur. Therefore, EUS-PD is a promising approach as a palliative treatment for patients with malignant strictures. However, EUS-guided puncture procedures should be avoided in patients with resectable tumors, as there are risks of tumor cell dissemination.

EUS-PD is a feasible and safe approach but is still a relatively primitive procedure with a high AE rate. It is very difficult to define the indications for EUS-PD, as pancreatic strictures can be caused by various complicated conditions. The technique, devices, and follow-up protocol of EUS-PD should be established in a future study.

Ethical Approval

This study was approved by the institutional review board of Okayama University. The study was registered in the UMIN protocol registration system (identification number UMIN000031756).

References

[1] M. Delhaye, M. Arvanitakis, G. Verset, M. Cremer, and J. Devière, "Long-term clinical outcome after endoscopic pancreatic ductal drainage for patients with painful chronic pancreatitis," *Clinical Gastroenterology and Hepatology*, vol. 2, no. 12, pp. 1096–1106, 2004.

[2] N. Eleftheriadis, F. Dinu, M. Delhaye et al., "Long-term outcome after pancreatic stenting in severe chronic pancreatitis," *Endoscopy*, vol. 37, no. 3, pp. 223–230, 2005.

[3] C. M. Wilcox and S. Varadarajulu, "Endoscopic therapy for chronic pancreatitis: An evidence-based review," *Current Gastroenterology Reports*, vol. 8, no. 2, pp. 104–110, 2006.

[4] G. B. Haber, "Double balloon endoscopy for pancreatic and biliary access in altered anatomy (with videos)," *Gastrointestinal Endoscopy*, vol. 66, no. 3, pp. S47–S50, 2007.

[5] G. Costamagna and M. Mutignani, "Pancreatic stenting for malignant ductal obstruction," *Digestive and Liver Disease*, vol. 36, no. 9, pp. 635–638, 2004.

[6] T. Wehrmann, A. Riphaus, M. B. Frenz, K. Martchenko, and N. Stergiou, "Endoscopic pancreatic duct stenting for relief of pancreatic cancer pain," *European Journal of Gastroenterology & Hepatology*, vol. 17, no. 12, pp. 1395–1400, 2005.

[7] Y. Kudo, N. Sato, T. Tamura, and K. Hirata, "Triple bypass for advanced pancreatic head cancer associated with biliary stricture, duodenal stenosis, and recurrent obstructive pancreatitis," *Surgical Case Reports*, vol. 2, no. 79, 2016.

[8] W. H. Nealon and J. C. Thompson, "Progressive loss of pancreatic function in chronic pancreatitis is delayed by main pancreatic duct decompression: A longitudinal prospective analysis of the modified puestow procedure," *Annals of Surgery*, vol. 217, no. 5, pp. 458–468, 1993.

[9] D. B. Adams, M. C. Ford, and M. C. Anderson, "Outcome after lateral pancreaticojejunostomy for chronic pancreatitis," *Annals of Surgery*, vol. 219, no. 5, pp. 481–489, 1994.

[10] G. Tessier, E. Bories, M. Arvanitakis et al., "EUS-guided pancreatogastrostomy and pancreatobulbostomy for the treatment of pain in patients with pancreatic ductal dilatation inaccessible for transpapillary endoscopic therapy," *Gastrointestinal Endoscopy*, vol. 65, no. 2, pp. 233–241, 2007.

[11] A. Ginès, S. Varadarajulu, and B. Napoleon, "EUS 2008 Working Group document: evaluation of EUS-guided pancreatic-duct drainage (with video)," *Gastrointestinal Endoscopy*, vol. 69, no. 2, pp. S43–S48, 2009.

[12] L. L. Fujii, M. D. Topazian, B. K. Abu Dayyeh et al., "EUS-guided pancreatic duct intervention: Outcomes of a single tertiary-care referral center experience," *Gastrointestinal Endoscopy*, vol. 78, no. 6, pp. 854–864, 2013.

[13] A. Tyberg, R. Z. Sharaiha, P. Kedia et al., "EUS-guided pancreatic drainage for pancreatic strictures after failed ERCP: a multicenter international collaborative study," *Gastrointestinal Endoscopy*, vol. 85, no. 1, pp. 164–169, 2017.

[14] D. Oh, D. H. Park, M. K. Cho et al., "Feasibility and safety of a fully covered self-expandable metal stent with antimigration properties for EUS-guided pancreatic duct drainage: Early and midterm outcomes (with video)," *Gastrointestinal Endoscopy*, vol. 83, no. 2, pp. 366–373, 2016.

[15] M. Ergun, T. Aouattah, C. Gillain, J.-F. Gigot, C. Hubert, and P. H. Deprez, "Endoscopic ultrasound-guided transluminal drainage of pancreatic duct obstruction: Long-term outcome," *Endoscopy*, vol. 43, no. 6, pp. 518–525, 2011.

[16] M. Shimatani, H. Hatanaka, H. Kogure et al., "Diagnostic and Therapeutic Endoscopic Retrograde Cholangiography Using a Short-Type Double-Balloon Endoscope in Patients with Altered Gastrointestinal Anatomy: A Multicenter Prospective Study in Japan," *American Journal of Gastroenterology*, vol. 111, no. 12, pp. 1750–1758, 2016.

[17] A. Irisawa, T. Hikichi, G. Shibukawa et al., "Pancreatobiliary drainage using the EUS-FNA technique: EUS-BD and EUS-PD," *Journal of Hepato-Biliary-Pancreatic Sciences*, vol. 16, no. 5, pp. 598–604, 2009.

[18] S. Varadarajulu and J. M. Trevino, "Review of EUS-guided pancreatic duct drainage (with video)," *Gastrointestinal Endoscopy*, vol. 69, no. 2, pp. S200–S202, 2009.

[19] T. Kurihara, T. Itoi, A. Sofuni, F. Itokawa, and F. Moriyasu, "Endoscopic ultrasonography-guided pancreatic duct drainage after failed endoscopic retrograde cholangiopancreatography in patients with malignant and benign pancreatic duct obstructions," *Digestive Endoscopy*, vol. 25, no. 2, pp. 109–116, 2013.

[20] M. Shimatani, M. Takaoka, M. Matsushita, and K. Okazaki, "Endoscopic approaches for pancreatobiliary diseases in patients with altered gastrointestinal anatomy," *Digestive Endoscopy*, vol. 26, pp. 70–78, 2014.

24

Maintenance of Remission with Partial Enteral Nutrition Therapy in Pediatric Crohn's Disease

Jacqueline M. Schulman,[1,2] Liat Pritzker,[2] and Ron Shaoul[2]

[1] *The Ruth and Bruce Rappaport Faculty of Medicine, Technion-Israel Institute of Technology, 3525433 Haifa, Israel*
[2] *Pediatric Gastroenterology & Nutrition Unit, Ruth Children's Hospital, Rambam Medical Center, 3109601 Haifa, Israel*

Correspondence should be addressed to Ron Shaoul; shaoul_r@012.net.il

Academic Editor: Jennifer Jones

Background. Partial enteral nutrition (PEN) may be helpful for the maintenance of remission in pediatric Crohn's disease patients. *Aims.* To evaluate the efficacy of PEN treatment for preventing clinical relapse. *Methods.* We retrospectively assessed 42 pediatric Crohn's disease patients who entered clinical remission on 4–12 weeks of exclusive enteral nutrition (EEN) and were maintained on PEN as a supplementary diet. We evaluated the efficacy of the treatment at different time points using the weighted Pediatric Crohn Disease Activity Index (wPCDAI), Physician Global Assessment, laboratory parameters, and growth of each patient. Additionally, we assessed the use of concomitant medications. *Results.* The median length of remission with PEN was 6 (0–36) months. Patients' remission was maintained on PEN without concomitant medications for a median time of zero months (0–16). The mean body mass index in the PEN group increased from 18.1 to 18.8 after six months of PEN. The median wPCDAI decreased from 30 at diagnosis to 5.0 after EEN and increased to 7.5 after three months of PEN. Overall, the median wPCDAI decreased by 26.2. *Conclusions.* PEN treatment was partially effective in maintaining remission and was able to increase BMI and lower wPCDAI. Most patients required concomitant medication after PEN initiation.

1. Introduction

Crohn's disease (CD) is a chronic disease that currently lacks a cure. Aside from the widespread prevalence of CD in adult patients, there is a rising incidence and prevalence in the pediatric population [1–3]. Treatment of CD patients involves a multidisciplinary approach that aims to induce and maintain clinical, laboratory, and mucosal remission and to ultimately prevent relapses. Current treatment of pediatric CD includes exclusive enteral nutrition (EEN), corticosteroids, immunomodulators, antibiotics, and biological agents together with psychological and psychiatric support.

Pediatric patients with CD are at constant risk of malnutrition, and, thus, proper nutrition is a vital aspect of the treatment of the disease. The liquid diet used in EEN was developed as an alternative to corticosteroid therapy for induction of remission and is gaining worldwide popularity in the medical community. Due to its excellent safety profile and its equipotential to corticosteroids in inducing remission, EEN is now considered a first-line agent to induce remission in children with active CD in many parts of the world [4]. EEN is associated with significantly fewer adverse effects, compared with corticosteroids. Using EEN instead of corticosteroids in pediatric patients has been shown to promote better linear growth, improve bone health, and achieve better mucosal healing [5–7].

As a supplement to their regular diet, partial enteral nutrition (PEN) has proven to be beneficial in the maintenance of remission in adults, especially after EEN treatment [8–13]. Long-term PEN has been shown to be an effective means of decreasing clinical relapse rates and in suppressing endoscopic disease activity [14]. A retrospective study by Wilschanski et al. that investigated the effects of PEN in the pediatric population showed that PEN treatment of children with CD is associated with prolonged remission and better linear growth after treatment with EEN. The patients were allowed a normal daytime diet and received the PEN diet through a nasogastric feeding tube at night [15]. Although several studies suggest that PEN may be helpful for the maintenance of remission in the pediatric population [15, 16], data on the long-term usage of PEN for remission maintenance in pediatric CD patients is still lacking.

We performed a retrospective study to investigate the efficacy of PEN treatment by analyzing the weighted Pediatric Crohn Disease Activity Index (wPCDAI), the Physician Global Assessment (PGA), and laboratory parameters, such as C-reactive protein (CRP) and albumin, as well as the growth of each patient. In particular, we aimed to gain more insight into PEN as a means of preventing clinical relapse, with the goal of improving the treatment for more effective maintenance of remission.

2. Materials and Methods

In our study, we retrospectively assessed pediatric CD patients treated in our clinic. The local ethics board at Rambam Medical Center approved the study and waived the requirement for informed consent. We reviewed the clinical records of 48 children aged 1–20 years diagnosed with CD during the period from January 2001 to June 2013. The patients entered clinical remission on 4–12 weeks of EEN and were subsequently maintained on PEN (50% of total calories as polymeric diet, usually Modulen® IBD) as a supplementary diet. We evaluated the efficacy of the treatment at different time points using the wPCDAI, PGA, laboratory parameters (CRP and albumin), and the growth of each patient in terms of weight, height, and body mass index (BMI). Also, we assessed the use of concomitant medication, such as corticosteroids, thiopurines, anti-TNF agents, methotrexate, and antibiotics in patients maintained on PEN. Children who were not treated with EEN followed by PEN, or for whom we lacked data, were excluded from the study. Six of the 48 patients were excluded from analysis, due to a lack of data, leaving a total of 42 patients to be included in the analysis. Children with CD who refused EN served as the control group, which consisted of 45 patients aged 1–18 years diagnosed with CD between August 2004 and June 2013. Patients in this group were evaluated at different time points using the wPCDAI, PGA, laboratory parameters (CRP and albumin), and the growth of each patient in terms of weight, height, and body mass index (BMI).

Anatomic location and behavior of the disease were evaluated using the Paris classification [17]. The wPCDAI [18] and PGA were used to assess the clinical activity of the disease, with the remission and relapses determined by the judgment of the physician.

Three types of EN were used: Modulen (Nestlé Health Science, Vevey, Switzerland) (90.7%), Ensure® (Abbott Nutrition, Columbus, Ohio) (7.0%), and PediaSure® (Abbott Nutrition, Columbus, Ohio) (2.3%). Further details on the different formulas can be found in the supporting information (Supplementary Table 1, in Supplementary Material available online at https://doi.org/10.1155/2017/5873158). The route of administration was oral, but if not tolerated, nasogastric feeding was used instead.

The patients were followed up regularly, with clinic appointments about once every 4–8 weeks.

Univariate analysis was done with Chi-square or Fisher's exact test for categorical data. Kolmogorov–Smirnov test was used for measuring normal distribution of the quantitative parameters. Based on the result obtained, we chose whether to use a nonparametric test (Mann–Whitney U test) or parametric test (t-test) for the assessment of differences between groups. A multivariate linear regression model was used for the prediction of length of remission with several independent parameters. A P value < 0.05 was considered to be statistically significant in a two-sided test. Statistical analyses were performed with the IBM® SPSS® Statistics software version 21.

3. Results and Discussion

3.1. Results. A total of 42 patients received EEN therapy to induce remission, followed by PEN therapy to maintain remission. Out of these, 30 (71%) were males, and the median age at diagnosis of the patients was 11.5 years (25–75% = 9.2–13.7 years). Patient characteristics at the time of diagnosis are illustrated in Table 1. The control group, which did not receive EN, consisted of 45 patients in total, of whom 31 (69%) were males. The median age at diagnosis in the control group was 14.7 years (25–75% = 12.7–16.3 years).

The median time between diagnosis of the disease and initiation of EEN was 2.0 months (range, 0–112 months). Thirty-seven patients (88%) received EN orally, whereas four patients (10%) required nasogastric feeding, and one patient received feeding via gastrostomy (2%).

Patients on PEN were followed up for a median time of 40 months (25–75% = 25.5–79 months) in the PEN group, while patients in the control group were followed for a median time of 63 months (25–75% = 52–87 months, $P = 0.005$). The resulting median length of remission with PEN was 6.0 months, and the longest remission period was 36 months. The median length of remission in the control group was 6.0 months, and the longest remission period achieved was 45 months ($P = 0.96$). Additional medications, including corticosteroids, thiopurines, anti-TNF agents, methotrexate, and antibiotics, were added to patients according to pediatric gastroenterologist discretion. Of the 42 patients on PEN, 26 (62%) received corticosteroids, 35 (83%) received thiopurines, 14 (33%) received anti-TNF agents, 7 (17%) received methotrexate, and 19 (45%) were given antibiotics at some point. Among the control subjects, 35 (78%) received corticosteroids, 30 (67%) received thiopurines, 10 (22%) received anti-TNF agents, 2 (4%) received methotrexate, and 19 (42%) were given antibiotics at some point. In more than 50% of the patients, remission could not be maintained with PEN alone without the addition of concomitant medications. Those who received concomitant medication in parallel to PEN were analyzed separately from those who received concomitant medication later. Although the parallel group had a longer remission (10.4 versus 8.6 months), the difference was not statistically significant. A summary of the remission rates and use of concomitant medication is presented in Table 2. In the multivariate analysis, there were no significant predictors for length of remission.

TABLE 1: Basic characteristics of the study population at the time of diagnosis.

Covariate	PEN group $N = 42$	Control group $N = 45$	P value*
Age (yr), median [25–75%]	11.5 [9.2–13.7]	14.7 [12.7–16.3]	0.001
Sex, male, n (%)	30 (71)	31 (69)	0.82
Disease location at presentation, n (%)			
L1 (distal ileum ± cecum)	21 (50)	28 (62)	0.28
L2 (colon)	12 (28)	20 (44)	0.18
L3 (ileocolon)	13 (31)	9 (20)	0.32
L4a (upper GI, proximal to ligament of Treitz)	28 (67)	29 (64)	1.00
L4b (upper GI, distal to ligament of Treitz)	1 (2)	5 (11)	0.20
Perianal disease	4 (10)	7 (16)	1.00

yr, years. *Calculated with Chi-square or Fisher's exact test for categorical data and independent samples t-test for continuous variables.

TABLE 2: Remission rates and concomitant medication.

Covariate	PEN group	Control group	P value
Time between diagnosis and EEN initiation (mo), median (range)	2.0 (0–112)		
Route of EN administration, n (%)			
Oral	37/42 (88)		
Nasogastric	4/42 (10)		
PEG	1/42 (2)		
Follow-up time (mo), median [25–75%]	40 [25.5–79]	63 [52–87]	0.005*
Length of remission (mo), median (range)	6.0 (0–36)	6.0 (range: 0–45)	0.96**
Concomitant medication, n (%)			
Corticosteroids	26 (62)	35 (78)	0.16*
Thiopurines	35 (83)	30 (67)	0.09*
Anti-TNF agents	14 (33)	10 (22)	0.34*
Methotrexate	7 (17)	2 (4)	0.08*
Antibiotics	19 (45)	19 (42)	0.83*
Time on PEN without concomitant medication (mo), median (range)**	0 (0–36)		
0	23/43 (55%)		
1–6	13/42 (31%)		
7–12	2/42 (5%)		
13+	4/42 (9%)		
Length of remission with PEN alone, without concomitant medication (mo), median (range)**	0 (0–16)		
0	25/42 (60%)		
1–6	14/42 (33%)		
7–12	2/42 (5%)		
13+	1/42 (2%)		

mo, months; EEN, exclusive enteral nutrition; PEN, partial enteral nutrition; EN, enteral nutrition; PEG, *Percutaneous endoscopic gastrostomy*; TNF, tumor necrosis factor. *Calculated with Chi-square or Fisher's exact test for categorical data and independent samples t-test for continuous variables. **Calculated with Mann–Whitney U tests.

Patients were followed up in terms of various laboratory parameters. In the PEN group, albumin and CRP were recorded before EEN initiation, at the end of EEN therapy, and after three months of PEN treatment. With EEN therapy, there was an increase in the mean albumin level and a decrease in the median CRP, followed by a decrease in albumin and an increase in CRP with PEN. In the control group, albumin and CRP were recorded at diagnosis, after eight weeks, and after five months. The mean albumin level increased after eight weeks and then remained the same

TABLE 3: Laboratory parameters.

Covariate	PEN group	Control group	P value
Albumin (g/L), mean ± SD			
Before EEN/at diagnosis*	35 ± 6	39 ± 6	0.008**
After EEN/eight weeks after diagnosis*	42 ± 5	42 ± 4	0.56**
After three months of PEN/five months after diagnosis*	39 ± 5	42 ± 3	0.007**
CRP (mg/L), median (range)			
Before EEN/at diagnosis*	21 (1–40)	10 (1–65)	0.03***
After EEN/eight weeks after diagnosis*	5 (0–107)	6.5 (1–48)	0.006***
After three months of PEN/ five months after diagnosis*	6.4 (0–180)	5 (1–84)	0.82***

EEN, exclusive enteral nutrition; PEN, partial enteral nutrition; CRP, C-reactive protein. *Control group. **Calculated with Chi-square or Fisher's exact test for categorical data and independent samples t-test for continuous variables. ***Calculated with Mann–Whitney U tests.

TABLE 4: Changes in weight, height, BMI, and wPCDAI over time.

Covariate	PEN group	Control group	P value
Weight (kg), mean ± SD			
Before EEN/at diagnosis*	40.4 ± 13.0	51.5 ± 20.5	$P = 0.002$
After EEN/eight weeks after diagnosis*	42.1 ± 13.2	52.2 ± 19.6	$P = 0.005$
After six months of PEN/eight months after diagnosis*	45.1 ± 13.9	55.5 ± 21.3	$P = 0.011$
Height (m), mean ± SD			
Before EEN/at diagnosis*	1.51 ± 0.17	1.58 ± 0.17	$P = 0.061$
After EEN/eight weeks after diagnosis*	1.51 ± 0.17	1.57 ± 0.17	$P = 0.12$
After six months of PEN/eight months after diagnosis*	1.53 ± 0.17	1.60 ± 0.17	$P = 0.065$
BMI, mean ± SD			
Before EEN/at diagnosis*	16.9 ± 2.3	20.3 ± 4.9	0.001**
After EEN/eight weeks after diagnosis*	18.1 ± 4.2	20.4 ± 5.4	0.03**
After six months of PEN/eight months after diagnosis*	18.8 ± 2.9	21.3 ± 4.8	0.006**
wPCDAI, median [25–75%]			
Before EEN/at diagnosis*	30.0 [20–40]	30.0 [25–42.5]	0.70***
After EEN/eight weeks after diagnosis*	5.0 [0–12.5]	10.0 [7.5–17.5]	0.005***
After three months of PEN/five months after diagnosis*	7.5 [0–17.5]	11.3 [5–27.5]	0.16***
After one year of PEN/one year after diagnosis*	3.8 [0–13.8]	10.0 [0–20]	0.12***
After two years of PEN/two years after diagnosis*	17.5 [10–20]	10.0 [2.5–23.8]	0.43***
After three years of PEN/three years after diagnosis*	17.5 [5–17.5]	15.0 [0–21.9]	0.88***

BMI, body mass index; EEN, exclusive enteral nutrition; PEN, partial enteral nutrition; wPCDAI, weighted Pediatric Crohn's Disease Activity Index. *Control group. **Calculated with Chi-square or Fisher's exact test for categorical data and independent samples t-test for continuous variables. ***Calculated with Mann–Whitney U tests.

after an additional three months, whereas the median CRP decreased after eight weeks and then further decreased after another three months. The laboratory parameters and their changes over time are listed in Table 3.

At each appointment, the height and weight of the patients were measured, and the BMI was calculated. The measurements were recorded and compared before EEN, after EEN, and after PEN in the PEN group. Similarly, in the control group, the measurements were recorded at diagnosis, eight weeks after diagnosis, and eight months after diagnosis. In the PEN group, the mean weight increased with EEN and then further increased with six months of PEN. The mean height did not change with EEN but did increase with six months of PEN. The mean BMI was higher after six months of PEN than before or after EEN. Among the control subjects, the mean weight increased eight weeks after diagnosis and then further increased after an additional six months. The mean height decreased eight weeks after diagnosis but then increased after another six months. The mean BMI was higher after eight months than at diagnosis or at eight weeks after diagnosis. The changes in mean weight, height, and BMI are illustrated in Table 4.

The wPCDAI was determined at the following time intervals in the PEN group: before EEN, after EEN, after three months of PEN, as well as after one, two, and three years of PEN. The results are shown in Table 4. The median wPCDAI decreased from 30.0 at diagnosis to 5.0 after completion of EEN and then increased to 7.5 after three months of PEN. The lowest median wPCDAI of 3.8 was achieved after completion of one year of PEN. In the control group, the wPCDAI was determined at diagnosis and then at eight weeks and five months after diagnosis, as well as at one, two, and three years after diagnosis. The median wPCDAI decreased from 30.0 at diagnosis to 10.0 after eight weeks and then increased to 11.3 after an additional three months. The lowest median wPCDAI was 10.0, which was achieved after eight weeks and at one year and two years after diagnosis. Overall, the median wPCDAI decreased by a total of 26.2 in the PEN group, as compared to a decrease of 20.0 in the control group. The changes in wPCDAI over time are summarized in Table 4.

4. Discussion

Currently, the main medications used for maintaining remission in pediatric CD are methotrexate and azathioprine. Both are associated with significant adverse effects. Methotrexate is associated with long-term liver injury, bone marrow depression, and occasionally significant nausea and vomiting around administration. Azathioprine is associated with pancreatitis, bone marrow depression, and long-term increased incidence of lymphoma. In addition, the one-year maintenance of remission is around 30% and 60% for methotrexate and azathioprine, respectively [4]. Therefore, we should aim for a safer and more efficient maintenance regimen, especially in children. PEN, after achievement of remission with EEN, seems a promising alternative. We have practiced this approach for the last several years. This retrospective study aimed to investigate the efficacy of PEN treatment in the maintenance of remission in the pediatric CD population. The total decrease in the mean wPCDAI was greater in the PEN group than in the control group, as was the total increase in BMI between the time of diagnosis and eight months after diagnosis. Laboratory parameters, such as albumin and CRP, also showed better improvement in the PEN group than in the control group. Although PEN was able to maintain short remission in patients initially treated with EEN, more than 50% of the patients required concomitant medications within two weeks of PEN initiation to maintain remission. Most patients required concomitant medication at some point after PEN initiation.

The use of PEN as a treatment for CD has been supported in numerous studies conducted by Yamamoto et al. A 2005 study confirmed that enteral nutrition can induce remission and produce mucosal healing of the intestines [19]. This study was followed by one in which the researchers investigated long-term EN and its effect on clinical and endoscopic disease activities, as well as mucosal tissue cytokines in quiescent CD patients [20]. Cytokines are thought to be important in the modulation of intestinal immune function. In particular, interleukin-1β (IL-1β), IL-6, and tumor necrosis factor-α (TNF-α) are thought to play a major role in the aggravation of intestinal inflammation in CD. In this 2007 prospective study, 40 CD patients in remission were divided into two groups. One group, the EN group, received the liquid diet as an infusion at night and a low-fat normal diet during the day, while the non-EN group did not receive the treatment and were not restricted in their diet. The two groups were followed for one year, with mucosal biopsies and ileocolonoscopy performed at entry, 6 months, and 12 months. They found that 5 patients (25%) of the EN group and 13 patients (65%) in the non-EN group relapsed ($P = 0.03$), and the non-EN group had significantly higher endoscopic inflammation (EI) scores at both 6 and 12 months ($P = 0.04$). In addition, while the EN group did not show a noteworthy increase in interleukin-1β (IL-1β), IL-6, and tumor necrosis factor-α (TNF-α) cytokine levels in the mucosal tissue, the non-EN group experienced a significant rise in these cytokines with time (IL-1β, $P = 0.02$; IL-6, $P = 0.002$; TNF- α, $P = 0.001$). These results led the researchers to conclude that long-term EN is effective in decreasing clinical relapse rates and in suppressing endoscopic disease activity, as well as mucosal cytokine levels in patients with quiescent CD.

In a comprehensive review, Yamamoto et al. evaluated the effect of EN on the maintenance of remission in CD patients who had achieved medically or surgically induced remission [14]. EN was associated with significantly higher remission rate and suppressive effects on endoscopic disease activity. Also, the efficacy of EN was shown to be dose-dependent, with higher amounts of enteral formula associated with higher remission rates.

While the available data suggests that EN is effective in maintaining remission in CD patients, the evidence level is not high. Its mechanism of action is not fully understood and remission is often short-lived, with many patients experiencing relapse and requiring upgrading of the therapy or surgery [21]. Furthermore, a significant portion of the studies have been conducted in Japan, as well as in adult populations, and their results may not always apply to pediatric patients in Western communities. A 2006 study by Johnson et al. comparing PEN with EEN suggested that PEN does not suppress inflammation and that EEN is more effective in inducing remission in children with active CD [22]. It is often, however, difficult for children to adhere to EEN in the long-term, resulting eventually in low compliance rates. Thus, the use of PEN for the maintenance of remission after induction with EEN becomes an important consideration.

Several recent studies have supported the findings of Wilschanski et al. that showed that long-term PEN treatment is an effective means of maintaining remission in pediatric CD patients [15]. Konno et al. concluded that EN therapy leads to a reduction in the rate of disease complications, such as intestinal surgeries. In contrast to our study, however, the authors found that EN treatment was capable of maintaining remission in pediatric CD patients for long periods of time without the concomitant use of corticosteroids and immunosuppressive medications [23]. In addition, Kang et al. showed in a prospective study that short-term PEN was effective in improving nutritional status in pediatric patients with severe CD [24]. The results of our study further support these findings. A potential approach to further improve the maintenance of remission in pediatric CD patients on PEN is to combine PEN with a carefully restricted diet. In a recent study, Sigall-Boneh et al. treated a group of children and young adults suffering from CD with a 6-week exclusion diet consisting of 50% PEN and whole foods, with restricted exposure to other dietary products. The dietary intervention resulted in induction of clinical remission and reduction of inflammatory markers in patients suffering from mild-to-moderate disease [25].

Several limitations of our study need to be acknowledged. First of all, the retrospective design of the study may increase the risk of selection bias. Furthermore, the number of EEN weeks needed to induce remission in the PEN group ranged from 4 to 12 and thus was not standardized. Three types of EN formula, Modulen, Ensure, and PediaSure, were used, introducing another degree of variability in the intervention. Nevertheless, almost all (90.7%) of the patients in the PEN group were treated with Modulen. We also acknowledge some key differences in the characteristics of the PEN group and control group. Namely, the median age of the control group was significantly older than that of the PEN group. There was also more colonic disease in the control group, although this was not statistically significant. Finally, the relatively small number of patients included in our investigation may introduce some bias and decrease the power of the study. Our study did include a control group, and therefore we were able to compare pediatric CD patients who were treated with long-term PEN with those who did not receive the treatment. It is important to note, however, that the control group did not receive a course of EEN prior to being maintained on their regular diet. This may cause a confounding effect on the results of the study. Additional studies that compare a study group receiving PEN following an EEN induction with a control group receiving a regular diet after EEN would be of significant value. Moreover, randomized clinical trials that compare treatment with PEN to treatment with medications only, such as corticosteroids and immunomodulators, are needed to identify the optimal management.

5. Conclusions

We conclude that PEN treatment was partially effective in maintaining remission in patients who were initially treated with EEN. Also, EN therapy was able to increase patients' BMI and lower their wPCDAI, further supporting its use over corticosteroids in pediatric patients. Most patients required concomitant medication at some point after PEN initiation. To better assess the efficacy of PEN for maintaining remission in children with CD, further prospective studies are required.

Disclosure

Findings from this paper have been briefly presented as an abstract presented to European Crohn's and Colitis Organization meeting. The abstract has been published in Journal of Crohn's and Colitis. The abstract can be found in the following URLs: https://academic.oup.com/ecco-jcc/article/9/suppl_1/S298/503942/P435-Maintenance-of-Remission-with-Partial-Enteral and https://www.ecco-ibd.eu/index.php/publications/congress-abstract-s/abstracts-2015/item/p435-maintenance-of-remission-with-partial-enteral-nutrition-therapy-in-pediatric-crohnaposs-disease-a-retrospective-study.html.

Acknowledgments

The authors would like to thank Ronit Leiba for her expertise and help with the statistical analysis in this study.

References

[1] M. D. Kappelman, K. R. Moore, J. K. Allen, and S. F. Cook, "Recent trends in the prevalence of Crohn's disease and ulcerative colitis in a commercially insured US population," *Digestive Diseases and Sciences*, vol. 58, no. 2, pp. 519–525, 2013.

[2] J. Askling, L. Grahnquist, A. Ekbom et al., "Incidence of paediatric Crohn's disease in Stockholm, Sweden," *The Lancet*, vol. 354, no. 9185, p. 1179, 1999.

[3] M. Cosgrove, R. F. Al-Atia, and H. R. Jenkins, "The epidemiology of paediatric inflammatory bowel disease," *Archives of Disease in Childhood*, vol. 74, no. 3, pp. 460–461, 1996.

[4] F. M. Ruemmele, G. Veres, K. L. Kolho et al., "Consensus guidelines of ECCO/ESPGHAN on the medical management of pediatric Crohn's disease," *Journal of Crohn's and Colitis*, vol. 8, no. 10, pp. 1179–1207, 2014.

[5] E. A. Newby, A. Sawczenko, A. G. Thomas et al., "Interventions for growth failure in childhood Crohn's disease," *Cochrane Database of Systematic Reviews*, no. 3, article CD003873, 2005.

[6] I. R. Sanderson, S. Udeen, P. S. W. Davies, M. O. Savage, and J. A. Walker-Smith, "Remission induced by an elemental diet in small bowel Crohn's disease," *Archives of Disease in Childhood*, vol. 62, no. 2, pp. 123–127, 1987.

[7] A. G. Thomas, F. Taylor, and V. Miller, "Dietary intake and nutritional treatment in childhood crohn's disease," *Journal of Pediatric Gastroenterology and Nutrition*, vol. 17, no. 1, pp. 75–81, 1993.

[8] A. K. Akobeng and A. G. Thomas, "Enteral nutrition for maintenance of remission in Crohn's disease," *Cochrane Database of Systematic Reviews*, no. 3, article CD005984, 2007.

[9] S. Takagi, K. Utsunomiya, S. Kuriyama et al., "Effectiveness of an 'half elemental diet' as maintenance therapy for Crohn's disease: a randomized-controlled trial," *Alimentary Pharmacology & Therapeutics*, vol. 24, no. 9, pp. 1333–1340, 2006.

[10] S. Verma, B. Kirkwood, S. Brown, and M. H. Giaffer, "Oral nutritional supplementation is effective in the maintenance of remission in Crohn's disease," *Digestive and Liver Disease*, vol. 32, no. 9, pp. 769–774, 2000.

[11] H. Hirakawa, Y. Fukuda, N. Tanida, M. Hosomi, and T. Shimoyama, "Home elemental enterai hyperalimentation (HEEH) for the maintenance of remission in patients with Crohn's disease," *Gastroenterologia Japonica*, vol. 28, no. 3, pp. 379–384, 1993.

[12] H. Koga, M. Iida, K. Aoyagi et al., "Long-term efficacy of low residue diet for the maintenance of remission in patients with Crohn's disease," *Nihon Shokakibyo Gakkai Zasshi*, vol. 90, no. 11, pp. 2882–2888, 1993.

[13] T. Yamamoto, M. Nakahigashi, S. Umegae, T. Kitagawa, and K. Matsumoto, "Impact of long-term enteral nutrition on clinical and endoscopic recurrence after resection for Crohn's disease: a prospective, non-randomized, parallel, controlled study," *Alimentary Pharmacology and Therapeutics*, vol. 25, no. 1, pp. 67–72, 2007.

[14] T. Yamamoto, M. Nakahigashi, S. Umegae, and K. Matsumoto, "Enteral nutrition for the maintenance of remission in Crohn's disease: a systematic review," *European Journal of Gastroenterol-*

ogy & Hepatology, vol. 22, no. 1, pp. 1–8, 2010.

[15] M. Wilschanski, P. Sherman, P. Pencharz, L. Davis, M. Corey, and A. Griffiths, "Supplementary enteral nutrition maintains remission in paediatric Crohn's disease," *Gut*, vol. 38, no. 4, pp. 543–548, 1996.

[16] D. C. Belli, E. Seidman, L. Bouthillier et al., "Chronic intermittent elemental diet improves growth failure in children with Crohn's disease," *Gastroenterology*, vol. 94, no. 3, pp. 603–610, 1988.

[17] A. Levine, A. Griffiths, J. Markowitz et al., "Pediatric modification of the Montreal classification for inflammatory bowel disease: the Paris classification," *Inflammatory Bowel Diseases*, vol. 17, no. 6, pp. 1314–1321, 2011.

[18] D. Turner, A. M. Griffiths, T. D. Walters et al., "Mathematical weighting of the pediatric Crohn's disease activity index (PCDAI) and comparison with its other short versions," *Inflammatory Bowel Diseases*, vol. 18, no. 1, pp. 55–62, 2012.

[19] T. Yamamoto, M. Nakahigashi, S. Umegae, T. Kitagawa, and K. Matsumoto, "Impact of elemental diet on mucosal inflammation in patients with active Crohn's disease: cytokine production and endoscopic and histological findings," *Inflammatory Bowel Diseases*, vol. 11, no. 6, pp. 580–588, 2005.

[20] T. Yamamoto, M. Nakahigashi, A. R. Saniabadi et al., "Impacts of long-term enteral nutrition on clinical and endoscopic disease activities and mucosal cytokines during remission in patients with Crohn's disease: a prospective study," *Inflammatory Bowel Diseases*, vol. 13, no. 12, pp. 1493–1501, 2007.

[21] A. M. Borowiec and R. N. Fedorak, "Predicting, treating and preventing postoperative recurrence of Crohn's disease: the state of the field," *Canadian Journal of Gastroenterology*, vol. 25, no. 3, pp. 140–146, 2011.

[22] T. Johnson, S. Macdonald, S. M. Hill, A. Thomas, and M. S. Murphy, "Treatment of active Crohn's disease in children using partial enteral nutrition with liquid formula: a randomised controlled trial," *Gut*, vol. 55, no. 3, pp. 356–361, 2006.

[23] M. Konno, M. Takahashi, N. Toita, S.-I. Fujiwara, and M. Nojima, "Long-term therapeutic effectiveness of maintenance enteral nutrition for Crohn's disease," *Pediatrics International*, vol. 57, no. 2, pp. 276–280, 2015.

[24] Y. Kang, S. Kim, S. Y. Kim, and H. Koh, "Effect of short-term partial enteral nutrition on the treatment of younger patients with severe Crohn's disease," *Gut and Liver*, vol. 9, no. 1, pp. 87–93, 2015.

[25] R. Sigall-Boneh, T. Pfeffer-Gik, I. Segal, T. Zangen, M. Boaz, and A. Levine, "Partial enteral nutrition with a Crohn's disease exclusion diet is effective for induction of remission in children and young adults with Crohn's disease," *Inflammatory Bowel Diseases*, vol. 20, no. 8, pp. 1353–1360, 2014.

25

Colon Epithelial MicroRNA Network in Fatty Liver

Paule V. Joseph,[1] Sarah K. Abey,[1] Dan Wang,[1] Nicolaas H. Fourie,[1] Natnael D. Kenea,[1] Tatyana G. Vishnyakova,[2] Jeffrey M. Robinson,[1] Kristen R. Weaver,[1] Christina M. Boulineaux,[1] Hannah R. Davidson,[1] LeeAnne B. Sherwin,[1] Onyinyechi Ozoji,[1] Ana F. Diallo,[1] Paul A. Smyser,[1] Amy P. Patterson,[3] and Wendy A. Henderson[1]

[1]*Digestive Disorder Unit, Division of Intramural Research, National Institute of Nursing Research, National Institutes of Health, Bethesda, MD 20892, USA*
[2]*Department of Laboratory Medicine, Clinical Center, National Institutes of Health, Bethesda, MD 20814, USA*
[3]*National Heart Lung and Blood Institute, Bethesda, MD 20814, USA*

Correspondence should be addressed to Wendy A. Henderson; hendersw@mail.nih.gov

Academic Editor: Salvatore Oliva

Background & Aims. Intestinal barrier alterations are associated with fatty liver (FL) and metabolic syndrome (MetS), but microRNA (miR) signaling pathways in MetS-FL pathogenesis remain unclear. This study investigates an epithelial-focused miR network in colorectal cell models based on the previously reported MetS-FL miR trio of hsa-miR-142-3p, hsa-miR-18b, and hsa-miR-890. *Methods.* Each miR mimic construct of MetS-FL miR trio was transfected into human colorectal cells, CRL-1790 or Caco-2. Global miRNome changes posttransfection were profiled (nCounter® Human v3 miRNA, NanoString Technologies). Changes in barrier (transepithelial electrical resistance, TEER) and epithelial cell junction structure (Occludin and Zona Occludens-1/ZO-1 immunofluorescence staining-confocal microscopy) were examined pre- and posttransfection in Caco-2 cell monolayers. A signaling network was constructed from the MetS-FL miR trio, MetS-FL miR-induced colorectal miRNome changes, ZO-1, and Occludin. *Results.* Transfection of CRL-1790 cells with each MetS-FL miR mimic led to global changes in the cellular miRNome profile, with 288 miRs being altered in expression by more than twofold. Eleven miRs with known cytoskeletal and metabolic roles were commonly altered in expression by all three miR mimics. Transfection of Caco-2 cell monolayers with each MetS-FL miR mimic induced barrier-associated TEER variations and led to structural modifications of ZO-1 and Occludin within epithelial cell junctions. Pathway analysis incorporating the MetS-FL miR trio, eleven common target miRs, ZO-1, and Occludin revealed a signaling network centered on TNF and AKT2, which highlights injury, inflammation, and hyperplasia. *Conclusions.* Colon-specific changes in epithelial barriers, cell junction structure, and a miRNome signaling network are described from functional studies of a MetS-FL miR trio signature.

1. Introduction

Metabolic Syndrome (MetS) arises from systemic metabolic perturbations characterized by dyslipidemia and central obesity [1]. MetS is associated with an increased risk of developing cardiovascular disease, liver fibrosis and cancer, colon cancer, and breast cancer [2–5]. MetS characteristics are highly prevalent among individuals with nonalcoholic fatty liver disease (NAFLD), particularly those who are obese (Body Mass Index or BMI ≥ 30) or have insulin resistance [6]. A meta-analysis of studies demonstrated that NAFLD patients had increased intestinal permeability compared to healthy controls. Intestinal inflammation and upregulation of tumor necrosis factor-α (TNFα), common in obese individuals with MetS and NAFLD, are also associated with intestinal leakage [7]. Pathophysiology of MetS and NAFLD has been attributed to changes in intestinal epithelial barriers, leading to altered intestinal permeability and translocation of microbes or microbial products, such as lipopolysaccharide (LPS) [8, 9]. Structural proteins, such as ZO-1 and Occludin, compose a cytoskeletal-supported cell junction network that maintains transport across the intestinal epithelial barrier and regulates permeability during normal physiology [10, 11]. Expression and localization of these structural proteins are known to be regulated by certain microRNAs (miRs), such as miR-142-3p, which regulates Rac1 [12]. We previously reported altered expression of miR-142-3p, miR-18b, and miR-890 in a cohort of patients with fatty liver (FL), who also met established criteria for MetS as defined by the International Diabetes Federation [1]. Also altered in this cohort were the expressions of mRNAs related to hepatocellular carcinoma progression pathways of adhesion, invasion, and metastasis [13]. Thus, these three miRs (hsa-miR-142-3p, hsa-miR-18b, and hsa-miR-890) may be indicators of epithelial barrier functional modifications in metabolically related MetS-FL.

The regulatory properties of miRs are unique in that a single miR can exert subtle effects on multiple mRNA targets simultaneously [14]. This property of miRs is increasingly recognized to be key in systemic metabolic disorders, as it allows multiple pathways to respond in concert when cells are faced with metabolic stress [15]. Furthermore, one mRNA species is susceptible to regulatory controls by several miRs; thus, a network of miRs is likely required to control a signaling pathway [16]. In MetS and NAFLD, a network of miRs is thought to act in concert across multiple organs to induce pathophysiological damage [15, 17]. Out of the three MetS-FL miRs identified in our previous cohort, the hsa-miR-142-3p has been shown to have functional multiplicity by being able to directly regulate structural proteins within the cell junction [18], participate in the initiation of LPS-induced inflammatory signaling in immune and dendritic cells [19], and be implicated in systemic metabolic stress through its upregulation in the adipose tissue of mice fed a high-fat diet [20] and in obese children [21]. Thus, a multifunctional signaling network that simultaneously affects metabolic stress and inflammation is likely involved in the regulation of genes encoding for epithelial cell junction proteins associated with altered barrier function in MetS and NAFLD.

The cytoskeletal structure that supports the intestinal epithelial cell junction consists of proteins regulated by a signaling network that responds to extracellular environments under normal physiological conditions or stress [10, 11]. In mice, a high-fat diet that induces higher levels of circulating LPS, insulin resistance, and obesity [22] also leads to altered levels of epithelial cell junction proteins, Zonula Occludens-1 (ZO-1), and Occludin, in the duodenum [23]. Altered expressions of ZO-1 and increased intestinal permeability have been observed in NAFLD patients [24]. While these observations suggest the involvement of microbial translocation and altered epithelial barriers in MetS and NAFLD, the underlying signaling network regulating these processes is not fully understood.

To facilitate the identification of an epithelial-focused functional miR network involved in altered epithelial barriers and cell junctions, we expressed each of our previously discussed MetS-FL miR trio (hsa-miR-142, hsa-miR-18b, and hsa-miR-890) in cultured epithelial cells [13, 25]. We utilized colorectal epithelial cells since our patient cohort also had evidence of altered permeability specific to the colon [26]. The human primary colorectal cell line CRL-1790 was chosen as a metabolically normal colon epithelial cell model for the following reasons: (1) CRL-1790 is a human primary, nontransformed, colorectal cell line [27], which therefore does not possess extraneously induced genetic alterations, including those related to metabolic adaptations found in immortalized cancer cell lines; (2) expression of beta-catenin (an inducer of cell migration) was shown to be very low for this cell line [28], prompting its utilization as a nonmetastatic cell line control for investigations of colorectal adenocarcinomas; (3) the cell line displays epithelial characteristics yet lacks keratin [27], a cytoskeletal protein which has been associated with many types of neoplasia [29]. Each of the miR mimics were transfected into CRL-1790 cells, and global miRNome expression profiling was performed (NanoString Technologies). In addition, we transfected each of the miR mimics into Caco-2 epithelial cell monolayers and analyzed changes in miR-induced epithelial barrier integrity by measuring transepithelial electrical resistance [30] pre- and posttransfection. Caco-2 cells have been shown to form epithelial monolayers *in vitro* resembling the intestinal barrier villi [31]. For this reason, Caco-2 cells have been found to be an excellent model for passive transcellular transport normally occurring *in vivo* [31] and to investigate intestinal barrier permeability in steatohepatitis [7]. Next, to evaluate the cytoskeletal proteins that may affect epithelial barrier function, we examined ZO-1 and Occludin structures in the epithelial cell junction and their mRNA levels post-miR mimic transfection. Finally, a signaling network was constructed from the MetS-FL miR trio, ZO-1, Occludin, and miR targets within the global miRNome affected by MetS-FL miR expressions.

2. Materials and Methods

2.1. Cell Cultures and Transfection of Cells with miR Mimics. Human colon epithelial cell lines Caco-2 and CRL-1790 were purchased from American Type Culture Collection (ATCC). Cells were cultured in Eagle's Minimum Essential Medium (EMEM; ATCC) containing 20% (Caco-2) or 10% (CRL-1790) Fetal Bovine Serum (FBS; ThermoFisher) at 37°C and 5% CO_2. Expression of miR mimics in Caco-2 and CRL-1790 cells was carried out using DharmaFect transfection reagent (GE Dharmacon) according to the manufacturer's protocols. Mature miRNA mimic constructs (miRIDIAN™, GE Dharmacon) were dissolved in siRNA buffer (GE Dharmacon) to achieve final concentrations of 100 nM. For RNA isolation from transfected CRL-1790 cells, transfection media containing miR mimics or vehicles (siRNA buffer) were replaced with fresh feeding media at 24 hours posttransfection and cells were incubated for an additional 24 hours. Total RNAs were isolated using a microRNA isolation kit (Qiagen). The *C.elegans* cel-miR-67 mimic (GE Dharmacon) was used as a nonmammalian miR control.

2.2. Analysis of the Global miRNome Signaling Network. Total RNA from miR mimic-transfected cells was evaluated using nCounter® Human v3 miRNA expression assays

(NanoString Technologies), as previously described (Fourie 2016). Endogenous changes of miRNAs in CRL-1790 cells expressing each of the MetS-FL miR mimics were analyzed using nSolver™ Analysis Software v3.0 (NanoString). Normalization of digital counts was performed using "Top 100" miRs with highest counts; only miRs with counts above the normalization threshold value of 43.17 (calculated from mean ±3 standard deviations of eight negative controls) were included in subsequent ratio calculations. The ratios of digital counts in cells expressing MetS-FL miR mimic to the digital counts in cells expressing control cel-miR mimic were determined. From this ratio calculation, only miRs with ratios of 2.0 or above, or -2.0 or below, were subjected to Venn analysis [33]. Venn analysis was performed with 288 miRs having these specified ratios and a diagram constructed to illustrate the number of miRs within the global cellular miRNome that were commonly targeted.

2.3. In Vitro Intestinal Permeability Assay. For each biological replicate, Caco-2 cells were seeded at 10^5 cells per well on Millicell filters (EMD Millipore) according to manufacturer instructions. Cells were allowed to polarize into apico-basolateral monolayers for 7 days prior to transfection, and feeding media (20% FBS) was replaced every 2 days. On day 8, cells were transfected with each of the MetS-FL miR mimics, control cel-miR-67 mimic, or vehicle (siRNA buffer). TEER values were measured every day pre- and posttransfection in replicate wells using Millicell ERS-2 and electrodes (EMD Millipore). TEER values in blank wells seeded with no cells were subtracted from these TEER values and then normalized against a 24-well plate surface area per well (values were shown as Ohm-cm^2). All TEER measurements were taken at room temperature in a tissue culture hood to maintain sterility.

2.4. Confocal Immunofluorescence Microscopy of Zona Occludens-1 and Occludin. Six days after transfection with miR mimics, polarized Caco-2 cells were washed with 1X phosphate-buffered saline (PBS) pH 7.4, fixed with 100% methanol, and blocked with 1% Bovine Serum Albumin (BSA) and with 5% goat serum/1% BSA in PBS. Fixed cells were permeabilized by two treatments of 0.2% Triton-X prior to staining with 2.5 μg/ml rabbit anti-ZO-1 (GE Life Technologies) or 20 μg/ml mouse anti-Occludin (GE Life Technologies). Subsequently, stained cells were washed in PBS and secondary antibodies were added: donkey anti-rabbit Alexa Fluor 594, donkey anti-mouse Alexa Fluor 488, control rabbit IgG, or control mouse IgG (GE Life Technologies). Images were acquired sequentially by using a 488-nm laser line and emission between 505 and 580 nm for Alexa Fluor 488, BODIPY 493/503, and BODIPY FL C12. A 594-nm laser line and emission >610 nm were used for Alexa 594. Z-series high-resolution (100 nm per pixel) images were obtained with a 63x, 1.4-numerical-aperture Plan-Apochromat oil-immersion objective under conditions avoiding bleed-through.

2.5. Quantitative Real-Time Polymerase Chain Reaction (qPCR). To obtain RNA for qPCR assays, cells were seeded on 24-well plates until they reached 80% confluence. miRIDIAN miR mimics (100 nM) were added with DharmaFect 1 transfection reagent according to manufacturer protocols (GE Dharmacon). The C. *elegans* cel-miR-67 mimic was used as a control (GE Dharmacon). After 24 hours, transfection media was replaced with fresh feeding media and cells were incubated for an additional 24 hours. Total cellular RNA from at least three independent biological replicates was isolated using a miRNeasy isolation kit (Qiagen). RNA concentration was measured using Nanodrop (Thermo Scientific). For qPCR of miRs, 100 ng total RNA was used for cDNA synthesis using TaqMan® MicroRNA Reverse Transcription Kit. qPCR was performed using sequence-specific TaqMan® qPCR microRNA assay primers (Thermo Scientific) and TaqMan® Universal Master Mix. Endogenous mature miRNA expression analysis was performed in triplicate and normalized to the expression level of hsa-miR-16 as a housekeeping control. For qPCR of mRNA, 450 ng total RNA was used for cDNA synthesis by the TaqMan® Reverse Transcription Reagents using oligo d(T) and random hexamers primer mixture (Thermo Scientific). cDNA then was subjected to qPCR analysis. Endogenous mRNA expression analysis was performed in triplicate with TaqMan® Gene Expression Master Mix using Zona Occludens-1 and Occludin TaqMan® gene expression assay primers (Thermo Scientific) and normalized to the expression level of GAPDH as a housekeeping control. Samples were run on the 7900HT Real-Time PCR System (Life Technologies-Applied Biosystems) platform in the following conditions: initial activation step of 2 min at 50°C, 10 min at 95°C, followed by 40 cycles of 15 s at 95°C, and extension for 1 min at 60°C. miRNA or mRNA fold expression relative to expression in untransfected (or cel-miR mimic-transfected) cells from each biological replicate was calculated based on the $\Delta\Delta$Ct method [34]. Means and standard deviations were reported from three biological replicates.

3. Results

3.1. Colorectal Cellular miRNome Is Globally Affected by MetS-FL miRs. In MetS and NAFLD, regulation of the intestinal barrier is essential as bacterial translocation and inflammation are thought to ensue following barrier breakage [8]. We tested whether the MetS-FL miR trio, found previously in patients with FL and altered colonic permeability, could be part of a signaling network in colon epithelial cells that form intestinal barriers. We transfected CRL-1790 cells with either the MetS-FL miR mimic or control cel-miR mimic and subjected the posttransfection RNA to a comprehensive 800 miR expression profiling (NanoString). A scatter plot shows miRs with altered digital counts of more than 2.0-fold in cells expressing MetS-FL miR mimics versus counts in control cells expressing the cel-miR mimic (see Figures 1(a)–1(c)). Two hundred and eighty-eight miRs in cells expressing MetS-FL miR mimics versus cells expressing cel-miR mimic, with count ratios $\geq$ 2.0 or $\leq$ -2.0, are listed in Supplementary Table S1. The three MetS-FL miRs were also found to significantly affect each other's expression levels

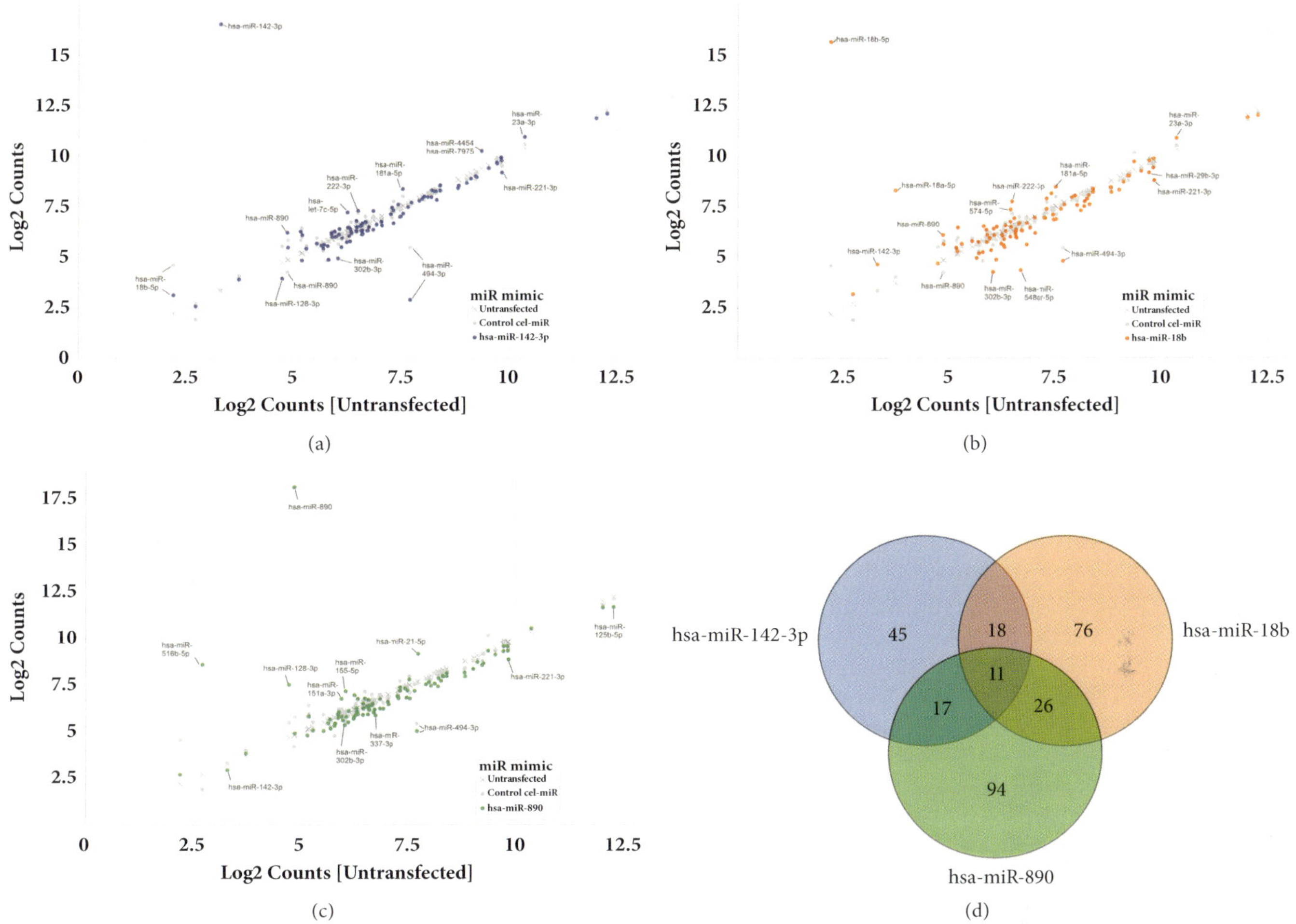

FIGURE 1: (a-c) Global alterations in colorectal cell miR levels in human epithelial CRL-1790 cells transfected with control cel-miR or MetS-FL miR mimics. (d) Common miR targets whose expression levels were altered by 2.0-fold or more following CRL-1790 cell transfection with each MetS-FL miR mimic. Eleven common miRs targeted by all three MetS-FL miRs are listed in Table 1.

(see Supplementary Table S2). The 288 miRs were subjected to Venn analysis, which revealed eleven commonly targeted miRs by the three MetS-FL miR mimics (see Figure 1(d) and Table 1). These eleven miRs have known functional roles in metabolic and cytoskeletal pathways (see Table 2).

3.2. MetS-FL miR Mimics Induce Barrier Changes and Modified Structural Appearance of Cell Junction, ZO-1, and Occludin. Global miRNome changes exerted by MetS-FL miR mimics include eleven target miRs with known metabolic and cytoskeletal signaling roles. To further investigate epithelial and cell junction effects exerted by the MetS-FL miR trio, Caco-2 cells were grown as polarized monolayers on a filter membrane. Apico-basolateral polarity across Caco-2 monolayers was examined by measuring TEER [30] daily. After a 7-day period of TEER stabilization, the polarized cells were transfected with individual MetS-FL miR mimic or control cel-miR mimic. Following cell transfection, changes in barrier integrity were captured by monitoring TEER daily for 6 days. Our data show that transient transfection of cells with each of the MetS-FL miR trio mimics leads to variable changes in TEER (see Figures 2(a)–2(c)). Notably, transfection of cells with hsa-miR-142-3p mimic led to a significant 19-29% reduction in TEER (see Figure 2(a)).

TEER values reflect epithelial cohesion and polarity, which are maintained by structural components within the epithelial cell junction [10, 30]. We investigated the cell junction architecture by staining some of the structural components, ZO-1 and Occludin, both of which had been previously associated with NAFLD patients [24] or animal models [23]. Following transfection of cells with each MetS-FL miR mimic, we found evidence of disruption of the continuous junctional appearance of both proteins (see Figure 2(d)). In particular, following transfection with hsa-miR-142-3p and hsa-miR-890, Occludin staining was absent along the cell junction locations where ZO-1 remained intact (see Figure 2(d)).

3.3. ZO-1 and Occludin mRNAs Are Not Significantly Altered in Cells Expressing MetS-FL miRs. We investigated whether any of the MetS-FL miRs had direct effects on the expression levels of ZO-1 mRNA or Occludin (OCLN) mRNA, with

TABLE 1: Eleven miRs commonly altered in expression levels (≥ 2.0-fold) in CRL-1790 cells transfected with MetS-FL miR mimics (miR-142-3p, miR-18b, and miR-890) compared with cells expressing control cel-miR mimic.

miR Name	miR-142-3p vs. cel-miR	P value of: miR-142-3p vs. cel-miR	miR-18b vs. cel-miR	P value of: miR-18b vs. cel-miR	miR-890 vs. cel-miR	P value of: miR-890 vs. cel-miR
hsa-miR-10b-5p	3.61	0.051	3.26	0.0736	4.06	0.0427
hsa-miR-1254	-3.8	0.0341	-2.55	0.0906	-1.96	0.3425
hsa-miR-1301-3p	2.14	0.3616	2.83	0.3184	3	0.1013
hsa-miR-18b-5p	-2.81	0.6243	2088.21	0.0454	-3.69	0.5328
hsa-miR-190a-3p	2.03	0.3964	2.16	0.3888	1.99	0.4261
hsa-miR-223-3p	2.9	0.05704	4.02	0.0266	2.03	0.1795
hsa-miR-342-5p	2.52	0.2326	3.12	0.2596	3.85	0.0781
hsa-miR-3614-3p	2.01	0.2026	2.35	0.0953	3.09	0.0476
hsa-miR-566	2.74	0.1073	2.38	0.3412	4.06	0.0151
hsa-miR-675-5p	5.41	0.022	2.79	0.0764	2.68	0.2566
hsa-miR-890	3.87	0.1851	3.57	0.386	15456.06	0.0031

[*] P-values are calculated from 3 independent (performed on separate dates) replicate transfection experiments.

expression levels of housekeeping gene GAPDH used as a control. Although target sequence alignments were predicted by a database (microrna.org; see Figure 3(c)), neither the endogenous ZO-1 nor Occludin mRNA levels were significantly altered by transient transfection of CRL-1790 cells with any of the MetS-FL miRs (see Figures 3(a) and 3(b)). Two of the miRs (miR-18b, miR-890) did exhibit a 2-3-fold increase in Occludin mRNA expression (see Figure 3(b)). While degradation of target transcripts is often the result of miR targeting [35, 36], cases of miR-mediated gene upregulation have also been identified [37]. A possible miR-mediated suppression of an Occludin transcriptional activator cannot be ruled out. We conclude that in normal colorectal cells, there is no observable direct effect of MetS-FL miRs on ZO-1 or Occludin cellular transcripts.

3.4. Signaling Networks and Canonical Pathways Are Predicted by hsa-miR-142-3p, hsa-miR-18b, hsa-miR-890, Eleven Common miR Targets, ZO1, and Occludin. To elucidate the potential signaling network affecting colorectal epithelial cells and the intestinal barrier based on the MetS-FL miR trio signature, we generated a network representation using QIAGEN's Ingenuity Pathway Analysis (IPA®, QIAGEN Redwood City, www.qiagen.com/ingenuity). IPA is a network database that integrates a broad variety of data from public databases and aggregates the data into network representations based on input nodes (usually genes). Data for the network architecture may be derived from protein-protein interactions, transcriptional activation or repression, or other regulatory interactions from human and other mammalian model systems. An integrated pathway analysis (IPA) was performed using the eleven common target miRs (see Table 1), MetS-FL miR trio, ZO-1, and Occludin. Pathway analysis revealed a signaling network centered on AKT2 and TNF (see Figure 4). The top canonical pathways reveal signaling related to cell-cell junction signaling, inflammation, injury, and hyperplasia. Using Pathway Designer (IPA), the hsa-miR-890 was added to the pathway based on global miRNome profiling presented in Figure 1(c). The hsa-miR-190, one of the eleven common miR targets, was also added to the pathway based on a recent literature report of its direct involvement in AKT signaling and inflammation [32].

4. Discussion

The present work demonstrates potential functional implications of our previously reported MetS-FL trio miR signature (hsa-miR-142-3p, hsa-miR-18b, and hsa-miR-890) [13, 25] upon colorectal epithelial cells and intestinal barrier function. Transient expression of each of the three miRs led to variable modifications of apico-basolateral polarity, which affects barrier cohesion and integrity. Although all miR expressions in the polarized epithelial model led to intermittent disappearance of ZO-1 and Occludin along the cell junction, none of the miRs had direct effects on Occludin or ZO1 mRNA levels. A global miRNome network that potentially exerts indirect effects on observed barrier changes was revealed, including a total of 288 miRs. Expression levels of the 288 miRs were altered by more than 2-fold in the human colon epithelial cells expressing the MetS-FL miR mimics, compared with the control cel-miR mimic. The MetS-FL miR mimics also affected each other's endogenous colorectal cell expressions. Of the 288 miRs, eleven miRs with known metabolic and cytoskeletal roles were found to be common targets of all three MetS-FL miRs. An epithelial-focused signaling network was assembled from the MetS-FL miR trio, the eleven common miR targets, ZO-1, and Occludin, which revealed cell junction signaling, inflammation, injury, and hyperplasia as major canonical pathways. In summary, our work suggests a MetS-FL miR signature to be associated with a functional epithelial cell junction and colorectal-specific signaling network.

Our network analysis revealed AKT and TNFα as mediators of this signaling pathway. TNFα is central to inflammation which mediates liver injury in the two-hit hypothesis proposed for NAFLD [38]. TNFα expression is enhanced

TABLE 2: Metabolic and cytoskeletal signaling roles of eleven common miR targets of the MetS-FL miR trio.

	Metabolic Role	Cytoskeletal or Cell Junction Role
hsa-miR-10b-5p	Striatal metabolism in Huntington's Disease [35]	Regulates cytoskeletal RhoC in glioblastoma [36]
hsa-miR-1254	Interacts with structured elements in cell cycle and apoptosis regulator 1 (CCAR1) 5' Untranslated Region [37]	Associated with miR export and processing between nuclear and cytoplasmic compartments [32]; Associated with invasive Retinoblastoma pathogenesis [38]
hsa-miR-1301-3p	Altered level in Low-Onset Hypogonadism [39]; Downregulates maternal circulating leptin levels [40]	Inhibits migration and invasion of HepG2 hepatic carcinoma cells [41]
hsa-miR-18b-5p	Interacts with insulin growth factor-1 to downregulate proliferation of human retinal endothelial cells grown in high-glucose media [12]; Increases plaque buildup, leading to atherosclerosis [42]	Modulates genes involved in cell migration and upregulated in breast cancer [43]
hsa-miR-190a-3p	Under regulation of estrogen receptor (ER) signaling [44]	Inhibits epithelial-mesenchymal transition of hepatoma cells [45]; Targets protease-activated-receptor 1 (PAR-1), which is a metastasis promoting protein [44]
hsa-miR-223-3p	Inversely correlated with insulin-like growth factor 1 levels [46]; Regulates osteoclast and osteoblast differentiation, leading to regulation of bone metabolism [47]; Downregulates glucose uptake controlled by insulin in the adipose tissue of insulin-resistant women [48]; Upregulates glucose uptake in cardiomyocytes via the glucose transporter 4 protein [49]; Regulates multiple pathways involved in cholesterol uptake and metabolism [50]; Downregulates high-density lipoprotein uptake [51]	Regulates epithelial mesenchymal transition [52]
hsa-miR-342-5p	Involved in regulatory T cell function in Type I Diabetes Mellitus [53]	Targets DNA methyltransferase 1 and inhibits colorectal cancer cell proliferation and invasion [54]
hsa-miR-3614-3p	Regulates the *OLR1* gene which encodes for the lectin-like oxidized low-density lipoprotein receptor-1 protein [55]	Involved in c-Myc-regulated migration and angiogenesis [56]
hsa-miR-566	Activates epidermal growth factor receptor signaling in glioblastoma cells [57]	Associated with metastatic colon cancer patient profile [58]
hsa-miR-675-5p	Inhibits the expression of insulin-like growth factor 1 receptor and insulin receptor in rhabdomyosarcoma cells [59]	Upregulates collagen proteins in the cartilage matrix of human articular chondrocytes [60]; Regulates tight junction proteins in intestinal epithelial barrier [61]
hsa-miR-890	Regulates tumor DNA repair [62]	Regulates autophagy and metastasis-associated Rad23B protein in prostate cancer [62]

under inflammasome deficiency due to activation of the TLR signaling pathways by microbial products, and this leads to exacerbation of liver steatosis and steatohepatitis [39]. In a Caco-2 monolayer model, TNFα has been shown to increase tight junction permeability and decrease TEER [40]. Such demonstrated roles in barrier maintenance in the context of the gut-liver axis have been the basis for anti-TNF therapy such as infliximab, which is effective in reversing liver steatosis and correcting insulin resistance in animal models [41]. More recently, TNF was shown as a mediator for the combinatorial effects of endoplasmic reticulum (ER) stress and hypernutrition in liver hyperplasia and hepatocellular carcinoma [42]. Whether injury or inflammation occurs prior to, or as a result of, altered barrier permeability is unclear; however, a clear role for both TNF and AKT in the unfolded protein response (UPR) and ER stress response is increasingly recognized [43]. The UPR and ER stress response are evolutionarily conserved cellular adaptations which balance survival versus death in response to stress, such as nutrient stress [43]. The critical role of AKT in the

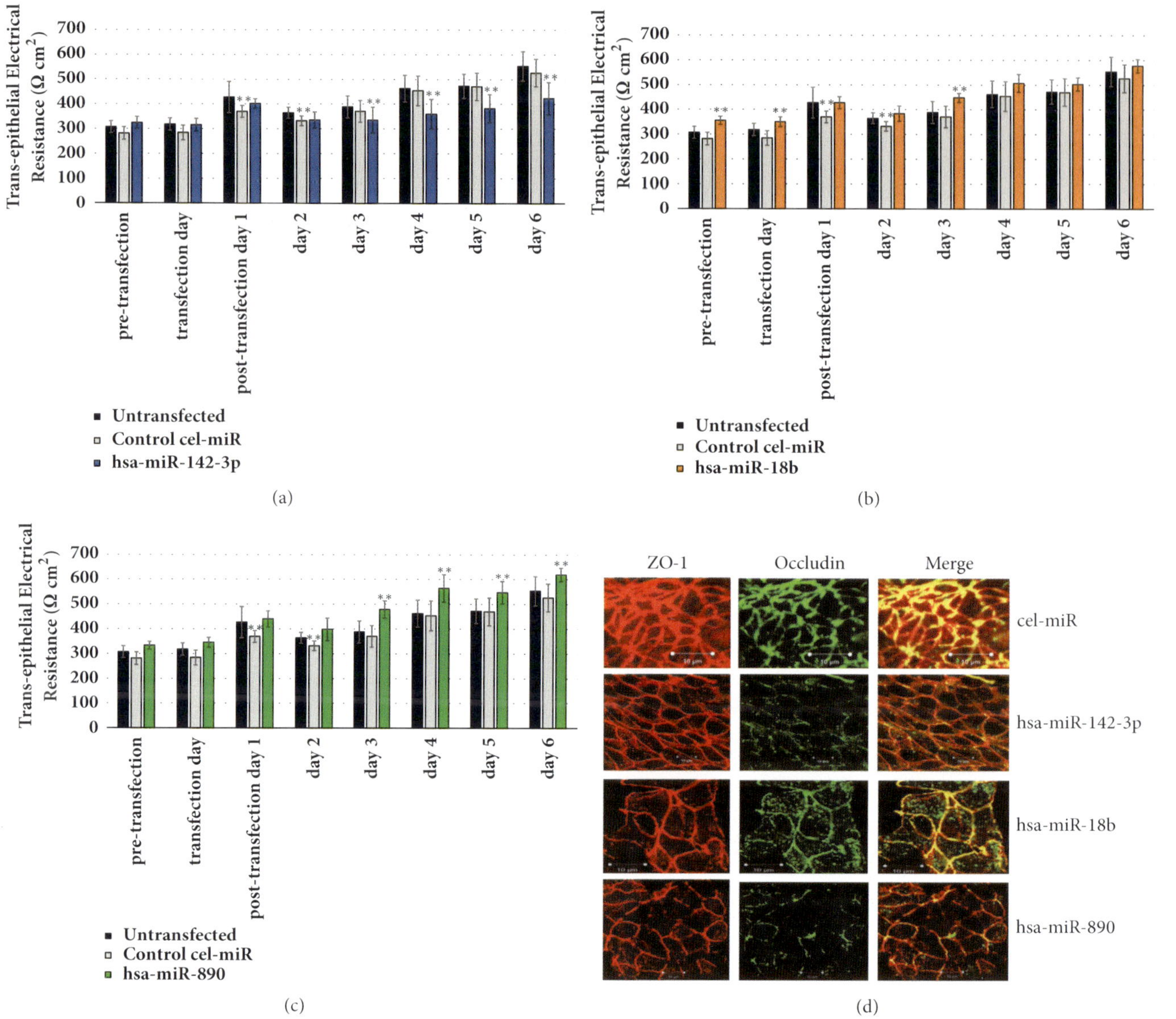

FIGURE 2: Transfection of MetS-FL miR mimics into Caco-2 colon epithelial monolayers leads to miR-specific changes in barrier integrity and epithelial cell junction. (a, b, c) Transepithelial electrical resistance (TEER) was measured daily pre- and posttransfection of cells with control miR mimic or MetS-FL miR mimics. Background TEER measurements in "blank" wells without cells were subtracted from TEER values in transfected cells. The subtracted TEER values are normalized against seeding surface area and expressed as Ohm-cm^2. Data are means ± standard deviations calculated from at least four biological replicates. Bar graphs show TEER values of untransfected cells and cells transfected with control *C.elegans* cel-miR-67 mimic or each of the MetS-FL miR mimics. ∗∗ indicates significant ($p < 0.05$) changes in barrier TEER in miR mimic-transfected compared to nontransfected cells. (d) Transfection of MetS-FL miR mimics into Caco-2 colon epithelial monolayers leads to altered appearance of Zona Occludens-1 (ZO-1) and Occludin within the cell junction. Images show immunofluorescence staining and confocal microscopy visualization of ZO-1 (red), Occludin (green), or both (yellow). Scale bars are 10 μm.

ER stress response is demonstrated by its ability to act both as an activator of metabolic pathways to increase de novo lipogenesis and glycolysis [44] and as an effector of nutrient signals such as metabolic stress induced by low glucose in the cell environment [45].

We have previously reported AKT as a predicted target in a signaling pathway constructed by peripheral miRs found in cohorts of patients with chronic gastrointestinal dysfunction and altered intestinal permeability [26, 46]. Of note, one of these peripheral miRs, miR-342, is one of the eleven common targets of MetS-FL miR trio in the present patient cohort. In addition to AKT and TNF, the present network also reveals MMP2 and hsa-miR-155, which we have previously reported to be altered in NAFLD (Longchamps 2012, Longchamps 2014) [13, 47]. Both Occludin and ZO-1, the two key protein components of the tight junction, are downstream to TNF signaling, with Matrix Metallo-Proteinases (MMP2, MMP1, and MMP3) appearing as intermediates. Thus, our network provides a generalized context for the hypothesis that dysregulation

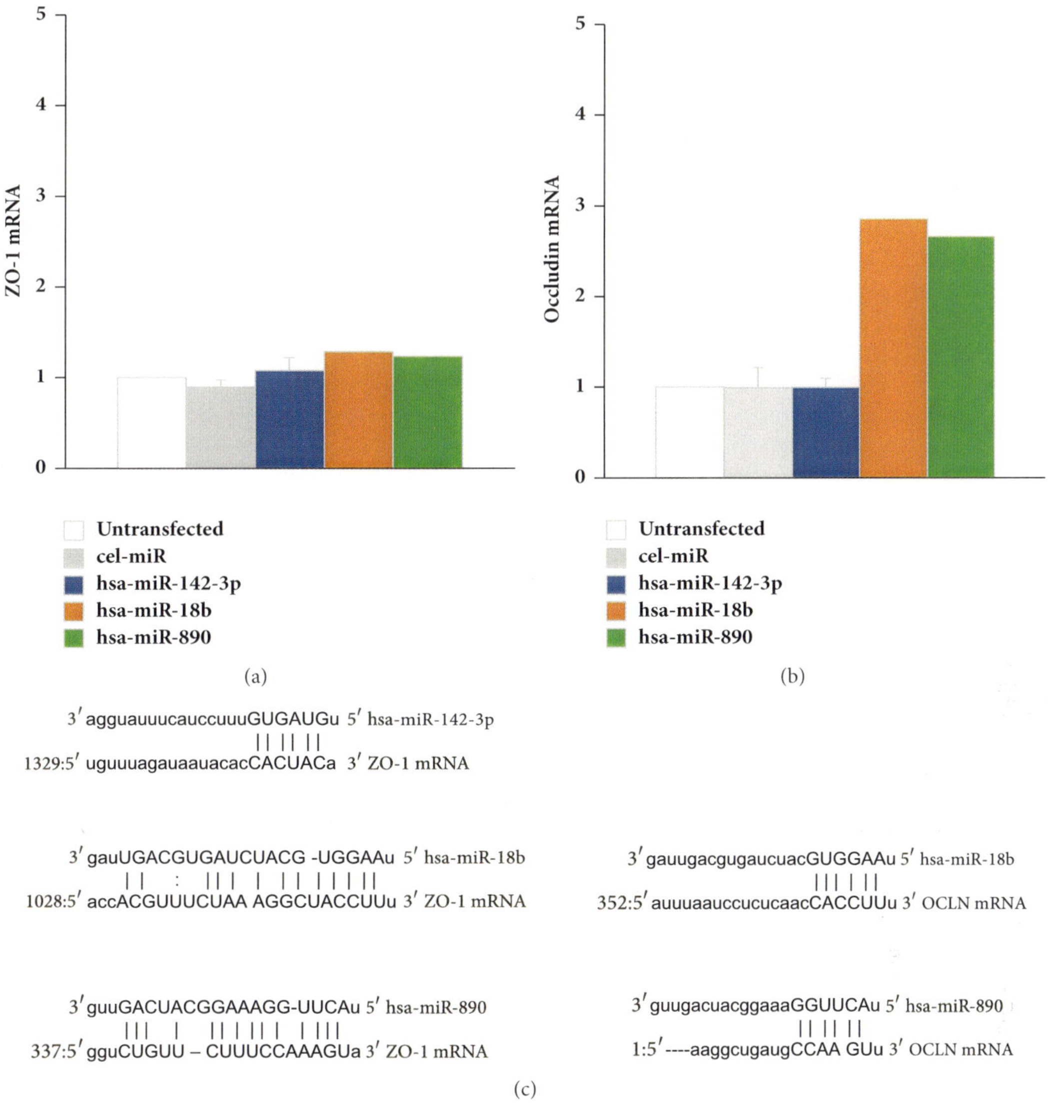

Figure 3: Transfection of MetS-FL miR mimics into CRL-1790 cells did not directly affect cellular ZO-1 (a) or Occludin (b) mRNA levels, although mRNA target sequence alignments with each of MetS-FL miRs were predicted (c).

of miRs may result in alteration of epithelial permeability via effects of TNF and AKT signaling.

Given that the MetS-FL miR trio and their common targets implicate TNF, AKT, injury, and hyperplasia as top canonical pathways and functions, our findings have implications for utilizing the miR trio signature as noninvasive biomarkers (see Table 3). First, the MetS-FL miR trio presents values for colon-specific context considerations when testing therapy directed against molecules such as TNF and AKT. Particularly for oral therapy, the demonstrated function on colon barrier modulation warrants considerations of its utilization as a biomarker before and during therapy. Second, current interest is rising on using miRs as targeted therapy. Anti-miR-155 has been suggested for hepatocellular carcinoma and alcoholic fatty liver disease [48, 49]. Our results lend support to miRNome network analysis, especially if a therapy is targeted at the colon. The current miR signature and network may also be considered in nutrient-derived molecule analysis such as resveratrol, which is suggested to promote intestinal health. While our current study is limited in sample size, the functional relevance and miR network signature could be incorporated in studies examining the role of intestinal health promoting nutrients such as resveratrol, a component of red wine and grape skin [50].

5. Conclusions

Based on the findings discussed, a working model for the MetS-FL miRs in the context of the gut barrier-liver axis is presented (see Figure 5). Changes in colon epithelial barrier structure from local and concerted effects of circulating MetS-FL miRs may be associated with increased intestinal permeability and microbial translocation. Serum LPS Binding Protein or LBP [51] has been shown by others [52–54] to be elevated as a correlate of microbial translocation and inflammatory response, which may be a signal of ongoing

TABLE 3: Top canonical pathways, top diseases and biological functions, and top toxicology functions revealed by the eleven common miR targets of the MetS-FL trio, ZO-1, and Occludin.

Top Canonical Pathways	p-value
Tight Junction Signaling	0.00255
Sertoli Cell-Sertoli Cell Junction Signaling	0.00277
Germ Cell-Sertoli Cell Junction Signaling	0.0763
Top Upstream Regulators	p-value
Gelatinase	5E-07
ERP29*	4.66E-06
MMP9*	0.000013
CAV1*	1.75E-05
MMP2*	2.54E-05
Top Diseases and Disorders	p-value
Inflammatory Response	0.00000116 - 0.0013
Cancer	0.00000659 - 0.0474
Hematological Disease	0.00000659 - 0.0316
Immunological Disease	0.00000659 - 0.0426
Organismal Injury and Abnormalities	0.00000659 - 0.0472
Top Molecular and Cellular Functions	p-value
Cell Death and Survival	0.000000194 - 0.0121
Cell-To-Cell Signaling and Interaction	0.00000116 - 0.0318
Cellular Function and Maintenance	0.00000116 - 0.0300
Energy Production	0.000190 - 0.000190
Molecular Transport	0.000190 - 0.000190
Top Tox Functions (Hepatotoxicity)	p-value
Liver Necrosis/Cell Death	0.00420 – 0.00420
Hepatocellular Carcinoma	0.345 – 0.345
Liver Hyperplasia/Hyperproliferation	0.345 – 0.596

*ERP29: endoplasmic reticulum protein 29; MMP: matrix metallo-proteinase; CAV1: caveolin-1.

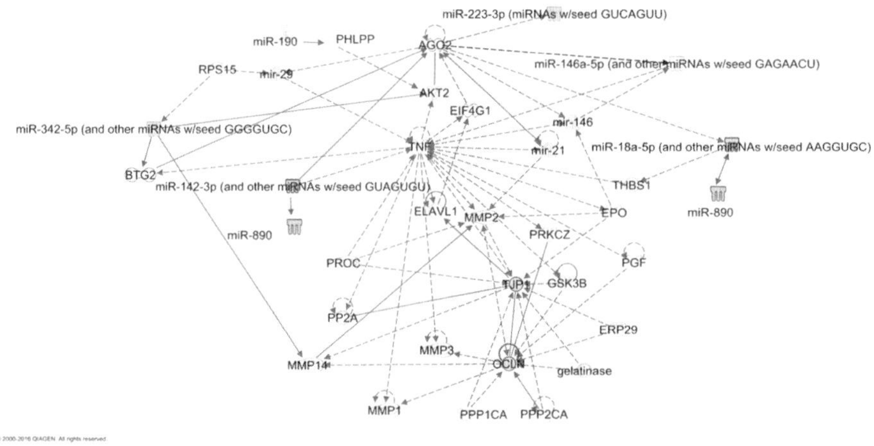

FIGURE 4: A signaling network was constructed by IPA core analysis from the MetS-FL miR trio, the eleven common miR targets of MetS-FL miRs, ZO1, and OCLN. Using Pathway Designer (IPA), miR-890 and miR-190 were added to the network based on present data (Figure 1) and literature [32].

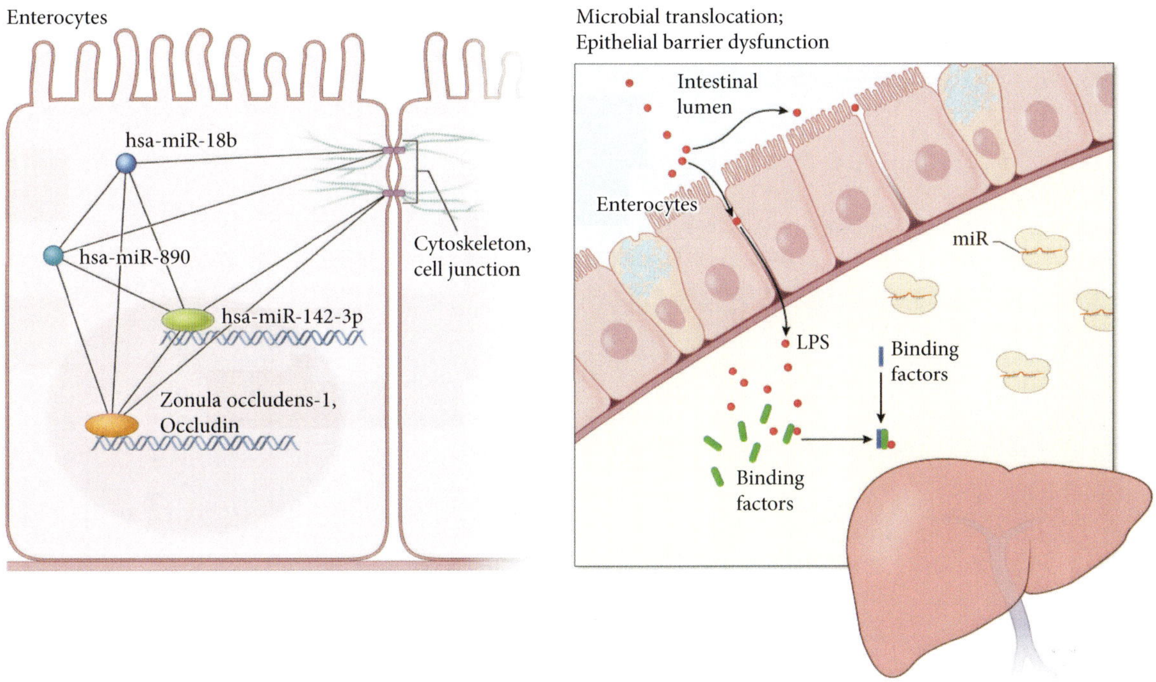

FIGURE 5: Working model of the MetS-FL miRs in colorectal epithelia. On left, signaling network in which the three miRs participate shows a global cellular miRNome network targeting the epithelial cell junction in colon enterocytes. On right, microbial translocation and epithelial barrier dysfunction are associated with the MetS-FL miR network. LPS: lipopolysaccharides. (Acknowledgment: A. Hoofring, NIH Medical Arts Branch).

metabolic stress or injury in the context of MetS and NAFLD. Overall, the present work supports the importance of miRs at the molecular level in MetS and fatty liver, and the *in vitro* data provides mechanistic support for the proposed gut-liver communication in NAFLD pathogenesis. Future work shall expand the present study in other models.

Authors' Contributions

Wendy A. Henderson and Sarah K. Abey designed research. Sarah K. Abey, Natnael D. Kenea, Tatyana G. Vishnyakova, Dan Wang, Nicolaas H. Fourie, and Paule V. Joseph performed experiments and collected data. Paule V. Joseph, Sarah K. Abey, Dan Wang, and Tatyana G. Vishnyakova analyzed data. Paule V. Joseph, Dan Wang, Tatyana G. Vishnyakova, Nicolaas H. Fourie, Christina M. Boulineaux, Kristen R. Weaver, and Jeffrey M. Robinson provided technical expertise. Paule V. Joseph and Dan Wang participated in intellectual discussions. Sarah K. Abey, Paule V. Joseph, and Wendy A. Henderson wrote the manuscript. All authors approved the final edited version. Alan Hoofring illustrated Figure 5 from NIH Medical Arts Branch.

Acknowledgments

This work was supported by the National Institute of Nursing Research (to Wendy A. Henderson, 1ZIANR000018-01-07, and Intramural Research Training Awards to Sarah K. Abey, Paule V. Joseph, Nicolaas H. Fourie, Natnael D. Kenea, Jeffrey M. Robinson, and Christina M. Boulineaux) and Office of Workforce Diversity NIH to PVJ, NIH, DHHS, Bethesda, Maryland, USA.

References

[1] K. G. M. M. Alberti, P. Zimmet, and J. Shaw, "Metabolic syndrome—a new world-wide definition. A consensus statement from the International Diabetes Federation," *Diabetic Medicine*, vol. 23, no. 5, pp. 469–480, 2006.

[2] E. Giovannucci, "Metabolic syndrome, hyperinsulinemia, and colon cancer: a review," *American Journal of Clinical Nutrition*, vol. 86, no. 3, pp. 836S–842S, 2007.

[3] G. C. Kabat, M. Kim, and R. T. Chlebowski, "A longitudinal study of the metabolic syndrome and risk of postmenopausal breast cancer," *Cancer Epidemiology, Biomarkers & Prevention*, vol. 18, no. 7, pp. 2046–2053, 2009.

[4] A. J. Sanyal, S. K. Yoon, and R. Lencioni, "The etiology of hepatocellular carcinoma and consequences for treatment.," *The Oncologist*, vol. 15, pp. 14–22, 2010.

[5] P. W. F. Wilson, R. B. D'Agostino, H. Parise, L. Sullivan, and J. B. Meigs, "Metabolic syndrome as a precursor of cardiovascular disease and type 2 diabetes mellitus," *Circulation*, vol. 112, no. 20, pp. 3066–3072, 2005.

[6] G. Marchesini, E. Bugianesi, G. Forlani et al., "Nonalcoholic fatty liver, steatohepatitis, and the metabolic syndrome," *Hepatology*, vol. 37, no. 4, pp. 917–923, 2003.

[7] J. Luther, J. J. Garber, H. Khalili et al., "Hepatic Injury in Nonalcoholic Steatohepatitis Contributes to Altered Intestinal Permeability," *Cellular and Molecular Gastroenterology and Hepatology*, vol. 1, no. 2, pp. 222–232.e2, 2015.

[8] C. Llorente and B. Schnabl, "The Gut Microbiota and Liver Disease," *Cellular and Molecular Gastroenterology and Hepatology*, vol. 1, no. 3, pp. 275–284, 2015.

[9] E. Spengler and R. Loomba, "The Gut Microbiota, Intestinal Permeability, Bacterial Translocation, and Nonalcoholic Fatty Liver Disease: What Comes First?" *Cellular and Molecular Gastroenterology and Hepatology*, vol. 1, no. 2, pp. 129-130, 2015.

[10] S. Ménard, N. Cerf-Bensussan, and M. Heyman, "Multiple facets of intestinal permeability and epithelial handling of dietary antigens," *Mucosal Immunology*, vol. 3, no. 3, pp. 247–259, 2010.

[11] C. Zihni, C. Mills, K. Matter, and M. S. Balda, "Tight junctions: From simple barriers to multifunctional molecular gates," *Nature Reviews Molecular Cell Biology*, vol. 17, no. 9, pp. 564–580, 2016.

[12] J.-H. Wu, Y.-H. Wang, W. Wang et al., "MIR-18b suppresses high-glucose-induced proliferation in HRECs by targeting IGF-1/IGF1R signaling pathways," *The International Journal of Biochemistry & Cell Biology*, vol. 73, pp. 41–52, 2016.

[13] R. J. Longchamps, S. Abey, A. C. Martino, AY. Del Valle-pinero, B. Majors, and W. A. Henderson, "Spred2, Cd24, and Mmp8 expression: Potential Markers for Fatty Liver Progression to Hepatocellular Carcinoma," *Hepatology*, vol. 56, pp. 892A–893A, 2012.

[14] W. Filipowicz, S. N. Bhattacharyya, and N. Sonenberg, "Mechanisms of post-transcriptional regulation by microRNAs: are the answers in sight?" *Nature Reviews Genetics*, vol. 9, no. 2, pp. 102–114, 2008.

[15] V. Rottiers and A. M. Näär, "MicroRNAs in metabolism and metabolic disorders," *Nature Reviews Molecular Cell Biology*, vol. 13, no. 4, pp. 239–250, 2012.

[16] J. S. Tsang, M. S. Ebert, and A. van Oudenaarden, "Genome-wide Dissection of MicroRNA Functions and Cotargeting Networks Using Gene Set Signatures," *Molecular Cell*, vol. 38, no. 1, pp. 140–153, 2010.

[17] C. Fernandez-Hernando, C. M. Ramírez, L. Goedeke, and Y. Suárez, "MicroRNAs in metabolic disease," *Arteriosclerosis, Thrombosis, and Vascular Biology*, vol. 33, no. 2, pp. 178–185, 2013.

[18] L. Wu, C. Cai, X. Wang, M. Liu, X. Li, and H. Tang, "MicroRNA-142-3p, a new regulator of RAC1, suppresses the migration and invasion of hepatocellular carcinoma cells," *FEBS Letters*, vol. 585, no. 9, pp. 1322–1330, 2011.

[19] Y. Sun, J. Sun, T. Tomomi et al., "PU.1-dependent transcriptional regulation of miR-142 contributes to its hematopoietic cell-specific expression and modulation of IL-6," *The Journal of Immunology*, vol. 190, no. 8, pp. 4005–4013, 2013.

[20] D. V. Chartoumpekis, A. Zaravinos, P. G. Ziros et al., "Differential expression of microRNAs in adipose tissue after long-term high-fat diet-induced obesity in mice," *PLoS ONE*, vol. 7, no. 4, Article ID e34872, 2012.

[21] A. Prats-Puig, F. J. Ortega, J. M. Mercader et al., "Changes in circulating MicroRNAs are associated with childhood obesity," *The Journal of Clinical Endocrinology & Metabolism*, vol. 98, no. 10, pp. E1655–E1660, 2013.

[22] P. D. Cani, J. Amar, M. A. Iglesias et al., "Metabolic endotoxemia initiates obesity and insulin resistance," *Diabetes*, vol. 56, no. 7, pp. 1761–1772, 2007.

[23] C. Sellmann, J. Priebs, M. Landmann et al., "Diets rich in fructose, fat or fructose and fat alter intestinal barrier function and lead to the development of nonalcoholic fatty liver disease over time," *The Journal of Nutritional Biochemistry*, vol. 26, no. 11, pp. 1183–1192, 2015.

[24] L. Miele, V. Valenza, G. La Torre et al., "Increased intestinal permeability and tight junction alterations in nonalcoholic fatty liver disease," *Hepatology*, vol. 49, no. 6, pp. 1877–1887, 2009.

[25] W. A. Henderson, A. C. Martino, A. Y. Del Valle-Pinero, R. M. Peace, and S. K. Abey, "The expression of miR-142-3p in fatty liver," *Gastroenterology*, vol. 142, no. 5S1, p. S-1021, 2012.

[26] A. Y. Del Valle-Pinero, H. E. Van Deventer, N. H. Fourie et al., "Gastrointestinal permeability in patients with irritable bowel syndrome assessed using a four probe permeability solution," *Clinica Chimica Acta*, vol. 418, pp. 97–101, 2013.

[27] A. A. Thompson, S. Dilworth, and R. J. Hay, "Isolation and culture of colonic epithelial cells in serum-free medium," *Journal of tissue culture methods*, vol. 9, no. 2, pp. 117–122, 1985.

[28] R. Mir, S. J. Pradhan, P. Patil, R. Mulherkar, and S. Galande, "Wnt/β-catenin signaling regulated SATB1 promotes colorectal cancer tumorigenesis and progression," *Oncogene*, vol. 35, no. 13, pp. 1679–1691, 2016.

[29] V. Karantza, "Keratins in health and cancer: more than mere epithelial cell markers," *Oncogene*, vol. 30, no. 2, pp. 127–138, 2011.

[30] B. Srinivasan, A. R. Kolli, M. B. Esch, H. E. Abaci, M. L. Shuler, and J. J. Hickman, "TEER measurement techniques for in vitro barrier model systems," *Journal of Laboratory Automation*, vol. 20, no. 2, pp. 107–126, 2015.

[31] P. Artursson, K. Palm, and K. Luthman, "Caco-2 monolayers in experimental and theoretical predictions of drug transport," *Advanced Drug Delivery Reviews*, vol. 46, no. 1-3, pp. 27–43, 2001.

[32] K. Beezhold, J. Liu, H. Kan et al., "miR-190-mediated downregulation of PHLPP contributes to arsenic-induced Akt activation and carcinogenesis," *Toxicological Sciences*, vol. 123, no. 2, pp. 411–420, 2011.

[33] J. Oliveros and C. Venny, "An interactive tool for comparing lists with Venn Diagrams," *Google Scholar*, 2007.

[34] K. J. Livak and T. D. Schmittgen, "Analysis of relative gene expression data using real-time quantitative PCR and the $2^{-\Delta\Delta CT}$ Method," *Methods*, vol. 25, no. 4, pp. 402–408, 2001.

[35] M. R. Fabian, N. Sonenberg, and W. Filipowicz, "Regulation of mRNA translation and stability by microRNAs," *Annual Review of Biochemistry*, vol. 79, pp. 351–379, 2010.

[36] E. Huntzinger and E. Izaurralde, "Gene silencing by microRNAs: contributions of translational repression and mRNA decay," *Nature Reviews Genetics*, vol. 12, no. 2, pp. 99–110, 2011.

[37] A. V. Orang, R. Safaralizadeh, and M. Kazemzadeh-Bavili, "Mechanisms of miRNA-mediated gene regulation from common downregulation to mRNA-specific upregulation," *International Journal of Genomics*, vol. 2014, Article ID 970607, 15 pages, 2014.

[38] H. Tilg and A. R. Moschen, "Evolution of inflammation in nonalcoholic fatty liver disease: the multiple parallel hits hypothesis," *Hepatology*, vol. 52, no. 5, pp. 1836–1846, 2010.

[39] J. Henao-Mejia, E. Elinav, C. Jin et al., "Inflammasome-mediated dysbiosis regulates progression of NAFLD and obesity," *Nature*, vol. 482, no. 7384, pp. 179–185, 2012.

[40] T. Y. Ma, M. A. Boivin, D. Ye, A. Pedram, and H. M. Said, "Mechanism of TNF-α modulation of Caco-2 intestinal epithelial tight junction barrier: role of myosin light-chain kinase protein

expression," *American Journal of Physiology-Gastrointestinal and Liver Physiology*, vol. 288, no. 3, pp. G422–G430, 2005.

[41] R. Barbuio, M. Milanski, M. B. Bertolo, M. J. Saad, and L. A. Velloso, "Infliximab reverses steatosis and improves insulin signal transduction in liver of rats fed a high-fat diet," *Journal of Endocrinology*, vol. 194, no. 3, pp. 539–550, 2007.

[42] H. Nakagawa, A. Umemura, K. Taniguchi et al., "ER Stress Cooperates with Hypernutrition to Trigger TNF-Dependent Spontaneous HCC Development," *Cancer Cell*, vol. 26, no. 3, pp. 331–343, 2014.

[43] B. J. Altman and J. C. Rathmell, "Metabolic Stress in Autophagy and Cell Death Pathways," *Cold Spring Harbor Perspectives in Biology*, vol. 4, no. 9, pp. a008763–a008763, 2012.

[44] K. Düvel, J. L. Yecies, S. Menon et al., "Activation of a metabolic gene regulatory network downstream of mTOR complex 1," *Molecular Cell*, vol. 39, no. 2, pp. 171–183, 2010.

[45] S. Shin, G. R. Buel, L. Wolgamott et al., "ERK2 Mediates Metabolic Stress Response to Regulate Cell Fate," *Molecular Cell*, vol. 59, no. 3, pp. 382–398, 2015.

[46] N. H. Fourie, R. M. Peace, S. K. Abey et al., "Elevated circulating miR-150 and miR-342-3p in patients with irritable bowel syndrome," *Experimental and Molecular Pathology*, vol. 96, no. 3, pp. 422–425, 2014.

[47] R. J. Longchamps, S. K. Abey, A. C. Martino, and W. A. Henderson, "Letter: Gender-associated cell-free microRNA profiles in non-alcoholic fatty liver disease," *Alimentary Pharmacology & Therapeutics*, vol. 39, no. 9, pp. 997-998, 2014.

[48] S. Bala, T. Csak, F. Momen-Heravi et al., "Biodistribution and function of extracellular miRNA-155 in mice," *Scientific Reports*, vol. 5, article 10721, 2015.

[49] M. Zhang, X. Zhou, B. Wang et al., "Lactosylated gramicidin-based lipid nanoparticles (Lac-GLN) for targeted delivery of anti-miR-155 to hepatocellular carcinoma," *Journal of Controlled Release*, vol. 168, no. 3, pp. 251–261, 2013.

[50] K.-H. Ling, M. L. Y. Wan, H. El-Nezami, and M. Wang, "Protective Capacity of Resveratrol, a Natural Polyphenolic Compound, against Deoxynivalenol-Induced Intestinal Barrier Dysfunction and Bacterial Translocation," *Chemical Research in Toxicology*, vol. 29, no. 5, pp. 823–833, 2016.

[51] R. R. Schumann, S. R. Leong, G. W. Flaggs et al., "Structure and function of lipopolysaccharide binding protein," *Science*, vol. 249, no. 4975, pp. 1429–1433, 1990.

[52] J. M. Brenchley, D. A. Price, T. W. Schacker et al., "Microbial translocation is a cause of systemic immune activation in chronic HIV infection," *Nature Medicine*, vol. 12, no. 12, pp. 1365–1371, 2006.

[53] J. Romaní, A. Caixàs, X. Escoté et al., "Lipopolysaccharide-binding protein is increased in patients with psoriasis with metabolic syndrome, and correlates with C-reactive protein," *Clinical and Experimental Dermatology*, vol. 38, no. 1, pp. 81–84, 2013.

[54] A. G. Ruiz, F. Casafont, J. Crespo et al., "Lipopolysaccharide-binding protein plasma levels and liver TNF-alpha gene expression in obese patients: evidence for the potential role of endotoxin in the pathogenesis of non-alcoholic steatohepatitis," *Obesity Surgery*, vol. 17, no. 10, pp. 1374–1380, 2007.

[55] E. Morini, B. Rizzacasa, S. Pucci et al., "The human rs1050286 polymorphism alters LOX-1 expression through modifying miR-24 binding," *Journal of Cellular and Molecular Medicine*, vol. 20, no. 1, pp. 181–187, 2016.

[56] H.-C. Chang, T.-H. Hsieh, Y.-W. Lee et al., "c-Myc and viral cofactor Kaposin B co-operate to elicit angiogenesis through modulating miRNome traits of endothelial cells," *BMC Systems Biology*, vol. 10, no. 1, 2016.

[57] K.-L. Zhang, X. Zhou, L. Han et al., "MicroRNA-566 activates EGFR signaling and its inhibition sensitizes glioblastoma cells to nimotuzumab," *Molecular Cancer*, vol. 13, no. 1, article no. 63, 2014.

[58] A. Drusco, G. J. Nuovo, N. Zanesi et al., "MicroRNA profiles discriminate among colon cancer metastasis," *PLoS ONE*, vol. 9, no. 6, p. e96670, 2014.

[59] M. Tarnowski, M. Tkacz, M. Czerewaty, A. Poniewierska-Baran, K. Grymuła, and M. Z. Ratajczak, "5-Azacytidine inhibits human rhabdomyosarcoma cell growth by downregulating insulin-like growth factor 2 expression and reactivating the H19 gene product miR-675, which negatively affects insulin-like growth factors and insulin signaling," *International Journal of Oncology*, vol. 46, no. 5, pp. 2241–2250, 2015.

[60] K. A. Dudek, J. E. Lafont, A. Martinez-Sanchez, and C. L. Murphy, "Type II collagen expression is regulated by tissue-specific miR-675 in human articular chondrocytes," *The Journal of Biological Chemistry*, vol. 285, no. 32, pp. 24381–24387, 2010.

[61] T. Zou, S. K. Jaladanki, L. Liu et al., "H19 long noncoding RNA regulates intestinal epithelial barrier function via microRNA 675 by Interacting with RNA-binding protein HuR," *Molecular and Cellular Biology*, vol. 36, no. 9, pp. 1332–1341, 2016.

[62] K. Hatano, B. Kumar, Y. Zhang et al., "A functional screen identifies miRNAs that inhibit DNA repair and sensitize prostate cancer cells to ionizing radiation," *Nucleic Acids Research*, vol. 43, no. 8, pp. 4075–4086, 2015.

26

Mesalazine for People with Diverticular Disease

Andrea Iannone,[1] Marinella Ruospo,[2,3] Germaine Wong,[4,5] Michele Barone,[1] Mariabeatrice Principi,[1] Alfredo Di Leo,[1] and Giovanni F. M. Strippoli[2,4,6,7]

[1]*Section of Gastroenterology, Department of Emergency and Organ Transplantation, University of Bari, Italy*
[2]*Diaverum Medical Scientific Office, Lund, Sweden*
[3]*Department of Translational Medicine, Amedeo Avogadro University of Eastern Piedmont, Novara, Italy*
[4]*Sydney School of Public Health, University of Sydney, Australia*
[5]*Centre for Transplant and Renal Research, Westmead Hospital, Sydney, Australia*
[6]*Diaverum Academy, Lund, Sweden*
[7]*Section of Nephrology, Department of Emergency and Organ Transplantation, University of Bari, Italy*

Correspondence should be addressed to Andrea Iannone; ianan@hotmail.it

Academic Editor: Salvatore Oliva

Background. Diverticular disease treatment is limited to fibres, antibiotics, and surgery. There is conflicting evidence on mesalazine benefits and harms. *Aim.* We systematically reviewed current evidence on benefits and harms of mesalazine versus all other treatments in people with diverticular disease. *Methods.* We searched MEDLINE, EMBASE, CENTRAL, ClinicalTrials.gov for studies published to July 2018. We estimated risk ratios (RR) for dichotomous outcomes (disease remission/recurrence, acute diverticulitis in symptomatic uncomplicated diverticular disease, need for surgery/hospitalization, all-cause/disease-related mortality, adverse events), mean differences (MD) or standardized MD (SMD) for continuous outcomes (quality of life, symptoms score, time to recurrence/remission), and their 95% confidence intervals (CI) using random-effects models. We quantified heterogeneity by Chi^2 and I^2 tests. We performed subgroup analyses by disease subtype, comparator, follow-up duration, mesalazine dose, and mode of administration. *Results.* We identified 13 randomized trials (n=3028 participants). There was a higher likelihood of disease remission with mesalazine than controls in acute uncomplicated diverticulitis (1 trial, 81 participants, RR=2.67, 95%CI=1.05-6.79), but not in symptomatic uncomplicated diverticular disease (1 trial, 123 participants, RR=1.04, 95%CI=0.81-1.34). There was a lower likelihood of disease recurrence with mesalazine than controls in symptomatic uncomplicated diverticular disease (2 trials, 216 participants, RR=0.52, 95%CI=0.28-0.97), but not in acute uncomplicated diverticulitis (7 trials, 2196 participants, RR=0.90, 95%CI=0.61-1.33). There was no difference in the likelihood of developing acute diverticulitis in symptomatic uncomplicated diverticular disease between the two groups (3 trials, 484 participants, RR=0.26, 95%CI=0.06-1.20). There was a higher global symptoms score reduction with mesalazine than controls in symptomatic uncomplicated diverticular disease (2 trials, 326 participants, SMD=-1.01, 95%CI=-1.51,-0.52) and acute uncomplicated diverticulitis (2 trials, 153 participants, SMD=-0.56, 95%CI=-0.88,-0.24). *Conclusions.* Mesalazine may reduce recurrences in symptomatic uncomplicated diverticular disease. There is uncertainty on the effect of mesalazine in achieving diverticular disease remission. Mesalazine may not prevent acute diverticulitis in symptomatic uncomplicated diverticular disease.

1. Introduction

The prevalence of colonic diverticulosis increases with age, ranging from approximately 30% in people aged 50-59 years to around 70% in those older than 80 years [1]. Some 20% of people with diverticulosis experience symptoms related to diverticular mucosa inflammation, ranging from mild abdominal pain to severe complications [2]; this condition is defined diverticular disease [3]. Low dietary fibre intake, gut microbiota alteration, obesity and changes in colonic motility, and sensitivity play a role in the development of symptoms and complications in diverticular disease [4]. About 2% of people with diverticular disease require hospital admission, 0.5% need surgery, and 1% die during hospitalization [5, 6].

Current management of diverticular disease focuses on dietary and pharmacological interventions, such as rifaximin and systemic antibiotics. Some guidelines [4, 7, 8] suggest the combination of high-fibre diet and rifaximin in symptomatic uncomplicated diverticular disease for symptoms relief and acute diverticulitis prevention. In case of acute diverticulitis, differently from early recommendations [3, 9–11], antibiotics are currently suggested only if complications arise and surgical interventions are required [4, 7, 8, 12–16]. No treatment prevents diverticular disease recurrences or complications (Supplementary Table 1).

Given the existing uncertainties, mesalazine, an anti-inflammatory drug, has been purported as a promising intervention in diverticular disease. Studies with different designs have investigated the use of mesalazine in diverticular disease and found contradicting results on achieving disease remission and preventing recurrences. Despite these individual conflicting findings, some clinical practice guidelines now recommend mesalazine for symptom relief in symptomatic uncomplicated diverticular disease [7, 14] or recurrence prevention in acute uncomplicated diverticulitis [12].

We systematically reviewed the totality of evidence on the benefits and harms of mesalazine versus all other treatments in people with diverticular disease, to inform clinical decisions.

2. Materials and Methods

The review was conducted according to the Preferred Reporting Items for Systematic Reviews and Meta-Analyses (PRISMA) statement [17].

2.1. Data Sources and Searches. A comprehensive literature search for randomized controlled trials of mesalazine in diverticular disease was performed in MEDLINE (1946 to July 2018), EMBASE (1996 to July 2018), the Cochrane Central Register of Controlled Trials (CENTRAL, from inception to July 2018), and ClinicalTrials.gov (searched on July 2018) using highly sensitive search strategies designed by an information specialist (RM). Searches were performed without language restriction. Relevant studies were also searched from reference lists of identified trials and guidelines. Search strategies are outlined in Supplementary Table 2.

2.2. Study Selection. Two reviewers (AI, MR) independently screened the searches by title and abstract, then the full text, to identify potentially eligible trials. We included any randomized controlled trials which compared mesalazine, at any dose, mode, and duration of administration with any intervention for the treatment of people with diverticular disease. Diverticular disease was defined as the presence of any colonic diverticula-related symptoms [3]. Considering the lack of a standardized definition of symptomatic uncomplicated diverticular disease, we considered this subtype of diverticular disease as the occurrence of nonspecific diverticular disease-related abdominal symptoms, such as lower abdominal pain and altered bowel habit, in the absence of macroscopic colonic mucosa alterations [4, 7, 14]. Acute uncomplicated diverticulitis was defined as the presence of macroscopic diverticula inflammation which causes symptoms, such as fever, lower abdominal pain, and leukocytosis in people with diverticular disease [4, 8, 14, 15]. The development of complications, such as abscess, perforation, obstruction, or bleeding, characterized by acute complicated diverticulitis [2]. We included studies in which colonic diverticulosis diagnosis was performed by endoscopy and/or radiologic imaging.

We excluded trials not involving any arm treated with mesalazine alone or comparing this treatment only with a combination therapy including mesalazine. We also excluded trials investigating mesalazine in people with segmental colitis associated with diverticulosis, a chronic inflammatory process involving the interdiverticular mucosa, since it is considered a distinct pathologic entity [4, 18].

2.3. Data Extraction and Quality Assessment. Two reviewers (AI, MR) independently assessed each randomized controlled trial for eligibility and extracted data on study, population, intervention (experimental and comparator treatments), and outcomes characteristics.

2.3.1. Outcomes Measures. We evaluated the number of participants achieving diverticular disease remission, developing diverticular disease recurrence, and experiencing acute diverticulitis in symptomatic uncomplicated diverticular disease. We considered disease remission as the disappearance of all diverticula-related symptoms after the beginning of treatment with mesalazine or other interventions; relapse of diverticula-related symptoms in asymptomatic participants, after the beginning of the treatment with mesalazine or other interventions, was defined as disease recurrence.

Other outcomes were quality of life and symptoms relief assessed by any instrument reported in the trials, the number of participants requiring surgery and needing hospitalization, all-cause and diverticular disease-related mortality, any adverse events and time to diverticular disease recurrence, diverticular disease remission, and surgery and acute diverticulitis onset in symptomatic uncomplicated diverticular disease. We extracted outcome data according to the maximum period of observation in each trial.

If published outcome data were not reported or provided in sufficient detail, an author (AI) contacted trial investigators one time by electronic mail requesting any relevant additional information. When obtained, information was included in the analyses.

2.3.2. Risk of Bias Assessment. We assessed the study level risk of bias with the Cochrane risk of bias tool, including the domains of random sequence generation, allocation concealment, blinding of participants or investigators, blinding of outcome assessment, completeness of outcome data, selective reporting, and other threats to validity.

Review authors resolved any disagreement in data extraction and quality assessment through discussion and involvement of an arbitrator (GFMS).

2.4. Data Synthesis and Analysis. We estimated risk ratios (RR) for dichotomous outcomes and mean differences (MD) for continuous outcomes, with their 95% confidence intervals (95%CI), in individual studies. If continuous outcomes were measured using different scales across individual studies, we calculated standardized mean differences (SMD) with 95%CI. We assessed pooled estimates using the DerSimonian and Laird random-effects model [19].

We formally estimated heterogeneity of intervention effects among studies with the Chi^2 (Cochran Q) and the I^2 statistics.

We performed prespecified subgroup analyses by subtype of diverticular disease (symptomatic uncomplicated diverticular disease, acute uncomplicated diverticulitis or acute complicated diverticulitis), type of comparator (probiotics, rifaximin, systemic antibiotics, placebo, or no treatment), follow-up duration (less than 3 months, 3 to 6 months, 6 to 12 months, or more than 12 months), mesalazine dose (800 to 1600 mg, more than 1600 to 2400 mg, or more than 2400 mg), and mode of administration (continuous or cyclic). All subgroup analyses were stratified by subtype of diverticular disease.

To avoid double-counting of participants in trials comparing mesalazine with more than one intervention, we divided the events and total number of participants allocated to the mesalazine arm according to the number of times that data from this group was used in each analysis. We used the same method for trials including more than one mesalazine arm, with different drug doses, dividing the events and total number of patients allocated to the comparator arm according to the number of times that data from this group was used in each analysis. We estimated differences among subgroups by the Mantel-Haenszel test. We planned to explore publication bias with funnel plots where at least 10 studies were included [20].

We rated quality of evidence according to the Grades of Recommendation, Assessment, Development and Evaluation (GRADE) approach [21].

All analyses were performed using RevMan 5.3 (The Cochrane Collaboration, Copenhagen, Denmark).

3. Results

3.1. Search Results. Of 245 articles identified electronically, 80 were duplicates and 131 were ineligible after abstract review (Figure 1). The remaining 34 articles were retrieved and reviewed in full text form, with 13 trials (11 publications) [22–32], enrolling a total of 3028 participants with diverticular disease, included. We received additional unpublished information from the authors of 3 trials [24, 25, 29]. Two trials published in 2007 by the same group [24, 25] had only 8 participants included in both studies; thus they were considered as separate trials.

3.2. Characteristics of Included Studies. Table 1 shows the characteristics of populations, intervention, and comparators in the included studies. Sample size in the trials varied from 43 to 592. Six trials (46%) [23–27, 30] enrolled people with symptomatic uncomplicated diverticular disease and 7 (54%) [22, 28, 29, 31, 32] enrolled people with acute uncomplicated diverticulitis. No study included patients with acute complicated diverticulitis. Mesalazine was compared with probiotics in 1 (8%) [23], rifaximin in 2 (15%) [24, 25], placebo in 8 (61%) [26–29, 31, 32], no treatment in 1 (8%) [22], and both probiotics and placebo in 1 (8%) trials [30]. No study compared mesalazine with systemic antibiotics.

3.3. Quality of Studies. The risk of bias of the 13 included trials is summarized in Supplementary Figure 1.

Random sequence generation was adequate in 7 (54%) trials and unclear in 6 (46%). Allocation concealment was adequate in 2 (15%) studies and unclear in 11 (85%). Blinding of participants and investigators was adequate in 8 (62%) trials, inadequate in 2 (15%), and unclear in the remaining 3 (23%). Seven (54%) trials had adequate blinding of outcome assessment, while in 6 (46%) this was unclear. Analysis was by intention-to-treat in 5 (38%) and both intention-to-treat and per protocol in 6 (46%) trials, while this was unclear in the remaining 2 (16%). Withdrawal of participants from analyses was <10% in 7 (54%) trials and >10% in 6 (46%).

Four (31%) out of 13 included trials were at low risk of bias for most of the quality domains [27, 30–32].

3.4. Outcomes. Table 2 summarizes key results of the comparison of mesalazine versus control interventions for diverticular disease, by disease subtype, and the grading of evidence assessment, according to the GRADE approach. Complete results of the comparison of mesalazine versus control interventions for diverticular disease are shown in Supplementary Table 3.

3.4.1. Disease Remission. There was no statistically significant difference in the likelihood of achieving diverticular disease remission between mesalazine and control interventions (2 trials, 204 participants, RR=1.51, 95%CI=0.57-3.98, and I^2=76%).

3.4.2. Disease Recurrence. There was no statistically significant difference in the likelihood of diverticular disease recurrence between mesalazine and control interventions (9 trials, 2414 participants, RR=0.83, 95%CI=0.58-1.19, and I^2=73%) (Figure 2). One trial [22] had participants treated only for 2 months and then followed up for 48 months, leading to uncertainty on the association between mesalazine and prevention of disease recurrence. Another trial [28] enrolled only people at their first diagnosis of acute uncomplicated diverticulitis, a condition with an increased response to mesalazine [2].

Table 1: Characteristics of the randomized controlled trials comparing mesalazine with control interventions for diverticular disease.

Study (reference)	Year	Number of patients	Mean age (SD)	Procedure used for diagnosis of diverticular disease		Characteristics of diverticular disease		First diagnosis of diverticular disease (%)	Mean time from last episode of diverticular disease (SD), *days*	Characteristics of experimental treatment (mesalazine)		Characteristics of control interventions			Treatment duration, *months*	Follow-up duration, *months*
				Endoscopy	Radiologic imaging	Subtype	Activity			Daily dose, *mg*	Mode of administration	Type	Daily dose	Mode of administration		
Trespi et al. [22]	1999	166	61.4 (6.4)	√	√	Acute uncomplicated diverticulitis	Remission	21.0	na	800	Continuous	No treatment	/	/	2	48
Tursi et al. [23]	2006	60[a]	67.5	√		Symptomatic uncomplicated diverticular disease	Remission	31.1	na	1600	Continuous	Lactobacillus casei sub-species DG	16 billion viable lyophilized bacteria	Cyclic (15 days/month)	12	12
Comparato et al. *a* [24]	2007	58[b]	67.3 (10.2)	√	√	Symptomatic uncomplicated diverticular disease	Active	na	na	800 or 1600	Cyclic (10 days/month)	Rifaximin	400 or 800 mg	Cyclic (10 days/month)	6	6
Comparato et al. *b* [25]	2007	268[b]	65.0 (7.2)–67.4 (9.1)	√	√	Symptomatic uncomplicated diverticular disease	Active	na	na	800 or 1600	Cyclic (10 days/month)	Rifaximin	400 or 800 mg	Cyclic (10 days/month)	12	12
Smith et al. [26]	2012	43	na	√		Symptomatic uncomplicated diverticular disease	Active	na	na	3000	Continuous	Placebo	/	Continuous	3	3
Kruis et al. [27]	2013	123	63.0 (8.6)-62.0 (8.6)	√		Symptomatic uncomplicated diverticular disease	Active	na	na	3000	Continuous	Placebo	/	Continuous	6 weeks	6 weeks
Parente et al. [28]	2013	92[c]	61.5 (11.1)	√	√	Acute uncomplicated diverticulitis	Remission	100.0	<12 months	1600	Cyclic (10 days/month)	Placebo	/	Cyclic (10 days/month)	24	24
Stollman et al. [29]	2013	81[d]	56.1 (11.1)-57.7 (12.8)		√	Acute uncomplicated diverticulitis	Active	49.6	na	2400	Continuous	Placebo	/	Continuous	3	12
Tursi et al. [30]	2013	156[e]	60-64[f]	√		Symptomatic uncomplicated diverticular disease	Remission	54.3	na	1600	Cyclic (10 days/month)	Placebo Lactobacillus casei sub-species DG	/ 24 billion viable lyophilized bacteria	Cyclic (10 days/month) Cyclic (10 days/month)	12	12
PREVENT1 [31][g]	2014	590	55.3 (11.4)	√	√	Acute uncomplicated diverticulitis	Remission	58.1	91.0[f]	1200 or 2400 or 4800	Continuous	Placebo	/	Continuous	24	24
PREVENT2 [31][g]	2014	592	56.1 (11.0)	√	√	Acute uncomplicated diverticulitis	Remission	59.7	115.5[f]	1200 or 2400 or 4800	Continuous	Placebo	/	Continuous	24	24
SAG-37 [32][h]	2017	345	58.6 (9.3)		√	Acute uncomplicated diverticulitis	Remission	55.0	87.0 (48.0)	3000	Continuous	Placebo	/	Continuous	12	12
SAG-51 [32][h]	2017	330	55.4 (10.6)		√	Acute uncomplicated diverticulitis	Remission	51.2	89.0 (44.0)	1500 or 3000	Continuous	Placebo	/	Continuous	24	24

SD, standard deviation; na, not assessed.
[a]The study includes 3 arms (mesalazine, probiotic, and mesalazine plus probiotic), but only the mesalazine and probiotic arms were considered in this analysis.
[b]8 participants were included in both studies.
[c]96 participants were randomized; 4 were excluded for no study drug assumption, but there is no mention on their study group. Thus, only 92 participants are included in our analysis.
[d]The study includes 3 arms (mesalazine, placebo, and mesalazine plus probiotic), but only the mesalazine and placebo arms were considered in this analysis.
[e]The study includes 4 arms (mesalazine, probiotic, mesalazine plus probiotic, and placebo), but only the mesalazine, probiotic, and placebo arms were considered in this analysis.
[f]Median value.
[g]The same publication includes two randomized trials with identical study design.
[h]The same publication includes two randomized trials.

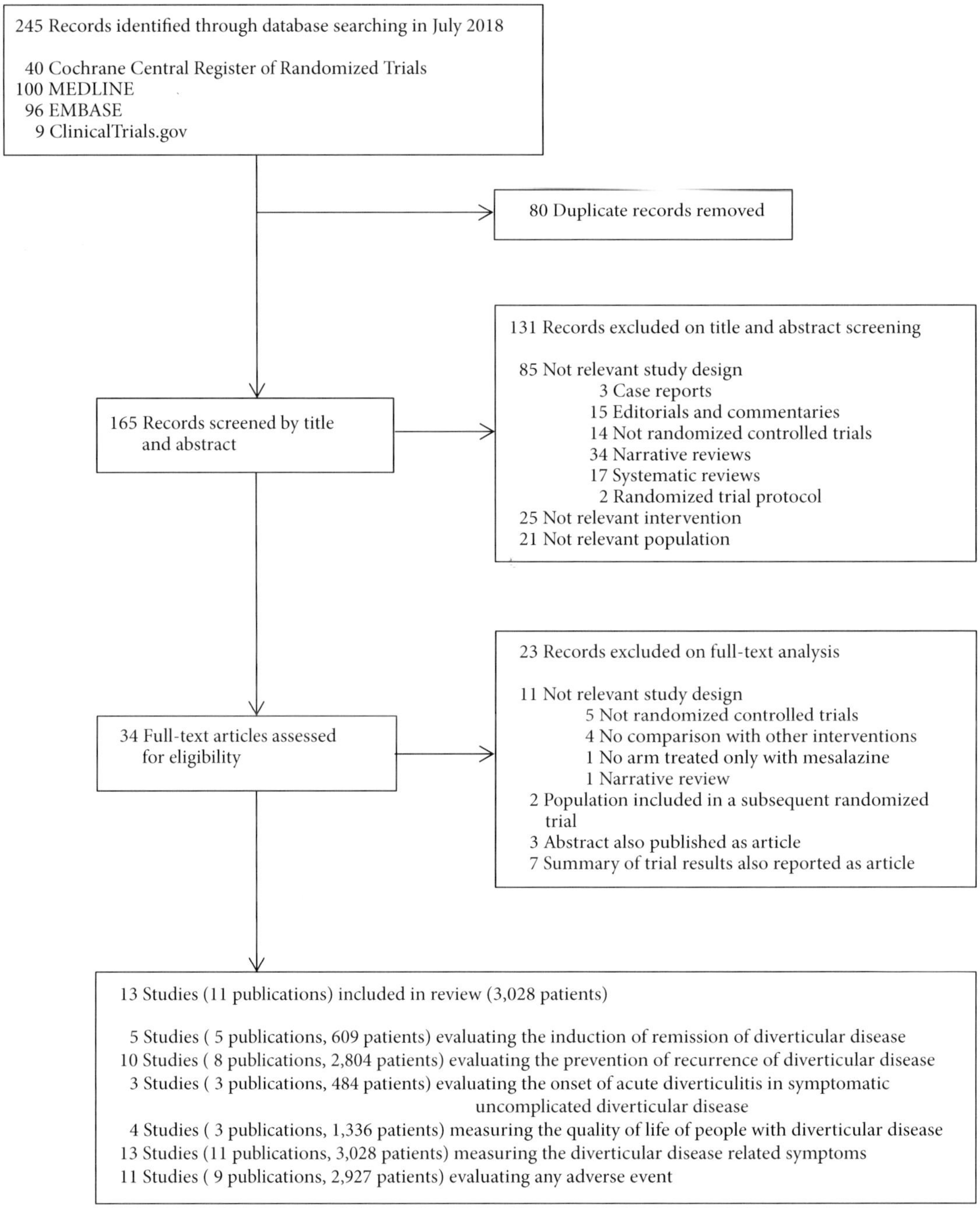

FIGURE 1: Flow diagram of search results and selection of included studies.

3.4.3. Acute Diverticulitis Onset in Symptomatic Uncomplicated Diverticular Disease. There was no statistically significant difference in the likelihood of developing acute diverticulitis in symptomatic uncomplicated diverticular disease between mesalazine and control interventions (3 trials, 484 participants, RR=0.26, 95%CI=0.06-1.20, and I^2=0%).

3.4.4. Quality of Life. Four trials [24, 28, 31] compared mesalazine with control interventions on quality of life (Table 3). One trial [24] included participants with symptomatic uncomplicated diverticular disease, while 3 [28, 31] included people with acute uncomplicated diverticulitis. There was a higher improvement of physical functioning ($p<0.05$) and general health ($p=0.01$) in the mesalazine than rifaximin group at 6 months in people with symptomatic uncomplicated diverticular disease [24]. Conversely, there was no significant difference in quality of life scores between the two groups in acute uncomplicated diverticulitis [28, 31].

3.4.5. Symptoms Relief. Thirteen trials [22–32] compared mesalazine with control interventions on symptoms relief (Supplementary Table 4). There was a statistically significant

TABLE 2: Summary of findings: mesalazine versus control interventions by subtype of diverticular disease.

Outcome	Subtype of diverticular disease	No. of participants (no. of studies)	Absolute effect (per 100 patients treated)	Relative effect (95% CI)	Certainty of the evidence (GRADE)	Conclusion
Achievement of disease remission	Symptomatic uncomplicated diverticular disease	123 (1)	3 more per 100 (95% CI: 14 fewer to 19 more)	1.04 (0.81 to 1.34)	Very Low ●○○○	It is uncertain whether mesalazine may lead to no difference in the achievement of disease remission.
	Acute uncomplicated diverticulitis	81 (1)	20 more per 100 (95% CI: 3 fewer to 38 more)	2.67 (1.05 to 6.79)	Very Low ●○○○	It is uncertain whether mesalazine may lead to the achievement of disease remission.
Disease recurrence	Symptomatic uncomplicated diverticular disease	216 (2)	13 fewer per 100 (95% CI: 23 to 2 fewer)	0.52 (0.28 to 0.97)	Low ●●○○	Mesalazine may decrease disease recurrence.
	Acute uncomplicated diverticulitis	2196 (7)	3 fewer per 100 (95% CI: 12 fewer to 6 more)	0.90 (0.61 to 1.33)	Low ●●○○	Mesalazine may lead to no difference in disease recurrence.
Acute diverticulitis onset in symptomatic uncomplicated diverticular disease	Symptomatic uncomplicated diverticular disease	484 (3)	3 fewer per 100 (95% CI: 7 fewer to 0)	0.26 (0.06 to 1.20)	Low ●●○○	Mesalazine may lead to no difference in the development of acute diverticulitis in patients with symptomatic uncomplicated diverticular disease.
Need for surgery	Symptomatic uncomplicated diverticular disease	424 (2)	No effect per 100 (95% CI: 1 fewer to 1 more)	0.68 (0.03 to 16.39)	Very Low ●○○○	It is uncertain whether mesalazine may lead to no difference in the need for surgery.
	Acute uncomplicated diverticulitis	1263 (3)	1 more per 100 (95% CI: 0 to 2 more)	1.41 (0.51 to 3.90)	Low ●●○○	Mesalazine may lead to no difference in the need for surgery.
Any adverse events	Symptomatic uncomplicated diverticular disease	391 (2)	1 fewer per 100 (95% CI: 5 fewer to 3 more)	1.04 (0.55 to 1.98)	Low ●●○○	Mesalazine may lead to no difference in any adverse events.
	Acute uncomplicated diverticulitis	2196 (7)	3 more per 100 (95% CI: 2 fewer to 7 more)	1.03 (0.96 to 1.11)	Moderate ●●●○	Mesalazine probably results in no difference in any adverse events.
All-cause mortality	Symptomatic uncomplicated diverticular disease	607 (4)	No effect per 100 (95% CI: 1 fewer to 1 more)	No event in included studies	Very Low ●○○○	It is uncertain whether mesalazine may lead to no difference in all-cause mortality.
	Acute uncomplicated diverticulitis	1512 (5)	No effect per 100 (95% CI: 1 fewer to 1 more)	0.52 (0.05 to 5.68)	Very Low ●○○○	It is uncertain whether mesalazine may lead to no difference in all-cause mortality.
Diverticular disease related mortality	Symptomatic uncomplicated diverticular disease	607 (4)	No effect per 100 (95% CI: 1 fewer to 1 more)	No event in included studies	Very Low ●○○○	It is uncertain whether mesalazine may lead to no difference in diverticular disease related mortality.
	Acute uncomplicated diverticulitis	1512 (5)	No effect per 100 (95% CI: 1 fewer to 1 more)	No event in included studies	Very Low ●○○○	It is uncertain whether mesalazine may lead to no difference in diverticular disease related mortality.
Global symptoms score[a]	Symptomatic uncomplicated diverticular disease	326 (2)	Standardized mean difference: 1.01 lower (95% CI: 1.51 to 0.52 lower)	-	Low ●●○○	Mesalazine may improve the global symptoms score.
	Acute uncomplicated diverticulitis	153 (2)	Standardized mean difference: 0.56 lower (95% CI: 0.88 to 0.24 lower)	-	Low ●●○○	Mesalazine may slightly improve the global symptoms score.
Time to recurrence (days)	Symptomatic uncomplicated diverticular disease	- (-)	No studies	-	Absent	No studies were found that evaluated the impact of mesalazine on time to disease recurrence of disease.
	Acute uncomplicated diverticulitis	91 (3)	Average difference in days: 30 lower (95% CI: 55 to 5 lower)	-	Very Low ●○○○	It is uncertain whether mesalazine may lead to a decrease in time to disease recurrence.

[a]The standardized mean difference was used because global symptoms were assessed using different scales across included studies: 0 to 33 [24], 0 to 36 [25], 0 to 60 [29], and 4 to 40 [28].

Study, year (reference)	Mesalazine Events	Mesalazine Total	Control interventions Events	Control interventions Total	Weight	Risk Ratio M-H, Random, 95% CI
Number of patients with recurrence of disease						
Symptomatic uncomplicated diverticular disease						
Tursi et al., 2006 [23]	4	30	6	30	6.1%	0.67 [0.21, 2.13]
Tursi et al., 2013 [30]	7	51	31	105	9.7%	0.46 [0.22, 0.98]
Subtotal (95% CI)	**11**	**81**	**37**	**135**	**15.7%**	**0.52 [0.28, 0.97]**
Heterogeneity: Tau² = 0.001; Chi² = 0.26, df = 1 (P = 0.61); I² = 0%						
Acute uncomplicated diverticulitis						
Parente et al., 2013 [28]	6	45	13	47	8.4%	0.48 [0.20, 1.16]
Stollman et al., 2013 [29]	12	40	12	41	10.5%	1.02 [0.52, 2.01]
Trespi et al., 1999 [22]	12	81	39	85	11.7%	0.32 [0.18, 0.57]
SAG-37, 2017 [32]	31	171	20	174	12.3%	1.58 [0.94, 2.66]
SAG-51, 2017 [32]	33	217	20	113	12.5%	0.86 [0.52, 1.43]
PREVENT2, 2014 [31]	122	446	28	146	14.2%	1.43 [0.99, 2.06]
PREVENT1, 2014 [31]	115	441	35	149	14.6%	1.11 [0.80, 1.54]
Subtotal (95% CI)	**331**	**1441**	**167**	**755**	**84.3%**	**0.90 [0.61, 1.33]**
Heterogeneity: Tau² = 0.20; Chi² = 25.02, df = 6 (P < 0.001); I² = 76%						
Total (95% CI)	**342**	**1522**	**204**	**890**	**100.0%**	**0.83 [0.58, 1.19]**
Heterogeneity: Tau² = 0.27; Chi² = 25.39, df = 6 (P < 0.001); I² = 76%						
Test for overall effect: Z = 1.34 (P = 0.18)						
Test for subgroup differences: Chi² = 1.02, df = 1 (P = 0.31), I² = 1.8%						

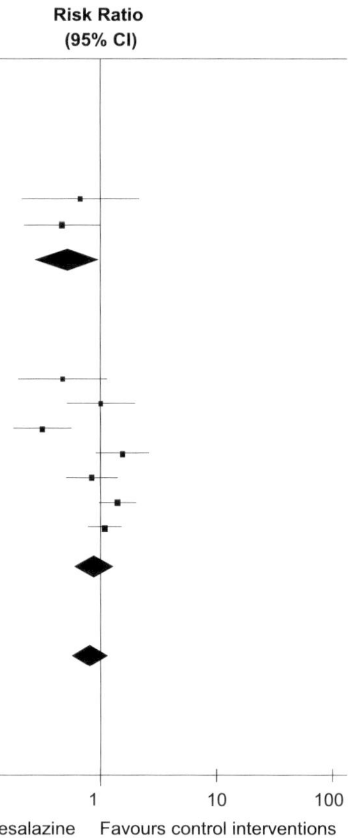

Figure 2: Comparative effectiveness of mesalazine versus control interventions by subtype of diverticular disease on the number of participants developing disease recurrence.

reduction of diverticula-related symptoms with mesalazine compared to control interventions in 4 out of 6 trials on symptomatic uncomplicated diverticular disease and in 2 out of 7 trials on acute uncomplicated diverticulitis. In the analysis of the 4 [24, 25, 28, 29] trials reporting a global symptoms score, there was a lower mean score at maximum follow-up with mesalazine than control interventions (4 trials, 479 participants, SMD=-0.79, 95%CI=-1.18,-0.39, and I^2=72%) (Figure 3). Baseline global symptoms score was not statistically different between mesalazine and control interventions arms in all included studies.

A summary of trial results for other outcomes is reported in Supplementary Table 3.

3.4.6. Subgroup Analyses. Subgroup analyses by subtype of diverticular disease, type of control intervention, follow-up duration, mesalazine dose, and mode of administration are reported in Supplementary Tables 3, 5, 6, 7, and 8, respectively.

Subtype of Diverticular Disease. There was a higher likelihood of achieving remission with mesalazine than control interventions in acute uncomplicated diverticulitis (1 trial, 81 participants, RR=2.67, and 95%CI=1.05-6.79), but not in symptomatic uncomplicated diverticular disease (1 trial, 123 participants, RR=1.04, and 95%CI=0.81-1.34). There was no significant interaction between subgroups (p=0.06). There was a lower likelihood of recurrence with mesalazine than control interventions in symptomatic uncomplicated diverticular disease (2 trials, 216 participants, RR=0.52, and 95%CI=0.28-0.97), but not in acute uncomplicated diverticulitis (7 trials, 2196 participants, RR=0.90, and 95%CI=0.61-1.33) (Figure 2). There was no significant interaction between subgroups (p=0.14). There was a lower mean score at maximum follow-up with mesalazine than control interventions in both symptomatic uncomplicated diverticular disease (2 trials, 326 participants, SMD=-1.01, and 95%CI=-1.51,-0.52) and acute uncomplicated diverticulitis (2 trials, 153 participants, SMD=-0.56, and 95%CI=-0.88,-0.24) (Figure 3). There was no significant interaction between subgroups (p=0.13).

Type of Comparator. There was a lower likelihood of symptomatic uncomplicated diverticular disease recurrence with mesalazine only in the comparison with placebo (1 trial, 101 participants, RR=0.33, and 95%CI=0.13-0.86). There was no significant interaction among subgroups (p=0.22). In acute uncomplicated diverticulitis, there was a lower likelihood of recurrence with mesalazine only in the comparison with no treatment (1 trial, 166 participants, RR=0.32, and 95%CI=0.18-0.57), with a statistically significant difference among subgroups (p=0.001). However, in the single study [22] comparing mesalazine with no treatment participants were treated only for 2 months and then followed up for 48

Table 3: Quality of life assessment of people enrolled in randomized trials comparing mesalazine with control interventions for diverticular disease.

Study, year (reference)	Quality-of-life instrument	Validation of the instrument	Time of assessment	Method of Reporting	Domains reported	Results
Comparato et al., 2007*a* [24]	Medical Outcome Study (MOS) 36-Item Short-Form Health Survey (SF-36, Italian version 1.6) questionnaire	Yes[a]	Baseline and 6 months	Mean change of each domain score between baseline and 6 months in the mesalazine and rifaximin group. Difference of the mean scores of each domain at baseline and 6 months between the two groups.	Physical health: Physical functioning Role limitation-physical Bodily pain General health Mental health: Role limitation-emotional Vitality Mental health Social functioning	In the mesalazine group there was a significant improvement of physical functioning (p=0.05), role limitation-physical (p=0.034), general health (p=0.01), and social functioning (p<0.01) at 6 months. In the rifaximin group there was a significant improvement of role limitation-physical (p=0.04) and social functioning (p=0.03) at 6 months. There was no statistically significant difference of SF-36 mean scores between the two groups at baseline. There was a higher improvement of physical functioning (p<0.05) and general health (p=0.01) in the mesalazine than rifaximin group at 6 months.
Parente et al., 2013 [28]	Therapy Impact Questionnaire (TIQ), quality-of-life sub-score[b]	No	Baseline and every 3 months until 24 months	Difference of the mean quality-of-life sub-scores at baseline and 24 months between mesalazine and placebo group.	Sleeping problem Physical status interfering with sexual activity Problem in out-door activities Problem in social activities Problem in in-house activities different from house works Problem in daily work activities Problem in free-time activities	There was no statistically significant difference of the total quality-of-life sub-score between the mesalazine and placebo group at baseline and 24 months.
PREVENT1, 2014 [31]	(1) EuroQol five dimensions questionnaire (EQ-5D) (2) Health Utilities Index Version Mark 2 (HUI2) questionnaire	Yes[a]	Baseline and 16, 52, 78, 104 weeks	Difference of the total EQ-5D and HUI2 scores at baseline and 104 weeks across study arms (mesalazine 1200mg, mesalazine 2400mg, mesalazine 4800mg, placebo).	EQ-5D questionnaire: Mobility Self-care Usual activities Pain/discomfort Anxiety/depression HUI2 questionnaire: Sensation Cognition Mobility Self-care Emotion Pain Fertility	There was no statistically significant difference of the total EQ-5D and HUI2 scores at baseline and 104 weeks across study arms.
PREVENT2, 2014 [31]	(1) EuroQol five dimensions questionnaire (EQ-5D) (2) Health Utilities Index Version Mark 2 (HUI2) questionnaire	Yes[a]	Baseline and 16, 52, 78, 104 weeks	Difference of the total EQ-5D and HUI2 scores at baseline and 104 weeks across study arms (mesalazine 1200mg, mesalazine 2400mg, mesalazine 4800mg, placebo).	EQ-5D questionnaire: Mobility Self-care Usual activities Pain/discomfort Anxiety/depression HUI2 questionnaire: Sensation Cognition Mobility Self-care Emotion Pain Fertility	There was no statistically significant difference of the total EQ-5D and HUI2 scores at baseline and 104 weeks across study arms.

EQ-5D, EuroQol five dimensions; HUI2, Health Utilities Index Version Mark 2.
[a]Instrument validated to measure generic health outcomes in all therapeutic areas.
[b]11-item questionnaire: the sum of items 1-4 defines the physical condition subscore, while the sum of items 5-11 defines the quality-of-life subscore.

Study, year (reference)	Mesalazine Patients, *n*	Mesalazine Mean (SD)	Control interventions Patients, *n*	Control interventions Mean (SD)	Weight	Standardized Mean Difference IV, Random, 95% CI
Global symptoms score*						
Symptomatic uncomplicated diverticular disease						
Comparato et al., 2007a [24]	31	5.77 (2.76)	27	8.04 (3.65)	21.6%	-0.70 [-1.23, -0.17]
Comparato et al., 2007b [25]	133	3.00 (1.86)	135	6.87 (4.07)	30.8%	-1.22 [-1.48, -0.96]
Subtotal (95% CI)	**164**		**162**		**52.3%**	**-1.01 [-1.51, -0.52]**
Heterogeneity: $Tau^2 = 0.09$; $Chi^2 = 2.93$, df = 1 (P = 0.09); $I^2 = 66\%$						
Acute uncomplicated diverticulitis						
Stollman et al., 2013 [29]	32	4.40 (6.05)	29	7.30 (7.00)	22.3%	-0.44 [-0.95, 0.07]
Parente et al., 2013 [28]	45	5.40 (2.70)	47	8.30 (5.70)	25.3%	-0.64 [-1.06, -0.22]
Subtotal (95% CI)	**77**		**76**		**47.7%**	**-0.56 [-0.88, -0.24]**
Heterogeneity: $Tau^2 = 0.001$; $Chi^2 = 0.36$, df = 1 (P = 0.55); $I^2 = 0\%$						
Total (95% CI)	**241**		**238**		**100.0%**	**-0.79 [-1.18, -0.39]**
Heterogeneity: $Tau^2 = 0.11$; $Chi^2 = 10.76$, df = 3 (P = 0.01); $I^2 = 72\%$						
Test for overall effect: Z = 3.91 (P < 0.001)						
Test for subgroup differences: $Chi^2 = 2.25$, df = 1 (P = 0.13), $I^2 = 55.5\%$						

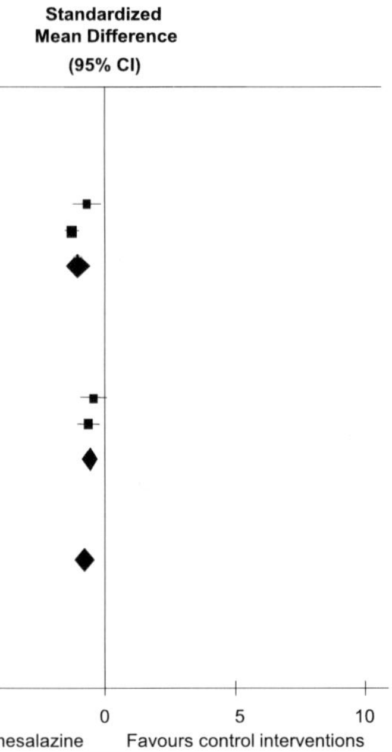

Figure 3: Comparative effectiveness of mesalazine versus control interventions by subtype of diverticular disease on global symptoms score. *There was not statistically significant difference in baseline global symptoms score between mesalazine and control interventions arms in all included studies.

months, leading to uncertainty on the association between mesalazine and prevention of disease recurrence.

Follow-Up Duration. In acute uncomplicated diverticulitis, there was a lower mean global symptoms score with mesalazine than control interventions only at long-term (more than 12 months) follow-up (1 trial, 92 participants, SMD=-0.64, and 95%CI=-1.06,-0.22). There was no significant interaction among subgroups (p=0.55).

Mode of Mesalazine Administration. There was a lower likelihood of symptomatic uncomplicated diverticular disease recurrence with mesalazine than control interventions only with cyclic administration (1 trial, 156 participants, RR=0.46, and 95%CI=0.22-0.98). There was no significant interaction among subgroups (p=0.61).

Publication bias could not be assessed due to the paucity of data.

4. Discussion

We found that mesalazine may decrease recurrences in symptomatic uncomplicated diverticular disease, but not in acute uncomplicated diverticulitis. Subgroup analyses confirmed an effect in symptomatic uncomplicated diverticular disease only when mesalazine was compared with placebo or cyclically administrated. Based on current evidence from randomized trials, there is uncertainty on the effect of mesalazine in achieving remission in both symptomatic uncomplicated diverticular disease and acute uncomplicated diverticulitis. The development of acute diverticulitis in people with symptomatic uncomplicated diverticular disease may not be reduced by mesalazine. Mesalazine may improve quality of life in symptomatic uncomplicated diverticular disease and the global symptoms score in both subtypes of diverticular disease, with a larger effect in symptomatic uncomplicated diverticular disease.

In acute uncomplicated diverticulitis, existing systematic reviews either suggest a role for mesalazine in symptoms relief [33, 34] and recurrence prevention [33–36] or find no evidence supporting mesalazine use in the prevention of disease relapse [37–39]. In symptomatic uncomplicated diverticular disease, three systematic reviews found that mesalazine has a role for symptoms relief [34, 36, 40], recurrence prevention [34, 36], and prevention of acute diverticulitis onset [36, 40].

Most of these analyses primarily described single study results without performing quantitative syntheses of data [33–36, 40]. In two of these reviews evidence is derived from both randomized trials and observational studies [33, 36], which are an inadequate study design to address intervention questions. Existing reviews also focused on one diverticular disease subtype only [33, 35, 37–40], with methodological limitations in search strategies and study selection or in outcomes analysis, considering selected outcomes rather than the full benefits-harms trade-off for mesalazine [33–40].

We found that mesalazine may not reduce acute uncomplicated diverticulitis recurrence but may possibly lead to its remission. This last finding is based only on one trial [29] enrolling a small sample of people with 1-3 previous episodes of acute diverticulitis, a condition with a high likelihood of response to mesalazine due to the low-grade intestinal fibrosis [41]. Thus, the certainty of evidence for this outcome was graded as "very low" and we could not provide any suggestions/recommendations on the use of mesalazine in the acute phase of acute uncomplicated diverticulitis. Our analysis confirms the role of mesalazine in symptomatic uncomplicated diverticular disease for the prevention of recurrences, but not for acute diverticulitis onset. We also found that mesalazine may produce a higher reduction in patients' symptoms compared to control interventions in both disease subtypes, with a large difference in symptomatic uncomplicated diverticular disease and a medium difference in acute uncomplicated diverticulitis.

Benchmarked with recommendations from key international guideline agencies, our findings support the more recently guidelines which do not recommend mesalazine for the prevention of acute uncomplicated diverticulitis recurrence [4, 7, 14, 15] and acute diverticulitis onset in symptomatic uncomplicated diverticular disease [4]. Guideline recommendations on mesalazine to achieve symptomatic uncomplicated diverticular disease remission are conflicting [4, 7, 14]. We found no benefit of mesalazine in this setting, although uncertainty persists since only one trial with a short-term follow-up assessed this outcome [27]. Finally, the Italian Group on Diverticular Diseases [4] states that there is no clear evidence on mesalazine use to achieve acute uncomplicated diverticulitis remission and prevent symptomatic uncomplicated diverticular disease recurrence. We show that mesalazine may decrease recurrences in symptomatic uncomplicated diverticular disease, while there is uncertainty on its effect in achieving acute uncomplicated diverticulitis remission.

Based on the analysis of 13 randomized trials, we can suggest the use of mesalazine for prevention of symptomatic uncomplicated diverticular disease relapse, a condition with no effective therapeutic alternatives, although results from long-term high-quality randomized trials and cost-effectiveness analyses are needed before extending the indications of this drug.

To the best of our knowledge, this is the first systematic review which compares mesalazine with other interventions for all diverticular disease subtypes, with a comprehensive evaluation of benefits and harms of this treatment and a quantitative synthesis of data. We evaluated the totality of evidence, including 13 trials versus 2-8 in existing systematic reviews [33–40], and only randomized trials compared to mixed use of both cohort and randomized designs in some previous reviews.

Our study has some limitations. Most of assessed outcomes had low/very low certainty of evidence due to the small number of included trials at low risk of bias (4 out of 13) and their heterogeneity. One trial [32] was stopped due to futility before the 24-month planned follow-up, leading to possible underestimation of events in mesalazine and control interventions arms. Moderate/high heterogeneity was found in some outcome analyses, which was mainly due to the different disease subtypes of primary studies populations. Anticipating this potential source of heterogeneity, we pre-planned to stratify all outcome and subgroup analyses by diverticular disease subtype. The criteria for the diagnosis of symptomatic uncomplicated diverticular disease varied across included studies, since the definition of this condition is not yet standardized. The diagnosis of diverticular disease was not standardized across included trials (use of endoscopy, radiologic imaging, or both). We could not analyze the impact of mesalazine formulations on the considered outcomes. Most included studies used pH-dependent preparations, with a similar drug release in the colon, while only two trials [31] used the multimatrix (MMX) mesalazine formulation. We could not evaluate the effect of mesalazine by diverticula localization. More than 90% of included patients in each trial had diverticula in the left colon and results based on disease localization were not provided. We could not evaluate some relevant outcomes (times to remission, acute diverticulitis development in symptomatic uncomplicated diverticular disease, surgery, and hospitalization), as these were not reported in included trials. Finally, we could not analyze the cost-effectiveness of the suggested therapeutic approach with mesalazine for the prevention of symptomatic uncomplicated diverticular disease recurrences because no trial provided data on costs.

There remains a need for high-quality randomized trials to further investigate the role of mesalazine in diverticular disease and, especially, its effects on achieving disease remission. These studies should also better clarify the impact of mesalazine on diverticular disease-related symptoms, quality of life, and costs in symptomatic uncomplicated diverticular disease. The role of mesalazine in acute complicated diverticulitis and the comparison between its cyclic versus continuous administration require further consideration. Finally, randomized trials including populations with right-sided disease, a condition with a described different pathogenesis from the left-sided disease, are warranted to evaluate any differences in benefits and harms of mesalazine.

5. Conclusions

Based on the totality of evidence, mesalazine may decrease symptomatic uncomplicated diverticular disease recurrence, whereas it may not prevent acute uncomplicated diverticulitis relapse. There is uncertainty on the effect of mesalazine in achieving remission in symptomatic uncomplicated diverticular disease and acute uncomplicated diverticulitis. The development of acute diverticulitis in people with symptomatic uncomplicated diverticular disease may not be reduced by mesalazine. Mesalazine may improve quality of life in symptomatic uncomplicated diverticular disease and patients' symptoms in both subtypes of diverticular disease, with a larger effect in symptomatic uncomplicated diverticular disease.

Acknowledgments

The authors acknowledge Ruth Mitchell, Trial Search Coordinator, for development of search strategies; Dr. Neil Stollman and Professor Francesco Di Mario for providing additional information; MAPI Institute (http://www.mapigroup.com) as reference for the assessment of the validation of the symptoms and quality of life tools used in included trials.

References

[1] J. E. Everhart and C. E. Ruhl, "Burden of Digestive Diseases in the United States Part II: Lower Gastrointestinal Diseases," *Gastroenterology*, vol. 136, no. 3, pp. 741–754, 2009.

[2] N. Stollman and J. B. Raskin, "Diverticular disease of the colon," *The Lancet*, vol. 363, no. 9409, pp. 631–639, 2004.

[3] L. Kohler, S. Sauerland, and E. Neugebauer, "Diagnosis and treatment of diverticular disease: results of a consensus development conference. The Scientific Committee of the European Association for Endoscopic Surgery," *Surgical Endoscopy*, vol. 13, no. 4, pp. 430–436, 1999.

[4] R. Cuomo, G. Barbara, F. Pace et al., "Italian consensus conference for colonic diverticulosis and diverticular disease," *United European Gastroenterology Journal*, vol. 2, no. 5, pp. 413–442, 2014.

[5] F. Sopeña and A. Lanas, "Management of colonic diverticular disease with poorly absorbed antibiotics and other therapies," *Therapeutic Advances in Gastroenterology*, vol. 4, no. 6, pp. 365–374, 2011.

[6] D. A. Etzioni, T. M. MacK, R. W. Beart, and A. M. Kaiser, "Diverticulitis in the United States: 1998-2005: changing patterns of disease and treatment," *Annals of Surgery*, vol. 249, no. 2, pp. 210–217, 2009.

[7] G. A. Binda, R. Cuomo, A. Laghi et al., "Practice parameters for the treatment of colonic diverticular disease: Italian Society of Colon and Rectal Surgery (SICCR) guidelines," *Techniques in Coloproctology*, vol. 19, no. 10, pp. 615–626, 2015.

[8] J. C. Andersen, L. Bundgaard, H. Elbrond et al., "Danish national guidelines for treatment of diverticular disease," *Danish Medical Journal*, vol. 59, 2012.

[9] N. H. Stollman and J. B. Raskin, "Diagnosis and management of diverticular disease of the colon in adults. Ad Hoc Practice Parameters Committee of the American College of Gastroenterology," *American Journal of Gastroenterology*, vol. 94, no. 11, pp. 3110–3121, 1999.

[10] T. Murphy, R. H. Hunt, M. Fried et al., *World Gastroenterology Organisation Practice Guidelines: Diverticular Disease*, World Gastroenterology Organisation, 2007, http://www.worldgastroenterology.org/guidelines/global-guidelines/diverticular-disease/diverticular-disease-english.

[11] J. B. J. Fozard, N. C. Armitage, J. B. Schofield, and O. M. Jones, "ACPGBI Position Statement on Elective Resection for Diverticulitis," *Colorectal Disease*, vol. 13, no. 3, pp. 1–11, 2011.

[12] C. S. Andeweg, I. M. Mulder, R. J. F. Felt-Bersma et al., "Guidelines of diagnostics and treatment of acute left-sided colonic diverticulitis," *Digestive Surgery*, vol. 30, no. 4-6, pp. 278–292, 2014.

[13] D. Feingold, S. R. Steele, S. Lee et al., "Practice parameters for the treatment of sigmoid diverticulitis," *Diseases of the Colon & Rectum*, vol. 57, no. 3, pp. 284–294, 2014.

[14] W. Kruis, C.-T. Germer, and L. Leifeld, "Diverticular disease: guidelines of the German society for gastroenterology, digestive and metabolic diseases and the German society for general and visceral surgery," *Digestion*, vol. 90, no. 3, pp. 190–207, 2014.

[15] N. Stollman, W. Smalley, and I. Hirano, "American Gastroenterological Association Institute Guideline on the Management of Acute Diverticulitis," *Gastroenterology*, vol. 149, no. 7, pp. 1944–1949, 2015.

[16] M. Sartelli, F. Catena, L. Ansaloni et al., "WSES Guidelines for the management of acute left sided colonic diverticulitis in the emergency setting," *World Journal of Emergency Surgery: WJES*, vol. 11, p. 37, 2016.

[17] D. Moher, A. Liberati, J. Tetzlaff, D. G. Altman, and The PRISMA Group, "Preferred reporting items for systematic reviews and meta-analyses: the PRISMA statement," *Annals of Internal Medicine*, vol. 151, no. 4, pp. 264–269, 2009.

[18] A. A. Sheth, W. Longo, and M. H. Floch, "Diverticular disease and diverticulitis," *American Journal of Gastroenterology*, vol. 103, no. 6, pp. 1550–1556, 2008.

[19] R. DerSimonian and N. Laird, "Meta-analysis in clinical trials," *Controlled Clinical Trials*, vol. 7, no. 3, pp. 177–188, 1986.

[20] J. A. C. Sterne, A. J. Sutton, J. P. A. Ioannidis et al., "Recommendations for examining and interpreting funnel plot asymmetry in meta-analyses of randomised controlled trials," *British Medical Journal*, vol. 343, no. 7818, Article ID d4002, 2011.

[21] D. Atkins, M. Eccles, S. Flottorp et al., "Systems for grading the quality of evidence and the strength of recommendations I: critical appraisal of existing approaches The GRADE Working Group," *BMC Health Services Research*, vol. 4, no. 38, 2004.

[22] E. Trepsi, C. Colla, P. Panizza et al., "Therapeutic and prophylactic role of mesalazine (5-ASA) in symptomatic diverticular disease of the large intestine. 4 year follow-up results," *Minerva Gastroenterol Dietol*, vol. 45, pp. 245–252, 1999.

[23] A. Tursi, G. Brandimarte, G. M. Giorgetti, and W. Elisei, "Mesalazine and/or Lactobacillus casei in preventing recurrence of symptomatic uncomplicated diverticular disease of the colon: A prospective, randomized, open-label study," *Journal of Clinical Gastroenterology*, vol. 40, no. 4, pp. 312–316, 2006.

[24] G. Comparato, L. Fanigliulo, G. Aragona et al., "Quality of life in uncomplicated symptomatic diverticular disease: Is it another good reason for treatment?" *Digestive Diseases*, vol. 25, no. 3, pp. 252–259, 2007.

[25] G. Comparato, L. Fanigliulo, L. G. Cavallaro et al., "Prevention of complications and symptomatic recurrences in diverticular disease with mesalazine: A 12-month follow-up," *Digestive Diseases and Sciences*, vol. 52, no. 11, pp. 2934–2941, 2007.

[26] J. Smith, D. Humes, K. Garsed et al., "OC-119 Mechanistic randomised control trial of mesalazine in symptomatic diverticular disease," *Gut*, vol. 61, pp. A51–A52, 2012.

[27] W. Kruis, E. Meier, M. Schumacher, O. Mickisch, R. Greinwald, and R. Mueller, "Randomised clinical trial: Mesalazine (Salofalk granules) for uncomplicated diverticular disease of the colon—a placebo-controlled study," *Alimentary Pharmacology & Therapeutics*, vol. 37, no. 7, pp. 680–690, 2013.

[28] F. Parente, S. Bargiggia, A. Prada et al., "Intermittent treatment with mesalazine in the prevention of diverticulitis recurrence: A randomised multicentre pilot double-blind placebo-controlled study of 24-month duration," *International Journal of Colorectal Disease*, vol. 28, no. 10, pp. 1423–1431, 2013.

[29] N. Stollman, S. Magowan, F. Shanahan, and E. M. M. Quigley, "A randomized controlled study of mesalamine after acute diverticulitis: Results of the DIVA trial," *Journal of Clinical Gastroenterology*, vol. 47, no. 7, pp. 621–629, 2013.

[30] A. Tursi, G. Brandimarte, W. Elisei et al., "Randomised clinical trial: Mesalazine and/or probiotics in maintaining remission of symptomatic uncomplicated diverticular disease - A double-blind, randomised, placebo-controlled study," *Alimentary Phar-*

macology & Therapeutics, vol. 38, no. 7, pp. 741–751, 2013.

[31] J. B. Raskin, M. A. Kamm, M. M. Jamal et al., "Mesalamine did not prevent recurrent diverticulitis in phase 3 controlled trials," *Gastroenterology*, vol. 147, no. 4, pp. 793–802, 2014.

[32] W. Kruis, V. Kardalinos, T. Eisenbach et al., "Randomised clinical trial: mesalazine versus placebo in the prevention of diverticulitis recurrence," *Alimentary Pharmacology & Therapeutics*, vol. 46, no. 3, pp. 282–291, 2017.

[33] A. M. Morris, S. E. Regenbogen, K. M. Hardiman, and S. Hendren, "Sigmoid diverticulitis: A systematic review," *Journal of the American Medical Association*, vol. 311, no. 3, pp. 287–297, 2014.

[34] L. Gatta, N. Vakil, D. Vaira et al., "Efficacy of 5-ASA in the treatment of colonic diverticular disease," *Journal of Clinical Gastroenterology*, vol. 44, no. 2, pp. 113–119, 2010.

[35] Ç. Ünlü, L. Daniels, B. C. Vrouenraets, and M. A. Boermeester, "Systematic review of medical therapy to prevent recurrent diverticulitis," *International Journal of Colorectal Disease*, vol. 27, no. 9, pp. 1131–1136, 2012.

[36] G. Maconi, G. Barbara, C. Bosetti, R. Cuomo, and B. Annibale, "Treatment of diverticular disease of the colon and prevention of acute diverticulitis: A systematic review," *Diseases of the Colon & Rectum*, vol. 54, no. 10, pp. 1326–1338, 2011.

[37] M. A. Khan, B. Ali, W. M. Lee, and C. W. Howden, "Mesalamine does not help prevent recurrent acute colonic diverticulitis: Meta-analysis of randomized, placebo-controlled trials," *American Journal of Gastroenterology*, vol. 111, no. 4, pp. 579–581, 2016.

[38] S. Urushidani, A. Kuriyama, and M. Matsumura, "5-aminosalicylic acid agents for prevention of recurrent diverticulitis: A systematic review and meta-analysis," *Journal of Gastroenterology and Hepatology*, vol. 33, no. 1, pp. 12–19, 2018.

[39] F. Carter, M. Alsayb, J. K. Marshall, and Y. Yuan, "Mesalamine (5-ASA) for the prevention of recurrent diverticulitis," *Cochrane Database of Systematic Reviews*, vol. 10, 2017.

[40] M. Picchio, W. Elisei, G. Brandimarte et al., "Mesalazine for the treatment of symptomatic uncomplicated diverticular disease of the colon and for primary prevention of diverticulitis: A systematic review of randomized clinical trials," *Journal of Clinical Gastroenterology*, vol. 50, pp. S64–S69, 2016.

[41] A. Tursi and M. Picchio, "Mesalazine in preventing acute diverticulitis occurrence: a meta-analysis of randomized, controlled trials," *Journal of Gastrointestinal and Liver Diseases*, vol. 25, no. 3, pp. 409-410, 2016.

Notch Signaling Pathway Is Inhibited in the Development of Barrett's Esophagus: An In Vivo and In Vitro Study

Yun-Cang Wang,[1,2] Zhi-Qiang Wang,[1] Yong Yuan,[1] Tao Ren,[3] Peng-Zhi Ni,[1] and Long-Qi Chen[1]

[1]*Department of Thoracic Surgery, West China Hospital, Sichuan University, Chengdu, China*
[2]*Department of Thoracic Surgery, Hospital of Chengdu Office of People's Government of Tibetan Autonomous Region, Chengdu, Sichuan, China*
[3]*Division of Gastroenterology, Hospital of Chengdu Office of People's Government of Tibetan Autonomous Region, Chengdu, Sichuan, China*

Correspondence should be addressed to Yong Yuan; yongyuan@scu.edu.cn

Academic Editor: Maikel P. Peppelenbosch

Objective. To explore the role of Notch signaling in the development of Barrett's esophagus. *Methods.* Patients with esophagectomy and gastric interposition were recruited as a human model of gastroesophageal reflux disease. The expressions of Notch signaling genes in normal esophagus from surgical specimen and columnar metaplasia in the esophageal remnant after esophagectomy were evaluated by real time quantitative Polymerase Chain Reaction (RT-qPCR) and immunohistochemistry (IHC). For in vitro experiments, Het-1A cells were treated with hydrochloric acid, deoxycholic acid, mixture of hydrochloric acid and deoxycholic acid, or Notch1-siRNA, and expressions of Notch1, Hes1, MUC2, and K13 were evaluated via RT-qPCR and western blot. *Results.* Samples were obtained from 36 patients with columnar metaplasia in the esophageal remnant. Both IHC and RT-qPCR indicated that Notch1 and Hes1 expressions were significantly higher in normal esophagus than that in metaplasia. Hydrochloric acid and deoxycholic acid suppressed Notch1, Hes1, and K13 expressions, in concert with increasing MUC2 expressions. Notch inhibition by Notch1-siRNA contributed to the downregulation of Notch1, Hes1, and K13 expressions, whereas MUC2 expression was enhanced. *Conclusions.* Both hydrochloric acid and deoxycholic acid could suppress Notch signaling pathway in esophageal epithelial cells, and inhibited Notch signaling has important functions in the development of Barrett's esophagus.

1. Introduction

Barrett's esophagus (BE), a condition wherein metaplastic columnar epithelium replaces normal stratified squamous epithelium, is a consequence of chronic esophageal mucosal injury caused by gastroesophageal reflux disease (GERD) [1]. GERD and Barrett's esophagus have clinical importance because they confer major risk factors for esophageal adenocarcinoma, one of the most deadly cancers worldwide [2]. Unfortunately, it remains unclear how GERD induces the BE and what molecular mechanism is involved. It has been proposed that some key developmental transcription factors might be involved in the development of reflux-related mucosal injury and Barrett's esophagus [3, 4].

Notch signaling pathway, a necessary intercellular signaling pathway for early development of multiple tissues and organs, is widely involved in regulating cell development, proliferation, differentiation, and apoptosis. It is generally regarded as an important signaling pathway for cell fate determination [5]. Some studies have shown that Notch signaling pathway regulates intestinal epithelial differentiation and decides the destiny and final outcomes of the intestinal epithelial cells. The Notch-knockout mice or the use of γ-secretase inhibitor will induce the metaplastic change of the goblet cells and inhibit the proliferation of intestinal epithelial cells, which might present as novel therapeutic target [6, 7]. A recent study compared the genome-wide expression in Barrett's esophagus and normal esophageal epithelium. The

TABLE 1: The sequences for the primers used for PCR.

Gene	Forward primer (5′→3′)	Reverse primer (5′→3′)	Tm	Amplicon size
β-Actin	GAAGATCAAGATCATTGCTCCT	TACTCCTGCTTGCTGATCCA	58	111 bp
Notch1	GCCACCACTGCGAGACCAACATCAA	AGGCAGAAGCAGAGGTAGGCGTTGT	68	100 bp
Hes1	CGTGCGAGGGCGTTAATACCGAGGT	GAGGTGCCGCTGTTGCTGGTGTAGA	69	385 bp
MUC2	AACACCCTGCTCGTCATC	CAAATGCTGGCATCAAAGTTGG	65	117 bp
K13	CGGGATGCTGAGGAATGGTT	CTGACGCTTCTTGGCGTCCT	60	110 bp

result showed that most of the genes related to the Notch signaling pathway were downregulated in Barrett's esophagus than in the normal esophageal epithelium [8]. Nevertheless, the role of Notch in the development of Barrett's esophagus is still controversial, which has not been systematically investigated both in vivo and in vitro experiment.

Esophagectomy with gastric interposition is usually indicated for patients with resectable esophageal cancer. Nevertheless, the normal antireflux mechanisms have to be damaged during operation. Patients with esophagectomy would inevitably suffer from significant reflux symptoms and reflux-related esophageal mucosal damage would eventually occur [9, 10]. Accordingly, esophagectomy and gastric interposition serve as an ideal human reflux model to study the molecular pathogenesis of reflux-induced esophageal mucosal damage. In the present study, we utilized this model to investigate the role of Notch signaling in the development of Barrett's esophagus. In vitro study was also conducted to explore the potential role of Notch pathway in Barrett's esophagus.

2. Materials and Methods

2.1. Study Population and Sample Preparation. This work was approved by the ethics committee of West China Hospital and informed consent was obtained from all patients. All experiments were performed in accordance with the relevant guidelines and regulations. From February 2011 to February 2016, patients with esophagectomy and gastric interposition for esophageal cancer were selected for upper gastrointestinal endoscopy and biopsies. We only included patients with newly diagnosis of columnar metaplasia in the residual esophagus after esophagectomy. Patients with preoperative history of gastroesophageal reflux disease, preoperative/postoperative adjuvant therapy for cancer, or evidence of tumor recurrence during the follow-up period were excluded from this study.

During operation, two pieces of normal esophageal mucosa from resected specimen were routinely obtained, one was flash frozen for Polymerase Chain Reaction (PCR), and the other was fixed into formalin for immunohistochemistry (IHC). For the postoperative endoscopy, four circumferential biopsies were taken by conventional forceps from suspected area of the esophageal remnant or at a distance of 2 cm away from the anastomotic site when there was no damage visualized. Two biopsies were fixed in formalin immediately for hematoxylin and eosin (HE) staining IHC, and the other two were flash frozen by liquid nitrogen for RT-qPCR.

2.2. Immunohistochemistry. The protein expression of Notch signaling pathway related genes (Notch1, Hes1) in samples was detected by immunohistochemical method. IHC staining was performed using formalin-fixed paraffin-embedded blocks as previously described [11]. The following primary antibodies were used: anti-Notch1, Santa Cruz, 1:100 dilution; anti-Hes1, Abcam, 1:200 dilution. Known positive controls using normal skin tissue were included for each run, and negative controls were done by omitting the primary antibodies. Two independent observers assessed immunoreactivity using a three-grade system, where 0 denoted negative staining; 1 denoted minimal and variable staining; 2 denoted obvious and intense staining. Sections with grade 2 were considered positive staining.

2.3. Real Time Quantitative Polymerase Chain Reaction (RT-qPCR). RT-qPCR was performed to detect mRNA expression levels of target genes in samples as previously described [12]. Trizol reagent (Invitrogen) was used to extract total RNA and complementary DNA (cDNA) was prepared using the QuantiTech Reverse Transcription kit (Qiagen). The RT-PCR was performed on Rotor Gene 3000 by using QuantiTect SYBR Green PCR kit, according to the instructions. β-Actin was used as reference gene, and results were expressed as the relative expression ratio of target gene to reference gene. The sequences and amplicon size for the primers are listed in Table 1.

2.4. Effects of Hydrochloric Acid and Deoxycholic Acid on the Notch Signaling Pathway. Human esophageal squamous cell line Het-1A (normal human esophageal squamous epithelial cell line immortalized by viral SV40 transfection) was purchased from China Center for Type Culture Collection (Wuhan, China). The cells were grown under standard conditions and treated with medium containing different concentrations of hydrochloric acid (pH4, pH5, and pH6), deoxycholic acid (DCA, 300 umol/L, 500 umol/L, and 1000 umol/L) or mixture of both (hydrochloric acid pH5 + DCA 500 umol/L), and blank controls were set up. Then cells were harvested at different time of incubation (24 h, 48 h, 72, and 96 h). Cell incubation time, hydrochloric acid, deoxycholic acid, and concentrations were chosen with reference to studies described elsewhere [12, 13]. Het-1A cells (5,000 cells/well) were seeded into 96-well plates and stimulated with hydrochloric acid (pH4, pH5, and pH6), deoxycholic acid (DCA, 300 umol/L, 500 umol/L, 1000 umol/L), or mixture of both (hydrochloric acid pH5 + DCA 500 umol/L).

TABLE 2: Antibodies used for western blotting.

Antibody	Company	Dilution
Notch1	Santa Cruz (sc-23299)	1:1000
Hes1	Abcam (ab49170)	1:2000
MUC2	Abcam (ab11197)	1:2000
K13	Abcam (ab92551)	1:1000
β-Actin	Abcam (ab8226)	1:5000

TABLE 3: Characteristics of patients.

Clinical characteristics	
Patients	$n = 36$
Age (years)	64 (51–68)
Gender	
Male	27 (75%)
Female	9 (25%)
Location of tumor	
Upper	3 (8%)
Middle	25 (69%)
Lower	8 (22%)
Pathological staging	
TisN0M0	5 (14%)
T1N0M0	9 (25%)
T2N0M0	22 (61%)
Adjuvant therapy	
None	36 (100%)
Yes	0 (0%)

MTT analysis was used to detect cell viability at 596 nm at 24, 48, 72, and 96 h after stimulation. Notch signal genes (Notch1 and downstream target Hes1), goblet cell-specific gene Mucin 2 (MUC2), and squamous keratin related gene (K13) were detected by RT-qPCR and western blot analysis as previously reported [14]; the antibodies used for western blotting are summarized in Table 2.

2.5. Small Interfering RNA (siRNA) Knockdown of Notch Signaling. The siRNA was used to silence Notch1 expression. The Notch1-siRNA was synthesized by Obio Technology (Shanghai, China). The sequences were as follows: 5′-GATCCTGGCGGGAAGTGTGAAGCGT-3′, 5′-AGACGCTTCACACTTCCCGCCATTA-3′. And the random sequences were used as negative control. Het-1A cells were transfected with Notch1-siRNA by using Lipofectamine 2000 according to the manufacturers' instructions. After incubation, cells were harvested and analyzed by RT-PCR and western blot as previously described [14].

2.6. Data Analysis. The measurement data with normal distribution were described as the mean ± standard deviation; otherwise they were expressed as median with interquartile range. The normal distribution data among multigroups were compared using single factor analysis of variance (ANOVA), and independent samples t-test was used to compare differences between groups. For the data with the nonnormal distribution, the Kruskal-Wallis test was used among multigroups and the Mann–Whitney U test was applied to compare differences between groups. Fisher's test was applied to compare categorical data between groups. The correlation between each gene was analyzed by Spearman correlation analysis. Two sides $p < 0.05$ were considered to be statistically significant, and data were processed using SPSS 19.0 (IBM, Inc., Chicago, Illinois, USA).

TABLE 4: Immunohistochemical results of Notch1.

Group	n	IHC Positive	IHC Negative	p
Normal	36	31	5	<0.001
Barrett	36	7	29	

TABLE 5: Immunohistochemical results of Hes1.

Group	n	IHC Positive	IHC Negative	p
Normal	36	28	8	<0.001
Barrett	36	10	26	

3. Results

3.1. Characteristics of Patients. From February 2011 to February 2016, 36 postesophagectomy patients with histologically confirmed columnar metaplasia in the esophageal remnant were included. All patients underwent esophagectomy with gastric interposition for esophageal squamous cell carcinoma. The mean follow-up period was 4.7 years. The main clinical characteristics of the included patients are shown in Table 3.

3.2. Immunohistochemical Analysis for Normal Esophageal Epithelium and Columnar Metaplasia. Normal esophageal mucosa from surgical specimen and columnar metaplastic samples in the esophageal remnant after esophagectomy were subject to IHC for Notch1 and Hes1. Histological evaluation of esophageal mucosa was done on sections with hematoxylin and eosin staining by independent pathologists. The results and representative pictures for immunohistochemical staining are shown in Tables 4 and 5, Figures 1 and 2. Notch1 protein was mainly expressed in cytoplasm of esophageal cells. The expression of Notch1 protein in normal esophageal epithelium was higher than that in metaplastic tissue ($p < 0.001$). As the Notch signaling downstream target gene, Hes1 expression was mainly located in cytoplasm and nucleus. It was significantly higher in normal esophagus than in metaplastic tissue ($p < 0.001$), which was in accordance with expression trend of Notch1. Furthermore, the protein expression of Notch1 was positively correlated with Hes1 protein expression ($p < 0.001$).

3.3. Real Time Quantitative Polymerase Chain Reaction (RT-qPCR) for Normal Esophagus, and Metaplastic Tissues. To analyze Notch1 and Hes1 mRNA expression levels in samples

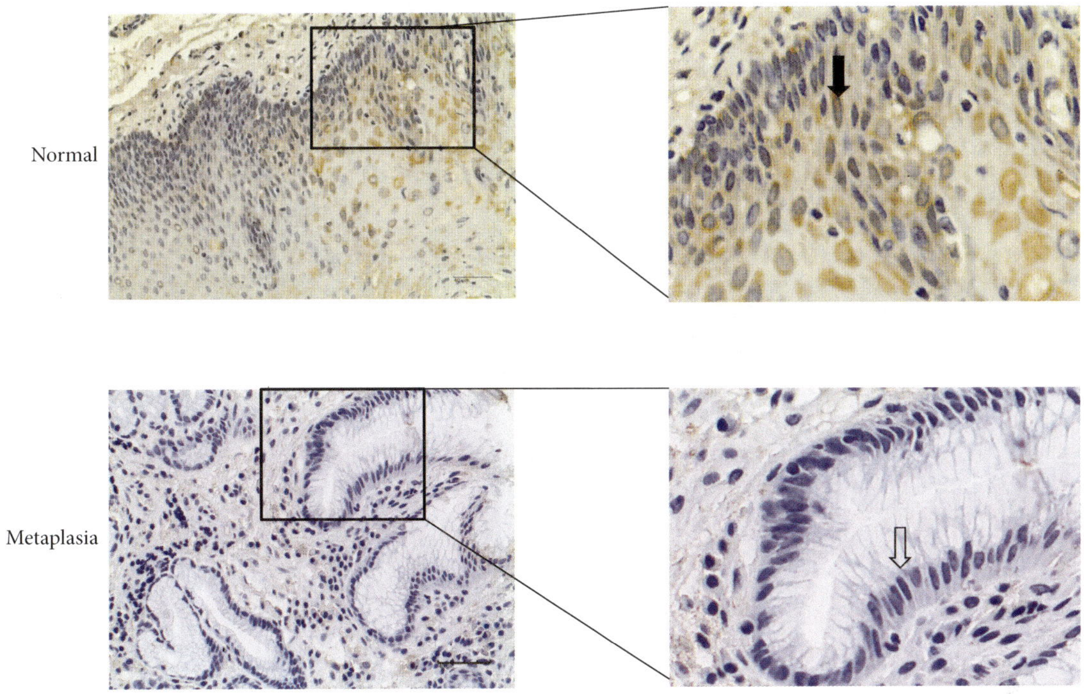

FIGURE 1: Representative Notch1 immunohistochemical staining in samples with different histological alterations. Notch1 protein was mainly expressed in cytoplasm of esophageal cells. Intense staining of Notch1 was mainly present in normal esophagus, and metaplastic columnar cells mainly exhibited negative staining (arrows). Scale bar in the figure is 40 μm. Magnified figures were shown in the right side.

with different histological alterations, RT-qPCR was performed (Figure 3). Notch1 mRNA expression level in normal esophageal epithelium was higher than that in columnar metaplastic tissues ($p < 0.001$). We also found a decreasing expression pattern of Hes1 mRNA from normal esophagus to columnar metaplasia ($p = 0.017$). Furthermore, Notch1 and Hes1 mRNA expressions were positively correlated ($p = 0.028$).

3.4. Effects of Hydrochloric Acid and Deoxycholic Acid on Notch1, Hes1, K13, and MUC2 Expressions. Hydrochloric acid and bile acid (deoxycholic acid) are known to play an important role in the development of reflux-related esophageal mucosal damage; we investigated their effects on Notch signaling (Notch1, Hes1), goblet cell-specific gene Mucin 2 (MUC2), and squamous keratin related gene (K13) expressions using Het-1A cells. Stimuli were added to the culture at different concentrations and indicated times. The cell proliferation was assessed by methyl thiazolyl tetrazolium (MTT) assay (Figure 4). The results showed cell proliferation was decreased with a more acidic pH. Het-1A cells could not survive when pH values are lower than 4. When the deoxycholic acid concentration was 300–400 umol/L, the cell proliferation rate decreased with the increasing deoxycholic acid concentration. From our study, it seemed that a prolonged incubation time of 3-4 days did not have negative effects on Het-1A cells. Concentration and pH of the stimuli were more important for cell viability and proliferation.

3.4.1. Effects of Hydrochloric Acid on Notch Signaling. Cells were stimulated with different concentrations of hydrochloric acid (pH4, pH5, and pH6); we found that Notch1 mRNA expression was suppressed in a concentration-dependent manner. And K13 mRNA expression was inhibited in a time-dependent manner, whereas Hes1 mRNA expression was decreased in concentration- and time-dependent manners. On the other hand, the expressions of MUC2 mRNA in Het-1A cells were increased in concentration- and time-dependent manners. We also investigated the effects of hydrochloric acid on Notch1, Hes1, MUC2, and K13 protein expressions, showing that expression patterns were consistent with their mRNAs. Representative pictures were shown in Figure 5.

3.4.2. Effects of Deoxycholic Acid on Notch Signaling. When Het-1A cells were cultured with deoxycholic acid (300 umol/L, 500 umol/L, and 1000 umol/L), both PCR and WB indicated that Notch1, Hes1, and K13 expressions were suppressed in concentration- and time-dependent manners. However, MUC2 expressions were augmented in concentration- and time-dependent manners. Representative pictures were shown in Figure 6.

3.4.3. Effects of Mixture of Hydrochloric Acid and Deoxycholic Acid on Notch Signaling. Both hydrochloric acid and deoxycholic acid may play important roles in development of reflux-related esophageal mucosa injury. We also evaluated effects of mixture of hydrochloric acid and deoxycholic acid on Notch signaling. According to our previous results, the mixture of hydrochloric acid (pH5) and deoxycholic acid (500 umol/L) was used for cell treatment. Our findings suggested that mixture of hydrochloric acid and deoxycholic

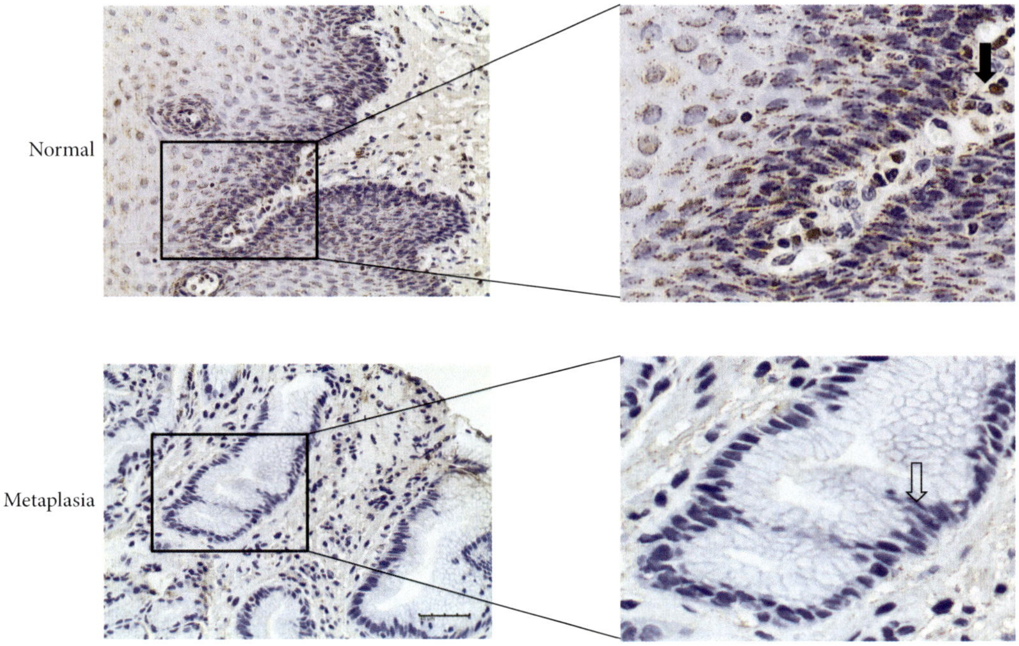

FIGURE 2: Representative Hes1 immunohistochemical staining in samples with different histological alterations. Intense Hes1 protein was mainly expressed in cytoplasm and nucleus of normal esophageal cells, and metaplastic columnar cells mainly exhibited negative staining (arrows). Scale bar in the figure is 40 μm. Magnified figures were shown in the right side.

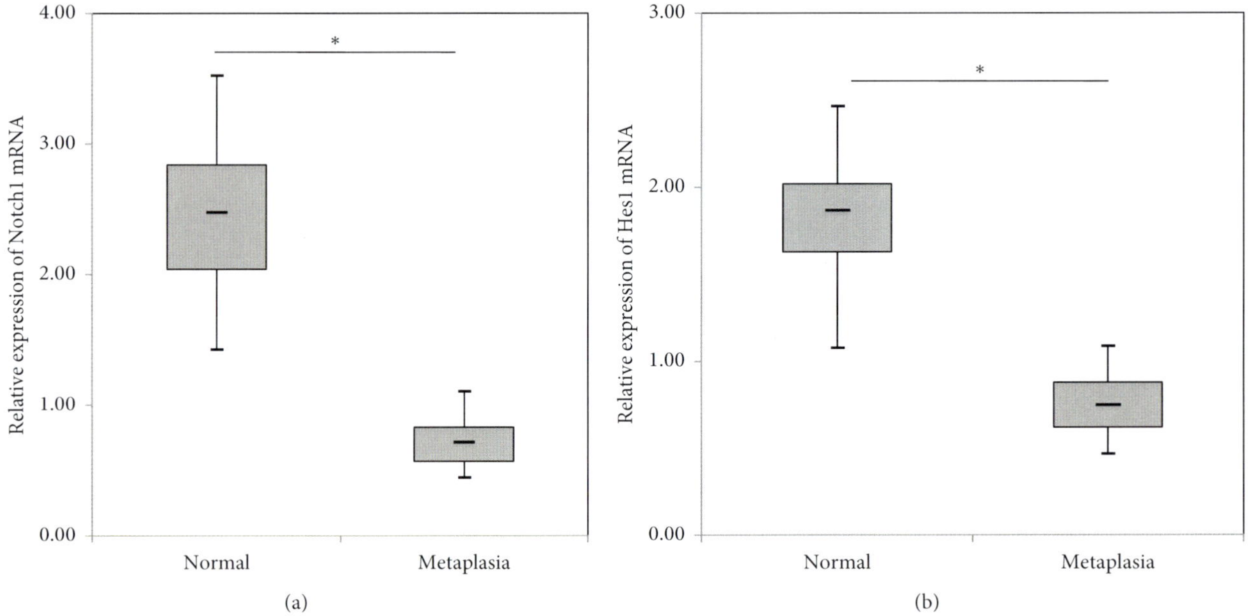

FIGURE 3: Relative expression of Notch1 (a) and Hes1 (b) mRNA in normal esophagus and metaplastic esophagus. Significant differences were detected in Notch1 mRNA and Hes1 mRNA expression values between normal squamous mucosa and metaplastic tissue. $^*p < 0.05$, statistically significant difference.

acid could suppress Notch1, Hes1, and K13 expressions in a time-dependent manner, in concert with increasing MUC2 expressions. Representative pictures were shown in Figure 7.

3.5. Effects of Notch Signaling Inhibition. In order to further investigate the effect of Notch knockdown on the expressions of goblet cell-specific gene MUC2 and squamous keratin related gene K13, Het-1A cells were used as in vitro models via Notch1-siRNA method. In our experiment, the Notch1 mRNA expression level showed a remarkable decrease in the Notch1-siRNA group as compared to that in control group. Western blot analysis also verified that Notch1 protein expression was significantly downregulated after Notch1-siRNA transinfection. In addition, the expressions of Notch1

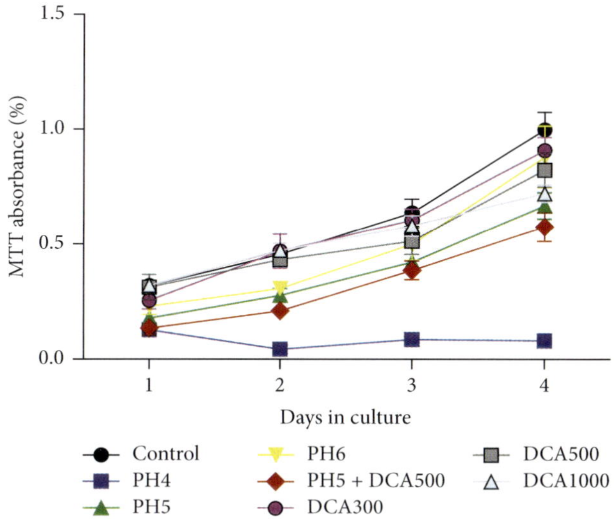

FIGURE 4: MTT assay was performed to detect cell viability at 24, 48, 72, and 96 h in Het-1A cells with different stimuli.

downstream target gene (Hesl) and squamous keratin related gene (K13) were remarkably inhibited in Notchl-siRNA group as evaluated by RT-PCR and western blot. On the contrary, inhibition of Notch signaling by Notchl-siRNA contributed to a significant increase of MUC2 expression. Representative pictures were shown in Figure 8.

4. Discussion

Studies on BE cover a variety of topics, among which gastroesophageal reflux is one of the most researched and understood. Many believe that BE is the results of adaptive metaplasia in an acid environment. The origin of newly generated columnar cells is still much disputed. The mainstream opinion holds that columnar cells originate from differentiation of basal layer of the esophagus or differentiation of esophageal submucosal glandular cells. Others believe that the columnar cells originate from the upward migration of the cells at the gastroesophageal junction to the esophageal mucosa. Regardless of the cellular origin for BE, it is generally believed that the refluxed contents alter the microenvironment of esophageal epithelial cells, which further leads to BE [15, 16]. However, the key molecular pathogenesis of this process is largely unknown.

It has been well documented that Notch signaling plays an important role in cell fate determination [5]. Whether Notch signaling pathway is involved in the development of BE is still controversial, which has not yet been systematically investigated in vivo and in vitro experiments. In our study, we firstly included patients with esophagectomy and gastric interposition as an ideal human model of gastroesophageal reflux. Normal esophagus from surgical specimen represented normal esophageal mucosa without reflux-related injury and postesophagectomy metaplasia in residual esophagus developed following long-term exposure to reflux. Expressions of Notchl and Hesl were evaluated for the biopsy specimens, and the expression levels of Notchl and Hesl had no correlation with the age, gender of the patients, and location and staging of tumor. Expression of Notch signaling was compared between normal esophageal mucosa and reflux-related columnar metaplasia. Both immunohistochemistry and PCR analyses indicated that Notchl expression levels were decreased from normal esophagus to columnar metaplasia. As the Notch signaling pathway downstream target gene, Hesl expression exhibited the same trend. For the first time, evidence from this in vivo human reflux model suggested that Notch signaling might be suppressed in the development of BE. Notably, Notch signaling has been investigated in rat and mouse models. They demonstrated that Notch inhibition could induce goblet cell differentiation and reduce cell proliferation, while cellular proliferation and progression of BE could be promoted by Notch activation, suggesting that Notch signaling might play binary roles in regulating Barrett metaplasia and its progression [4]. In this human reflux model, we also found Notch inhibition in the development of BE metaplasia. However, it is still unclear if Notch plays a role in the progression of BE in this in vivo model. It would be very interesting to continue to follow up our patients for further exploring the role of Notch signaling on cellular proliferation and BE progression.

BE is considered to be caused by chronic gastroesophageal reflux. We further investigated effects of reflux contents on the expressions of Notching signaling via in vitro experiments. It has been confirmed that both gastric acid and bile acid are composed of the gastric contents refluxing up to the esophagus, though in varying proportions. The gastric fluid is usually mixed with bile, and both play a synergistic role in esophageal mucosal damage [17–19]. In the current study, esophageal cells (Het-1A) were stimulated with hydrochloric acid, deoxycholic acid, or mixture of the two. We found that both hydrochloric acid and deoxycholic acid suppressed Notch signaling (Notchl and Hesl), and deoxycholic acid exhibited a stronger effect as compared with hydrochloric acid. Previously, Tamagawa et al. [19] evaluated expression and function of Notch signaling pathway in the development of BE. Firstly, they compared Notch expressions between human normal esophagus and BE, and then some esophageal cell lines were stimulated with bile acid or gamma-secretase inhibitor. They found Hesl expression was significantly lower in BE than in normal esophageal specimens, with no significant difference between BE and normal esophagus for Notchl expression. This result was further validated by the in vitro experiments using deoxycholic acid incubation (DCA 200 uM, 6–12 hours). However, both in vivo and in vitro experiments in our study revealed that expressions of Notchl and Hesl were decreased in the development of BE. One possible explanation for this discrepancy might be that Notchl antibodies used in the experiments were different. Tamagawa et al. used Notchl C-terminus antibody or cleaved Notchl antibody which detects Notchl intracellular domain and does not recognize extracellular domain. Besides, different cell culture and stimulation conditions might result in different gene expressions.

BE is featured by replacement of squamous cells with columnar cells, typically with the presence of goblet cells. Squamous cells contain squamous keratin and K13 is a

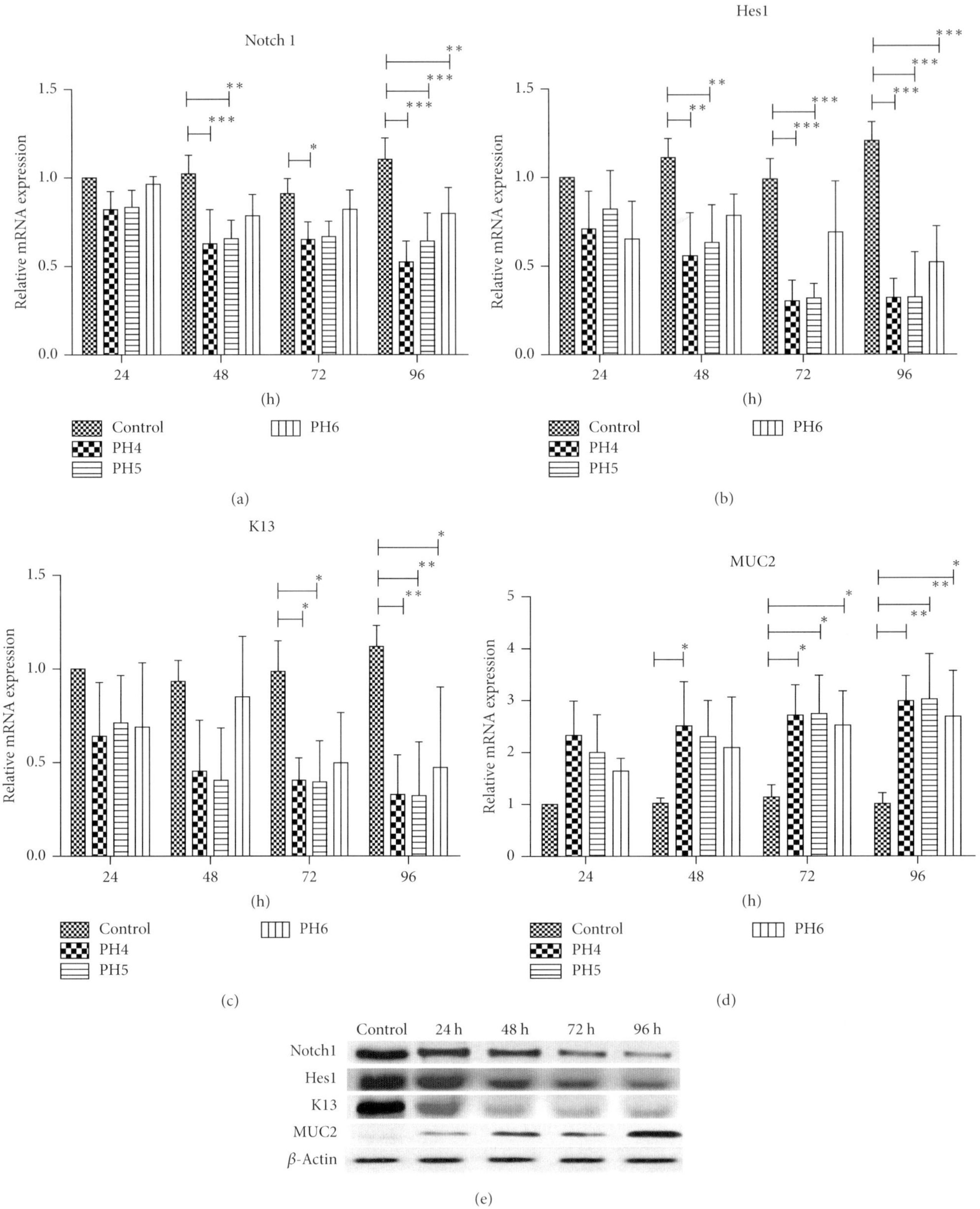

FIGURE 5: Effects of hydrochloric acid on Notch1, Hes1, K13, and MUC2 expressions. Cells were treated with different concentrations of hydrochloric acid (pH4, pH5, and pH6) for 24 h, 48 h, 72 h, and 96 h, respectively. (a–d) Notch1, Hes1, K13, and MUC2 mRNA expression levels in Het-1A cells exposing to different concentrations of hydrochloric acid for different time periods. $^{*}p < 0.05$, statistically significant difference. $^{**}p < 0.01$, statistically significant difference. $^{***}p < 0.001$, statistically significant difference. (e) Representative western blot results of Notch1, Hes1, K13, and MUC2 protein expressions in Het-1A cells treated with hydrochloric acid (pH5) for different time periods.

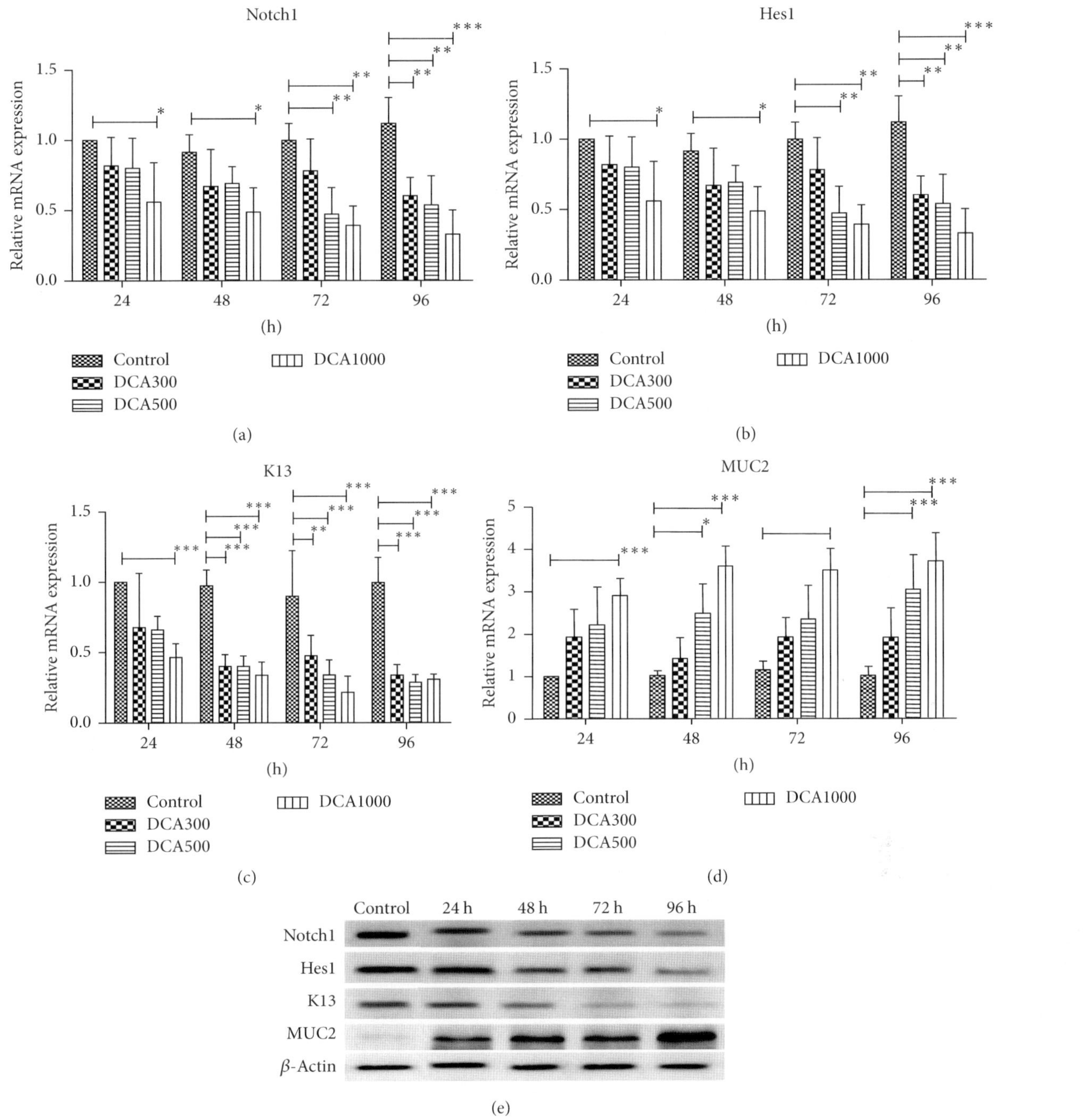

FIGURE 6: Effects of deoxycholic acid on Notch1, Hes1, K13, and MUC2 expressions. Cells were treated with different concentrations of deoxycholic acid (300 umol/L, 500 umol/L and 1000 umol/L) for 24 h, 48 h, 72 h, and 96 h, respectively. (a–d) Notch1, Hes1, K13, and MUC2 mRNA expression levels in Het-1A cells exposing to different concentrations of deoxycholic acid for different time periods. $^{*}p < 0.05$, statistically significant difference. $^{**}p < 0.01$, statistically significant difference. $^{***}p < 0.001$, statistically significant difference. (e) Representative western blot results of Notch1, Hes1, K13, and MUC2 protein expressions in Het-1A cells treated with deoxycholic acid (500 umol/L) for different time periods.

common protein for detecting squamous keratin. Mucin 2 (MUC2) is considered specific to the goblet cells, and the secretory function of the cells can be characterized by MUC2 [7, 20–22]. In this experiment, MUC2 and K13 were used as gene markers for determining different functional inclinations of cells. Our findings indicated that both hydrochloric acid and deoxycholic acid would inhibit Notch signaling, in concert with increased expression of MUC2 and downregulated K13 expression, implying that Notch signaling inhibition by hydrochloric acid and bile acid could promote transdifferentiation of esophageal epithelial cells toward columnar-like cells.

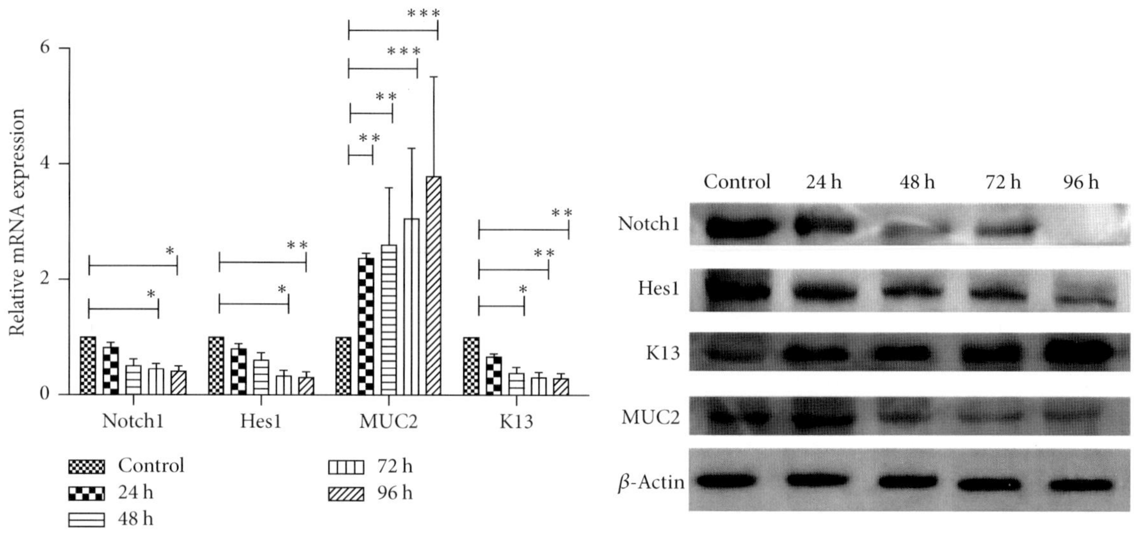

FIGURE 7: Effects of mixture of hydrochloric acid and deoxycholic acid on Notch1, Hes1, K13, and MUC2 expressions. Cells were treated with mixture of hydrochloric acid (pH = 5) and deoxycholic acid (500 umol/L) for 24 h, 48 h, 72 h, and 96 h, respectively. (a) Notch1, Hes1, K13, and MUC2 mRNA expression levels in Het-1A cells exposing to mixture of hydrochloric acid and deoxycholic acid for different time periods. $^{*}p < 0.05$, statistically significant difference. $^{**}p < 0.01$, statistically significant difference. $^{***}p < 0.001$, statistically significant difference. (b) Representative western blot results of Notch1, Hes1, K13, and MUC2 protein expressions in Het-1A cells treated with mixture of hydrochloric acid (pH = 5) and deoxycholic acid (500 umol/L) for different time periods.

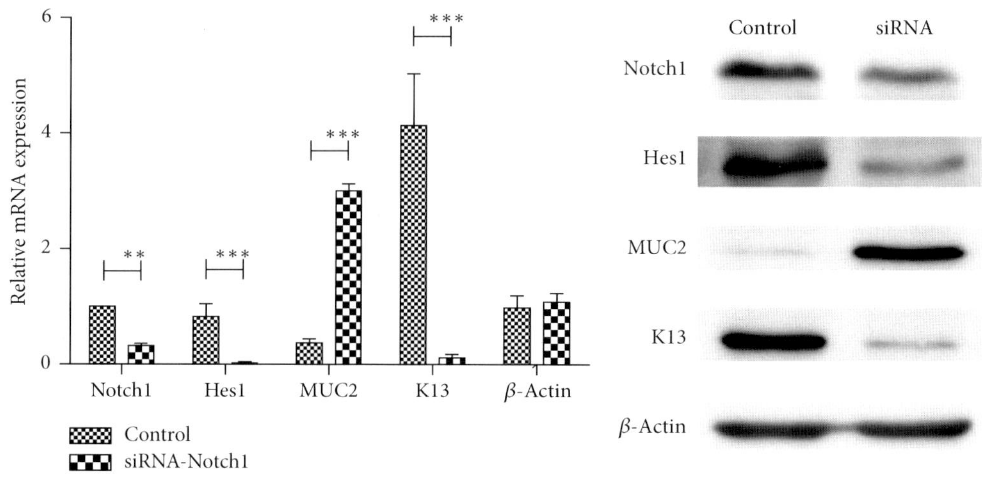

FIGURE 8: Effects of Notch signaling inhibition. Expressions of Notch1, Hes1, and K13 were significantly downregulated in cells transfected with Notch1-siRNA, in concert with significant increase of MUC2 expression. (a) Notch1, Hes1, K13, and MUC2 mRNA expression levels by RT-qPCR in Het-1A cells transfected with Notch1-siRNA. $^{**}p < 0.01$, statistically significant difference. $^{***}p < 0.001$, statistically significant difference. (b) Notch1, Hes1, K13, and MUC2 protein expressions by western blot analysis in Het-1A cells after Notch signaling inhibition by Notch1-siRNA.

To further evaluate whether K13 downregulation and MUC2 upregulation were induced by Notch signaling inhibition, we employed treatment of Notch1-siRNA in Het-1A cells. Both PCR and WB confirmed effective inhibition of Notch1 expression by specific Notch1-siRNA. The Notch downstream target gene Hes1 was also decreased, in concert with inhibition of K13 expression and elevation of MUC2 expression. In addition, inhibition of Notch signaling was correlated well with K13 downregulation and MUC2 upregulation. Consistent with our study, Tamagawa et al. used gamma-secretase inhibitor to inhibit Notch signaling in human esophageal cells and revealed that Hes1 expression was suppressed, while MUC2 expression was augmented following stimulation with gamma-secretase inhibitor [19]. These findings indicated that Notch signaling inhibition has the potential role to promote transdifferentiation of esophageal epithelial cells toward columnar-like cells as demonstrated by increased expression of glandular Mucin (MUC2) and decreased expression of squamous keratin (K13). One limitation for our in vitro study which needs to be mentioned is that only one cell line was investigated, two or more cell lines need to be further investigated to verify the findings. In Krishnadath's study, they compared gene expression profile for the BE and squamous esophagus by serial analysis of gene expression (SAGE), they found 72 tags were more than 10-fold up-regulated, and 26 tags were more than 10-fold downregulated. But they did not report a decreased expression of Notch signaling [23]. However, another study by Vega et al. also performed Affymetrix gene expression microarray on BE tissues and showed decreased Notch signaling for BE samples. Furthermore, via 3D organotypic culture technique, they observed elongated cells in the basal layer of epithelium after inhibition of Notch signaling. And they concluded that esophageal epithelial transdifferentiation might promote the evolution of BE [7].

5. Conclusion

In conclusion, findings from this in vivo and in vitro study suggest that both hydrochloric acid and deoxycholic acid could suppress Notch signaling pathway in esophageal epithelial cells and inhibited Notch signaling has important functions in the development of Barrett's esophagus.

Disclosure

This study was orally presented at 24th ESTS Annual Meeting (Naples, Italy, 2016). It was also orally presented at 15th World Congress of the International Society for Diseases of the Esophagus (ISDE) (Singapore, September, 2016).

Authors' Contributions

Yun-Cang Wang and Zhi-Qiang Wang contributed equally to this work.

Acknowledgments

This work was supported by National Natural Science Foundation of China (Grant no. 81500419). This study was granted the ESTS-DGT Travel Grant.

References

[1] S. J. Spechler and R. F. Souza, "Barrett's esophagus," *The New England Journal of Medicine*, vol. 371, no. 9, pp. 836–845, 2014.

[2] K. B. Dunbar and S. J. Spechler, "Controversies in Barrett esophagus," *Mayo Clinic Proceedings*, vol. 89, no. 7, pp. 973–984, 2014.

[3] D. Croagh, R. J. S. Thomas, W. A. Phillips, and P. Kaur, "Esophageal stem cells - A review of their identification and characterization," *Stem Cell Reviews and Reports*, vol. 4, no. 4, pp. 261–268, 2008.

[4] M. Quante, J. A. Abrams, Y. Lee, and T. C. Wang, "Barrett esophagus: What a mouse model can teach us about human disease," *Cell Cycle*, vol. 11, no. 23, pp. 4328–4338, 2012.

[5] S. Fre, M. Huyghe, P. Mourikis, S. Robine, D. Louvard, and S. Artavanis-Tsakonas, "Notch signals control the fate of immature progenitor cells in the intestine," *Nature*, vol. 435, no. 7044, pp. 964–968, 2005.

[6] V. Menke, J. H. van Es, W. de Lau et al., "Conversion of metaplastic Barrett's epithelium into post-mitotic goblet cells by -secretase inhibition," *Disease Models & Mechanisms*, vol. 3, no. 1-2, pp. 104–110, 2010.

[7] M. E. Vega, V. Giroux, M. Natsuizaka et al., "Inhibition of notch signaling enhances transdifferentiation of the esophageal squamous epithelium towards a Barrett's-like metaplasia via KLF4," *Cell Cycle*, vol. 13, no. 24, article no. A15, pp. 3857–3866, 2014.

[8] P. L. Hyland, N. Hu, M. Rotunno et al., "Global Changes in Gene Expression of Barrett's Esophagus Compared to Normal Squamous Esophagus and Gastric Cardia Tissues," *PLoS ONE*, vol. 9, no. 4, p. e93219, 2014.

[9] R. V. N. Lord, K. Wickramasinghe, J. J. Johansson, S. R. DeMeester, J. Brabender, and T. R. DeMeester, "Cardiac mucosa in the remnant esophagus after esophagectomy is an acquired epithelium with Barrett's-like features," *Surgery*, vol. 136, no. 3, pp. 633–640, 2004.

[10] X. B. D'Journo, J. Martin, G. Rakovich et al., "Mucosal damage in the esophageal remnant after esophagectomy and gastric transposition," *Annals of Surgery*, vol. 249, no. 2, pp. 262–268, 2009.

[11] R. W. Phillips, H. F. Frierson Jr., and C. A. Moskaluk, "Cdx2 as a marker of epithelial intestinal differentiation in the esophagus," *The American Journal of Surgical Pathology*, vol. 27, no. 11, pp. 1442–1447, 2003.

[12] D. J. Morrow, N. E. Avissar, L. Toia et al., "Pathogenesis of Barrett's esophagus: Bile acids inhibit the Notch signaling pathway with induction of CDX2 gene expression in human esophageal cells," *Surgery*, vol. 146, no. 4, pp. 714–722, 2009.

[13] Y. Hu, V. A. Williams, O. Gellersen, C. Jones, T. J. Watson, and J. H. Peters, "The pathogenesis of Barrett's esophagus: secondary bile acids upregulate intestinal differentiation factor CDX2 expression in esophageal cells," *Journal of Gastrointestinal Surgery*, vol. 11, no. 7, pp. 827–834, 2007.

[14] Y. Tamagawa, N. Ishimura, G. Uno et al., "Notch signaling pathway and Cdx2 expression in the development of Barrett's esophagus," *Laboratory Investigation*, vol. 92, no. 6, pp. 896–909, 2012.

[15] R. F. Souza, K. Krishnan, and S. J. Spechler, "Acid, Bile, and CDX: The ABCs of making Barrett's metaplasia," *American Journal of Physiology-Gastrointestinal and Liver Physiology*, vol. 295, no. 2, pp. G211–G218, 2008.

[16] X. Wang, H. Ouyang, Y. Yamamoto et al., "Residual embryonic cells as precursors of a Barrett's-like metaplasia," *Cell*, vol. 145, no. 7, pp. 1023–1035, 2011.

[17] N. E. Avissar, L. Toia, Y. Hu et al., "Bile acid alone, or in combination with acid, induces CDX2 expression through activation of the epidermal growth factor receptor (EGFR)," *Journal of Gastrointestinal Surgery*, vol. 13, no. 2, pp. 212–222, 2009.

[18] G. Burnat, T. Rau, E. Elshimi, E. G. Hahn, and P. C. Konturek, "Bile acids induce overexpression of homeobox gene CDX-2 and vascular endothelial growth factor (VEGF) in human Barrett's esophageal mucosa and adenocarcinoma cell line,"

Scandinavian Journal of Gastroenterology, vol. 42, no. 12, pp. 1460–1465, 2007.

[19] Y. Tamagawa, N. Ishimura, G. Uno et al., "Bile acids induce Delta-like 1 expression via Cdx2-dependent pathway in the development of Barrett's esophagus," *Laboratory Investigation*, vol. 96, no. 3, pp. 325–337, 2016.

[20] Y. Hu, C. Jones, O. Gellersen, V. A. Williams, T. J. Watson, and J. H. Peters, "Pathogenesis of Barrett esophagus deoxycholic acid up-regulates goblet-specific gene MUC2 in concert with CDX2 in human esophageal cells," *JAMA Surgery*, vol. 142, no. 6, pp. 540–544, 2007.

[21] J. H. B. Van De Bovenkamp, A. M. Korteland-Van Male, C. Warson et al., "Gastric-type mucin and TFF-peptide expression in Barrett's oesophagus is disturbed during increased expression of MUC2," *Histopathology*, vol. 42, no. 6, pp. 555–565, 2003.

[22] H. Steininger, D. A. Pfofe, H. Müller, G. Haag-Sunjic, and V. Fratianu, "Expression of CDX2 and MUC2 in Barrett's mucosa," *Pathology - Research and Practice*, vol. 201, no. 8-9, pp. 573–577, 2005.

[23] J. W. van Baal, F. Milano, A. M. Rygiel et al., "A Comparative Analysis by SAGE of Gene Expression Profiles of Barrett's Esophagus, Normal Squamous Esophagus, and Gastric Cardia," *Gastroenterology*, vol. 129, no. 4, pp. 1274–1281, 2005.

28

Reduced Incidence and Better Liver Disease Outcomes among Chronic HCV Infected Patients Who Consume Cannabis

Adeyinka Charles Adejumo,[1,2,3] Oluwole Muyiwa Adegbala,[4] Kelechi Lauretta Adejumo,[3] and Terence Ndonyi Bukong[2,5]

[1]*Department of Medicine, North Shore Medical Center, Salem, MA, USA*
[2]*Department of Medicine, University of Massachusetts Medical School, Worcester MA, USA*
[3]*School of Public Health, University of Massachusetts Lowell, Lowell, MA, USA*
[4]*Department of Medicine, Englewood Hospital and Medical Center, Englewood, NJ, USA*
[5]*INRS-Institut Armand-Frappier, Institut National de la Recherche Scientifique, Laval, QC, Canada*

Correspondence should be addressed to Terence Ndonyi Bukong; terencendonyi.bukong@iaf.inrs.ca

Academic Editor: Pierluigi Toniutto

Background and Aim. The effect of cannabis use on chronic liver disease (CLD) from Hepatitis C Virus (HCV) infection, the most common cause of CLD, has been controversial. Here, we investigated the impact of cannabis use on the prevalence of CLD among HCV infected individuals. *Methods.* We analyzed hospital discharge records of adults (age ≥ 18 years) with a positive HCV diagnosis. We evaluated records from 2007 to 2014 of the Nationwide Inpatient Sample (NIS). We excluded records with other causes of chronic liver diseases (alcohol, hemochromatosis, NAFLD, PBC, HBV, etc.). Of the 188,333 records, we matched cannabis users to nonusers on 1:1 ratio (4,728:4,728), using a propensity-based matching system, with a stringent algorithm. We then used conditional regression models with generalized estimating equations to measure the adjusted prevalence rate ratio (aPRR) for having liver cirrhosis (and its complications), carcinoma, mortality, discharge disposition, and the adjusted mean ratio (aMR) of total hospital cost and length of stay (LOS) [SAS 9.4]. *Results.* Our study revealed that cannabis users (CUs) had decreased prevalence of liver cirrhosis (aPRR: 0.81[0.72-0.91]), unfavorable discharge disposition (0.87[0.78-0.96]), and lower total health care cost ($39,642[36,220-43,387] versus $45,566[$42,244-$49,150]), compared to noncannabis users (NCUs). However, there was no difference among CUs and NCUs on the incidence of liver carcinoma (0.79[0.55-1.13]), in-hospital mortality (0.84[0.60-1.17]), and LOS (5.58[5.10-6.09] versus 5.66[5.25-6.01]). Among CUs, dependent cannabis use was associated with lower prevalence of liver cirrhosis, compared to nondependent use (0.62[0.41-0.93]). *Conclusions.* Our findings suggest that cannabis use is associated with decreased incidence of liver cirrhosis, but no change in mortality nor LOS among HCV patients. These novel observations warrant further molecular mechanistic studies.

1. Introduction

Globally chronic Hepatitis C Infection (HCV), followed by alcoholic and nonalcoholic-fatty liver diseases (ALD and NAFLD), represents the most common cause of chronic liver disease (CLD) that can progress to liver fibrosis and hepatic cellular carcinoma (HCC) [1]. In the United States of America (USA), HCV imposes significant financial and utilization burden on the healthcare system [2]. Fortunately, with recent advances in HCV therapy using direct-acting antivirals (DAA) [3], sustained virologic response (SVR) has been achieved in about 95% of infected individuals [4], resulting in gradual decline in the burden of HCV [1]. However, the remaining 5% with uncontrolled SVR might still progress to CLD. Furthermore, individuals who develop resistance to or do not have access to DAA such as individuals with modest incomes or from less developed countries are more likely to still suffer from CLD [5, 6].

Cannabis, the most commonly used illicit drug [7], has been shown to modulate inflammatory and fibrotic processes in the liver in preclinical studies [8, 9]. These preclinical observations have additionally been confirmed by recent population studies on ALD and NAFLD [10, 11]. However, the relationship between cannabis use and HCV has been controversial and remains unclear. While earlier studies suggested that cannabis use resulted in increased steatosis, fibrosis, and worsening of HCV disease [12–14], recent observations are now advancing that cannabis use has no effect on HCV disease progression [15–17]. A recent reports even revealed that cannabis use was associated with reduced steatosis in HCV infected individuals [18]. However, most of these studies had significant limitations given that evaluations were made from a single center. Further, these studies were limited in size and lacked diversity in study individuals. Additionally, these studies often included subjects with other chronic liver diseases, which might impact the effects of cannabis on HCV disease study outcomes. Interestingly, a recent study revealed that cannabidiol (CBD), the main nonpsychoactive agent in cannabis, induced cell death in approximately 85% of HCV infected cells in vitro, similar to interferon alpha-2b treatment [19].

In this study, we examined a large, nationally representative sample of over 900,000 subjects with chronic HCV infection. We used propensity-matched analysis with the objective of eliminating differences in demographics and comorbid characteristics of study participants. We additionally investigated the relationships between cannabis versus noncannabis use on the prevalence of liver cirrhosis and liver carcinoma in our study population. Furthermore, we estimated how cannabis use affected hospitalization outcomes: mortality, discharge disposition, cost, and length of stay (LOS).

Our investigations revealed that, among HCV infected individuals, cannabis use was associated with decreased prevalence of liver cirrhosis and lower overall treatment cost.

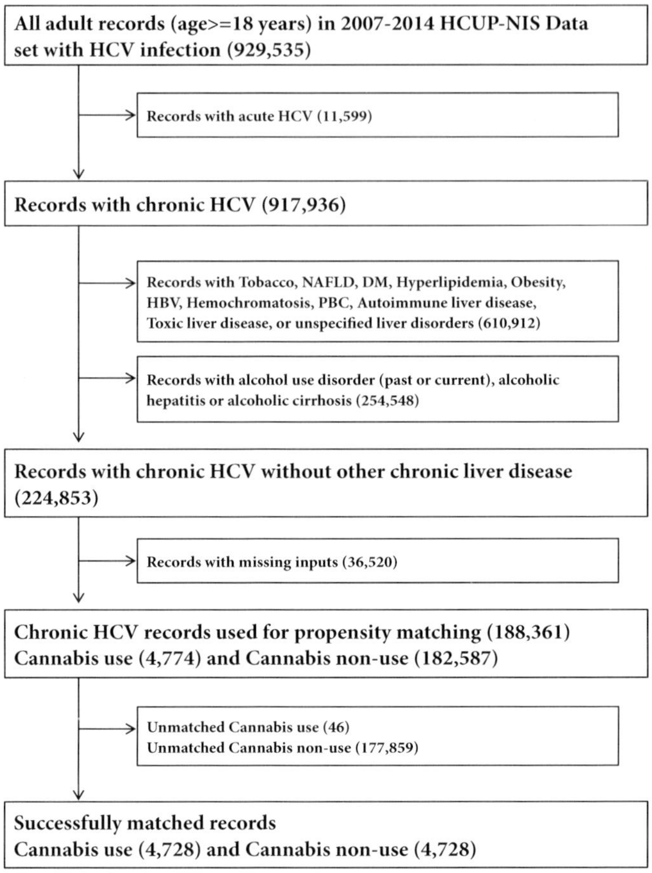

Figure 1: **Selection flow chart of study populations.** Illustrative flow chart of how our study population was grouped for statistical analysis to determine the impact and disease outcomes among HCV infected individuals who use cannabis.

2. Materials and Methods

2.1. Study Population and Design. Our study data included hospital discharge records of adults (≥18 years old) with a diagnosis of HCV infection (HCV+). These records are comprised of hospitalized patients in the USA from 2007 to 2014, archived in the Healthcare Cost and Utilization Project Nationwide Inpatient Sample (HCUP-NIS) database. HCUP-NIS is the largest inpatient database in the USA, produced and maintained by the Agency for Healthcare Research and Quality (AHRQ) [20]. HCUP-NIS contains about 7-8 million records from over 3,000 nonfederal hospitals across more than 30 states in the US [20]. Each record has up to 30 different clinical diagnoses, encoded with the International Classification of Diseases, Ninth Edition, Clinical Modification (ICD-9-CM). Our study design is a propensity-matched cohort study. As the HCUP-NIS is a completely deidentified and the data is readily available publicly, we did not require an Institutional Review Board approval.

2.2. Selection of Cannabis Cohort and Propensity Matching Variables. All clinical attributes were either identified as variables (demographics, region, and hospital factors) in the dataset or retrieved from containing variables using the International Classification of Diseases, Ninth Revision, Clinical Modification (ICD-9-CM). After pooling records collected from January 1, 2007, to December 31, 2014, in the HCUP-NIS, we first identified HCV+ (acute and chronic) records and then eliminated records with acute HCV+, chronic HCV+ individuals with a history of abusive alcohol use and diagnosis of alcoholic liver diseases. We also excluded records with risk factors for CLD or those having other potential causes of CLD (tobacco use, nonalcoholic fatty liver disease, diabetes mellitus, hyperlipidemia, obesity, HBV, PBC, autoimmune liver disease, toxic liver diseases, chronic passive congestion of the liver, hepatic infarction, hepatitis from other viral illnesses, and unspecified liver disorders) (Figure 1). The ICD-9-CM codes used have been utilized to identify HCV infections and outcomes from the HCUP-NIS by numerous studies [10, 11, 21–23].

Cannabis users were identified using ICD-9-CM codes, and this code selects patients using Indian hemp, marijuana, and different varieties of cannabinoid-containing substances. We then retrieved data from the NIS on demographics features including age, gender (male, female), race (White, Black, Hispanics, and other races), primary health insurance (Medicare, Medicaid, private, self-pay, and others), income, region, and hospital teaching status. Income was stratified into four based on average household income of the zip-code of residence. Region was stratified into four based on US Census Bureau: Northeast, Midwest, South, and West. Hospital teaching status was classified into three: rural, urban nonteaching, and urban teaching.

In order to develop a logistic model to predict cannabis use, we used ICD-9-CM codes to identify various factors/comorbidities that might be associated with cannabis usage: peripheral vascular disease, chronic heart failure, hypertension, chronic lung disease, valvular heart disease, cardiac arrhythmias, chronic kidney disease, cerebral vascular disease, ischemic heart disease, hypothyroidism, hyperthyroidism, acquired immune deficiency syndrome, other substance abuse, and malignancies. Some of these variables were either identified in literature to be associated with cannabis use or included as general comorbid disorders common among inpatients.

2.3. Outcome Variables. After matching, we identified 13 outcomes: three primary and ten secondary. Our primary outcomes were having a diagnosis of liver cirrhosis, liver carcinoma, and in-hospital mortality. Six of our ten secondary outcomes are known complications of liver cirrhosis including ascites, variceal bleeding, hepatorenal syndrome, hepatic encephalopathy, portal hypertension, and jaundice. The seventh secondary outcome assessed the proportion of individuals with decompensated versus nondecompensated cirrhosis. We deduced cirrhotic decompensation by using the complications of cirrhosis mentioned above, to stratify patients based on the Baveno4 methodology. The three other outcomes were length of stay (LOS), total hospital cost, and disposition on discharge. All pre-2014 total hospital cost values were escalated to the 2014 numbers with the inflation rate. Unfavorable disposition on discharge was defined as discharge to secondary health facilities versus others (discharged home with/without home health care aide). Besides mortality, LOS, total hospital cost, and discharge disposition, which were variables in the dataset, all the other outcomes were identified using ICD-9-CM codes. The liver cirrhosis and the Baveno4 system codes have been extensively used and validated in the NIS [24, 25].

2.4. Statistical Analysis. Continuous variables were represented with a mean (standard deviation) or median (interquartile range), depending on the underlying distribution, compared with Mann-Whitney U test; categorical variables are presented with percentages, compared with Rao-Scott Chi-square.

After selecting our chronic HCV+ population, we identified cannabis users and developed a multivariate logistic regression model, with stepwise negative selection, to generate propensity scores for cannabis use versus noncannabis use. With a caliper less than 0.2 of the standard deviation of the logit of the propensity scores, we used a greedy-match algorithm (gmatch macro) to match cannabis users to nonusers in a 1:1 ratio [26]. Propensity matching has been shown to eliminate a large percentage of residual confounding in observational studies, such as ours, and to generate effect estimates that are comparable with a randomized clinical control trial in the magnitude and outcomes [27, 28]. After matching, paired equivalents of the tests above such as Paired T-test, Wilcoxon signed-rank test, and McNemar's test were used to compare differences in outcomes between cannabis users versus nonusers.

Next, we developed conditional Poisson regression models, with robust modification of the error variance, to estimate the adjusted prevalence rate ratio (adjusted by matching) [aPRR] of having liver cirrhosis, the complications of liver cirrhosis including ascites, variceal bleeding, hepatorenal syndrome, hepatic encephalopathy, portal hypertension, and jaundice, and other noncirrhotic outcomes: liver carcinoma, mortality, cost, LOS, and unfavorable discharge to secondary health facilities [29]. For the noncirrhotic outcomes, we additionally adjusted for presence of cirrhosis, to eliminate the confounding effect of cirrhosis on health care utilization, as cirrhosis has been shown to be the major pathologic pathway of liver cancer in HCV+ livers and to also contribute to a significant healthcare utilization. Among individuals with liver cirrhosis, we designed additional Poisson models for aPRR for having decompensated versus compensated cirrhosis with respect to cannabis exposure, using the Baveno4 classification system. The models were specified to match the outcomes: gamma for total hospital cost and negative binomial for LOS to generate the adjusted mean ratios (aMR).

To investigate if the amount of cannabis used had an impact on the prevalence of liver cirrhosis, we performed additional analyses. Using the ICD-9-CM codes, we categorized cannabis users into two groups (dependent and nondependent users), to loosely approximate the quantity and frequency of use, since the HCUP-NIS data does not contain such information. Then we recalculated the effect of cannabis use on cirrhosis, with Bonferroni adjustment of the confidence intervals to account for the grouping of cannabis users. Because our result revealed that the frequency of cirrhosis remained lower among cannabis users after matching, we redesigned the propensity matching factors to include liver cirrhosis, to completely eliminate a possible confounding effect of cirrhosis in the matched cohort. Then, we reestimated the health care utilization outcomes, with respect to cirrhosis. All models used a p-value of <0.05, reported with a 95% confidence intervals (CI), and were performed using Statistical Analysis System (SAS V.9.4, SAS Institute Inc., Cary, NC, US). We plotted the estimates with GraphPad Prism 7.

3. Results

3.1. Study Population before and after Matching. After eliminating records with acute HCV+, abusive alcohol use, alcoholic liver disorders, other etiologies of chronic liver diseases, and records with missing inputs, there were 4,774 records with cannabis use disorder out of a total of 188,361 records (Figure 1). Cannabis users were younger (mean age of 40 years versus 53 years for nonusers), more likely to be White, to be on Medicaid or Self-pay/Uninsured, and to be from the lower income quartiles (Table 1). Besides having higher frequency of other substance abuse and similar

Table 1: Baseline characteristics of chronic hepatitis C infected patients, by cannabis use status (before propensity matching).

	No Cannabis use	Cannabis use	p-value
n (~weighted)	182587 (~887,975)	4774 (~23,371)	
Age, mean (SD)	53.06 (14.15)	40 (12.96)	<0.0001
Gender			0.3599
Male	53.86	54.60	
Female	46.14	45.40	
Race			<0.0001
White	59.90	66.23	
Black	21.63	18.92	
Hispanics	12.74	10.73	
Others	5.74	4.12	
Health insurance			<0.0001
Medicare	33.91	20.92	
Medicaid	30.91	46.10	
Private	21.00	12.05	
Self-pay & others	14.18	20.93	
Income			<0.0001
Lowest Quartile	38.04	45.92	
Second Quartile	24.42	25.41	
Third Quartile	20.99	18.50	
Highest Quartile	16.55	10.17	
Hospital region			<0.0001
Northeast	24.99	22.23	
Midwest	11.72	15.18	
South	39.69	39.21	
West	23.60	23.38	
Hospital teaching status			<0.0001
Rural	7.06	10.35	
Urban non-teaching	32.71	33.34	
Urban teaching	60.23	56.31	
Peripheral vascular disease	2.43	1.05	<0.0001
Congestive heart failure	6.23	2.59	<0.0001
Hypertension	35.92	22.34	<0.0001
Chronic lung disease	16.49	16.21	0.6303
Valvular heart disease	3.14	1.74	<0.0001
Cardiac arrhythmias	10.24	5.29	<0.0001
Chronic kidney disease	12.64	4.49	<0.0001
Cerebral vascular disease	3.45	1.71	<0.0001
Ischemic heart disease	8.68	4.77	<0.0001
Hypothyroidism	7.32	3.65	<0.0001
Hyperthyroidism	0.38	0.38	0.9553
Other substance abuse	15.83	65.38	<0.0001
Malignancies	9.95	3.55	<0.0001
AIDS	2.89	2.59	0.2394

frequencies for hyperthyroidism and AIDS, cannabis users had lower percentages for all the other comorbidities. The frequency of the outcomes of the study including liver cirrhosis, complications of cirrhosis, mortality, liver cancer, and unfavorable discharge disposition were all lower among patients with cannabis use (Table S1).

During propensity matching, 4,728 of 4,774 cannabis users were successfully matched to an equal number of nonusers (Table S2). The frequencies of demographic and comorbid characteristics became statistically identical among the matched cannabis versus noncannabis users. Furthermore, matching eliminated the aOR for having cannabis use disorder with respect to different factors (Table S3).

3.2. Outcomes among Propensity-Matched Cohort. After matching, cannabis users had lower frequencies for liver cirrhosis and its complications, lower frequencies of higher Baveno4 scores, and unfavorable discharges. But the frequency of mortality and liver cancer were similar between cannabis users and nonusers (Table 2). On regression analysis (Table 3 and Figure 2), when compared to nonusers, cannabis users had lower prevalence rate ratio for liver cirrhosis (aPRR:0.81[0.72-0.91]). They had a cirrhosis prevalence rate of 40.18 per 1,000 hospitalizations versus 49.72 per 1,000 hospitalizations among nonusers (Table 4). Furthermore, cannabis users had decreased frequencies of ascites and portal hypertension, while other complications of cirrhosis were similar across noncannabis users. The adjusted prevalence of liver cancer and in-hospital mortality was similar across both cannabis and noncannabis user groups. While the LOS was similar among both groups (5.57[5.10-6.09] versus 5.66[5.25-6.10] days), cannabis users had decreased total hospital cost ($39,642[36,220-43,387] versus $45,566[$42,244-$49,150]) and less unfavorable discharge disposition (0.87[0.78-0.96]).

3.3. Post Hoc Analyses. After categorizing cannabis users into two groups (dependent and nondependent users), we found that the prevalence of liver cirrhosis decreased by 15% and 48% among nondependent (0.85[0.73-0.99], p-value: 0.0272) and dependent users (0.52[0.35-0.79], p-value: 0.0004), respectively. Further, compared to nondependent cannabis users, dependent users had a 38% decreased prevalence of liver cirrhosis (0.62[0.41-0.93], p-value: 0.0156).

After redesigning the propensity matching with cirrhosis as a predictor of cannabis use, the associations between cannabis use and healthcare utilization was similar to the previous model, which did not match with cirrhosis, but adjusted for cirrhosis as a predictor (Table S4).

4. Discussion

Our study utilizing a large dataset spanning records from 2007 to 2014 of NIS revealed novel associations between cannabis use and chronic liver disease among HCV infected individuals. Using propensity matching to effectively eliminate many confounding differences, our studies revealed that cannabis use was associated with more favorable HCV infection outcomes. Compared to other population studies performed before 2010, which all suggested that cannabis use resulted in steatosis and cirrhosis among HCV [12–14], our results revealed the contrary. These three earlier studies had limited sample sizes (204, 270, and 315 subjects) and included patients with alcohol and tobacco use, which might have resulted in a different outcome compared to our study.

Cannabinoids act through CB-1 and CB-2 receptors, with pro- and antifibrotic effects respectively. Early studies mostly rationalized with the fact that HCV was associated with a significant induction in hepatic CB-1 receptor expression [30]. However, later studies between 2013 and 2016 among HCV [16] or HCV+HIV [15, 17] coinfected individuals concluded that cannabis had no effect on liver disease from HCV. Although these three newer studies had larger samples sizes (550, 575, and 690 subjects), they did not eliminate many chronic liver diseases from diverse etiologies. Further, a more recent study on HCV+HIV coinfected patients in 2017 [18] used an even larger sample size (838 subjects) and revealed that cannabis use was associated with a decrease in hepatic steatosis. Our analysis extended on these previous studies in an attempt to overcome limitations of sample size and inclusions of liver disease from non-HCV infection and other synergistic etiologies. We also excluded other causes of CLD and used a more recent nationally representative dataset. Further, we additionally investigated a larger array of clinical outcomes and health care utilization indicators.

Cannabinoids have been demonstrated to kill profibrotic hepatic stellate cells [31] and reverse liver fibrosis/cirrhosis in preclinical models after chronic administration [32]. These actions might explain our findings of decreased hepatic cirrhosis and its attendant complications, which are all secondary to portal hypertension from cirrhosis. Likewise, cannabigerol, a nonpsychotropic component of cannabis thwarts the growth of colorectal cancer cells [33], and tetrahydrocannabinol inhibited glioblastoma cell growth both in vitro and in patients [34]. Both of these mechanisms and decreased prevalence of cirrhosis might explain why cannabis users had lower prevalence of liver carcinoma.

We reveal that cannabis was associated with reduced unfavorable discharge and hospital cost. These outcomes might be due to less burden of CLD because of the smaller frequency of cirrhosis and carcinoma. Cannabis has been shown to be related to lower mortality among hospitalized cancer patients [35].

In summary, the effect of cannabis on HCV disease might be multifaceted. First, cannabis might be directly toxic to hepatitis virus in vivo, as is recently shown in vitro [19]. Second, cannabis users might make HCV patients feel less nauseous and more motivated to take their other antiviral medications and another medical regimen [36]. Third, cannabis might be associated with decreased hepatic cirrhosis and complications of cirrhosis, thereby resulting in the lower cost and better discharge disposition outcomes among cannabis users. Thee potential roles played by cannabis use on liver disease progression in HCV positive patients will require additional complementary evaluation by way of prospective studies.

4.1. Study Strengths and Limitations. The major weaknesses in our study are the cross-sectional design, recall biases, coding errors in the ICD-9-CM application, lack of information

TABLE 2: Outcome characteristics by cannabis use status, after propensity matching.

	No Cannabis use	Cannabis use	p-value
n	4728	4728	
Liver cirrhosis	10.55	8.52	0.0014
Ascites	4.51	2.79	<0.0001
Variceal bleeding	1.57	1.61	0.0258
Hepatorenal syndrome	0.49	0.38	0.4329
Hepatic encephalopathy	0.59	0.40	0.1964
Portal hypertension	2.92	2.07	0.0108
Jaundice	0.53	0.34	0.158
Baveno4 scoring			0.0019
0: No cirrhosis	89.45	91.48	
1: Compensated cirrhosis	5.31	4.72	
2: Decompensated cirrhosis	5.25	3.81	
Mortality	1.65	1.27	0.119
Liver cancer	1.31	1.04	0.2282
Discharge disposition			0.0014
Favourable discharge	80.71	83.27	
Unfavourable discharge	19.29	16.73	

TABLE 3: Comparison of liver disease and outcomes among HCV patients.

	aPRR/aMR	LCL	UCL	p-value
Liver cirrhosis	0.81	0.72	0.91	0.0004
Liver cancer*	0.79	0.55	1.13	0.2013
Complications of cirrhosis				
Ascites	0.62	0.50	0.76	<0.0001
Variceal bleeding	1.03	0.75	1.40	0.8658
Hepatorenal syndrome	0.78	0.42	1.45	0.436
Hepatic encephalopathy	0.68	0.38	1.20	0.1824
Portal hypertension	0.71	0.56	0.91	0.0065
Jaundice	0.64	0.34	1.20	0.1633
Baveno4	0.97	0.93	1.02	0.2167
Health care utilization				
Inpatient mortality*	0.84	0.60	1.17	0.298
Length of stay*	0.99	0.93	1.05	0.6319
Total hospital cost*	0.87	0.80	0.95	0.0012
Unfavourable discharge*	0.85	0.77	0.95	0.0025

aPRR: adjusted prevalence rate ratio; aMR: adjusted mean ratio (LOS and total hospital cost). LCL and UCL: lower and upper confidence limit; *: effects are after adjusting for cirrhosis.

TABLE 4: Adjusted estimates of liver disease, mortality, and outcomes of HCV patients.

	Cannabis use			No Cannabis use		
	Prevalence	LCL	UCL	Prevalence	LCL	UCL
Cirrhosis	54.8	48.29	62.18	67.85	60.66	75.89
Cancer*	3.265	1.819	5.859	4.131	2.356	7.243
Mortality*	1.741	1.194	2.536	2.078	1.486	2.907
	Mean	**LCL**	**UCL**	**Mean**	**LCL**	**UCL**
LOS, days	5.5762	5.104	6.092	5.6611	5.251	6.103
Charge, $	39642	36220	43387	45566	42244	49150
	Percentage	**LCL**	**UCL**	**Percentage**	**LCL**	**UCL**
Unfavourable discharge	25.18	22.28	28.46	29.57	26.3	33.26

LCL and UCL: lower and upper confidence limit.

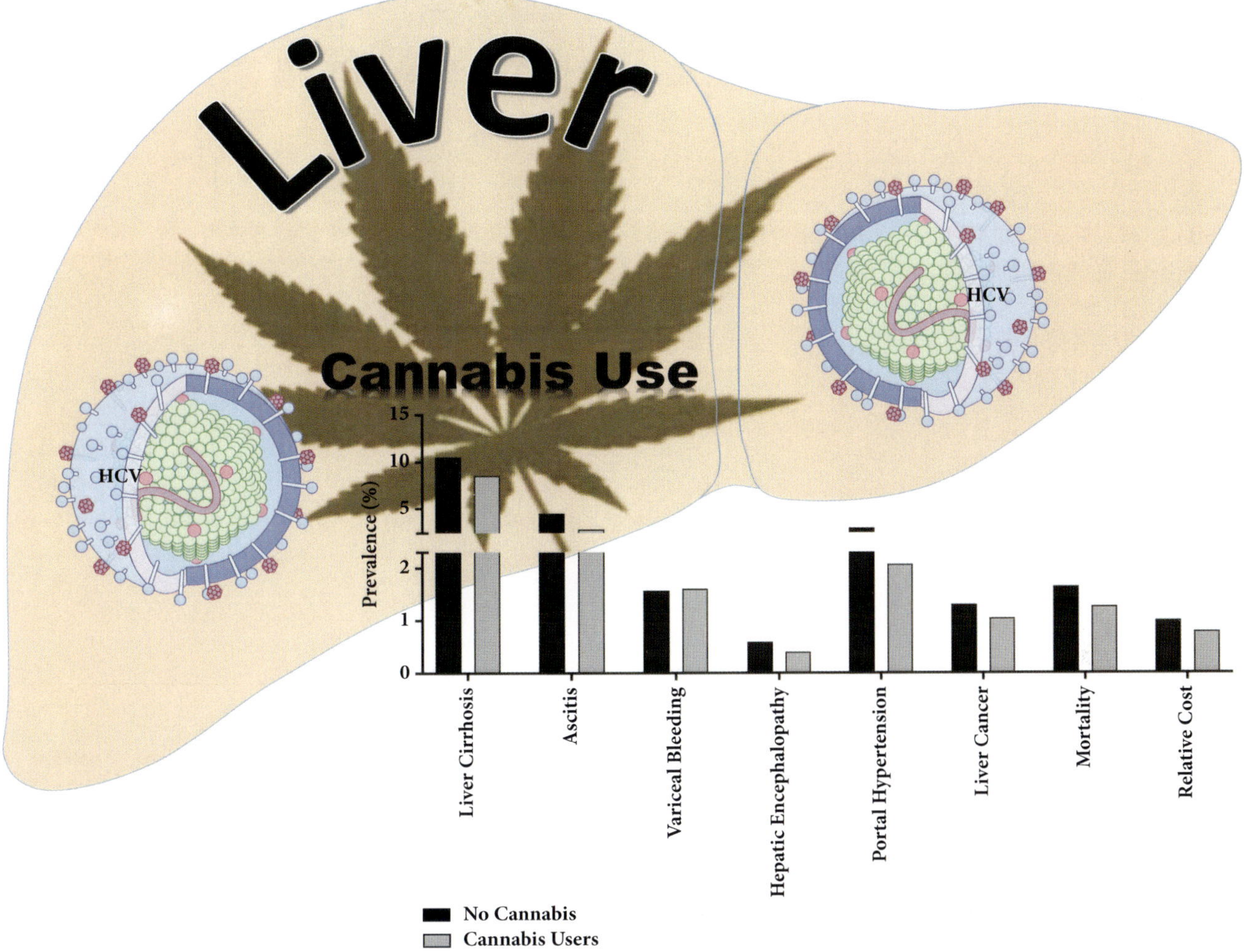

Figure 2: **Summary schematic of the effects of cannabis use by HCV infected individuals and liver disease associated parameters.** Our observations suggest that cannabis use by HCV infected individuals is associated with significant reduction in adverse progressive disease associated pathologies. Further, cannabis users had an overall lower cost of disease management compared to noncannabis users. Schematic illustrations made use of some motifolio templates (http://www.motifolio.com/).

on medications such as antiviral therapies, type of cannabis ingested, mode of cannabis use (oral versus inhalation), and sensitivity and specificity of ICD-9-CM coding for cannabis use disorder. Absence of data on which patients received the new direct-acting antiviral therapy is a significant limitation, given that these medications are extremely effective and significantly modulate the progress of HCV liver disease. We mitigated many of these errors by first eliminating other causes of CLD and using a propensity-matched analysis, which directly balanced and eliminated the effect of factors associated with cannabis use in the NIS and allowed a less biased estimation of our outcomes. However, it is possible that additional unmeasured confounding factors might still impact our observations. These errors are likely to similarly impact both cannabis and noncannabis use groups and would likely decrease our observed effects on cannabis use and the incidence of CLD. Therefore, the true effect of cannabis use on HCV might be stronger than observed estimates in our current study. Furthermore, the large size of the NIS data allowed us to conduct a very efficient propensity matching and to capture subjects from all over the USA, making our result more generalizable.

5. Conclusions

Our novel study to the best of our knowledge represents the largest population-based study to assess the effect of cannabis use on CLD associated with HCV infection. Our observations suggest cannabis use might have a positive impact in alleviating complications of portal hypertension, liver cancer, and disease outcomes among HCV infected individuals. These novel findings require additional prospective and translational molecular research studies to decipher which specific active components of cannabis impact liver disease development during chronic HCV infection.

Abbreviations

AC: Alcoholic cirrhosis
AH: alcoholic hepatitis
ALD: Alcoholic liver disease
AS: Alcoholic steatosis
CBD: Cannabidiol
CLD: Chronic liver disease
CU: Cannabis use
HBV: Hepatitis b viral infection
HCC: Hepatocellular carcinoma
HCV: Hepatitis c viral infection
THC: Tetrahydrocannabinol.

Disclosure

The funders had no role in the project design, execution, data interpretation, or decision to publish.

Authors' Contributions

Adeyinka Charles Adejumo and Terence Ndonyi Bukong conceived and designed the study. Adeyinka Charles Adejumo, Kelechi Lauretta Adejumo, Oluwole Muyiwa Adegbala, and Terence Ndonyi Bukong acquired, analyzed, and interpreted the data. Adeyinka Charles Adejumo and Terence Ndonyi Bukong drafted the manuscript, and Adeyinka Charles Adejumo, Kelechi Lauretta Adejumo, Oluwole Muyiwa Adegbala, and Terence Ndonyi Bukong edited the manuscript.

Acknowledgments

This work was funded by a start-up grant to Terence Ndonyi Bukong by INRS-Institut Armand-Frappier, Institut National de la Recherche Scientifique, 531 Boulevard des Prairies, Laval (Quebec) H7V 1B7, Canada.

References

[1] D. Goldberg, I. C. Ditah, K. Saeian et al., "Changes in the Prevalence of Hepatitis C Virus Infection, Nonalcoholic Steatohepatitis, and Alcoholic Liver Disease Among Patients With Cirrhosis or Liver Failure on the Waitlist for Liver Transplantation," *Gastroenterology*, vol. 152, no. 5, pp. 1090–1099.e1, 2017.

[2] "Snapshot," 2017, http://onlinelibrary.wiley.com/doi/10.1111/jvh.12262/abstract.

[3] C. Welsch, A. Jesudian, S. Zeuzem, and I. Jacobson, "New direct-acting antiviral agents for the treatment of hepatitis C virus infection and perspectives," *Gut*, vol. 61, no. 1, pp. i36–i46, 2012.

[4] S. Zeuzem, R. Ghalib, K. R. Reddy et al., "Grazoprevir-elbasvir combination therapy for treatment-naive cirrhotic and noncirrhotic patients with chronic hepatitis C virus genotype 1, 4, or 6 infection: a randomized trial," *Annals of Internal Medicine*, vol. 163, no. 1, pp. 1–13, 2015.

[5] K. A. Forde, O. Tanapanpanit, and K. R. Reddy, "Hepatitis B and C in African Americans: Current status and continued challenges," *Clinical Gastroenterology and Hepatology*, vol. 12, no. 5, pp. 738–748, 2014.

[6] M. Lemoine, S. Nayagam, and M. Thursz, "Viral hepatitis in resource-limited countries and access to antiviral therapies: Current and future challenges," *Future Virology*, vol. 8, no. 4, pp. 371–380, 2013.

[7] A. Azofeifa, M. E. Mattson, G. Schauer, T. McAfee, A. Grant, and R. Lyerla, "National Estimates of Marijuana Use and Related Indicators — National Survey on Drug Use and Health, United States, 2002–2014," *MMWR Surveillance Summaries*, vol. 65, no. 11, pp. 1–28, 2016.

[8] E. Gabbay, Y. Avraham, Y. Ilan, E. Israeli, and E. M. Berry, "Endocannabinoids and liver disease - Review," *Liver International*, vol. 25, no. 5, pp. 921–926, 2005.

[9] E. Patsenker, P. Sachse, A. Chicca et al., "Elevated levels of endocannabinoids in chronic hepatitis c may modulate cellular immune response and hepatic stellate cell activation," *International Journal of Molecular Sciences*, vol. 16, no. 4, pp. 7057–7076, 2015.

[10] A. C. Adejumo, S. Alliu, T. O. Ajayi et al., "Cannabis use is associated with reduced prevalence of non-alcoholic fatty liver disease: A cross-sectional study," *PLoS ONE*, vol. 12, no. 4, 2017.

[11] A. C. Adejumo, T. O. Ajayi, O. M. Adegbala et al., "Cannabis use is associated with reduced prevalence of progressive stages of alcoholic liver disease," *Liver International*, 2018.

[12] C. Hézode, F. Roudot-Thoraval, S. Nguyen et al., "Daily cannabis smoking as a risk factor for progression of fibrosis in chronic hepatitis C," *Hepatology*, vol. 42, no. 1, pp. 63–71, 2005.

[13] C. Hézode, E. S. Zafrani, F. Roudot-Thoraval et al., "Daily cannabis Use: a novel risk factor of steatosis severity in patients with chronic hepatitis C," *Gastroenterology*, vol. 134, no. 2, pp. 432–439, 2008.

[14] J. H. Ishida, M. G. Peters, C. Jin et al., "Influence of Cannabis Use on Severity of Hepatitis C Disease," *Clinical Gastroenterology and Hepatology*, vol. 6, no. 1, pp. 69–75, 2008.

[15] L. Brunet, E. E. M. Moodie, K. Rollet et al., "Marijuana smoking does not accelerate progression of liver disease in HIV-hepatitis C coinfection: A longitudinal Cohort analysis," *Clinical Infectious Diseases*, vol. 57, no. 5, pp. 663–670, 2013.

[16] Theresa Liu, G. T. Howell, Lucy Turner, Kimberley Corace, Gary Garber, and Curtis Cooper, "Marijuana Use in Hepatitis C Infection does not Affect Liver Biopsy Histology or Treatment Outcomes," *Canadian Journal of Gastroenterology and Hepatology*, vol. 28, Article ID 804969, 4 pages, 2014.

[17] E. Kelly, J. Dodge, M. Sarkar et al., "Marijuana Use Is Not Associated With Progression to Advanced Liver Fibrosis in HIV/Hepatitis C Virus–coinfected Women," *Clin Infect Dis*, vol. 63, no. 4, pp. 512–518, 2016.

[18] S. Nordmann, A. Vilotitch, P. Roux et al., "Daily cannabis and reduced risk of steatosis in human immunodeficiency virus and hepatitis C virus-co-infected patients (ANRS CO13-HEPAVIH)," *Journal of Viral Hepatitis*, vol. 25, no. 2, pp. 171–179, 2018.

[19] H. Lowe, N. Toyang, and W. McLaughlin, "Potential of cannabidiol for the treatment of viral hepatitis," *Pharmacognosy Research*, vol. 9, no. 1, pp. 116–118, 2017.

[20] "Citations for HCUP Databases and Tools," 2017, https://www.hcup-us.ahrq.gov/tech_assist/citations.jsp.

[21] Z. M. Younossi, M. Otgonsuren, L. Henry et al., "Inpatient

resource utilization, disease severity, mortality and insurance coverage for patients hospitalized for hepatitis C virus in the United States," *Journal of Viral Hepatitis*, vol. 22, no. 2, pp. 137–145, 2015.

[22] A. N. Ananthakrishnan, E. L. McGinley, J. Fangman, and K. Saeian, "Hepatitis C/HIV co-infection is associated with higher mortality in hospitalized patients with Hepatitis C or HIV," *Journal of Viral Hepatitis*, vol. 17, no. 10, pp. 720–729, 2010.

[23] R. Rajbhandari, C. J. Danford, R. T. Chung, and A. N. Ananthakrishnan, "HBV infection is associated with greater mortality in hospitalised patients compared to HCV infection or alcoholic liver disease," *Alimentary Pharmacology & Therapeutics*, vol. 41, no. 10, pp. 928–938, 2015.

[24] A. J. Kruger, K. Mumtaz, A. Anaizi et al., "Cirrhosis Is Associated with Increased Mortality in Patients with Diverticulitis: A Nationwide Cross-Sectional Study," *Digestive Diseases and Sciences*, vol. 62, no. 11, pp. 3149–3155, 2017.

[25] H. Wu and G. C. Nguyen, "Liver cirrhosis is associated with venous thromboembolism among hospitalized patients in a nationwide US study," *Clinical Gastroenterology and Hepatology*, vol. 8, no. 9, pp. 800–e1, 2010.

[26] B. Hammill, "GMATCH SAS macro: computerized matching of cases to controls using the greedy matching algorithm with a fixed number of controls per case," 2015, http://people.duke.edu/~hammill/software/gmatch.sas.

[27] I. J. Dahabreh, R. C. Sheldrick, J. K. Paulus et al., "Do observational studies using propensity score methods agree with randomized trials? A systematic comparison of studies on acute coronary syndromes," *European Heart Journal*, vol. 33, no. 15, pp. 1893–1901, 2012.

[28] G. D. Kitsios, I. J. Dahabreh, S. Callahan, J. K. Paulus, A. C. Campagna, and J. M. Dargin, "Can We Trust Observational Studies Using Propensity Scores in the Critical Care Literature? A Systematic Comparison with Randomized Clinical Trials," *Critical Care Medicine*, vol. 43, no. 9, pp. 1870–1879, 2015.

[29] D. Spiegelman and E. Hertzmark, "Easy SAS calculations for risk or prevalence ratios and differences," *American Journal of Epidemiology*, vol. 162, no. 3, pp. 199-200, 2005.

[30] D. van der Poorten, M. Shahidi, E. Tay et al., "Hepatitis C Virus Induces the Cannabinoid Receptor 1," *PLoS ONE*, vol. 5, no. 9, p. e12841, 2010.

[31] B. Julien, P. Grenard, F. Teixeira-Clerc et al., "Antifibrogenic role of the cannabinoid receptor CB2 in the liver," *Gastroenterology*, vol. 128, no. 3, pp. 742–755, 2005.

[32] J. Muñoz-Luque, J. Ros, G. Fernández-Varo et al., "Regression of fibrosis after chronic stimulation of cannabinoid CB2 receptor in cirrhotic rats," *The Journal of Pharmacology and Experimental Therapeutics*, vol. 324, no. 2, pp. 475–483, 2008.

[33] F. Borrelli, E. Pagano, B. Romano et al., "Colon carcinogenesis is inhibited by the TRPM8 antagonist cannabigerol, a Cannabis-derived non-psychotropic cannabinoid," *Carcinogenesis*, vol. 35, no. 12, pp. 2787–2797, 2014.

[34] M. Guzman, M. J. Duarte, C. Blázquez et al., "A pilot clinical study of Δ9-tetrahydrocannabinol in patients with recurrent glioblastoma multiforme," *British Journal of Cancer*, vol. 95, no. 2, pp. 197–203, 2006.

[35] N. Vin-Raviv, T. Akinyemiju, Q. Meng, S. Sakhuja, and R. Hayward, "Marijuana use and inpatient outcomes among hospitalized patients: analysis of the nationwide inpatient sample database," *Cancer Medicine*, vol. 6, no. 1, pp. 320–329, 2017.

[36] D. L. Sylvestre, B. J. Clements, and Y. Malibu, "Cannabis use improves retention and virological outcomes in patients treated for hepatitis C," *European Journal of Gastroenterology & Hepatology*, vol. 18, no. 10, pp. 1057–1063, 2006.

Effect of a Cooperation Strategy between Primary Care Physicians and Hospital Liver Units on HBV Care in Campania, Italy

Rosa Zampino ,[1,2] Nicolina Capoluongo,[3] Adriana Boemio ,[1] Margherita Macera,[3] Martina Vitrone ,[1] Luigi Elio Adinolfi,[1] Pietro Filippini,[3] Evangelista Sagnelli,[3] Caterina Sagnelli ,[4] Emanuele Durante-Mangoni,[2,4] and Nicola Coppola[3]

[1] *Department of Medical, Surgical, Neurological, Metabolic and Geriatric Sciences, University of Campania "L. Vanvitelli", Italy*
[2] *Unit of Infectious & Transplant Medicine, "V. Monaldi" Hospital, AORN dei Colli, Naples, Italy*
[3] *Infectious Diseases Unit, Department of Mental and Physical Health and Preventive Medicine, University of Campania "L. Vanvitelli", Italy*
[4] *Department of Precision Medicine, University of Campania "L. Vanvitelli", Italy*

Correspondence should be addressed to Rosa Zampino; rosa.zampino@unicampania.it

Academic Editor: Alessandro Granito

Aims. This study is aimed at assessing the efficacy of an active search and treat strategy for HBV-infected subjects in an endemic area (Campania, Italy). To do this, we created a cooperation bundle between 24 General Practitioners (GPs) and 3 Hospital Liver Units (HLU). We assessed whether this strategy improved the detection of HBV infection in patients at risk and the overall quality of care, with the aim of reducing liver disease progression. *Methods.* We estimated that, among about 20,000 patients cared for by the 24 GPs, approximately 280 patients unaware of or underestimating HBV infection would be found. Identified patients were to be referred to the HLU for clinical evaluation and treatment from February 2016 for 12 months. *Results.* Unexpectedly, screening and enrolment were poor (48 patients only). GP workloads, patient financial difficulties, and patients' refusal were the major causes of enrolment failure according to GPs. All patients referred to HLU completed the program; most of them were HBV inactive carriers. *Conclusions.* This program failed to scavenge chronic HBV-infected patients in an endemic area and establish a successful clinical collaboration between GPs and HLU. Underlying reasons are diverse and call for new strategies to implement cooperation between primary care providers and hospital specialists.

1. Introduction

In recent decades, a progressive reduction in the incidence of acute hepatitis B (AHB) and the prevalence of HBV-related chronic hepatitis has been observed in endemic areas, such as the Campania region of Italy, as a result of improved socioeconomic conditions and universal vaccination [1–3]. The current incidence of AHB is about 1/100,000 inhabitants per year, 15% of cases involving the immigrant population [4], and the prevalence of HBsAg carriers is estimated at nearly 1% in the native population and 3-10% in documented immigrants (regular immigrants who arrived in Italy for economic reasons and have now stable work and residency). It is estimated that 600,000 Italians and nearly 250,000 immigrants are chronic carriers of HBV infection, of whom 50% and 70%, respectively, are unaware of their virological condition [4]. These subjects may transmit HBV infection and remain untreated, even when treatment is warranted [4].

Italian General Practitioners (GPs) are the physicians providing primary care and are usually overwhelmed by a considerable number of patients with symptomatic diseases, leaving them little time for asymptomatic patients, such as most HBsAg-positive patients. Consequently, most of them are not referred to a hepatologist for screening, follow-up, treatment (when necessary), and the implementation of preventive measures [5, 6]. Previous experience showed the benefit of GP involvement in screening strategies to reduce the number of undiagnosed hepatic infections and clarify the prevalence and correlates of the different risk factors [7, 8]. This cooperation could improve the quality of care and the cost-benefit ratio.

We applied a clinical bundle to first actively screen, identify, and treat HBV infection in subjects unaware of their virological condition in Campania, Italy, and refer them to a Hospital Liver Unit (HLU) for clinical evaluation and antiviral treatment, when indicated. A second aim was to create a network between GPs and hepatology specialists to improve the quality of care (diagnosis, clinical evaluation, follow-up, and treatment). The ultimate aim was to reduce the progression of liver disease to cirrhosis, the development of hepatocellular carcinoma (HCC), the risk of in-house and sexual transmission of HBV infection, and the cost of management.

2. Methods

We contacted two GP associations in Naples and a group of GPs in Caserta to illustrate the program and seek their participation. One of the GP associations did not join the program because of excessive prior workload, while other GPs gave their full availability to participate. In Caserta, of 15 GPs invited, 5 joined the program. GPs use a database for their clinical records, which we thought would be useful tool to screen data and identify patients' anthropometric measures, clinical history, and current pharmacologic treatment.

Within this network, we tried to apply to a large primary care population methods similar to those successfully used in an ongoing study performed to identify and manage HBV infection in irregular immigrants and refugees [9].

2.1. Study Design. The planned duration of the program was one year. On the basis of chronic HBV infection prevalence in Campania [4] and the number of subjects cared for by the GPs participating in this program, we estimated that in a cohort of about 20,000 subjects (at least 20 GPs randomly involved) approximately 280 citizens with HBV infection would be found. An educational meeting with participating GPs was held to discuss the study protocol and review HBV epidemiology, pathophysiology, and treatment. Posters illustrating the "Scavenge HBV in Campania" program were put up in the GPs' offices to inform subjects and sensitize them towards HBV infection. The essential role of the GPs in alerting HBV carriers was stressed. A financial support to participate in the program was given to the GP association.

Each GP was to extrapolate from his/her database subjects cared for with risk factors for HBV infection and/or ALT abnormalities and refer them for screening for serum HBsAg. Each known HBV carrier was to fill out a questionnaire recording age, sex, geographical origin, level of education, religion, family history, cohabitation conditions, sexual habits, history of previous surgery, dental care, tattooing, piercing, drug addiction, blood transfusion, abortion for females, and (when applicable) time of immigration and tribal rituals. GPs had to refer patients with known HBsAg positivity, if not already cared by other HLU.

Family members of subjects found to be HBsAg-positive were to be screened for HBV serum markers. All subjects found to be HBsAg-positive were to be referred at the nearest HLU involved in the program, for clinical examination and the determination of liver function tests, liver ultrasound scan, and HBeAg, anti-HBe, HBV DNA, anti-HDV, anti-HCV, and anti-HIV testing. Fibrosis assessment by non-invasive method (transient elastography, TE; Fibro Scan®, EchoSens, Paris, France) or liver biopsy was to be performed and treatment offered when indicated, in accordance with patient's compliance and current guidelines [10, 11]. Comorbidities and coinfections were to be investigated in depth and treated when indicated.

Figure 1 shows the fundamental steps of the program.

All patients, either treated or untreated, were to be followed up with a personalized educational and clinical program. Particular attention was to be given to patients with an advanced liver disease. Cooperation between the GP and the HLU specialist was to be long-lasting to ensure qualified assistance to the HBV subjects and their family members. To favor patient enrolment and adherence, a junior doctor of the investigator's team met with each patient at GP's office and assisted them at their first HLU visit. Moreover, an administrative assistant coordinated visit schedules and kept telephone contacts with doctors and patients to ease required encounters.

Statistical analysis of data was performed using the statistical package STATA to identify risk factors independently associated with HBsAg positivity. The outcome of HBV patients (both treated and untreated) was evaluated according to the criteria suggested in the current AASLD and EASL guidelines [10, 11].

In addition, continued cooperation between GPs and specialists after the project was also assessed.

The study was conducted in accordance with the rules of the Good Clinical Practice and the protocol and procedures were approved by the Ethics Committee of the University of Campania "L. Vanvitelli".

3. Results

The program started in February 2016 with the involvement of 25 randomly selected GPs. As only 33 patients from 15 of 25 GP offices were enrolled during the initial 4 months of study, we decided to extend the bundle to all 116 GPs included in the GP association (Figure 2).

3.1. Enrolment. The analysis of the GP databases at the beginning of the study identified 282 known HBsAg-positive patients. However, many of these patients either were not involved by GPs or were misclassified as HBsAg. Moreover, less than 50% of patients who were anticipated to have risk factors for HBV infection and/or elevated ALT were screened. The reasons for such a low enrolment rate

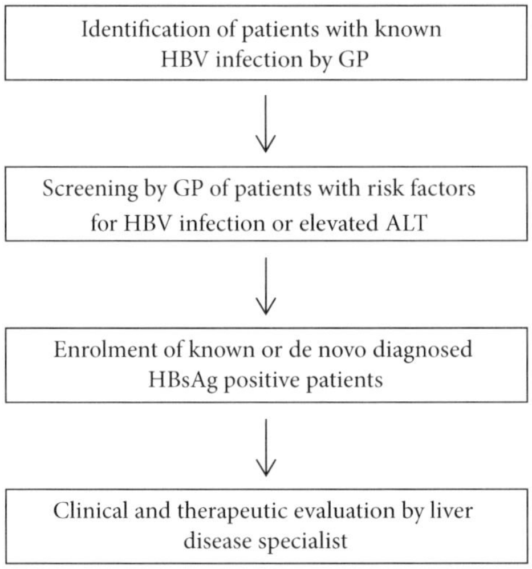

FIGURE 1: Flowchart of the fundamental phases of the program.

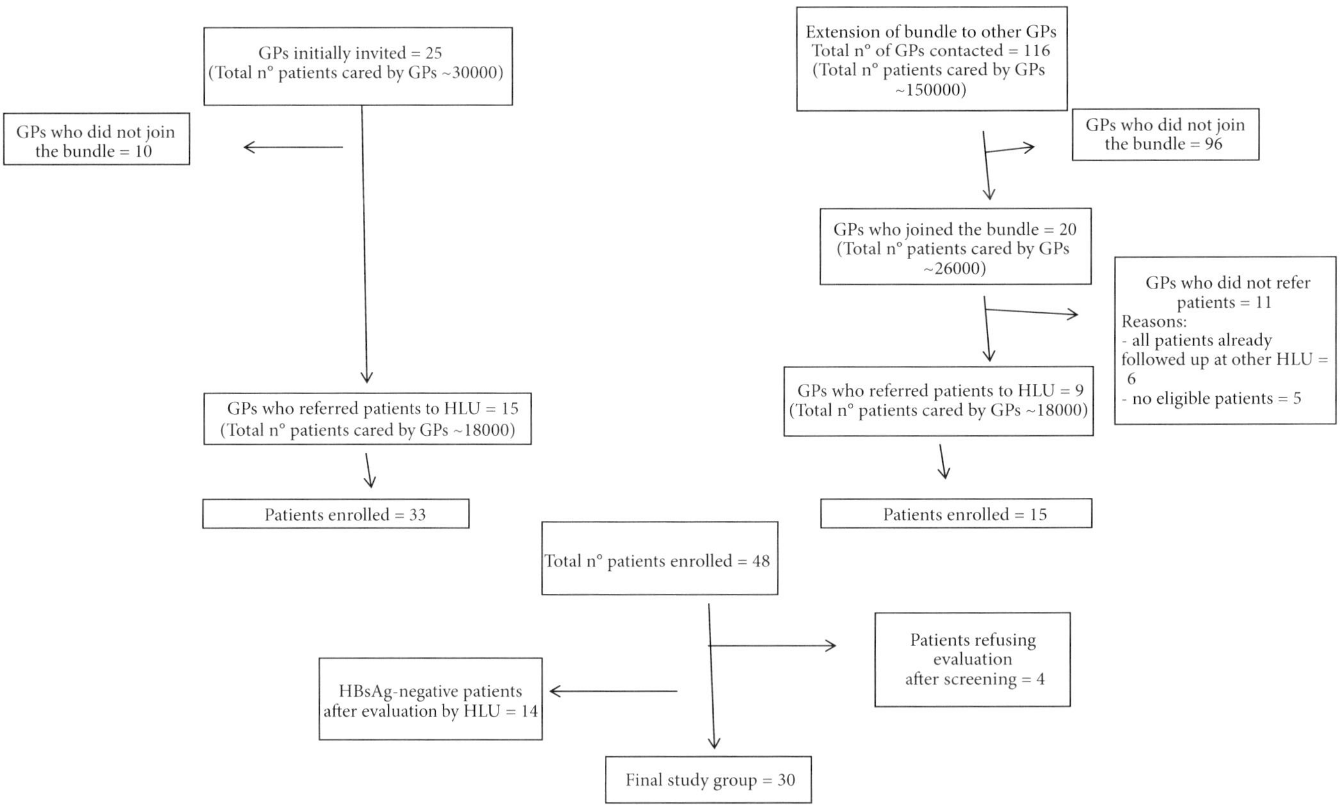

FIGURE 2: GP involvement in the program.

were reported only by a small number of GPs and are summarized in Table 1. GP workloads (many patients with different symptomatic disorders to follow), patients' financial difficulties, and simple refusal to participate were the most frequently reported. Furthermore, diabetes mellitus and oncohematologic diseases were considered a priority by some GPs compared to possible or asymptomatic liver disease.

Eleven GPs did not refer patients to the specialist liver units stating these were already followed up at other HLU (6 GPs) or due to lack of any HBsAg-positive subject in their patient population (5 GPs) (Figure 2).

An analysis performed by a member of the HLU specialists' team, who was in direct contact with GPs, revealed common mistakes in the GP databases, with patient misclassification regarding ALT values or HBV status or failure to update past test results. In particular, 30% of patients who were meant to be HBsAg-positive were in fact HBsAg-negative. This likely caused the initial overestimation of the number of patients available for the study.

TABLE 1: Declared reasons for low enrolment by the 20 GPs participating in the program.

	N (%)
Patients' refusal	2 (10)
High workload	5 (25)
Involvement in other projects	4 (20)
Patient's contribution costs	9 (45)

3.2. Referral to Hospital Liver Units. Although the percentage of HBsAg-positive subjects referred was much lower than expected, among the identified patients, only 4 declined to continue HLU follow-up after screening.

Overall, 44 referred patients as known or presumed HBsAg-positive started screening at the HLU. Of them, 14 (32%) were actually found to be HBsAg-negative when tested at the HLU laboratory and were instead anti-HBs-positive. Thus, 30 HBsAg-positive patients were finally included in the HLU follow-up.

3.3. Specialist Follow-Up. Specialist follow-up was highly successful, as all 30 HBsAg-positive subjects referred concluded the diagnostic, clinical, and therapeutic (where indicated) course. A clinical and laboratory report for the GP was given to each patient at the end of the evaluation and a schedule for the following appointments.

3.4. Data of HBsAg Patients Enrolled. Table 2 summarizes clinical, biochemical, and virological data of the 30 patients enrolled. Twenty-seven patients were Italian and 3 were immigrants (2 from Benin and 1 from Brasil). They had a median age of 59.5 years and a median BMI of 27 and were mostly free of significant comorbidities. Among them, a high prevalence of HBV inactive carriers was observed, defined as presence of serum antibodies to HBeAg (anti-HBe), undetectable or low (< 2,000 IU/ml) HBV DNA levels, and normal ALT [11]. HBVDNA was undetectable in 8 patients. No patient showed HCV or HDV coinfection. Liver disease was generally mild, with liver function tests within normal values and no signs of liver disease progression and/or HCC. Liver fibrosis assessment was performed by transient elastography in 15 patients (median 5.4 kPa, range 4.0 - 12). This test was not performed in patients with undetectable HBVDNA or in those who refused. However, all patients started a standard clinical follow-up. Ultrasound evaluation was performed in all patients: a bright liver echo-pattern was observed in 6 patients, a coarse pattern was observed in 2 patients, and signs of portal hypertension (increased portal vein and/or spleen diameter) were present in 3 patients. No other clear alteration in the liver echo-pattern was described in the remaining patients.

Household spread of the virus or surgery and dental procedures were the most common risk factors for HBV infection. More than 30% of the analysed patients consumed alcohol daily. Only 2 patients needed antiviral treatment and were started on entecavir and tenofovir, respectively.

TABLE 2: Characteristics of 30 patients enrolled.

General parameters	
Median age (range)	59.5 (32-85)
Males, n° (%)	15 (50%)
Median BMI (range)	27 (22-40)
Daily alcohol consumers N (%)	10 (33.3%)
Biochemical data	
Glucose (mean±SD) mg/dl	93.5±35.6
AST (mean±SD) IU/dl	21.75±10.9
ALT (mean±SD) IU/dl	24.14±16.1
GGT (mean±SD) mg/dl	24.3±13.7
Bilirubin total(mean±SD) mg/dl	0.66±0.26
Bilirubin direct(mean±SD) mg/dl	0.2±0.07
Cholesterol(mean±SD) mg/dl	180.9±53.6
Triglycerides(mean±SD) mg/dl	88.13±35.5
Albumin(mean±SD) mg/dl	4.3±0.4
Cholinesterase (mean±SD) mg/dl	10707±3883
Creatinine(mean±SD) mg/dl	0.8±0.24
Median WBC/mmc (range)	7.6 (3.0 – 8.7)
Median PLT/mmc (range)	203000 (50000- 315000)
Virological data	
HBeAg+ number (%)	1 (3)
antiHBe+ number (%)	29 (97)
Median HBV DNA (range) IU/ml	100 (0-1x10^7)
Risk Factors for HBV infection	
Intravenous drug use, n° (%)	0
Household contact, n° (%)	7 (23.3%)
Surgery, n° (%)	23 (76.6%)
Dental treatment, n° (%)	22 (73.3%)
Piercing, n° (%)	5 (16.6%)
Blood transfusion, n° (%)	0
At risk sexual contact, n° (%)	0
Hepatocellular Carcinoma, n°(%)	0

4. Discussion

This study shows that, despite our structured attempt to establish a cooperation between GPs and HLU specialists, we failed to effectively identify all HBsAg-positive cared subjects and significantly reduce the number of those not receiving specialist care. In fact, our results highlight the obstacles to an effective primary care detection of hepatitis B infection in an endemic area, the Campania region of Italy.

The major drawback of our bundle was the poor effectiveness of HBV screening. GPs reported that enrolment failure was related to their "excessive workload", consisting in too many patients to care for with different and complex diseases, coupled with difficulties in practical organization and simultaneous engagement with other ongoing projects in unrelated fields of medicine. After early detecting these difficulties, we extended the number of GPs involved in the program, in the hope that additional GPs would be more successful in their screening efforts. As a matter of fact, only

48 of the 282 anticipated HBV-positive patients were referred overall and only 30 were finally assessed.

Current patients' costs for HBsAg screening in Italy are about 20 euros and have to be paid by those without a formal prior diagnosis of hepatitis B. Only after a formal HBV diagnosis, subsequent costs are covered by the National Health Service. However, considering the number of the GP cared subjects and the metropolitan area involved, it is hardly credible that so few subjects were able to afford these costs. It is instead more likely that patients did not perceive the importance of the health problem we aimed to actively search, possibly due to unfocused information.

When referred, patients were successfully taken on by the HLU. Interestingly, they were mostly found to be HBV inactive carriers. This suggests that most HBV-infected patients who are unaware of their condition have a mild or inactive disease. Notwithstanding, they remain at risk of progressing to a more severe form of liver disease as well as developing hepatocellular carcinoma [12, 13]. In accordance with the latest international guidelines [11], follow-up and possible antiviral treatment should be extended to these patients for whom treatment was previously considered optional. Furthermore, one-third of our patients consumed alcohol on a daily basis. This was probably due to the fact that they were unaware of their liver infection. However, alcohol consumption can definitely increase the risk of liver disease progression and could be prevented by timely diagnosis and management.

In the "scavenged" HBV patients, the most frequent risk factors were related to iatrogenic transmission; this is in agreement with the senior age of most patients and an infection acquired many years before.

Cooperation with GPs is necessary to "scavenge" asymptomatic diseases in the general population. Studies in other settings reported variable results in the screening and evaluation of liver diseases of different etiologies. Some studies identified problems in screening or basic knowledge [7, 8, 14–18], and others obtained very good results [19, 20].

Although our experience was not entirely satisfactory, we are firmly convinced that the involvement of primary care providers in the management of HBV infection is pivotal. Starting from the results of this study, we hypothesize some approaches to implement the outcome of such studies.

(i) Organizing periodic (i.e., every 2-3 months) educational meetings to raise GPs awareness on specific epidemiologic and clinical problems

(ii) Organizing periodic hospital meetings between GPs and specialists to discuss the results obtained and critically assess the ongoing programs

(iii) Alerting the population through media information campaigns, so that they, themselves, ask their GPs for screening and subsequent clinical investigation

(iv) Offering GPs public financial incentives proportional to their enrolment commitment

(v) Offering free screening tests for indigent subjects

(vi) Strengthening the idea of patient well-being and scientific and/or social gratification to stimulate study participation.

GPs could be also selected on the basis of their scientific interest and expertise, making their role more stimulating, as well as their prior workload. Although this could lead to a selection bias, in our current experience, in the absence of a specific interest, the studies could not be feasible and, even if suboptimal, these criteria should be considered when other strategies have failed.

These approaches could be diversely applied in the different geographical settings on the basis of available means and the results obtained could be subsequently evaluated.

Recently, to overcome the difficulties related to the possible involvement of primary care physicians in anti-HCV treatment, it has been proposed to choose subgroups of more expert GPs to help hepatologists and increase the numbers of patients treated [14, 21]. Certainly, treatment calls for a more complex approach than simple screening, and perhaps in some geographical areas we need to work on more basic levels of intervention.

Further studies using new strategies of cooperation are needed to verify the best options for the management of health problems, HBV infection included.

5. Conclusions

This program failed in its intent to scavenge chronic HBV-infected patients in the Campania area and to establish a close clinical collaboration between GPs and liver units. GP work pressure, economic difficulties of the patients, and their refusal to participate were the causes most frequently stated by GPs to justify poor enrolment.

The patients referred to the liver units completed their program and most of them were HBV inactive carriers.

New strategies to implement cooperation between GPs and hospital specialists are suggested.

Acknowledgments

This work has been supported by an unrestricted grant from Gilead Science Ltd., goShape Program 2015 (Grant no. 000/IHQ/15-09//1686]).

References

[1] G. Giusti, E. Sagnelli, C. Gallo, F. Piccinino, B. Galanti, and G. B. Gaeta, "The Etiology of Chronic Hepatitis in Italy: A Multicenter Study," *Hepato-Gastroenterology*, vol. 41, no. 4, pp. 397–400, 1994.

[2] G. B. Gaeta, G. Stornaiuolo, D. F. Precone et al., "Epidemiological and clinical burden of chronic hepatitis B virus/hepatitis C virus infection. A multicenter Italian study," *Journal of Hepatology*, vol. 39, no. 6, pp. 1036–1041, 2003.

[3] E. Sagnelli, C. Sagnelli, M. Pisaturo, M. Macera, and N. Coppola, "Epidemiology of acute and chronic hepatitis B and delta over the last 5 decades in Italy," *World Journal of Gastroenterology* vol. 20, no. 24, pp. 7635–7643, 2014.

[4] http://www.epicentro.iss.it/problemi/epatite/EpidemiologiaItalia.asp. Accessed Jan 2018.

[5] I. El-Hamad, M. C. Pezzoli, E. Chiari et al., "Point-of-care screening, prevalence, and risk factors for hepatitis B infection among 3,728 mainly undocumented migrants from non-EU countries in northern Italy," *Journal of Travel Medicine*, vol. 22, pp. 78–86, 2015.

[6] B. Heidrich, A. Cetindere, M. Beyaz et al., "High prevalence of hepatitis markers in immigrant populations: A prospective screening approach in a real-world setting," *European Journal of Gastroenterology & Hepatology*, vol. 26, no. 10, pp. 1090–1097, 2014.

[7] I. Wolffram, D. Petroff, O. Bätz et al., "Prevalence of elevated ALT values, HBsAg, and anti-HCV in the primary care setting and evaluation of guideline defined hepatitis risk scenarios," *Journal of Hepatology*, vol. 62, no. 6, article no. 5514, pp. 1256–1264, 2015.

[8] A. Sharifian, N. Naderi, A. Sanati et al., "The Early Results of a New Health Care Program Implementation in HBV Screening: an Iranian Experience," *Middle East Journal of Digestive Diseases*, vol. 7, pp. 226–232, 2015.

[9] N. Coppola, L. Alessio, L. Gualdieri et al., "Hepatitis B virus, hepatitis C virus and human immunodeficiency virus infection in undocumented migrants and refugees in southern Italy," *Eurosurveillance*, vol. 20, article 30009, 2015.

[10] N. A. Terrault, N. H. Bzowej, K.-M. Chang, J. P. Hwang, M. M. Jonas, and M. H. Murad, "AASLD guidelines for treatment of chronic hepatitis B," *Hepatology*, vol. 63, no. 1, pp. 261–283, 2016.

[11] European Association for the Study of the Liver, "EASL Clinical Practice Guidelines: Management of Chronic Hepatitis B Virus Infection," *Journal of Hepatology*, vol. 67, pp. 370–398, 2017.

[12] J. Bruix, M. Sherman, and Association for the Study of Liver Diseases, "Management of hepatocellular carcinoma: an update," *Hepatology*, vol. 53, no. 3, pp. 1020–1022, 2011.

[13] H. B. El-Serag, "Erratum: Epidemiology of viral hepatitis and hepatocellular carcinoma," *Gastroenterology*, vol. 142, no. 1, pp. 1246–1273, 2012.

[14] M. Thomson, M. A. Konerman, H. Choxi, and A. S. Lok, "Primary care physician perspectives on hepatitis C management in the era of direct-acting antiviral therapy," *Digestive Diseases and Sciences*, vol. 61, no. 12, pp. 3460–3468, 2016.

[15] N. Upadhyaya, R. Chang, C. Davis, M. C. Conti, D. Salinas-Garcia, and H. Tang, "Chronic hepatitis B: Perceptions in Asian American communities and diagnosis and management practices among primary care physicians," *Postgraduate Medical Journal*, vol. 122, no. 5, pp. 165–175, 2010.

[16] P. Blais, N. Husain, J. R. Kramer, M. Kowalkowski, H. El-Serag, and F. Kanwal, "Nonalcoholic fatty liver disease is underrecognized in the primary care setting," *American Journal of Gastroenterology*, vol. 110, no. 1, pp. 10–14, 2015.

[17] A. Said and J. H. Jou, "Hepatitis B vaccination and screening awareness in primary care practitioners," *Hepatitis Research and Treatment*, vol. 2014, 7 pages, 2014.

[18] M. Salinas, M. López-Garrigós, E. Flores, J. Uris, C. Leiva-Salinas, and Pilot Group of the Appropriate Utilization of Laboratory Tests (REDCONLAB) working group, "Request of laboratory liver tests in primary care in Spain: Potential savings if appropriateness indicator targets were achieved," *European Journal of Gastroenterology & Hepatology*, vol. 27, no. 10, pp. 1130–1136, 2015.

[19] I. Cacciola, R. Scoglio, A. Alibrandi et al., "Evaluation of liver enzyme levels and identification of asymptomatic liver disease patients in primary care," *Internal and Emergency Medicine*, vol. 12, no. 2, pp. 181–186, 2017.

[20] D. J. McLernon, P. T. Donnan, F. M. Sullivan et al., "Prediction of liver disease in patients whose liver function tests have been checked in primary care: Model development and validation using population-based observational cohorts," *BMJ Open*, vol. 4, no. 6, Article ID e004837, 2014.

[21] R. Fox, "Going Viral: Why Eliminating the Burden of Hepatitis C Requires Enhanced Cooperation Between Specialists and Primary Care Providers," *Digestive Diseases and Sciences*, vol. 61, no. 12, pp. 3381–3383, 2016.

30

Percutaneous Ablation for Hepatocellular Carcinoma: Comparison of Various Ablation Techniques and Surgery

Shuichiro Shiina ,[1] Koki Sato,[1] Ryosuke Tateishi,[2] Motonori Shimizu,[1] Hideko Ohama,[1] Takeshi Hatanaka,[1] Masashi Takawa,[1] Hiroaki Nagamatsu,[1] and Yasuharu Imai[1]

[1]*Department of Gastroenterology, Juntendo University School of Medicine, Japan*
[2]*Department of Gastroenterology, The University of Tokyo, Japan*

Correspondence should be addressed to Shuichiro Shiina; ivo@juntendo.ac.jp

Academic Editor: Tatsuo Kanda

Image-guided percutaneous ablation is considered best in the treatment of early-stage hepatocellular carcinoma (HCC). Ablation is potentially curative, minimally invasive, and easily repeatable for recurrence. Ethanol injection used to be the standard in ablation. However, radiofrequency ablation has recently been the most prevailing ablation method for HCC. Many investigators have reported that radiofrequency ablation is superior to ethanol injection, from the viewpoints of treatment response, local tumor curativity, and overall survival. New-generation microwave ablation can create a larger ablation volume in a shorter time period. Further comparison studies are, however, mandatory between radiofrequency ablation and microwave ablation, especially in terms of complications and long-term survival. Irreversible electroporation, which is a non-thermal ablation method that delivers short electric pulses to induce cell death due to apoptosis, requires further studies, especially in terms of long-term outcomes. It is considerably difficult to compare outcomes in ablation with those in surgical resection. However, radiofrequency ablation seems to be a satisfactory alternative to resection for HCC 3 cm or smaller in Child-Pugh class A or B cirrhosis. Furthermore, radiofrequency ablation may be a first-line treatment in HCC 2 cm or smaller in Child-Pugh class A or B cirrhosis. Various innovations would further improve outcomes in ablation. Training programs may be effective in providing an excellent opportunity to understand basic concepts and learn cardinal skills for successful ablation. Sophisticated ablation would be more than an adequate alternative of surgery for small- and possibly middle-sized HCC.

1. Introduction

Hepatocellular carcinoma (HCC) is the sixth in prevalence and the second in mortality among malignant neoplasms in the world [1]. Currently, almost 80% of victims are found in Asia, and the global incidence of HCC is increasing steadily [2, 3]. Surgical resection can be applicable in only 20 % of HCC patients [4]. Furthermore, HCC frequently recurs even after apparently curative resection. Liver transplantation, which is the best therapeutic option in some patients because it can be a treatment not only for HCC but also for cirrhosis, plays a limited role by organ donor shortage. Thus, various nonsurgical therapies have developed [3, 5, 6]. Among these, image-guided percutaneous ablation is regarded as best in the treatment of early-stage HCC. It includes ethanol injection [7–9], microwave ablation (MWA) [10], radiofrequency ablation (RFA) [11–13], irreversible electroporation (IRE), and cryoablation. Ablation can be curative, minimally invasive, and easily repeatable for recurrence. Ablation is generally indicated on patients with small HCC, preferably for those with Child-Pugh class A or B liver dysfunction, up to three tumors each 3 cm or smaller in diameter [14, 15].

2. Ethanol Injection

Percutaneous ethanol injection was first described in the early 1980s [7–9] and had long been the standard in ablation. It is a well-tolerated, low-cost, and considerably safe treatment. Survival of patients who underwent ethanol injection has been reported to be 38–60% at 5 years [16–19]. In our study of 685 primary HCC patients on whom we performed 2,147 ethanol injection treatments, with a median follow-up of 51.6

months, survival rates were 49.0%, 17.9%, and 7.2% at 5, 10, and 20 years, respectively [19]. It has been reported that local tumor progression rates after percutaneous ethanol injection were 6–31%, which were significantly related to the size of tumor [16, 18, 20, 21]. There has been a general agreement that percutaneous ethanol injection is a safe procedure, with mortality and morbidity of 0–3.2% and 0–0.4%, respectively [18–20, 22]. Nowadays, ethanol injection is a treatment of choice only in cases in which RFA cannot be feasible because of either enterobiliary reflux, adhesion of the tumor with the gastrointestinal tract, or other reasons [15].

3. RFA

RFA uses high-frequency alternating current to destroy solid tumor tissue. Radiofrequency energy emitted from the exposed tip of the electrode is converted into heat. Heat is conducted considerably homogeneously in all directions; the capsule or septa of the lesion may not be a barrier of the conduction to a great degree. There are three types of electrodes: multitined expandable electrodes, internally cooled ones, and perfusion ones. RFA has recently been the most prevailing ablation technique for HCC [15]. It has been reported that survival at 5 years was 39.9–68.5% [14, 23–27]. In our study of 1,170 primary HCC patients on whom we performed 2,982 RFA treatments, with a median follow-up of 38.2 months, survival rates were 60.2 % and 27.3 % at 5 and 10 years, respectively [14]. It has been reported that local tumor progression rates after RFA were 2.4–27.0% [14, 23–27]. It has been reported that mortality and morbidity of RFA were 0.9–7.9% and 0–1.5%, respectively [14, 23–26]. Various clinical attempts, such as combination of transcatheter arterial chemoembolization followed by RFA [28] and hepatic arterial balloon occlusion during RFA [29], have been conducted to increase the ablation volume by decreasing the cooling effect of the arterial flow. There have also been some studies in which they say that multipolar RFA would be useful to increase the volume of ablation and reduce local tumor progression [30].

4. MWA

In MWA, tumor tissue is destroyed by direct hyperthermic injury produced by electromagnetic wave emitted from the noninsulated portions of the antenna. Microwave coagulation has been used in transaction of the liver to control bleeding from planes during resection. The first-generation MWA for clinical practice was reported in the 1990s [10]. However, its necrotic volume was small. It was prolate spheroid, 1.5 cm in short diameter and 2.5 cm in long diameter. Still worse, antenna shaft became hot from reflected power in the first-generation MWA, which results in development of pleural effusion or skin burn at the insertion site. We shifted from ethanol injection and the first-generation MWA to RFA in Japan [31].

MWA is, however, considered to have physical advantages in comparison with RFA. These advantages include a larger volume of active heating resulting in shorter procedure times, insensitivity to carbonization, higher tissue temperatures beyond the threshold of water vaporization, and less susceptibility to the heat sink effect of blood flow which results in incomplete ablation [32–34]. Thus, new-generation MWA systems incorporating water or gas antenna cooling and high-power generation have been developed and have recently been attracting large attention [35]. New-generation MWA may create a more predictable ablation zone and a larger ablation volume in a shorter time period. However, its clinical data have been insufficient compared with that of RFA. Further studies are mandatory especially in terms of long-term survival [36, 37].

5. IRE

IRE is a non-thermal ablation treatment that delivers short electric pulses to induce cell death due to apoptosis. The basic principle of IRE is to create irreversible pores in cellular bilipid membranes by subjecting them to a series of high voltage (>640 V/cm) and high intensity (>20 A) electrical pulses of short duration (70–100 μsec) [38]. With this method, the skeleton of connective tissue, vessels, and bile ducts are largely preserved [39]. IRE seems to be an attractive alternative option for tumors near the porta hepatis or others in which thermal ablations are risky to be performed [40, 41]. However, IRE is more invasive and troublesome because general anesthesia with muscular blockade is needed. In addition, IRE also produces some degree of thermal effects which can injure bile ducts and other structures. Further studies are mandatory in IRE especially in terms of long-term outcomes.

6. Cryoablation

In contrast to RFA and MWA, cryoablation uses extremely low temperature to kill tumors. Tumor tissue is destroyed by both direct and indirect effects. The direct effect is a result of intra-and extracellular ice crystal formation and solute-solvent shifts, which induce cell dehydration and rupture. The indirect effect resulted from the vascular injury which would result in ischemic hypoxia. Apoptosis and immunomodulation may also play a role in cell injury [42]. Cryoablation has an advantage of its precise monitoring of ablated area during the procedure by various imaging modalities, such as CT, MRI, or ultrasound [43], therefore optimally controlling the treatment effects. A meta-analysis concluded that RFA is superior to cryoablation from the viewpoints of complications, local recurrence of patient, and local recurrence of tumor although there was no significant difference in mortality [44]. However, a randomized controlled trial said that local tumor progression is significantly less frequent in cryoablation than in RFA, although complications, tumor-free survival rates, and overall survival rates were not significantly different between the two techniques [45].

7. Comparison among Percutaneous Ablation Therapies

Six randomized controlled trials have been reported to compare RFA with ethanol injection. Superiority of RFA to ethanol injection, from the viewpoints of treatment response, local tumor curativity, and overall survival, has been found in four of them [13, 46–48], while the other two trials showed that the overall survival was not significantly different between them [49]. Ethanol injection, however, does not need special instruments and is inexpensive [50]. Ethanol injection may be an option in very small HCC.

Regarding the first-generation MWA, a randomized controlled trial to compare it with RFA demonstrated that the number of treatment sessions was smaller in RFA, although there was no statistically significant difference in terms of complete therapeutic effect, major complication, and local tumor progression between them [51]. A cohort study to compare the first-generation MWA with RFA for HCC of up to 2 cm in diameter showed that RFA was more effective than the first-generation MWA, because there was a significant difference in terms of treatment sessions, size of necrotic area, local recurrence rate, cumulative survival rate, adverse events of pain, fever, biliary injury, pleural effusion, and ascites between the two therapies [52].

Regarding new-generation MWA, many studies failed to show that new-generation MWA is superior to RFA from the viewpoint of local control and overall survival. A cohort study to compare it with RFA showed that there was no significant difference in complete therapeutic response, residual foci of untreated disease rate, recurrence rate, or progression-free survival between the two therapies [53]. Another cohort study to compare new-generation MWA with RFA for HCC up to 5 cm in diameter showed that there was no significant difference in complete ablation, local tumor progression, overall survival, or disease-free survival rates [54]. Another study also failed to show that there was a significant difference in terms of complete ablation, local recurrence, major adverse events, disease-free survival, or overall survival rates between the two therapies [55]. Another study to compare the two therapies for HCC within the Milan criteria did not demonstrate that complete ablation, local recurrence, disease-free survival, cumulative survival, or major complication rates were different between them, either [56]. Another comparative study showed that there was no significant difference in complete ablation, complication, de novo lesions, portal vein thrombosis, abdominal lymphadenopathy, and overall survival rates between the two therapies, while local recurrence rates were significantly lower in MWA [57]. Further comparison studies are mandatory between RFA and new-generation MWA, especially in terms of adverse events and long-term survival.

8. Comparison between Percutaneous Ablation Therapies and Surgical Resection

Comparison of ablation with surgical resection is considerably difficult; the indications are somewhat different between the two treatments. Patients of multiple lesions, advanced age, or more deteriorated liver function tend to undergo ablation while those of a large tumor tend to receive surgical resection. Furthermore, both treatments are highly operator-dependent and their indications may be different from institution to institution. Thus, a patient who is decided by medical professionals to undergo ablation or surgical resection at an institution may not be given the same treatment at others.

There have been four randomized controlled trials to compare RFA with surgical resection. Three of them demonstrated that overall survival was not significantly different between the two treatments. A study on patients with a solitary HCC up to 5 cm in diameter showed that overall survival and disease-free survival were not statistically different between the two treatments, but adverse events were more frequent and severe in surgical resection [58]. Another study on patients with nodular diameters of less than 4 cm and one or two nodules showed that there were no significant differences between the two treatments in overall survival and recurrence-free survival [59]. In another trial on patients with HCC up to 3 cm in diameter, there was no significant difference of the disease-free and overall survival between the two treatments, although the postoperative adverse events were significantly more frequent and hospital stay was significantly longer in surgical resection [60]. Only the remaining study on patients within the Milan criteria showed that there was a significant difference in overall survival and recurrence-free survival between the two treatments [61]. There was a randomized controlled trial to compare chemoembolization plus RFA with partial hepatectomy for HCC within the Milan criteria, which said that partial hepatectomy had better overall and recurrence-free survival than the combination of chemoembolization with RFA [61, 62]. However, it does not seem to be widely used to combine chemoembolization with RFA for HCC within the Milan criteria.

Concerning overall survival, some nonrandomized comparative studies reported that RFA had similar outcomes to resection [63–76] while others found that resection had better survival [74, 77–82]. There was a study in which RFA showed a better long-term survival than surgical resection after propensity score analysis [83]. There was another study which reported that, in HCC cases of 2 cm or smaller, major adverse events occurred significantly more often in surgical resection than in RFA and overall survival was better in RFA than in surgical resection [84]. Even in studies in which surgical resection was reported to be superior to RFA, there were no significant differences in overall survival between the two treatments in patients with HCC 2 cm or smaller [80] or 3 cm or smaller in diameter [74, 78, 79]. RFA was associated with less frequent adverse events [71, 79] and shorter hospital stay [71]. From the viewpoint of cost-effectiveness, RFA may be superior to surgical resection [85]. RFA seems to be a satisfactory alternative to resection for HCC up to 3 cm in diameter in Child-Pugh class A or B cirrhosis. Furthermore, RFA may be a first-line treatment in HCC up to 2 cm in diameter in Child-Pugh class A or B cirrhosis.

Most studies reported that recurrence-free survival was better in surgical resection than in RFA, although overall survival was not significantly different between the two treatments. This is probably because surgical resection sacrifices a much larger volume of non-cancerous liver tissue. It may remove some latent metastases and reduce new carcinogenesis, resulting in lower recurrence rates. However, it may lead to liver decompensation in some cases. In addition, most recurrence can be treated curatively by iterative RFA but not

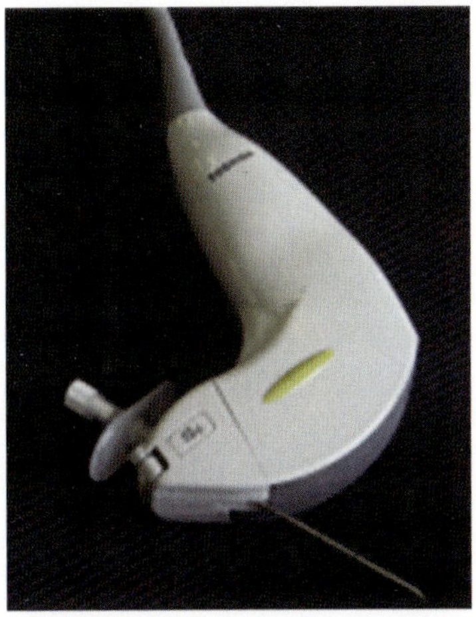

FIGURE 1: We participated in development of a dedicated ultrasonic transducer and have used it in 12,000 procedures of radiofrequency ablation. The dedicated ultrasonic transducer has the following advantages: (1) needle slot is located inside the transducer, (2) a puncture angle of 100 degrees is available in addition to 55, 70, and 85 degrees, (3) the same image is obtained as a regular convex transducer generates, (4) a puncture attachment is unified with the transducer, and (5) it is capable of multimodality fusion imaging.

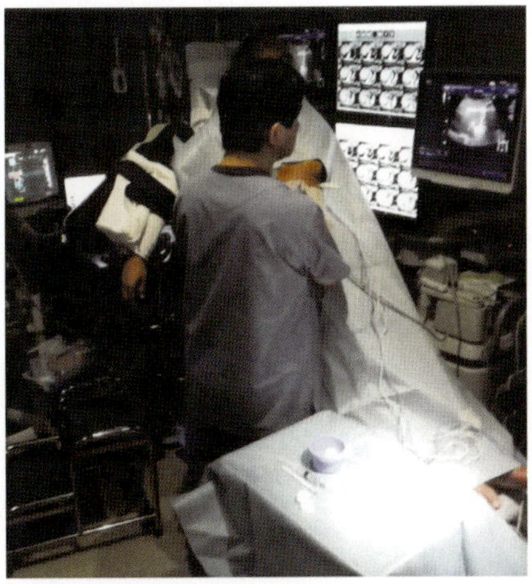

FIGURE 2: We developed a dedicated procedure bed. Using this bed, we can keep a patient in an optimal position, such as right hemilateral decubitus position, left hemilateral decubitus position, head-up position, sitting position, and almost standing position.

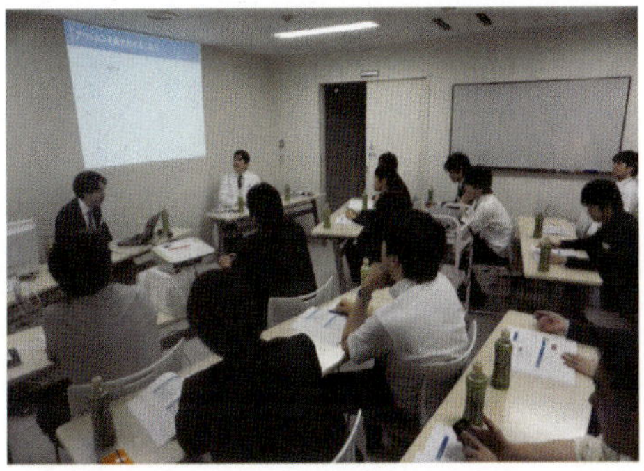

FIGURE 3: Lecture topics are current status of ablation, ablation systems, ultrasound systems, various techniques in ablation, and others.

by repeated surgical resection. In our study, the first recurrence was treated by iterative RFA in 659 (88.9 %) of the 741 patients. In the remaining, transarterial chemoembolization in 69 (9.3 %), systemic chemotherapy in 4 (0.5 %), surgical resection in 3 (0.4 %), radiation therapy in 2 (0.3 %), and supportive care in 4 (0.5 %) were chosen [14]. On the other hand, repeated surgical resection can be an option in only 20-30% of patients with recurrent HCC.

9. Various Innovations and Sophisticated Instruments

We developed a dedicated ultrasound transducer for puncture (PVT-350BTP, Toshiba, Japan) (Figure 1) in corporation with Toshiba. We have performed RFA over 10,000 cases of liver tumors using this dedicated ultrasound probe. Contrast-enhanced ultrasound is useful to detect viable tumor persistence following locoregional treatment (either ablation or chemoembolization). There are cases in which B-mode ultrasound cannot clearly identify a viable portion of the tumor. Using ultrasound contrast agents, vascular imaging shows a hypervascular area which represents the residual cancer tissue. We developed a dedicated procedure bed (Figure 2). Using this bed, we can keep a patient in an optimal position. Multimodality fusion imaging is also useful to detect tumors not clearly identified by ultrasound. It is a system in which fused CT or MR images created from previously acquired imaging data demonstrate the same plane and move synchronously with **real-time** ultrasound images. Various innovations would further improve outcomes in percutaneous ablation.

10. Training Programs

Because ablation appears a simple procedure, it may be done without sufficient training. However, ablation is considerably operator-dependent. Its skills and outcomes differ much from operator to operator. In order to disseminate skills and know-hows, there are some training programs for ablation. For example, our training programs are composed of comprehensive lectures (Figure 3), live demonstrations (Figure 4), and case studies (Figure 5). We have held domestic training programs 10 times, and a total of 170 doctors attended. We also have had international ones 4 times, which were successfully completed with 49 participants in total. Training programs may be effective in providing an excellent opportunity to understand basic concepts and learn cardinal skills for successful ablation.

11. Conclusions

Ablation has been widely performed in the treatment of HCC. Ablation is potentially curative, minimally invasive,

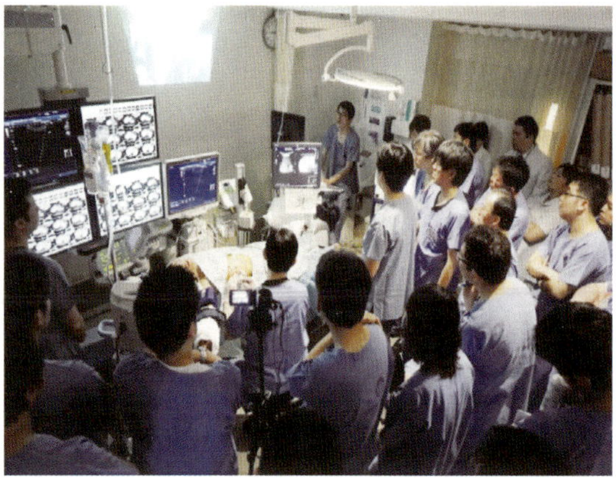

Figure 4: In live demonstrations, we perform ablation on various cases: a case of first diagnosed cancer not difficult to ablate judging from its size and location, a case of a tumor beneath the diaphragm requiring artificial ascites, a case of a tumor in the caudate lobe, a case of a tumor adjacent to the heart, a case of a tumor next to portal vein or hepatic vein at porta hepatis, a case of a tumor over 5 cm in diameter, a case of more than five tumors, cases of hepatic metastasis from the colorectal cancer or the gastric cancer, a case of simple nodular type HCC with extranodular growth or confluent multinodular type HCC, a case of a tumor with unclear boundaries on ultrasound which requires contrast-enhanced ultrasound to perform RFA, a case in which a tumor cannot be detected on ultrasound and requires support of fusion imaging, and others. From these cases, we demonstrate the importance of appropriate patient posture, usefulness of our original dedicated probe for interventional procedures and our RFA dedicated operation table, and the way to carry out ablation under contrast-enhanced ultrasound guidance and with multimodality fusion imaging.

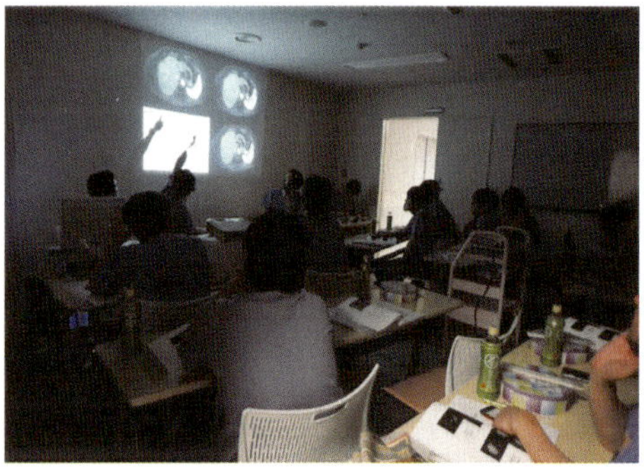

Figure 5: In case studies, difficult to ablate cases from participants' institutions are presented and discussed.

and easily repeatable for recurrence. In RFA, outcomes in over 10-year period clearly show that RFA is a curative treatment and enables long-term survival. There are still arguments regarding whether it is proper to perform ablation on resectable cases or not. The number of patients treated by ablation, however, has been increasing. Various innovations would further improve outcomes in ablation. Training programs may be effective in acquiring necessary skills, knowledge, and experience for successful ablation. Sophisticated ablation would be more than an adequate alternative of surgery for small- and possibly middle-sized HCC.

References

[1] D. Maxwell Parkin, F. Bray, J. Ferlay, and P. Pisani, "Estimating the world cancer burden: Globocan 2000," *International Journal of Cancer*, vol. 94, no. 2, pp. 153–156, 2001.

[2] D. Poon, B. O. Anderson, L.-T. Chen et al., "Management of hepatocellular carcinoma in Asia: consensus statement from the Asian Oncology Summit 2009," *The Lancet Oncology*, vol. 10, no. 11, pp. 1111–1118, 2009.

[3] S. D. Ryder, "Guidelines for the diagnosis and treatment of hepatocellular carcinoma (HCC) in adults," *Gut*, vol. 52, no. 3, pp. iii1–iii8, 2003.

[4] F. Borie, A.-M. Bouvier, A. Herrero et al., "Treatment and prognosis of hepatocellular carcinoma: A population based study in France," *Journal of Surgical Oncology*, vol. 98, no. 7, pp. 505–509, 2008.

[5] J. M. Llovet, A. Burroughs, and J. Bruix, "Hepatocellular carcinoma," *The Lancet*, vol. 362, no. 9399, pp. 1907–1917, 2003.

[6] J. Bruix and M. Sherman, "Management of *Hepatocellular carcinoma*," *Hepatology*, vol. 42, no. 5, pp. 1208–1236, 2005.

[7] N. Sugiura, "Ultrasound image-guided percutaneous intratumor ethanol injection for small hepatocellular carcinoma," *Acta Hepatologica Japonica*, pp. 24–920, 1983 (Japanese).

[8] T. Livraghi, D. Festi, F. Monti, A. Salmi, and C. Vettori, "US-guided percutaneous alcohol injection of small hepatic and abdominal tumors," *Radiology*, vol. 161, no. 2, pp. 309–312, 1986.

[9] S. Shiina, H. Yasuda, H. Muto et al., "Percutaneous ethanol injection in the treatment of liver neoplasms.," *AJR. American journal of roentgenology*, vol. 149, no. 5, pp. 949–952, 1987.

[10] T. Seki, M. Wakabayashi, T. Nakagawa et al., "Ultrasonically guided percutaneous microwave coagulation therapy for small hepatocellular carcinoma," *Cancer*, vol. 74, no. 3, pp. 817–825, 1994.

[11] S. Rossi et al., "Percutaneous radiofrequency interstitial thermal ablation in the treatment of small hepatocellular carcinoma," *Cancer J Sci Am*, vol. 1, no. 1, pp. 73–81, 1995.

[12] T. Livraghi, S. N. Goldberg, S. Lazzaroni, F. Meloni, L. Solbiati, and G. S. Gazelle, "Small hepatocellular carcinoma: treatment with radio-frequency ablation versus ethanol injection," *Radiology*, vol. 210, no. 3, pp. 655–661, 1999.

[13] S. Shiina, T. Teratani, S. Obi et al., "A randomized controlled trial of radiofrequency ablation with ethanol injection for small hepatocellular carcinoma," *Gastroenterology*, vol. 129, no. 1, pp. 122–130, 2005.

[14] S. Shiina, R. Tateishi, T. Arano et al., "Radiofrequency ablation for hepatocellular carcinoma: 10-Year outcome and prognostic factors," *American Journal of Gastroenterology*, vol. 107, no. 4, pp. 569–577, 2012.

[15] M. Omata, A.-L. Cheng, N. Kokudo et al., "Asia–Pacific clinical practice guidelines on the management of hepatocellular carcinoma: a 2017 update," *Hepatology International*, vol. 11, no. 4, pp. 317–370, 2017.

[16] M. Ebara, S. Okabe, K. Kita et al., "Percutaneous ethanol injection for small hepatocellular carcinoma: Therapeutic efficacy based on 20-year observation," *Journal of Hepatology*, vol. 43, no. 3, pp. 458–464, 2005.

[17] S. Shiina, K. Tagawa, Y. Niwa et al., "Percutaneous ethanol injection therapy for hepatocellular carcinoma: Results in 146 patients," *American Journal of Roentgenology*, vol. 160, no. 5, pp. 1023–1028, 1993.

[18] Y. M. Sung et al., "Long-term results of percutaneous ethanol injection for the treatment of hepatocellular carcinoma in Korea," *Korean J Radiol*, vol. 7, no. 3, pp. 187–192, 2006.

[19] S. Shiina, R. Tateishi, M. Imamura et al., "Percutaneous ethanol injection for hepatocellular carcinoma: 20-year outcome and prognostic factors," *Liver International*, vol. 32, no. 9, pp. 1434–1442, 2012.

[20] T. Livraghi, A. Giorgio, G. Marin et al., "Hepatocellular carcinoma and cirrhosis in 746 patients: Long-term results of percutaneous ethanol injection," *Radiology*, vol. 197, no. 1, pp. 101–108, 1995.

[21] H. Ishii, *Local recurrence of hepatocellular carcinoma after percutaneous ethanol injection*, vol. 77, Cancer, 1996.

[22] M. Di Stasi, L. Buscarini, T. Livraghi et al., "Percutaneous ethanol injection in the treatment of hepatocellular carcinoma: A multicenter survey of evaluation practices and complication rates," *Scandinavian Journal of Gastroenterology*, vol. 32, no. 11, pp. 1168–1173, 1997.

[23] R. Lencioni, D. Cioni, L. Crocetti et al., "Early-stage hepatocellular carcinoma in patients with cirrhosis: long-term results of percutaneous image-guided radiofrequency ablation," *Radiology*, vol. 234, no. 3, pp. 961–967, 2005.

[24] R. Tateishi, S. Shiina, T. Teratani et al., "Percutaneous radiofrequency ablation for hepatocellular carcinoma. An analysis of 1000 cases," *Cancer*, vol. 103, no. 6, pp. 1201–1209, 2005.

[25] T. Livraghi, F. Meloni, M. Di Stasi et al., "Sustained complete response and complications rates after radiofrequency ablation of very early hepatocellular carcinoma in cirrhosis: is resection still the treatment of choice?" *Hepatology*, vol. 47, no. 1, pp. 82–89, 2008.

[26] K. Yan, "Radiofrequency ablation of hepatocellular carcinoma: long-term outcome and prognostic factors," *Eur J Radiol*, vol. 67, no. 2, pp. 336–347, 2008.

[27] Y.-S. Kim, H. K. Lim, H. Rhim et al., "Ten-year outcomes of percutaneous radiofrequency ablation as first-line therapy of early hepatocellular carcinoma: analysis of prognostic factors," *Journal of Hepatology*, vol. 58, no. 1, pp. 89–97, 2013.

[28] M. Morimoto, K. Numata, M. Kondou, A. Nozaki, S. Morita, and K. Tanaka, "Midterm outcomes in patients with intermediate-sized hepatocellular carcinoma: A randomized controlled trial for determining the efficacy of radiofrequency ablation combined with transcatheter arterial chemoembolization," *Cancer*, vol. 116, no. 23, pp. 5452–5460, 2010.

[29] M. Kobayashi, K. Ikeda, Y. Kawamura et al., "Randomized controlled trial for the efficacy of hepatic arterial occlusion during radiofrequency ablation for small hepatocellular carcinoma - Direct ablative effects and a long-term outcome," *Liver International*, vol. 27, no. 3, pp. 353–359, 2007.

[30] V. Cartier, J. Boursier, J. Lebigot, F. Oberti, I. Fouchard-Hubert, and C. Aubé, "Radiofrequency ablation of hepatocellular carcinoma: Mono or multipolar?" *Journal of Gastroenterology and Hepatology*, vol. 31, no. 3, pp. 654–660, 2016.

[31] S. Shiina, T. Teratani, S. Obi, K. Hamamura, Y. Koike, and M. Omata, "Nonsurgical treatment of hepatocellular carcinoma: From percutaneous ethanol injection therapy and percutaneous microwave coagulation therapy to radiofrequency ablation," *Oncology*, vol. 62, no. 1, pp. 64–68, 2002.

[32] C. L. Brace, P. F. Laeseke, L. A. Sampson, T. M. Frey, D. W. Van Der Weide, and F. T. Lee Jr., "Microwave ablation with a single small-gauge triaxial antenna: In vivo porcine liver model," *Radiology*, vol. 242, no. 2, pp. 435–440, 2007.

[33] G. D. Dodd III, N. A. Dodd, A. C. Lanctot, and D. A. Glueck, "Effect of variation of portal venous blood flow on radiofrequency and microwave ablations in a blood-perfused bovine liver model," *Radiology*, vol. 267, no. 1, pp. 129–136, 2013.

[34] W. Fan, X. Li, L. Zhang, H. Jiang, and J. Zhang, "Comparison of microwave ablation and multipolar radiofrequency ablation in vivo using two internally cooled probes," *American Journal of Roentgenology*, vol. 198, no. 1, pp. W46–W50, 2012.

[35] M. G. Lubner, C. L. Brace, J. L. Hinshaw, and F. T. Lee Jr., "Microwave tumor ablation: mechanism of action, clinical results, and devices," *Journal of Vascular and Interventional Radiology*, vol. 21, no. 8, pp. S192–S203, 2010.

[36] R. T. Groeschl, C. H. C. Pilgrim, E. M. Hanna et al., "Microwave ablation for hepatic malignancies: A multiinstitutional analysis," *Annals of Surgery*, vol. 259, no. 6, pp. 1195–1200, 2014.

[37] Y. Liu, Y. Zheng, S. Li, B. Li, Y. Zhang, and Y. Yuan, "Percutaneous microwave ablation of larger hepatocellular carcinoma," *Clinical Radiology*, vol. 68, no. 1, pp. 21–26, 2013.

[38] E. W. Lee, C. Chen, V. E. Prieto, S. M. Dry, C. T. Loh, and S. T. Kee, "Advanced hepatic ablation technique for creating complete cell death: Irreversible electroporation," *Radiology*, vol. 255, no. 2, pp. 426–433, 2010.

[39] J. F. Edd, L. Horowitz, R. V. Davalos, L. M. Mir, and B. Rubinsky, "In vivo results of a new focal tissue ablation technique: irreversible electroporation," *IEEE Transactions on Biomedical Engineering*, vol. 53, no. 7, pp. 1409–1415, 2006.

[40] R. Cannon, S. Ellis, D. Hayes, G. Narayanan, and R. C. G. Martin II, "Safety and early efficacy of irreversible electroporation for hepatic tumors in proximity to vital structures," *Journal of Surgical Oncology*, vol. 107, no. 5, pp. 544–549, 2013.

[41] T. P. Kingham, A. M. Karkar, M. I. D'Angelica et al., "Ablation of perivascular hepatic malignant tumors with irreversible electroporation," *Journal of the American College of Surgeons*, vol. 215, no. 3, pp. 379–387, 2012.

[42] N. E. Hoffmann and J. C. Bischof, "The cryobiology of cryosurgical injury," *Urology*, vol. 60, no. 2, pp. 40–49, 2002.

[43] A. Orlacchio, G. Bazzocchi, D. Pastorelli et al., "Percutaneous cryoablation of small hepatocellular carcinoma with US guidance and CT monitoring: Initial experience," *CardioVascular and Interventional Radiology*, vol. 31, no. 3, pp. 587–594, 2008.

[44] Y.-Z. Huang, S.-C. Zhou, H. Zhou, and M. Tong, "Radiofrequency ablation versus cryosurgery ablation for hepatocellular carcinoma: A meta-analysis," *Hepato-Gastroenterology*, vol. 60, no. 125, pp. 1131–1135, 2013.

[45] C. Wang, H. Wang, W. Yang et al., "Multicenter randomized controlled trial of percutaneous cryoablation versus radiofrequency ablation in hepatocellular carcinoma," *Hepatology*, vol. 61, no. 5, pp. 1579–1590, 2015.

[46] R. A. Lencioni, H.-P. Allgaier, D. Cioni et al., "Small hepatocellular carcinoma in cirrhosis: Randomized comparison of radio-frequency thermal ablation versus percutaneous ethanol injection," *Radiology*, vol. 228, no. 1, pp. 235–240, 2003.

[47] S.-M. Lin, C.-J. Lin, C.-C. Lin, C.-W. Hsu, and Y.-C. Chen, "Radiofrequency ablation improves prognosis compared with ethanol injection for hepatocellular carcinoma ≤4 cm," *Gastroenterology*, vol. 127, no. 6, pp. 1714–1723, 2004.

[48] S.-M. Lin, C.-J. Lin, C.-C. Lin, C.-W. Hsu, and Y.-C. Chen, "Randomised controlled trial comparing percutaneous radiofrequency thermal ablation, percutaneous ethanol injection, and percutaneous acetic acid injection to treat hepatocellular carcinoma of 3 cm or less," *Gut*, vol. 54, no. 8, pp. 1151–1156, 2005.

[49] F. Brunello, A. Veltri, P. Carucci et al., "Radiofrequency ablation versus ethanol injection for early hepatocellular carcinoma: A randomized controlled trial," *Scandinavian Journal of Gastroenterology*, vol. 43, no. 6, pp. 727–735, 2008.

[50] A. Giorgio, A. Di Sarno, G. De Stefano et al., "Percutaneous radiofrequency ablation of hepatocellular carcinoma compared to percutaneous ethanol injection in treatment of cirrhotic patients: An Italian randomized controlled trial," *Anticancer Reseach*, vol. 31, no. 6, pp. 2291–2295, 2011.

[51] T. Shibata, Y. Iimuro, Y. Yamamoto et al., "Small hepatocellular carcinoma: Comparison of radio-frequency ablation and percutaneous microwave coagulation therapy," *Radiology*, vol. 223, no. 2, pp. 331–337, 2002.

[52] K. Ohmoto, N. Yoshioka, Y. Tomiyama et al., "Comparison of therapeutic effects between radiofrequency ablation and percutaneous microwave coagulation therapy for small hepatocellular carcinomas," *Journal of Gastroenterology and Hepatology*, vol. 24, no. 2, pp. 223–227, 2009.

[53] T. J. Vogl, P. Farshid, N. N. N. Naguib et al., "Ablation therapy of hepatocellular carcinoma: a comparative study between radiofrequency and microwave ablation," *Abdominal Imaging*, vol. 40, no. 6, pp. 1829–1837, 2015.

[54] L. Zhang, N. Wang, Q. Shen, W. Cheng, and G.-J. Qian, "Therapeutic efficacy of percutaneous radiofrequency ablation versus microwave ablation for hepatocellular carcinoma," *PLoS ONE*, vol. 8, no. 10, Article ID e76119, 2013.

[55] M.-D. Lu, H.-X. Xu, X.-Y. Xie et al., "Percutaneous microwave and radiofrequency ablation for hepatocellular carcinoma: A retrospective comparative study," *Journal of Gastroenterology*, vol. 40, no. 11, pp. 1054–1060, 2005.

[56] J. Ding, X. Jing, J. Liu et al., "Comparison of two different thermal techniques for the treatment of hepatocellular carcinoma," *European Journal of Radiology*, vol. 82, no. 9, pp. 1379–1384, 2013.

[57] A. Abdelaziz, T. Elbaz, H. I. Shousha et al., "Efficacy and survival analysis of percutaneous radiofrequency versus microwave ablation for hepatocellular carcinoma: an egyptian multidisciplinary clinic experience," *Surgical Endoscopy*, vol. 28, no. 12, pp. 3429–3434, 2014.

[58] M. S. Chen et al., "A prospective randomized trial comparing percutaneous local ablative therapy and partial hepatectomy for small hepatocellular carcinoma," *Ann Surg*, vol. 243, no. 3, pp. 321–328, 2006.

[59] K. Feng, J. Yan, X. Li et al., "A randomized controlled trial of radiofrequency ablation and surgical resection in the treatment of small hepatocellular carcinoma," *Journal of Hepatology*, vol. 57, no. 4, pp. 794–802, 2012.

[60] Y. Fang, W. Chen, X. Liang et al., "Comparison of long-term effectiveness and complications of radiofrequency ablation with hepatectomy for small hepatocellular carcinoma," *Journal of Gastroenterology and Hepatology*, vol. 29, no. 1, pp. 193–200, 2014.

[61] J. Huang, Y. Zeng, H. Wu, Z. Chen, and Q. Lu, "A Randomized Trial Comparing Radiofrequency Ablation and Surgical Resection For HCC Conforming to the Milan Criteria," *Annals of Surgery*, vol. 254, no. 5, p. 839, 2011.

[62] H. Liu, Z. G. Wang, S. Y. Fu et al., "Randomized clinical trial of chemoembolization plus radiofrequency ablation versus partial hepatectomy for hepatocellular carcinoma within the Milan criteria," *British Journal of Surgery*, vol. 103, no. 4, pp. 348–356, 2016.

[63] S. N. Hong et al., "Comparing the outcomes of radiofrequency ablation and surgery in patients with a single small hepatocellular carcinoma and well-preserved hepatic function," *J Clin Gastroenterol*, vol. 39, no. 3, pp. 247–252, 2005.

[64] K. Yamagiwa, K. Shiraki, K. Yamakado et al., "Survival rates according to the Cancer of the Liver Italian Program scores of 345 hepatocellular carcinoma patients after multimodality treatments during a 10-year period in a retrospective study," *Journal of Gastroenterology and Hepatology*, vol. 23, no. 3, pp. 482–490, 2008.

[65] K. Yamakado, A. Nakatsuka, H. Takaki et al., "Early-stage hepatocellular carcinoma: Radiofrequency ablation combined with chemoembolization versus hepatectomy," *Radiology*, vol. 247, no. 1, pp. 260–266, 2008.

[66] G.-A. Kim, J. H. Shim, M.-J. Kim et al., "Radiofrequency ablation as an alternative to hepatic resection for single small hepatocellular carcinomas," *British Journal of Surgery*, vol. 103, no. 1, pp. 126–135, 2016.

[67] L. Jiang, L. Yan, T. Wen et al., "Comparison of Outcomes of Hepatic Resection and Radiofrequency Ablation for Hepatocellular Carcinoma Patients with Multifocal Tumors Meeting the Barcelona-Clinic Liver Cancer Stage A Classification," *Journal of the American College of Surgeons*, vol. 221, no. 5, pp. 951–961, 2015.

[68] T. W. Kang, J. M. Kim, H. Rhim et al., "Small hepatocellular carcinoma: Radiofrequency ablation versus nonanatomic resection - Propensity score analyses of long-term outcomes," *Radiology*, vol. 275, no. 3, pp. 908–919, 2015.

[69] H. Yang, J. Lee, D. H. Lee et al., "Small Single-Nodule Hepatocellular Carcinoma: Comparison of Transarterial Chemoembolization, Radiofrequency Ablation, and Hepatic Resection by Using Inverse Probability Weighting," *Radiology*, vol. 271, no. 3, pp. 909–918, 2014.

[70] A. Cucchetti, F. Piscaglia, M. Cescon et al., "An explorative data-analysis to support the choice between hepatic resection and radiofrequency ablation in the treatment of hepatocellular carcinoma," *Digestive and Liver Disease*, vol. 46, no. 3, pp. 257–263, 2014.

[71] Z. Zhou and et al., "Liver resection and radiofrequency ablation of very early hepatocellular carcinoma cases (single nodule <2 cm): a single-center study," *Eur J Gastroenterol Hepatol*, vol. 26, no. 3, pp. 339–344, 2014.

[72] S. Tohme, D. A. Geller, J. S. Cardinal et al., "Radiofrequency ablation compared to resection in early-stage hepatocellular carcinoma," *HPB*, vol. 15, no. 3, pp. 210–217, 2013.

[73] T. Takayama, M. Makuuchi, and K. Hasegawa, "Single HCC smaller than 2 cm: Surgery or ablation? Surgeon's perspective," *Journal of Hepato-Biliary-Pancreatic Sciences*, vol. 17, no. 4, pp. 422–424, 2010.

[74] H. Hung, Y. Chiou, C. Hsia et al., "Survival Rates Are Comparable After Radiofrequency Ablation or Surgery in Patients With Small Hepatocellular Carcinomas," *Clinical Gastroenterology and Hepatology*, vol. 9, no. 1, pp. 79–86, 2011.

[75] R. Santambrogio, E. Opocher, M. Zuin et al., "Surgical resection versus laparoscopic radiofrequency ablation in patients with hepatocellular carcinoma and child-pugh class a liver cirrhosis," *Annals of Surgical Oncology*, vol. 16, no. 12, pp. 3289–3298, 2009.

[76] K.-M. Wong, M.-L. Yeh, S.-C. Chuang et al., "Survival comparison between surgical resection and percutaneous radiofrequency ablation for patients in Barcelona Clinic Liver Cancer early stage hepatocellular carcinoma," *Indian Journal of Gastroenterology*, vol. 32, no. 4, pp. 253–257, 2013.

[77] M. Vivarelli, A. Guglielmi, A. Ruzzenente et al., "Surgical resection versus percutaneous radiofrequency ablation in the treatment of hepatocellular carcinoma on cirrhotic liver," *Annals of Surgery*, vol. 240, no. 1, pp. 102–107, 2004.

[78] A. Guglielmi, A. Ruzzenente, A. Valdegamberi et al., "Radiofrequency ablation versus surgical resection for the treatment of hepatocellular carcinoma in cirrhosis," *Journal of Gastrointestinal Surgery*, vol. 12, no. 1, pp. 192–198, 2008.

[79] I. Gory, M. Fink, S. Bell et al., "Radiofrequency ablation versus resection for the treatment of early stage hepatocellular carcinoma: a multicenter Australian study," *Scandinavian Journal of Gastroenterology*, vol. 50, no. 5, pp. 567–576, 2015.

[80] K. Hasegawa, N. Kokudo, M. Makuuchi et al., "Corrigendum to: "Comparison of resection and ablation for hepatocellular carcinoma: A cohort study based on a Japanese nationwide survey" [J Hepatol 2013;58:724–729]," *Journal of Hepatology*, vol. 59, no. 3, p. 641, 2013.

[81] W. K. Yun, M. S. Choi, D. Choi et al., "Superior long-term outcomes after surgery in child-pugh class a patients with single small hepatocellular carcinoma compared to radiofrequency ablation," *Hepatology International*, vol. 5, no. 2, pp. 722–729, 2011.

[82] J. Desiderio, S. Trastulli, R. Pasquale et al., "Could radiofrequency ablation replace liver resection for small hepatocellular carcinoma in patients with compensated cirrhosis? A 5-year follow-up," *Langenbeck's Archives of Surgery*, vol. 398, no. 1, pp. 55–62, 2013.

[83] Y.-H. Lee, C.-Y. Hsu, C.-W. Chu et al., "Radiofrequency ablation is better than surgical resection in patients with hepatocellular carcinoma within the Milan criteria and preserved liver function: A retrospective study using propensity score analyses," *Journal of Clinical Gastroenterology*, vol. 49, no. 3, pp. 242–249, 2015.

[84] Z.-W. Peng, X.-J. Lin, Y.-J. Zhang et al., "Radiofrequency ablation versus hepatic resection for the treatment of hepatocellular carcinomas 2 cm or smaller: A retrospective comparative study," *Radiology*, vol. 262, no. 3, pp. 1022–1033, 2012.

[85] A. Cucchetti, F. Piscaglia, M. Cescon et al., "Cost-effectiveness of hepatic resection versus percutaneous radiofrequency ablation for early hepatocellular carcinoma," *Journal of Hepatology*, vol. 59, no. 2, pp. 300–307, 2013.

Risk Evaluation of Endoscopic Retrograde Cholangiopancreatography-Related Contrast Media Allergic-Like Reaction: A Single Centre Experience

Félix Trottier-Tellier, Laurence Harvey, and Jean-Daniel Baillargeon

Gastroenterology, Department of Medicine, CHUS, Sherbrooke, QC, Canada

Correspondence should be addressed to Félix Trottier-Tellier; trottife@gmail.com

Academic Editor: Salvatore Oliva

Background and Aims. Few cases of endoscopic retrograde cholangiopancreatography- (ERCP-) related contrast media (CM) adverse reactions have been reported in the current literature. There is a lack of standardisation in practice regarding premedication prophylaxis for at-risk patients undergoing ERCP and there are few data to guide the practitioners. Our goal is to evaluate the risk of CM adverse reaction in a group of patients with a past history of allergic-like reaction to iodine product undergoing ERCP. *Methods.* A retrospective chart review study was performed of patients who underwent ERCP at our single centre from January 2010 to December 2015. *Results.* 2295 ERCPs were performed among 1766 patients. No anaphylactoid or severe adverse reaction occurred. One (0.04%) ERCP-related CM benign reaction was reported in a patient known for penicillin allergy. Among 127 ERCPs performed on patients with a prior adverse reaction to iodine, 121 procedures were done without and 6 with a premedication prophylaxis. In both groups, no ERCP-related CM reaction occurred. *Conclusions.* To our knowledge, we report the largest cohort of iodine allergic patients undergoing ERCP ever published. These results suggest that ERCP-related CM adverse reactions are very rare even among patients at risk for CM reaction.

1. Introduction

A few cases of ERCP-related CM adverse reactions have been reported in large cohort series [1]. The exact incidence rate of ERCP-related CM reaction is unknown but seems very low [2]. Several studies have documented that systemic absorption of CM occurs after ERCP and it has been shown that there is a rise in serum iodine concentration following ERCP, increasing concerns about possible post-ERCP systemic CM adverse reaction [3–7]. The paucity of data concerning post-ERCP CM reaction has lead clinicians to look up to radiologic literature and the risk of intravenous (IV) CM reaction in an attempt to better understand possible post-ERCP CM reaction. Systemic CM adverse reactions after IV CM injection are classified as acute (within 1 hour) or delayed (even after 10 days) [8]. The underlying mechanism is sometime chemotoxic, but the majority of cases are anaphylactoid or pseudoallergic [9]. They are mainly due to the release of histamine from basophils and mast cells which can cause diffuse vasodilation and bronchospasm [8]. CM adverse reactions are mostly mild or moderate, but when rare life-threatening reactions occur, they arise minutes after CM injection. Adverse CM reactions after IV injection are hard to predict but many large scale studies identified risk factors including a prior allergic-like reaction to CM, an allergic diathesis, and asthma [10–12]. Of these, the strongest risk factor identified is a prior allergic-like reaction to CM justifying a premedication prophylaxis before IV CM injection and raising the question: Should we use a prophylaxis for ERCP in patients known for a prior CM reaction?

There is a controversy concerning the prevention of ERCP-related CM reaction. The American Society for Gastrointestinal Endoscopy (ASGE) issued a guideline on the topic of radiographic contrast media used in ERCP and reported that there is no evidence-based standard of practice

Table 1: Definition of CM adverse reaction severity.

Severity	Included reactions
Mild	Limited urticaria or pruritus Limited cutaneous oedema Nasal flushing Conjunctivitis
Moderate	Diffuse urticaria Facial oedema Diffuse cutaneous erythema Bronchospasm without hypoxia
Severe	Anaphylactoid shock Bronchospasm with hypoxia Laryngeal oedema with stridor or hypoxia Diffuse erythema with hypotension Diffuse or facial oedema with dyspnea

for prophylaxis against contrast reactions during performance of ERCP [2]. They conclude that prophylaxis against ERCP-related CM reaction might be considered for high risk patients based on theoretical considerations. Despite the lack of clinical evidence supporting prophylaxis for ERCP-related CM reaction, recent surveys among a small sample ($n = 44$) of American ERCP practitioners show that a majority (82%) use prophylaxis in patients with prior reactions to IV contrast medium [13]. Considering these, there seem to be a gap in current guidelines and confusion among practitioners as to whether we should use premedication prophylaxis for iodine allergic patients undergoing ERCP. To address this question, the goal of our study was to evaluate the risk of ERCP-related CM acute adverse reaction among patients known for iodine allergic-like reactions. Our hypothesis is that these reactions are very rare in this category of patients and may not justify prophylaxis.

2. Methods

This single centre retrospective study was approved by the University of Sherbrooke Research Ethics Board. Two reviewers analysed all the identified medical records for data extraction. All patients who underwent ERCP at our centre from January 2010 to December 2015 were identified for the study. Patients not exposed to iodine containing CM during ERCP were excluded. Collected data for all patients included demographics, reported allergic diathesis, reported iodine allergy, ERCP indication, and severe ERCP-related CM reaction. Severity of CM adverse reaction was defined as described in Table 1 [14]. Since it is our main study group, additional data were collected for patients known for iodine allergy: hospitalisation status, premedication prophylaxis, use of corticosteroid and antihistaminic, type of contrast media used, biliary manipulation during ERCP, post-ERCP duration of observation, and any ERCP-related CM adverse reaction. Patients who received corticosteroid with or without antihistaminic before ERCP were considered to have had premedication prophylaxis.

3. Results

From January 2010 to December 2015, 2295 ERCPs among 1766 patients were included in our study. Study population is described in Table 2. 828 ERCPs were performed in high risk of CM adverse reaction patients including 127 ERCPs among patients with prior adverse reaction to iodine containing product and 701 in patients reporting any other allergic diathesis. Results are described in Table 3. In our total study population, following 2295 ERCPs performed, no anaphylactoid or severe adverse reaction occurred. Only 1 (0.12%) ERCP-related CM moderate reaction was reported in a patient known for penicillin allergy. He had a delayed diffuse pruritic rash 24 hours following ERCP that was attributed to CM reaction after medical evaluation by the attending gastroenterology team and review of possible drug cause by the hospital pharmacist. This rash delayed the patient departure from the hospital but had a favorable response to medical treatment with IV corticosteroid and antihistaminic. 127 ERCPs were performed on 75 iodine allergic patients. Among these 75 high risk patients, prior reactions to CM were 10 (13.3%) severe reactions, 22 (29.3%) rashes, 16 (21.3%) oedema-angioedema reactions, and 27 (36.0%) others or unknown. CM used for ERCPs among iodine allergic patients were mostly low osmolality CM Omnipaque 240 (82.7%). Six (4.7%) ERCPs were done with prior premedication prophylaxis and 121 (95.3%) without. In both groups, no ERCP-related CM reaction occurred.

4. Discussion

As expected our study suggests that ERCP-related CM adverse reaction is very rare even among patients deemed to be at high risk. We found no severe adverse reaction after 2295 ERCPs performed including 127 ERCPs in patients with prior reaction to iodine product and 828 ERCPs in patients with any allergic diathesis. Only one moderate adverse reaction was reported. These results are similar to prior studies showing that ERCP-related CM reactions are very rare. Draganov and Forsmark prospectively studied 601 patients undergoing ERCP including 80 patients with a prior documented reactions to IV CM and 215 with other history of allergic reaction [15]. In their study, no adverse reactions associated with the administration of CM at the time of ERCP were observed in any of the patients. They concluded that prophylactic regimen against CM reaction before ERCP is unnecessary. Similarly, Moreira et al. reported performing ERCP in 16 patients with a previous history of minor reactions to radiological CM. None of them developed adverse reaction during ERCP or one hour after [16]. Catalano and Schwartz reported 25 patients with documented allergy to iodine undergoing ERCP [17]. No patients developed severe adverse reaction following CM injection during ERCP, but one patient known for a prior severe reaction to IV CM developed moderate nausea-vomiting and pruritus following ERCP even though he received premedication prophylaxis in the form of IV corticosteroid. Moreover, in a voluntary survey of more than 10,000 ERCP cases, Bilbao et al. reported no cases of serious adverse reaction to CM but 3 cases of

TABLE 2: Characteristic of study patients.

Characteristics	All patients (N = 1766)	Iodine allergic patients (N = 75)
Endoscopic procedure, no	2295	127
Age (years), mean ± SD	66.2 ± 28.1	69.6 ± 24.3
Gender		
(i) Male, no (%)	1067 (46.5)	46 (36.2)
(ii) Female, no (%)	1228 (53.5)	81 (63.8)
Year of the procedure		
(i) 2010, no (%)	345 (15.0)	-
(ii) 2011, no (%)	338 (14.7)	-
(iii) 2012, no (%)	349 (15.2)	-
(iv) 2013, no (%)	403 (17.6)	-
(v) 2014, no (%)	411 (17.9)	-
(vi) 2015, no (%)	449 (19.6)	-
Allergy		
(i) Yes, no (%)	828 (36.1)	127 (100.0)
(ii) No, no (%)	1467 (63.9)	0 (0.0)
Iodine Allergy		
(i) Yes, no (%)	127 (5.5)	127 (100.0)
(ii) No, no (%)	2168 (94.5)	0 (0.0)
History of severe iodine allergic reaction		
(i) Yes, no (%)	0 (0.0)	17 (13.3)
Prior iodine allergic reaction reported		
(i) Rash, no (%)	-	36 (28.3)
(ii) Oedema-angioedema, no (%)	-	34 (26.7)
(iii) Others-unknown, no (%)	-	57 (44.8)
ERCP indication		
(i) Lithiasis, no (%)	978 (42.6)	40 (31.5)
(ii) Cholangitis, no (%)	442 (19.3)	35 (27.5)
(iii) Main biliary obstructive lesion, no (%)	508 (22.1)	30 (23.6)
(iv) Stent manipulation, no (%)	228 (9.9)	14 (11.0)
(v) Chronic pancreatitis, no (%)	24 (1.0)	0 (0.0)
(vi) Biliary leak, no (%)	26 (1.1)	1 (0.8)
(vii) Other, no (%)	89 (3.9)	7 (5.5)
Hospitalised for ERCP		
(i) Yes, no (%)	-	77 (60.6)
(ii) No, no (%)	-	47 (37.0)
(iii) Unknown, no (%)	-	3 (2.4)

erythema following CM injection during ERCP [1]. These results cannot be considered exact, however, due to the survey nature of the report.

Taken together these results suggest that minor or moderate ERCP-related CM reactions are possible but very rare. None of these studies reported a severe adverse reaction after CM injection during ERCP. The risk of a severe reaction would certainly argue for the use of premedication prophylaxis, and even though such reactions might be possible, we conclude on the basis of available clinical data that they must be exceedingly rare. Such a low risk certainly does not seem to justify premedication prophylaxis.

A cost-effectiveness study regarding CM premedication prophylaxis management strategies for ERCP is not available and will likely never exist since it seems unrealistic to prove any benefit with such rare and mostly benign adverse effect. It would still be valuable to know the costs of prophylaxis related to medication cost, ERCP procedures delays, and prophylaxis side effects as it could add arguments against premedication prophylaxis.

Our study main strength is the large cohort size. It is, to our knowledge, the largest cohort of CM reaction high risk patients undergoing ERCP. A large number of patients is necessary when looking for rare events. As such, we can conclude that among 828 patients with allergic diathesis, no serious adverse CM reaction occurred but 1 moderate CM reaction occurred. Also, among 127 patients with iodine product allergy undergoing ERCP no CM-related adverse

TABLE 3: Study results.

Results	All patients ($N = 1766$)	Iodine allergic patients ($N = 75$)
Endoscopic procedure included, no	2295	127
Post-ERCP anaphylaxis		
(i) Yes, no (%)	0 (0.0)	0 (0.0)
(ii) No, no (%)	2294 (99.9)	127 (100.0)
(iii) Not available, no (%)	1 (0.04)	-
Reported allergic reaction		
(i) Yes, no (%)	1 (0.0004)	0 (0.0)
(ii) No, no (%)	2294 (99.9)	127 (100.0)
Contrast induced adverse reaction		
(i) Rash, pruritus, no (%)	1 (0.0004)	0 (0.0)
(ii) Other, no (%)	0 (0.0)	0 (0.0)
ERCP details		
(i) Cholangiography, no (%)	-	124 (97.6)
(ii) Pancreatography, no (%)	-	66 (51.9)
(iii) Sphincterotomy, no (%)	-	67 (52.7)
(iv) Lithiasis extraction, no (%)	-	49 (38.5)
(v) Stent placement, no (%)	-	61 (48.0)
(vi) Biliary biopsy, no (%)	-	16 (12.6)
(vii) Brush cytology, no (%)	-	10 (7.8)
Contrast media		
(i) Omnipaque 240, no (%)	-	105 (82.7)
(ii) Visipaque 320, no (%)	-	19 (15.0)
(iii) Visipaque 270, no (%)	-	3 (2.4)
Observation period		
(i) 4 hours and less, no (%)	-	47 (37.0)
(ii) 4 to 24 hours, no (%)	-	20 (15.7)
(iii) More than a day, no (%)	-	60 (47.2)

event occurred. These results reinforce the safety of CM injection during ERCP even among high risk patients without premedication prophylaxis.

Our study has many limitations. The retrospective nature of the study made it impossible to have complete data and limited the characterization of allergic diathesis. It is likely that some patients had previous adverse reaction to IV CM contrast although they were not identified as such and it is likely that some were falsely identified as iodine allergic-like patients. Another limit of the study is the limited data on follow-up after ERCP for patients not known for iodine reaction. We chose to focus data collection on iodine allergic-like patients to achieve the study goal as well as possible. In this group, 52.7% had a follow-up time of 24 hours or less (and we presume that this proportion should be the same for the rest of the whole cohort). It is therefore possible that some delayed CM reactions were missed in data collection due to short follow-up time. Nevertheless, most delayed CM reactions are mild self-limited cutaneous reactions, and the vast majority of life-threatening reactions occur within minutes after CM injection. Severe adverse CM reaction would then certainly have not been missed. Finally, any monocentric study offers a limited external validity. Even though a retrospective study has inevitable flaws, it also allowed us to study a very large cohort which makes the strength of our study.

To conclude, our study results suggest that ERCP-related CM adverse reactions are very rare even among patients perceived at high risk for CM reaction. Therefore, we suggest that CM premedication prophylaxis for ERCP should not be given routinely neither in the general population, nor among patients with a past history of CM reaction.

Disclosure

An abstract of the present study has previously been published for the poster session of the Canadian Digestive Disease week 2017 [18].

References

[1] M. K. Bilbao, C. T. Dotter, T. G. Lee, and R. M. Katon, "Complications of endoscopic retrograde cholangiopancreatography (ERCP). A study of 10,000 cases," *Gastroenterology*, vol. 70, no. 3, pp. 314–320, 1976.

[2] D. Mishkin, S. Carpenter, J. Croffie et al., "ASGE technology status evaluation report: radiographic contrast media used in ERCP," *Gastrointestinal Endoscopy*, vol. 62, no. 4, pp. 480–484, 2005.

[3] K. Mann, J. Rendl, R. Busley et al., "Systemic iodine absorption during endoscopic application of radiographic contrast agents for endoscopic retrograde cholangiopancreaticography," *European Journal of Endocrinology*, vol. 130, no. 5, pp. 498–501, 1994.

[4] K. D. Hopper, S. J. Wegert, and S. E. Hallgren, "Renal excretion of endoscopic retrograde cholangiopancreatography injected contrast a common phenomenon," *Investigative Radiology*, vol. 24, no. 5, pp. 394–396, 1989.

[5] S. D. Ladas, T. Rokkas, J. Kaskarelis, J. Hatzioannou, and S. Raptis, "Absorption of iodized contrast media during ERCP," *Gastrointestinal Endoscopy*, vol. 32, no. 5, p. 376, 1986.

[6] M. H. Roszler and W. L. Campbell, "Post-ERCP pancreatitis: Association with urographic visualization during ERCP," *Radiology*, vol. 157, no. 3, pp. 595–598, 1985.

[7] R. A. Sable, W. S. Rosenthal, J. Siegel, R. Ho, and R. H. Jankowski, "Absorption of contrast medium during ERCP," *Digestive Diseases and Sciences*, vol. 28, no. 9, pp. 801–806, 1983.

[8] J.-J. Pan and P. V. Draganov, "Adverse reactions to iodinated contrast media administered at the time of endoscopic retrograde cholangiopancreatography (ERCP)," *Inflammation & Allergy - Drug Targets*, vol. 8, no. 1, pp. 17–20, 2009.

[9] S. K. Morcos and H. S. Thomsen, "Adverse reactions to iodinated contrast media," *European Radiology*, vol. 11, no. 7, pp. 1267–1275, 2001.

[10] M. A. Bettmann, T. Heeren, A. Greenfield, and C. Goudey, "Adverse events with radiographic contrast agents: results of the SCVIR contrast agent registry," *Radiology*, vol. 203, no. 3, pp. 611–620, 1997.

[11] K. J. Mortelé, M.-R. Oliva, S. Ondategui, P. R. Ros, and S. G. Silverman, "Universal use of nonionic iodinated contrast medium for CT: evaluation of safety in a large urban teaching hospital," *American Journal of Roentgenology*, vol. 184, no. 1, pp. 31–34, 2005.

[12] A. F. Kopp, K. J. Mortele, Y. D. Cho, P. Palkowitsch, M. A. Bettmann, and C. D. Claussen, "Prevalence of acute reactions to iopromide: postmarketing surveillance study of 74,717 patients," *Acta Radiologica*, vol. 49, no. 8, pp. 902–911, 2008.

[13] P. V. Draganov, A. L. Suarez, and P. B. Cotton, "Variability in management of ERCP-related contrast media reaction," *Gastrointestinal Endoscopy*, vol. 82, no. 5, pp. 973-974, 2015.

[14] Committee on drugs and contrast media of the american college of radiology, "ACR Manual on Contrast Media Version 10.1," 2015.

[15] P. V. Draganov and C. E. Forsmark, "Prospective evaluation of adverse reactions to iodine-containing contrast media after ERCP," *Gastrointestinal Endoscopy*, vol. 68, no. 6, pp. 1098–1101, 2008.

[16] V. F. Moreira, E. Merono, J. L. Larraona et al., "ERCP and allergic reactions to iodized contrast media," *Gastrointestinal Endoscopy*, vol. 31, no. 4, p. 293, 1985.

[17] M. F. Catalano and E. Schwartz, "Use of iodine-based contrast during ERCP in patients with iodine allergy," *The American Journal of Gastroenterology*, pp. 88–1528, 1993.

[18] F. Trottier-Tellier, L. Harvey, H. Bernard, and J. Baillargeon, *Risk evaluation of endoscopic retrograde cholangiopancreatography related contrast media allergic reaction among patients known for adverse reaction to iodine containing product*, 2018, https://www.cag-acg.org/publications/cag-scientific-publications/2017-cddw-abstracts/abstract-library/abstracts/poster-presentation/a325.html.

32

Bacterial Infection and Predictors of Mortality in Patients with Autoimmune Liver Disease-Associated Acute-On-Chronic Liver Failure

Xuan Zhang,[1] Ping Chen,[2] Hainv Gao,[2] Shaorui Hao,[1] Meifang Yang,[1] Hong Zhao,[1] Jianhua Hu,[1] Weihang Ma,[1] and Lanjuan Li[1]

[1]*State Key Laboratory for Diagnosis and Treatment of Infectious Diseases, Collaborative Innovation Center for Diagnosis and Treatment of Infectious Diseases, The First Affiliated Hospital, College of Medicine, Zhejiang University, Hangzhou 310003, China*
[2]*Infectious disease department, Shulan (Hangzhou) Hospital, Hangzhou, China*

Correspondence should be addressed to Lanjuan Li; ljli@zju.edu.cn

Academic Editor: Yu-Chen Fan

Objective. To date, few studies are available on autoimmune liver disease-associated acute-on-chronic liver failure (ACLF). The aim of this study is to investigate bacterial infection and predictors of mortality in these patients. *Methods.* We retrospectively studied patients with autoimmune liver disease from August 2012 to August 2017. Clinical data of the patients were retrieved for analysis. *Results.* There were 53 ACLF patients and 53 patients without ACLF in this study. The ACLF group had a higher prevalence of complications ($P < 0.05$). The 28-day and 90-day mortality rates were also obviously high in patients with ACLF (38.3% and 74.5%, resp.) ($P < 0.05$). No predictor was significantly associated with 28-day and 90-day transplant-free mortality. In 53ACLF patients, 40 (75.5%) patients showed bacterial infection. ACLF patients with bacterial infection showed high Child-Pugh score, MELD score, CLIF-SOFA score, 28-day mortality, and 90-day mortality ($P > 0.05$). Moreover, C-reactive protein (CRP) using 12.15 mg/L cut-off value proved to be more accurate than procalcitonin in identifying patients with infection. *Conclusions.* Autoimmune liver disease-associated ACLF showed more complications and high mortality. Bacterial infection patients displayed a more severe condition than those without infection. Elevated CRP is an accurate marker for diagnosing bacterial infection in autoimmune liver disease-associated ACLF patients.

1. Introduction

In recent years, acute-on-chronic liver failure (ACLF) as a specific clinical form of liver failure has attracted increasing attention. In fact, ACLF is considered a syndrome that occurs on the background of chronic liver disease, and previously diagnosed cirrhosis is not required, which is characterized by acute hepatic decompensation resulting in liver failure (jaundice and prolongation of the international normalized ratio [INR]) and one or more extrahepatic organ failures that are associated with increased mortality within a period of 28 days and up to three months from onset [1, 2]. Moreover, ACLF can rapidly progress, requiring an urgent need for assessment and referral for liver transplantation [3]. Therefore, recognition and intervention of the predictors of mortality in ACLF patients can prevent or reverse the process and improve the survival rate.

Several patients with ACLF have been recently reported [3–7]. Moreau et al. found that bacterial infection is the trigger of 33% ACLF and is the most commonly identifiable trigger of this syndrome [4]. Some studies considered hepatic encephalopathy, low-serum sodium, and high INR as predictors of poor outcome in ACLF patients [3, 5]. However, few studies about autoimmune liver disease-induced ACLF patients are available to date. Except for the known predictors, possible risk factors have also received less attention. Moreover, bacterial infection in the population is not largely known. The aim of this study is, therefore, to collect data about autoimmune liver disease-associated ACLF patients to investigate bacterial infection and predictors of mortality to reduce the mortality in this population.

2. Materials and Methods

2.1. Study Population and Data Collection. We retrospectively analyzed the data of all patients admitted at the infectious disease wards of the First Affiliated Hospital, College of Medicine, Zhejiang University, China, and diagnosed with autoimmune liver disease-associated ACLF from August 2012 to August 2017. Patients with autoimmune liver disease who satisfied the 13th Asia-Pacific Congress of Clinical Microbiology and Infection (APCCMI) Consensus Guidelines for diagnosis and treatment of liver failure [8], but not diagnostic criteria of the European Association for the Study of the Liver (EASL) [4], were as control group (i.e., no ACLF group). All of the patients in our study had oral care after they admitted to hospital. Patients showing the following were excluded: coinfections with other viruses, including hepatitis A virus, hepatitis B virus, hepatitis C virus, hepatitis D virus, hepatitis E virus, and human immunodeficiency virus; concomitant liver diseases, such as Wilson's disease; coexisting liver cancer or extrahepatic malignancy; usage of hepatotoxic drugs. We used the composite of death or liver transplantation as our endpoint.

The research protocol was reviewed and approved by the Ethics Committee of the First Affiliated Hospital of Zhejiang University. The need for consent was waived because the study was retrospective and data were analyzed anonymously.

The following data were collected from hospital information system and medical documents: age, gender, diabetes, coexisting other autoimmune diseases, steroid exposure, laboratory findings, symptoms, the presence of bacterial infection at admission or during hospitalization, and mortality at 28 and 90 days. The chronic liver failure-sequential organ failure assessment (CLIF-SOFA) score, Child-Pugh score, and model for end-stage liver disease (MELD) score were calculated from the collected data.

2.2. Definitions. Diagnostic criteria of primary biliary cholangitis (PBC), autoimmune hepatitis (AIH), and primary sclerosing cholangitis (PSC) were defined by American Association for the Study of Liver Diseases (AASLD) [9–11]. Diagnosis of AIH-PBC overlap syndrome referenced the standard which was proposed by Chazouillères et al. in 1998 [12].

Diagnostic criteria and grades of ACLF were defined according to EASL definition [4], as follows.

ACLF Grade 1. This group includes 3 subgroups: (1) patients with single kidney failure, (2) patients with single failure of the liver, coagulation, circulation, or respiration who had a serum creatinine level ranging from 1.5 to 1.9 mg/dL and/or mild to moderate hepatic encephalopathy, and (3) patients with single cerebral failure who had a serum creatinine level ranging from 1.5 and 1.9 mg/dL.

ACLF Grade 2. This group includes the patients with 2 organ failures.

ACLF Grade 3. This group includes the patients with 3 organ failures or more.

The patients as control group satisfied the following criteria specified by the 13th APCCMI Consensus Guidelines for diagnosis and treatment of liver failure [8] as follows.

Patients with chronic liver diseases have acute or subacute deterioration of liver function. ACLF usually exhibits the following symptoms: (a) fatigue with gastrointestinal tract symptoms; (b) rapidly deepening jaundice, with total bilirubin 10 times higher than the upper limit of normal or a daily increase $\geq$ 17.1 μmol/L; (c) hemorrhagic tendency with INR $\geq$ 1.5 or prothrombin activity $\leq$ 40% and other causes which have been excluded; (d) progressive reduction in liver size; and (e) hepatic encephalopathy occurrence.

Bacterial infection in parts of the body was defined as follows [13]. Bacterial pneumonia was defined as the association of clinical and radiological signs of lung infection observed in chest radiographs. Spontaneous bacterial peritonitis was diagnosed when ascites culture was positive or polymorphonuclear count was no less than 250 cells/μL in ascites, excluding other inflammations such as pancreatitis, peritoneal carcinosis, tuberculosis, and bloody ascites. Urinary tract infection was diagnosed using bacterial culture positive or urine leukocyte count >15 cells/high power field and >10^6 bacteria/μL. Fever and cellulitis associated with leukocytosis were used to diagnose skin and soft tissue infection. Septicemia was defined as clinical signs of infection and two consecutive blood cultures yielding the same organism, when a blood culture yielding an organism was considered as bacteremia. Patients considered for bacterial infections but without positive culture or evidence of organ involvement were considered as undetermined infection.

2.3. Statistical Analyses. Statistical analysis was performed using SPSS version 18.0 (SPSS, Chicago, IL, USA). Categorical variables were expressed in percentages and frequencies. Continuous variables were expressed as means and standard deviation. Continuous variables were analyzed with independent-sample t-test when they in line with the normal distribution otherwise Mann–Whitney U test was used. The chi-square test was performed to analyze categorical variables. The 90-day mortality prediction was carried out with univariate and multivariate logistic regression. P value < 0.05 was considered statistically significant.

3. Result

3.1. Characteristics of the Study Cohort. During the study period, 53 patients with autoimmune liver disease-associated ACLF who were admitted to the infectious disease ward of our hospital were included in this study. Fifty-three patients were included as control group. The clinical features and laboratory results of the ACLF patients and no ACLF patients are shown in Table 1. From these 53 ACLF patients, 30 patients (56.6%) showed PBC, 21 (39.6%) displayed AIH, 1 (1.9%) had PSC, and one (1.9%) patients had AIH-PBC overlap

Table 1: Comparison of clinical features and laboratory results among the overall study collective.

Characteristics	No ACLF (n = 53)	ACLF (n = 53)	P value	ACLF Infection group (n = 40)	ACLF Noninfection group (n = 13)	P value
Age	56.34 ± 11.64	58.23 ± 11.86	0.410	58.88 ± 13.18	56.23 ± 6.29	0.336
Female	46 (86.8%)	47 (88.7%)	0.767	34 (85.0%)	13 (100%)	0.317
Diabetes mellitus	9 (17.0%)	6 (11.3%)	0.403	5 (12.5%)	1 (7.7%)	0.635
Coexisting other autoimmune diseases	7 (13.2%)	7 (13.2%)	1.000	4 (10.0%)	3 (23.1%)	0.460
Steroid exposure	8 (15.1%)	11 (20.8%)	0.447	7 (17.5%)	4 (30.8%)	0.528
Complications						
Ascites	25 (47.2%)	41 (77.4%)	0.001	32 (80%)	9 (69.2%)	0.710
Gastrointestinal bleeding	3 (5.7%)	12 (14.0%)	0.026	8 (20%)	4 (30.8%)	0.671
Hepatic encephalopathy	2 (3.8%)	29 (54.7%)	≤0.001	21 (52.5%)	8 (61.5%)	0.570
Hepatorenal syndrome	2 (3.8%)	16 (30.2%)	0.001	15 (37.5%)	1 (7.7%)	0.092
Bacterial infection	27 (50.9%)	40 (75.5%)	0.005			
Laboratory data						
Leukocyte counts (×10 * 9/L)	6.32 ± 3.93	10.43 ± 6.40	≤0.001	12.20 ± 6.34	4.97 ± 2.01	≤0.001
Hemoglobin (g/L)	99.06 ± 21.09	89.32 ± 19.51	0.015	86.30 ± 19.91	98.62 ± 15.39	0.047
Platelet (×10 * 9/L)	108.83 ± 65.32	87.25 ± 52.30	0.063	89.70 ± 56.43	79.69 ± 37.68	0.472
CRP (mg/L)	19.25 ± 15.71	25.51 ± 19.05	0.071	30.49 ± 18.83	8.89 ± 5.93	≤0.001
PCT (ng/ml)	0.43 ± 0.44	1.25 ± 1.65	0.007	1.44 ± 1.76	0.33 ± 0.14	0.136
ALT (U/L)	227.06 ± 302.30	258.34 ± 331.79	0.613	177.15 ± 210.97	508.15 ± 492.74	0.034
AST (U/L)	288.42 ± 352.18	310.58 ± 290.45	0.724	270.48 ± 244.16	434.00 ± 387.24	0.172
AKP (U/L)	197.77 ± 105.19	1879.09 ± 104.54	0.361	176.05 ± 100.90	188.46 ± 118.91	0.714
GGT (U/L)	185.15 ± 199.38	143.72 ± 165.20	0.247	161.15 ± 183.58	90.08 ± 67.81	0.045
Total bilirubin (mg/dL)	20.44 ± 8.21	26.68 ± 8.20	0.005	26.16 ± 8.49	21.37 ± 6.21	0.067
Albumin (g/L)	27.53 ± 5.98	26.71 ± 3.30	0.372	26.59 ± 3.61	26.97 ± 2.22	0.723
Creatinine (mg/dL)	0.65 ± 0.19	1.22 ± 0.88	≤0.001	1.39 ± 0.91	0.72 ± 0.56	0.004
Fasting blood glucose (mmol/L)	4.68 ± 1.52	3.99 ± 1.99	0.119	3.80 ± 0.90	4.57 ± 3.74	0.471
Serum sodium (mmol/L)	136.60 ± 5.12	133.81 ± 5.59	0.009	133.03 ± 5.88	136.23 ± 3.79	0.072
INR	1.76 ± 0.29	3.04 ± 1.23	≤0.001	3.33 ± 1.54	2.95 ± 1.11	0.328
Child-Pugh score	9.53 ± 1.19	11.79 ± 1.46	≤0.001	11.06 ± 1.49	10.47 ± 1.85	0.055
MELD score	18.72 ± 3.15	29.60 ± 8.72	≤0.001	29.47 ± 7.06	27.37 ± 5.35	0.109
CLIF-SOFA score	7.43 ± 0.77	10.74 ± 2.22	≤0.001	11.03 ± 2.38	10.23 ± 1.54	0.266
ACLF grade						
Grade 1	42 (79.2%)	6 (11.3%)	0.186	4 (20.0%)	2 (15.4%)	0.678
Grade 2	0	30 (56.6%)	≤0.001	22 (55.0%)	8 (61.5%)	0.003
Grade 3	0	17 (32.1%)	≤0.001	14 (35.0%)	3 (23.1%)	0.008
28-day transplant-free mortality	4 (8.9%)	18 (38.3%)	0.001	15 (39.5%)	3 (33.3%)	0.733
90-day transplant-free mortality	6 (13.3%)	35 (74.5%)	≤0.001	27 (71.1%)	5 (55.6%)	0.618

CRP, C-reactive protein; PCT, procalcitonin; ALT, alanine transaminase; AST, aspartate aminotransferase; AKP, alkaline phosphatase; GGT, gamma glutamyl transpeptidase; INR, international normalized ratio; MELD, model for end-stage liver disease; CLIF-SOFA, chronic liver failure-sequential organ failure assessment.

TABLE 2: Significant univariate and multivariate logistic regression analyses of 28-day transplant-free mortality.

Variable	Univariate			Multivariate		
	OR	95% CI	*P* value	OR	95% CI	*P* value
Gastrointestinal bleeding	5.000	1.225–20.409	0.025	3.406	0.687–16.894	0.134
Hepatic encephalopathy	3.683	1.036–13.100	0.044	2.349	0.461–11.972	0.304
CLIF-SOFA score	1.362	1.023–1.812	0.034	1.093	0.741–1.613	0.653

CLIF-SOFA, chronic liver failure-sequential organ failure assessment.

TABLE 3: Significant univariate and multivariate logistic regression analyses of 90-day transplant-free mortality.

Variable	Univariate			Multivariate		
	OR	95% CI	*P* value	OR	95% CI	*P* value
Hepatic encephalopathy	8.800	2.024–38.253	0.004	36.714	0.085–15810.528	0.244
Leukocyte counts	1.160	1.003–1.342	0.046	1.328	0.962–1.832	0.085
Hemoglobin	0.964	0.930–1.000	0.048	0.912	0.808–1.029	0.135
AST	0.997	0.995–1.000	0.021	0.998	0.992–1.004	0.477
Creatinine	5.426	1.362–21.612	0.016	160.487	0.049–527959.376	0.219
INR	2.935	1.192–7.224	0.019	50.782	0.415–6206.850	0.109
MELD score	1.232	1.070–1.418	0.004	0.664	0.309–1.430	0.295
Child-Pugh score	2.003	1.169–3.430	0.011	0.595	0.114–2.457	0.473
CLIF-SOFA score	2.936	1.532–5.630	0.001	1.578	0.350–7.117	0.553

AST, aspartate aminotransferase; INR, international normalized ratio; MELD, model for end stage liver disease; CLIF-SOFA, chronic liver failure-sequential organ failure assessment.

syndrome. The control group included 26 (49.1%) patients of PBC, 24 (45.3%) patients of AIH, and 3 (5.7%) cases of PSC. Compared to patients without ACLF, the ACLF group had a higher prevalence of complications ($P < 0.05$), such as hepatic encephalopathy (54.7% and 3.8%, $P \leq 0.001$) and bacterial infection (75.5% and 50.9%, $P = 0.005$). The 28-day and 90-day mortality rates were also obviously high in patients with ACLF ($P < 0.05$).

3.2. Risk Factors Associated with 28-Day and 90-Day Mortality. In the study, 6 (11.3%) patients underwent liver transplantation. In the remaining 47 patients, 28-day mortality and 90-day mortality were 38.3% (18) and 74.5% (35), respectively. For the 28-day transplant-free mortality, in univariate analysis, gastrointestinal bleeding ($P = 0.025$), hepatic encephalopathy ($P = 0.044$), and CLIF-SOFA score ($P = 0.034$) were significant factors (Table 2). However, in multivariate analysis, there was no predictor associated with increased mortality. In addition, for the 90-day transplant-free mortality, in univariate analysis, hepatic encephalopathy ($P = 0.004$), leukocyte counts ($P = 0.046$), hemoglobin ($P = 0.048$), aspartate aminotransferase (AST) ($P = 0.021$), serum creatinine ($P = 0.016$), serum sodium ($P = 0.017$), INR ($P = 0.019$), MELD score ($P = 0.004$), Child-Pugh score ($P = 0.011$), and CLIF-SOFA score ($P = 0.001$) were significant factors (Table 3). In multivariate logistic regression analysis, no predictor was significantly associated with 90-day transplant-free mortality (Table 3).

3.3. Clinical Features of Bacterial Infection in Patients with Autoimmune Liver Disease-Associated ACLF. In our study, 40 (75.5%) patients had bacterial infection, and 14 (35.0%) patients were diagnosed with bacterial coinfection in the first 72 h of admission. The demographic and clinical characteristics of ACLF patients with and without bacterial infection are detailed in Table 1.

ACLF patients with bacterial infection showed high Child-Pugh score, MELD score, CLIF-SOFA score, 28- day mortality, and 90-day mortality. Meanwhile, no statistical significance was observed ($P > 0.05$). However, in laboratory findings, bacterial infection patients displayed high leukocyte counts and C-reactive protein (CRP) ($P < 0.05$). High serum levels of serum creatinine and gamma glutamyl transpeptidase (GGT), low levels of hemoglobin, and alanine transaminase (ALT) were also observed in bacterial infection patients ($P < 0.05$) (Table 1).

In 40 ACLF patients with bacterial infection, the most common site of bacterial infection was in the respiratory tract (17, 42.5%), followed by the peritoneum, bloodstream, biliary tract, urinary tract, intestinal tract, skin and soft tissue, and undetermined site with percentage values of 22.5% (9), 7.5% (3), 7.5% (3), 5.0% (2), 5.0% (2), 2.5% (1), and 7.5% (3), respectively. The bacteriological evidence of infection was 7 cases (17.5%). The pathogens that caused bacterial infections were *Escherichia coli* in three cases, two of which produced extended spectrum β lactamase (ESBL); *Klebsiella pneumoniae* in two cases; *Staphylococcus aureus* in two cases, one of which involved methicillin-resistant *S. aureus*; and *Enterococcus faecalis* in one case.

3.4. Comparison of CRP and PCT in ACLF Patients with Bacterial Infection. CRP and PCT levels were obtained in 52 and 37 patients, respectively, among 53 patients. Thirty-seven patients had both biomarkers measured simultaneously.

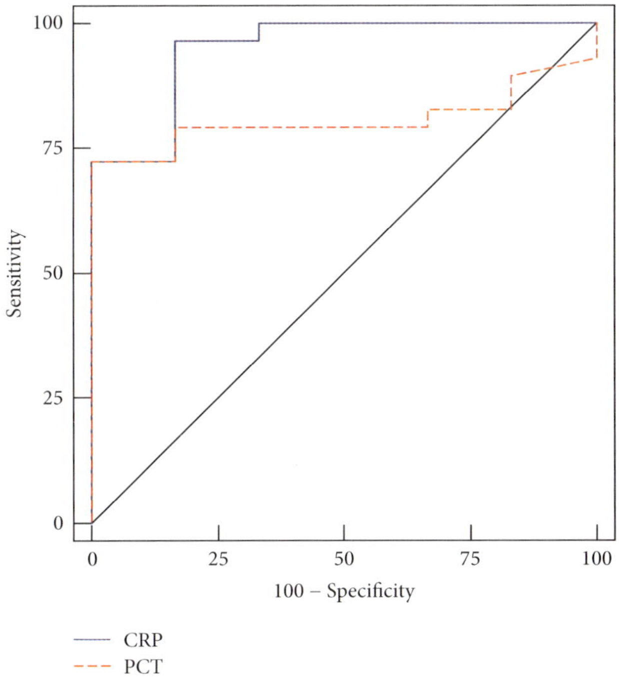

FIGURE 1: Using receiver operating characteristic analysis, comparison of C-reactive protein (CRP) and procalcitonin (PCT) in acute-on-chronic liver failure patients with bacterial infection.

Using receiver operating characteristic analysis, area under curve (AUC) to diagnose bacterial infection was 0.948 (95% confidence interval [CI]: 0–1.000) for CRP ($P = 0.001$) compared with 0.807 (95% CI: 0.668–0.947) for PCT ($P = 0.019$) (Figure 1). For diagnosis of bacterial infection in CRP at a cut-off value of 12.15 mg/L, the sensitivity and specificity were 96.6% and 83.3%, respectively. For diagnosis of bacterial infection in PCT at a cut-off value of 0.57 ng/mL, the sensitivity and specificity were 72.4% and 100% respectively.

4. Discussion

ACLF is a hotspot issues; however, it is lack of uniform diagnostic criteria. Different diagnostic criteria could lead to different patient prognosis. In our study, ACLF patients satisfied the EASL definition, and patients who met APCCMI definition but not EASL definition were included as control group. The 28-day transplantation-free mortality of autoimmune liver disease-associated ACLF was 38.3%, and 90-day transplantation-free mortality was 74.5%. Of note, a great number of critically ill patients were included in the ACLF group; ACLF grades 2 and 3 (56.6% and 36.1%, resp.) were dominant. Moreover, similar to the CANONIC study [4], the ACLF group had a higher prevalence of complications and higher 28-day and 90-day mortality rates.

Several studies were available about predictors of mortality in ACLF patients [5, 14–19]. Yu et al. [14] found that age, etiology, serum sodium, and ascites are independently associated with mortality. Cárdenas et al. [5] considered that the presence of hyponatremia is an independent predictive factor of survival in patients with ACLF. In Mücke's study, infection-triggered ACLF was considered as an independent predictors associated with increased mortality [19]. In our study, no predictor was significantly associated with 28-day and 90-day transplant-free mortality. Small size of study population may cause the situation.

In this study, among the 53 patients with autoimmune liver disease-associated ACLF, 40 (75.5%) patients had bacterial infection. Bacterial infection in liver disease had been reported by previous documents, and the incidence was 24.4%–90% [13, 20–23]. However, study populations were different. Although bacterial infection in ACLF had been studied, autoimmune liver disease-associated ACLF received minimal attention.

In bacterial infection patients with ACLF, Child-Pugh score, MELD score, CLIF-SOFA score, 28-day mortality, and 90-day mortality were high in bacterial infection patients although no statistical significance was observed ($P > 0.05$). ACLF patients with bacterial infection showed a more severe condition than those without infection; this finding was consistent with that of previous study [13].

In recent years, serum CRP and PCT have been suggested for diagnosis and prediction of bacterial infection in chronic liver disease, with or without cirrhosis [13, 24–26]. Papp et al. [25] reported that CRP using a 10 mg/L cut-off value proved to be more accurate than PCT in identifying patients with infection (AUC: 0.93). In this study, we also revealed that CRP levels are more effective than PCT in the diagnosis of bacterial infection in autoimmune liver disease-associated ACLF. The optimal cut-off value of CRP for bacterial infection diagnosis is 12.15 mg/L (96.6% sensitivity and 83.3% specificity), with an AUC of 0.948, which is similar to previous report [25].

Several limitations were observed in this study. First, this work was a retrospective study at a single center. Some data collections were limited, and bacterial infection might be affected by specific circumstance of our institution. Second, some patients had been treated by antibacterial agents before admission, which might affect the accuracy of bacterial infection rate. Third, immunosuppressor except corticosteroid was not used in our study population. Thus, further studies are needed to investigate bacterial infection and predictors of mortality in autoimmune liver disease-associated ACLF patients using immunosuppressor.

5. Conclusions

In conclusion, autoimmune liver disease-associated ACLF displayed high mortality and had more complications. ACLF patients with bacterial infection showed a more severe condition than those without infection. CRP levels higher than 12.15 mg/L suggested bacterial infection in autoimmune liver disease-associated ACLF patients. No predictor was significantly associated with 28-day and 90-day transplant-free mortality. Further prospective and intervention studies on bacterial infection and predictors of mortality in autoimmune liver disease-associated ACLF patients with large sample numbers are thus needed.

Abbreviations

ACLF: Acute-on-chronic liver failure
PBC: Primary biliary cholangitis
AIH: Autoimmune hepatitis
PSC: Primary sclerosing cholangitis
CLIF-SOFA: Chronic liver failure-sequential organ failure assessment
APPCCMI: Asia-Pacific Congress of Clinical Microbiology and Infection
EASL: European Association for the Study of the Liver
CRP: C-reactive protein
PCT: Procalcitonin
GGT: Gamma glutamyl transpeptidase
ALT: Alanine transaminase
INR: International normalized ratio
MELD: End-stage liver disease
AUC: Area under curve
CI: Confidence interval.

Authors' Contributions

Xuan Zhang and Ping Chen contribute equally to the study.

Acknowledgments

This work was supported by the National Science and Technology Major Project (2017ZX10204401002002) and the Zhejiang Provincial Natural Science Foundation (LQ15H030004).

References

[1] R. Jalan, P. Gines, J. C. Olson et al., "Acute-on chronic liver failure," *Journal of Hepatology*, vol. 57, no. 6, pp. 1336–1348, 2012.

[2] R. Jalan, C. Yurdaydin, J. S. Bajaj et al., "Toward an improved definition of acute-on-chronic liver failure," *Gastroenterology*, vol. 147, no. 1, pp. 4–10, 2014.

[3] H. Garg, A. Kumar, V. Garg, P. Sharma, B. C. Sharma, and S. K. Sarin, "Clinical profile and predictors of mortality in patients of acute-on-chronic liver failure," *Digestive and Liver Disease*, vol. 44, no. 2, pp. 166–171, 2012.

[4] R. Moreau, R. Jalan, P. Gines et al., "Acute-on-chronic liver failure is a distinct syndrome that develops in patients with acute decompensation of cirrhosis," *Gastroenterology*, vol. 144, no. 7, pp. 1426.e9–1437.e9, 2013.

[5] A. Cárdenas, E. Solà, E. Rodríguez et al., "Hyponatremia influences the outcome of patients with acute-on-chronic liver failure: an analysis of the CANONIC study," *Critical Care (London, England)*, vol. 18, no. 6, p. 700, 2014.

[6] R. Jalan, F. Saliba, M. Pavesi et al., "Development and validation of a prognostic score to predict mortality in patients with acute-on-chronic liver failure," *Journal of Hepatology*, vol. 61, no. 5, pp. 1038–1047, 2014.

[7] Y. Shi, M. Zheng, and Y. Yang, "Increased delayed mortality in patients with acute-on-chronic liver failure who have prior decompensation," *Journal of Gastroenterology Hepatology*, vol. 30, no. 4, pp. 712–718, 2015.

[8] L.-J. Li, "13th Asia-Pacific congress of clinical microbiology and infection consensus guidelines for diagnosis and treatment of liver failure," *Hepatobiliary & Pancreatic Diseases International*, vol. 12, no. 4, pp. 346–354, 2013.

[9] E. J. Heathcote, "Management of primary biliary cirrhosis. The American Association for the Study of Liver Diseases practice guidelines," *Hepatology*, vol. 31, no. 4, pp. 1005–1013, 2000.

[10] M. P. Manns, A. J. Czaja, J. D. Gorham et al., "Diagnosis and management of autoimmune hepatitis," *Hepatology*, vol. 51, no. 6, pp. 2193–2213, 2010.

[11] R. Chapman, J. Fevery, A. Kalloo et al., "Diagnosis and management of primary sclerosing cholangitis," *Hepatology*, vol. 51, no. 2, pp. 660–678, 2010.

[12] O. Chazouillères, D. Wendum, L. Serfaty, S. Montembault, O. Rosmorduc, and R. Poupon, "Primary biliary cirrhosis-autoimmune hepatitis overlap syndrome: clinical features and response to therapy," *Hepatology*, vol. 28, no. 2, pp. 296–301, 1998.

[13] J. K. Park, C. H. Lee, I. H. Kim et al., "Clinical characteristics and prognostic impact of bacterial infection in hospitalized patients with alcoholic liver disease," *Journal of Korean Medical Science*, vol. 30, no. 5, pp. 598–605, 2015.

[14] J.-W. Yu, G.-Q. Wang, and S.-C. Li, "Prediction of the prognosis in patients with acute-on-chronic hepatitis using the MELD scoring system," *Journal of Gastroenterology and Hepatology*, vol. 21, no. 10, pp. 1519–1524, 2006.

[15] S. Alam, B. Lal, V. Sood, and et al., "Pediatric Acute-on-chronic Liver Failure in a Specialized Liver Unit: Prevalence, Profile, Outcome and Predictive Factors," *Journal of Pediatric Gastroenterology & Nutrition*, vol. 63, no. 4, pp. 400–405, 2016.

[16] C. Dominguez, E. Romero, J. Graciano, J. L. Fernandez, and L. Viola, "Prevalence and risk factors of acute-on-chronic liver failure in a single center from Argentina," *World Journal of Hepatology*, vol. 8, no. 34, pp. 1529–1534, 2016.

[17] T. Bruns, R. Nuraldeen, M. Mai et al., "Low serum transferrin correlates with acute-on-chronic organ failure and indicates short-term mortality in decompensated cirrhosis," *Liver International*, vol. 37, no. 2, pp. 232–241, 2017.

[18] K. A. Wlodzimirow, S. Eslami, A. Abu-Hanna, M. Nieuwoudt, and R. A. F. M. Chamuleau, "A systematic review on prognostic indicators of acute on chronic liver failure and their predictive value for mortality," *Liver International*, vol. 33, no. 1, pp. 40–52, 2013.

[19] M. M. Mücke, T. Rumyantseva, V. T. Mücke et al., "Bacterial infection-triggered acute-on-chronic liver failure is associated with increased mortality," *Liver International*, 2017.

[20] N. Rolando, F. Harvey, J. Brahm et al., "Prospective study of bacterial infection in acute liver failure: An analysis of fifty patients," *Hepatology*, vol. 11, no. 1, pp. 49–53, 1990.

[21] N. Rolando, J. Philpott-Howard, and R. Williams, "Bacterial and fungal infection in acute liver failure," *Seminars in Liver Disease*, vol. 16, no. 4, pp. 389–402, 1996.

[22] A. D. Zider, R. Zopey, R. Garg, X. Wang, T. S. Wang, and J. C. Deng, "Prognostic significance of infections in critically ill adult patients with acute liver injury: a retrospective cohort study," *Liver International*, vol. 36, no. 8, pp. 1143–1150, 2016.

[23] R. Moreau and V. Arroyo, "Acute-on-Chronic Liver Failure: A New Clinical Entity," *Clinical Gastroenterology and Hepatology*, vol. 13, no. 5, pp. 836–841, 2015.

[24] A. Tsiakalos, A. Karatzaferis, P. Ziakas, and G. Hatzis, "Acute-phase proteins as indicators of bacterial infection in patients with cirrhosis," *Liver International*, vol. 29, no. 10, pp. 1538–1542, 2009.

[25] M. Papp, Z. Vitalis, I. Altorjay et al., "Acute phase proteins in the diagnosis and prediction of cirrhosis associated bacterial infections," *Liver International*, vol. 32, no. 4, pp. 603–611, 2012.

[26] C. Lazzarotto, M. F. Ronsoni, L. Fayad et al., "Acute phase proteins for the diagnosis of bacterial infection and prediction of mortality in acute complications of cirrhosis.," *Annals of Hepatology*, vol. 12, no. 4, pp. 599–607, 2013.

Permissions

All chapters in this book were first published in CJGH, by Hindawi Publishing Corporation; hereby published with permission under the Creative Commons Attribution License or equivalent. Every chapter published in this book has been scrutinized by our experts. Their significance has been extensively debated. The topics covered herein carry significant findings which will fuel the growth of the discipline. They may even be implemented as practical applications or may be referred to as a beginning point for another development.

The contributors of this book come from diverse backgrounds, making this book a truly international effort. This book will bring forth new frontiers with its revolutionizing research information and detailed analysis of the nascent developments around the world.

We would like to thank all the contributing authors for lending their expertise to make the book truly unique. They have played a crucial role in the development of this book. Without their invaluable contributions this book wouldn't have been possible. They have made vital efforts to compile up to date information on the varied aspects of this subject to make this book a valuable addition to the collection of many professionals and students.

This book was conceptualized with the vision of imparting up-to-date information and advanced data in this field. To ensure the same, a matchless editorial board was set up. Every individual on the board went through rigorous rounds of assessment to prove their worth. After which they invested a large part of their time researching and compiling the most relevant data for our readers.

The editorial board has been involved in producing this book since its inception. They have spent rigorous hours researching and exploring the diverse topics which have resulted in the successful publishing of this book. They have passed on their knowledge of decades through this book. To expedite this challenging task, the publisher supported the team at every step. A small team of assistant editors was also appointed to further simplify the editing procedure and attain best results for the readers.

Apart from the editorial board, the designing team has also invested a significant amount of their time in understanding the subject and creating the most relevant covers. They scrutinized every image to scout for the most suitable representation of the subject and create an appropriate cover for the book.

The publishing team has been an ardent support to the editorial, designing and production team. Their endless efforts to recruit the best for this project, has resulted in the accomplishment of this book. They are a veteran in the field of academics and their pool of knowledge is as vast as their experience in printing. Their expertise and guidance has proved useful at every step. Their uncompromising quality standards have made this book an exceptional effort. Their encouragement from time to time has been an inspiration for everyone.

The publisher and the editorial board hope that this book will prove to be a valuable piece of knowledge for researchers, students, practitioners and scholars across the globe.

List of Contributors

Lachlan R. Ayres
Poole Hospital NHS Foundation Trust, Poole, UK

Elizabeth K. Kmiotek
Jagiellonian University Medical College, Krakow, Poland

Eric Lam and Jennifer J. Telford
Division of Gastroenterology, St. Paul's Hospital, University of British Columbia, Vancouver, BC, Canada

Zhang Hao, Yang Ling and Zeng Wenting
Department of Infectious Diseases,The First Affiliated Hospital of Guangzhou Medical University, Guangzhou Medical University, Yanjiang Road 151, Guangzhou 510120, China

Zhu Biqing
Guangzhou Kingmed Center for Clinical Laboratory Co., Ltd., Guangzhou International Biological Island, Spiral Three Road 10, Guangzhou 510330, China

Fátima Higuera-de-la-Tijera, Francisco Salas-Gordillo, José L. Pérez-Hernández and Juan M. Abdo-Francis
Gastroenterology and Hepatology Department, Mexico's General Hospital, Mexico City 06726, Mexico

Alfredo I. Servín-Caamaño and Jaime Camacho-Aguilera
Internal Medicine Department, Mexico's General Hospital, Mexico City 06726,Mexico

Sai N. Alla and Fiacro Jiménez-Ponce
Research Department, Chief of the Medical Direction of "Instituto de Seguridad y Servicios Sociales de los Trabajadores del Estado" (ISSSTE), Mexico City 14050, Mexico
Cognitive Science A.C., Mexico City 10700,Mexico

Peter C. Church
Division of Gastroenterology, Hepatology and Nutrition, The Hospital for Sick Children, Department of Paediatrics, University of Toronto, Toronto, Canada

Anne M. Griffiths
Division of Gastroenterology, Hepatology and Nutrition, The Hospital for Sick Children, Department of Paediatrics, University of Toronto, Toronto, Canada
Sick Kids Inflammatory Bowel Disease Centre, The Hospital for Sick Children, Toronto, Canada

Jeffrey Hyams
Division of Digestive Diseases, Hepatology, and Nutrition, Connecticut Children's Medical Center, Hartford, CT, USA
University of Connecticut School of Medicine, Farmington, CT, USA

Frank Ruemmele
Université Sorbonne Paris Citę Université Paris Descartes and Assistance Publique-Hôpitaux de Paris Hôpital Necker-Enfants malades, Service de Gastroentérologie Pédiatrique, Paris, France

Lissy de Ridder
Department of Pediatric Gastroenterology,The Erasmus MC Sophia Children's Hospital, Rotterdam, Netherlands

Dan Turner
The Juliet Keidan Institute of Pediatric Gastroenterology and Nutrition, Shaare Zedek Medical Center, The Hebrew University of Jerusalem, Jerusalem, Israel

Chunqing Zhang
Department of Gastroenterology, Shandong Provincial Hospital Affiliated t o Shandong University, Jinan, China

Xiaolong Qi
Department of Gastroenterology, Shandong Provincial Hospital Affiliated to Shandong University, Jinan, China
CHESS, Hepatic Hemodynamic Lab, Institute of Hepatology, Nanfang Hospital, Southern Medical University Guangdong Provincial Research Center for Liver Fibrosis, Guangzhou, China

Tongwei Wu and Deke Jiang
CHESS, Hepatic Hemodynamic Lab, Institute of Hepatology, Nanfang Hospital, Southern Medical University Guangdong Provincial Research Center for Liver Fibrosis, Guangzhou, China

Min An
The Second School of Clinical Medicine, Southern Medical University, Guangzhou, China

Mengyun Peng and Jing Wang
Department of Hepatobiliary Disease,The Affiliated (T.C.M) Hospital of Southwest Medical University, Luzhou, China

Weidong Wang
Department of Hepatobiliary Surgery, Shunde Hospital, Southern Medical University, Foshan, China

Barry J. Hall
Leeds Gastroenterology Institute, St. James's University Hospital, Leeds, UK

P. John Hamlin, David J. Gracie and Alexander C. Ford
Leeds Gastroenterology Institute, St. James's University Hospital, Leeds, UK
Leeds Institute of Biomedical and Clinical Sciences, University of Leeds, Leeds, UK

Jorge Maldonado-Hernández, Gabriela E. Saldaña-Dávila, Mónica I. Piña-Aguero, Benjamín A. Núñez-García and Mardia G. López-Alarcón
Laboratorio de Espectrometría de Masas, Unidad de Investigaci´on Médica en Nutrición, Hospital de Pediatría, Centro Médico Nacional Siglo XXI, IMSS, Ciudad de México, Mexico

Laura E. Dowsett, Stephanie Coward, Gail MacKean and Fiona Clement
The Department Community Health Sciences, Teaching, Research andWellness Building, 3280 Hospital Drive NW, Calgary, AB, Canada T2N 4N1
O'Brien Institute for Public Health, Teaching, Research andWellness Building, 3280 Hospital Drive NW, Calgary, AB, Canada T2N 4N1

Diane L. Lorenzetti
The Department Community Health Sciences, Teaching, Research andWellness Building, 3280 Hospital Drive NW, Calgary, AB, Canada T2N 4N1
O'Brien Institute for Public Health, Teaching, Research andWellness Building, 3280 Hospital Drive NW, Calgary, AB, Canada T2N 4N1
Institute of Health Economics, 1200, 10405 Jasper Avenue, Edmonton, AB, Canada T5J 3N4

Marta Flisiak-Jackiewicz, Anna Bobrus-Chociej and Dariusz Marek Lebensztejn
Department of Pediatrics, Gastroenterology and Allergology, Medical University of Białystok, Białystok, Poland

Eugeniusz Tarasów
Department of Radiology, Medical University of Białystok, Białystok, Poland

MaBgorzata Wojtkowska
Department of Radiology, University Children Hospital, Białystok, Poland

Irena BiaBokoz-Kalinowska
Łom˙za State University of Applied Sciences, Łom˙za, Poland

Hikmet Akkiz, Sedef Kuran, Ümit KaraoLullarJndan, Oguz Üsküdar, Salih Tokmak, Burcu Arslan, Figen Doran, Hüseyin Tugsan Balli, Abdulalh Ülkü, Tolga AtJlgan Akçam, and AnJl Delik,
Çukurova University Gastroenterology Department, Adana, Turkey

Brian I. Carr
Izmir Biomedicine and Genome Institute, Dokuz Eyl¨ul University, ˙Izmir, Turkey

Halil Ebrahim Bahçeci
Fırat University, Turkey

Kamil YalçJn Polat
˙Istanbul Memorial Hospital, Turkey

Necati Örmeci
Ankara University, Turkey

Halis FimGek
Hacettepe University, Turkey

Abdullah Sonsuz
Istanbul Cerrahpaşa University, Turkey

Ali Demir
Konya Necmettin Erbakan University, Turkey

Engin AltıntaG
Mersin University, Turkey

Mehmet Demir
Hatay Mustafa Kemal University, Turkey

Kendal Yalçın and Nazım Ekinci
Dicle University, Turkey

Ayşegül Harmancı Özakyol
Eskişehir Osmangazi University, Turkey

Mehmet Yücesoy
Erciyes University, Turkey

Ahmet Uygun
Haydarpaşa Sultan Abd¨ulhamid E˘gitim Araştırma Hospital, Turkey

Vito Guerra
Trials Centre, National Institute for Digestive Diseases, IRCCS "Saverio de Bellis", Castellana, Bari, Italy

Yaman Tokat
Florence Nightingale Hospital, ˙Istanbul, Turkey

Sezai Yilmaz
Inonu University, Malatya, Turkey

Ahmet BektaG
Ondokuz Mayıs University, Turkey

Murat KJlJç
Izmir Kent Hospital, Turkey

Saranya Kittanakom
Department of Pathology and Molecular Medicine, McMaster University, Hamilton, ON, Canada L8S 4K1
Pathology and Laboratory Medicine, Schulich School of Medicine and Dentistry,Western University, London, ON, Canada

Md. Sharif Shajib
Department of Pathology and Molecular Medicine, McMaster University, Hamilton, ON, Canada L8S 4K1
Farncombe Family Digestive Health Research Institute, Hamilton, ON, Canada

Waliul I. Khan
Department of Pathology and Molecular Medicine, McMaster University, Hamilton, ON, Canada L8S 4K1
Farncombe Family Digestive Health Research Institute, Hamilton, ON, Canada
Hamilton Regional Laboratory Medicine Program, Hamilton Health Sciences, Hamilton, ON, Canada

V. Tony Chetty and Joseph Macri
Department of Pathology and Molecular Medicine, McMaster University, Hamilton, ON, Canada L8S 4K1
Hamilton Regional Laboratory Medicine Program, Hamilton Health Sciences, Hamilton, ON, Canada

Robert Issenman
Farncombe Family Digestive Health Research Institute, Hamilton, ON, Canada
Division of Pediatric Gastroenterology, McMaster University, Hamilton, ON, Canada

Kristine Garvie, Joceline Turner and Dan Brooks
Hamilton Regional Laboratory Medicine Program, Hamilton Health Sciences, Hamilton, ON, Canada

Sufian Odeh
Division of Pediatric Gastroenterology, McMaster University, Hamilton, ON, Canada

Hideki Kamada, Hideki Kobara, Naohito Uchida, Kiyohito Kato, Takayuki Fujimori Kiyoyuki Kobayashi, Takuma Yamashita, Masahiro Ono, Yuichi Aritomo, Kunihiko Tsutsui and Tsutomu Masaki
Department of Gastroenterology and Neurology, Faculty of Medicine, Kagawa University, Kagawa, Japan

Keiichi Okano and Yasuyuki Suzuki,
Department of Gastroenterological Surgery, Faculty of Medicine, Kagawa University, Kagawa, Japan

Junya Sato, Kazunari Nakahara, Ryo Morita, Nozomi Morita, Keigo Suetani, Yosuke Michikawa and Fumio Itoh
Department of Gastroenterology and Hepatology, St. Marianna University School of Medicine, 2-16-1 Sugao, Miyamae-ku, Kawasaki 216-8511, Japan

Shinjiro Kobayashi
Department of Gastroenterological and General Surgery, St. Marianna University School of Medicine, 2-16-1 Sugao, Miyamae-ku, Kawasaki 216-8511, Japan

Masanori Sato, Koji Miyanishi, Shingo Tanaka, Akira Sakurada, Hiroki Sakamoto, Yutaka Kawano, Kohichi Takada and Junji Kato
Department of Medical Oncology, Sapporo Medical University School of Medicine, South-1, West-16, Chuo-Ku, Sapporo 060-8543, Japan

Masayoshi Kobune
Department of Medical Hematology, Sapporo Medical University School of Medicine, South-1, West-16, Chuo-Ku,Sapporo 060-8543, Japan

Yi Shen, Ruoting Men, Tinghong Ye and Li Yang
Department of Gastroenterology and Hepatology,West China Hospital, Sichuan University, Chengdu, Sichuan 610041, China

Changli Lu and Jianping Liu
Department of Pathology,West China Hospital, Sichuan University, Chengdu, Sichuan 610041, China

Chunyan Wu, Ying Zhu and Mengqian Yu The First Affiliated Hospital of Dalian Medical University, Dalian 116011, China

Tracy Davyduke
Alberta Health Services, 8440 112 Street, Edmonton, AB, Canada T6G 2B7

Michelle Carbonneau
Alberta Health Services, 8440 112 Street, Edmonton, AB, Canada T6G 2B7
Cirrhosis Care Clinic, 8540 112 Street, Zeidler Ledcor Centre, Edmonton, AB, Canada T6G 2X8

Puneeta Tandon
Cirrhosis Care Clinic, 8540 112 Street, Zeidler Ledcor Centre, Edmonton, AB, Canada T6G 2X8
University of Alberta, Faculty of Medicine, 2J2.00Walter C Mackenzie Health Sciences Centre, 8440 112 St.,Edmonton, AB, Canada T6G 2R7

Jude Spiers
University of Alberta, Faculty of Nursing, 3-141 Edmonton Clinic Health Academy (ECHA) 11405 87 Avenue,Edmonton, AB, Canada T6G 1C9

Kathleen Ismond
University of Alberta, Faculty of Medicine, 2J2.00Walter C Mackenzie Health Sciences Centre, 8440 112 St.,Edmonton, AB, Canada T6G 2R7

Amanda Brisebois
University of Alberta, Faculty of Medicine, 2J2.00Walter C Mackenzie Health Sciences Centre, 8440 112 St.,Edmonton, AB, Canada T6G 2R7
University of Alberta, Department of Oncology, Division of Palliative Care, 2J2.00Walter C Mackenzie Health Sciences Centre, 8440 112 St., Edmonton, AB, Canada T6G 2R7

Kianoosh Dadashzadeh
Department of Medical Laboratory Sciences, Marand Branch, Islamic Azad University, Marand, Iran

Maikel P. Peppelenbosch and Akyala Ishaku Adamu
Erasmus MC Cancer Institute, Erasmus University Rotterdam, Rotterdam, Netherlands

Mohammad Golriz, Maryam Ashra i, Elias Khajeh, Ali Majlesara and Arianeb Mehrabi
Department of General, Visceral, and Transplantation Surgery, University of Heidelberg, Heidelberg, Germany

Christa Flechtenmacher
Department of General Pathology, University of Heidelberg, Heidelberg, Germany

Jersey Heitor da S.Maués
Human Cytogenetics Laboratory, Institute of Biological Sciences, Federal University of Pará, Belém, Brazil

Helem Ferreira Ribeiro
Human Cytogenetics Laboratory, Institute of Biological Sciences, Federal University of Pará, Belém, Brazil
Center of Biological and Health Sciences, Department of Biomedicine, University of Amazon, Beléem, Brazil

Giovanny R. Pinto and Luana de Oliveira Lopes
Department of Biomedicine, Federal University of Piauí, Parnaíba, Brazil

Let-cia M. Lamarão
Laboratory of Nucleic Acids, State Center of Hematology and Hemotherapy, Belém, Brazil

Carla Mariana F. Pessoa and Paulo P. Assumpção
Oncology Research Nucleus, University Hospital João de Barros Barreto, Federal University of Pará, Belém, Brazil

Caroline de Fátima Aquino Moreira-Nunes
Laboratory of Pharmacogenetics, Drug Research and Development Center, Federal University of Ceará, Fortaleza, Brazil

Raimundo Miranda de Carvalho and Rommel M. Rodr-guez Burbano
Laboratory of Molecular Biology, Ophir Loyola Hospital, Bel´em, Brazil

Juan A. Rey
Molecular Oncogenetics Laboratory, Research Unit, Hospital Universitario La Paz, Madrid, Spain

Milica Stojkovic Lalosevic, Nevena Jocic, Sanja Dragasevic and Ivana Jovicic
Clinic of Gastroenterology and Hepatology, Clinical Center of Serbia, 11000 Belgrade, Serbia

Tamara Milovanovic Alempijevic, Aleksandra Pavlovic Markovic, Snezana Lukic, Dragan Popovic and Tomica Milosavljevic
Clinic of Gastroenterology and Hepatology, Clinical Center of Serbia, 11000 Belgrade, Serbia
Faculty of Medicine, University of Belgrade, 11000 Belgrade, Serbia

Igor Dumic
Mayo Clinic College of Medicine and Sciences, Rochester, MN, USA
Mayo Clinic Health System, Eau Claire,WI, USA

Jiawei Li, Jaslyn Gan and Paul Cordero,
Institute for Liver and Digestive Health, University College London, Royal Free Hospital, Rowland Hill Street, London NW3 2PF, UK

Vi Nguyen, Shuvra Ray and Jude A. Oben
Institute for Liver and Digestive Health, University College London, Royal Free Hospital, Rowland Hill Street, London NW3 2PF, UK
Department of Gastroenterology and Hepatology, Guy's and StThomas' Hospital, NHS Foundation Trust, Westminster Bridge Rd., London SE1 7EH, UK

Alessandro Solis-Cuevas and Mai Khatib
Department of Biological Sciences, University College London, Gower St., Bloomsbury, London-WC1E 6BT, UK

Daisuke Uchida, Hironari Kato, Yosuke Saragai, Saimon Takada, Sho Mizukawa, Shinichiro Muro, Yutaka Akimoto, Takeshi Tomoda, Kazuyuki Matsumoto, Shigeru Horiguchi and Hiroyuki Okada
Department of Gastroenterology, Okayama University Hospital, 2-5-1 Shikata-cho, Kita-ku, Okayama 700-8558, Japan

Jacqueline M. Schulman
The Ruth and Bruce Rappaport Faculty of Medicine, Technion-Israel Institute of Technology, 3525433 Haifa, Israel
Pediatric Gastroenterology and Nutrition Unit, Ruth Children's Hospital, Rambam Medical Center, 3109601 Haifa, Israel

Liat Pritzker and Ron Shaoul
Pediatric Gastroenterology and Nutrition Unit, Ruth Children's Hospital, Rambam Medical Center, 3109601 Haifa, Israel

Paule V. Joseph, Sarah K. Abey, Dan Wang, Nicolaas H. Fourie, Natnael D. Kenea, JeffreyM. Robinson, Kristen R.Weaver, ChristinaM. Boulineaux, Hannah R. Davidson, LeeAnne B. Sherwin, Onyinyechi Ozoji, Ana F. Diallo, Paul A. Smyser and Wendy A. Henderson
Digestive Disorder Unit, Division of Intramural Research, National Institute of Nursing Research, National Institutes of Health, Bethesda, MD 20892, USA

Tatyana G. Vishnyakova
Department of Laboratory Medicine, Clinical Center, National Institutes of Health, Bethesda, MD 20814, USA

Amy P. Patterson
National Heart Lung and Blood Institute, Bethesda, MD 20814, USA

Andrea Iannone, Michele Barone, Mariabeatrice Principi and Alfredo Di Leo
Section of Gastroenterology, Department of Emergency and Organ Transplantation, University of Bari, Italy

Marinella Ruospo
Diaverum Medical Scientific Office, Lund, Sweden
Department of Translational Medicine, Amedeo Avogadro University of Eastern Piedmont, Novara, Italy

Giovanni F. M. Strippoli
Diaverum Medical Scientific Office, Lund, Sweden
Sydney School of Public Health, University of Sydney, Australia
Diaverum Academy, Lund, Sweden
Section of Nephrology, Department of Emergency and Organ Transplantation, University of Bari, Italy

Germaine Wong
Sydney School of Public Health, University of Sydney, Australia
Centre for Transplant and Renal Research,Westmead Hospital, Sydney, Australia

Zhi-Qiang Wang, Yong Yuan , Peng-Zhi Ni and Long-Qi Chen
Department of Thoracic Surgery, West China Hospital, Sichuan University, Chengdu, China

Yun-Cang Wang
Department of Thoracic Surgery, West China Hospital, Sichuan University, Chengdu, China
Department of Thoracic Surgery, Hospital of Chengdu Office of People's Government of Tibetan Autonomous Region, Chengdu, Sichuan, China

Tao Ren
Division of Gastroenterology, Hospital of Chengdu Office of People's Government of Tibetan Autonomous Region, Chengdu, Sichuan, China

Adeyinka Charles Adejumo
Department of Medicine, North Shore Medical Center, Salem, MA, USA
Department of Medicine, University of Massachusetts Medical School,Worcester MA, USA
School of Public Health, University of Massachusetts Lowell, Lowell,MA, USA

Terence Ndonyi Bukong
Department of Medicine, University of Massachusetts Medical School,Worcester MA, USA
INRS-Institut Armand-Frappier, Institut National de la Recherche Scientifique, Laval, QC, Canada

Kelechi Lauretta Adejumo
School of Public Health, University of Massachusetts Lowell, Lowell,MA, USA

Oluwole Muyiwa Adegbala
Department of Medicine, Englewood Hospital and Medical Center, Englewood, NJ, USA

Adriana Boemio, Martina Vitrone and Luigi Elio Adinolfi
Department of Medical, Surgical, Neurological, Metabolic and Geriatric Sciences, University of Campania "L. Vanvitelli", Italy

Rosa Zampino
Department of Medical, Surgical, Neurological, Metabolic and Geriatric Sciences, University of Campania "L. Vanvitelli", Italy
Unit of Infectious and Transplant Medicine, "V. Monaldi" Hospital, AORN dei Colli, Naples, Italy

Emanuele Durante-Mangoni
Unit of Infectious and Transplant Medicine, "V. Monaldi" Hospital, AORN dei Colli, Naples, Italy
Department of Precision Medicine, University of Campania "L. Vanvitelli", Italy

Nicolina Capoluongo, Margherita Macera, Pietro Filippini, Evangelista Sagnelli and Nicola Coppola
Infectious Diseases Unit, Department of Mental and Physical Health and Preventive Medicine, University of Campania "L. Vanvitelli", Italy

Caterina Sagnelli
Department of Precision Medicine, University of Campania "L. Vanvitelli", Italy

Shuichiro Shiina, Koki Sato, Motonori Shimizu, Hideko Ohama, Takeshi Hatanaka, Masashi Takawa, Hiroaki Nagamatsu and Yasuharu Imai
Department of Gastroenterology, Juntendo University School of Medicine, Japan

Ryosuke Tateishi
Department of Gastroenterology,The University of Tokyo, Japan

Félix Trottier-Tellier, Laurence Harvey and Jean-Daniel Baillargeon
Gastroenterology, Department of Medicine, CHUS, Sherbrooke, QC, Canada

Xuan Zhang, Shaorui Hao, Meifang Yang, Hong Zhao, Jianhua Hu, Weihang Ma and Lanjuan Li
State Key Laboratory for Diagnosis and Treatment of Infectious Diseases, Collaborative Innovation Center for Diagnosis and Treatment of Infectious Diseases, The First Affiliated Hospital, College of Medicine, Zhejiang University, Hangzhou 310003, China

Ping Chen and Hainv Gao
Infectious disease department, Shulan (Hangzhou) Hospital, Hangzhou, China

Index